NURSING RESEARCH

Methods and Critical Appraisal for Evidence-Based Practice

NURSING RESEARCH

Methods and Critical Appraisal for Evidence-Based Practice

10th Edition

GERI LOBIONDO-WOOD, PhD, RN, FAAN

Bette P. Thomas Distinguished Professor for Innovative Healthcare Delivery
Director, PhD in Nursing Program
University of Texas Health Science Center
Cizik School of Nursing
Houston, Texas

JUDITH HABER, PhD, RN, APRN, FAAN

Ursula Springer Leadership Professor in Nursing
New York University
Rory Meyers College of Nursing
New York, New York

ELSEVIER

Elsevier

3251 Riverport Lane
St. Louis, Missouri 63043

NURSING RESEARCH: METHODS AND CRITICAL APPRAISAL
FOR EVIDENCE-BASED PRACTICE, TENTH EDITION

ISBN: 978-0-323-76291-5

Notice

Practitioners and researchers must always rely on their own experience and knowledge in evaluating and using any information, methods, compounds or experiments described herein. Because of rapid advances in the medical sciences, in particular, independent verification of diagnoses and drug dosages should be made. To the fullest extent of the law, no responsibility is assumed by Elsevier, authors, editors or contributors for any injury and/or damage to persons or property as a matter of products liability, negligence or otherwise, or from any use or operation of any methods, products, instructions, or ideas contained in the material herein.

Previous editions copyrighted 2018, 2014, 2010, 2006, 2002, 1998, 1994, 1990, 1986.

Library of Congress Control Number: 2021931862

Executive Content Strategist: Lee Henderson
Senior Content Development Manager: Lisa Newton
Content Development Specialist: Melissa Rawe/Danielle Frazier
Publishing Services Manager: Shereen Jameel
Senior Project Manager: Kamatchi Madhavan
Design Direction: Renee Duenow

Printed in India

Last digit is the print number: 9 8 7 6 5 4 3 2 1

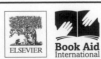

Working together
to grow libraries in
developing countries

www.elsevier.com • www.bookaid.org

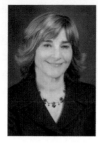

Geri LoBiondo-Wood, PhD, RN, FAAN, is the Bette P. Thomas Distinguished Professor for Innovative Healthcare Delivery and the director of the PhD Nursing Program at the University of Texas Health Science Center (UTHSC) Cizik School of Nursing at Houston and holds a joint appointment with MD Anderson Cancer Center, Houston, Texas, to advance the nursing research agenda. She received her diploma in nursing at St. Mary's Hospital School of Nursing in Rochester, New York; bachelor's and master's degrees from the University of Rochester; and a PhD in nursing theory and research from New York University (NYU) Meyers College of Nursing. Dr. LoBiondo-Wood teaches and mentors doctoral students. She has extensive national and international experience guiding nurses and other health care professionals in the development and utilization of research. Dr. LoBiondo-Wood is an editorial board member of *Progress in Transplantation* and a reviewer for *Nursing Research*, *Oncology Nursing Forum*, and *Oncology Nursing.* Her research and publications focus on chronic illness and oncology nursing. Dr. LoBiondo-Wood has received research funding from the National Institutes of Health (NIH) and funding for the PhD Nursing Program at the UTHSC Cizik School of Nursing from the Robert Wood Johnson Foundation. Dr. LoBiondo-Wood was the primary editor of *Evidence-Base Practice for Nursing & Health Care Quality Improvement* (2019) with Dr. Judith Haber and Dr. Marita Titler.

Dr. LoBiondo-Wood has been active locally and nationally in many professional organizations, including the Oncology Nursing Society, the Southern Nursing Research Society, the Midwest Nursing Research Society, and the North American Transplant Coordinators Organization. She has received local and national awards for teaching and contributions to nursing, including the Distinguished Alumnus Award from NYU Meyers College of Nursing. In 2001, she was inducted as a Fellow of the American Academy of Nursing and in 2007 as a Fellow of the University of Texas Academy of Health Science Education. In 2012, she was appointed as a Distinguished Teaching Professor of the University of Texas System, and in 2015, she received the John McGovern Outstanding Teacher Award from the UTHSC Cizik School of Nursing.

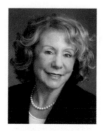

Judith Haber, PhD, RN, APRN, FAAN, is the Ursula Springer Leadership Professor in Nursing at the Rory Meyers College of Nursing at NYU. She received her undergraduate nursing education at Adelphi University in New York; she holds a master's degree in adult psychiatric–mental health nursing and a PhD in nursing theory and research from NYU. Dr. Haber is internationally recognized as a clinician and educator in psychiatric–mental health nursing. She was the editor of the award-winning classic textbook *Comprehensive Psychiatric Nursing,* published for eight editions and translated into five languages. She has extensive clinical experience in psychiatric nursing, having been an advanced practice psychiatric nurse in private practice for over 30 years, specializing in the treatment of families coping with the psychosocial impact of acute and chronic illness. Her NIH-funded program of research addressed physical and psychosocial adjustment to illness, focusing specifically on women with breast cancer and their partners and, more recently, breast cancer survivorship and lymphedema prevention and risk reduction. Dr. Haber is also committed to an interprofessional program of clinical scholarship related to interprofessional education and improving oral-systemic health outcomes, and is the executive director of a national nursing oral health initiative, the Oral Health Nursing Education and Practice (OHNEP) program, funded by the DentaQuest Partnership and Arcora Foundation.

Dr. Haber is the recipient of numerous awards, including the 1995 and 2005 American Psychiatric Nurses Association (APNA) Psychiatric Nurse of the Year Award, the 2005 APNA Outstanding Research Award, and the 1998 American Nurses Association (ANA) Hildegarde Peplau Award. She received the 2007 NYU Distinguished Alumnae Award, the 2011 Distinguished Teaching Award, the 2014 NYU Meritorious Service Award, and the 2020 NYU Changemaker Award. In 2015, Dr. Haber received the Sigma Theta Tau International Marie Hippensteel Lingeman Award for Excellence in Nursing Practice; she also received the 2017 DentaQuest Health Equity Heroes Award and the 2019 American Academy of Nursing Edgerunner Award. Dr. Haber is a Fellow in the American Academy of Nursing and the New York Academy of Medicine. Dr. Haber has consulted, presented, and published widely on evidence-based practice, interprofessional education and practice, and oral-systemic health issues.

CONTRIBUTORS

Karla M. Abela, PhD, RN, CCRN-K, CPN
Assistant Professor
University of Texas Health Science Center
Cizik School of Nursing
Houston, Texas

Dian P. Baker, PhD, RN, APRN-BC
Professor
Nursing
California State University, Sacramento
Sacramento, California

Julie Barroso, PhD, RN, FNAP, FAAN
Blair Chenault Professor of Nursing
Vanderbilt University School of Nursing
Nashville, Tennessee

Carol Bova, PhD, RN, ANP
Professor
Graduate School of Nursing
University of Massachusetts Medical School
Worcester, Massachusetts

Abraham A. Brody, PhD, RN, FAAN
Associate Professor of Nursing and Medicine
Associate Director, Hartford Institute for
    Geriatric Nursing
New York University
Rory Meyers College of Nursing
New York, New York

**Carolynn Spera Bruno, PhD, RN, APRN,
    CNS, FNP-C**
Clinical Associate Professor
New York University
Rory Meyers College of Nursing
New York, New York

Brynne A. Campbell, BA, MS
Health Sciences Reference Associate
Coles Science Center
New York University
Rory Meyers College of Nursing
New York, New York

Dona M. Rinaldi, EdD, RN
Professor and Chairperson
Nursing
University of Scranton
Scranton, Pennsylvania

Maja Djukic, PhD, RN, FAAN
John P. McGovern Distinguished Professor in
    Nursing
Associate Professor
University of Texas Health Science Center
Cizik School of Nursing
Houston, Texas

Dalmacio Dennis Flores III, PhD, ACRN
Assistant Professor
Family and Community Health
University of Pennsylvania
School of Nursing
Pennsylvania, Philadelphia

Mattia J. Gilmartin, PhD, RN, FAAN
Executive Director
Nurses Improving Care for Healthsystem
    Elders
New York University
Rory Meyers College of Nursing
New York, New York

Judith Haber, PhD, RN, APRN, FAAN
Ursula Springer Leadership Professor in
    Nursing
New York University
Rory Meyers College of Nursing
New York, New York

Tonda L. Hughes, PhD, RN, FAAN
Henik H. Bendixen Professor of International
    Nursing
Associate Dean, Global Health Nursing
Columbia University School of Nursing
New York, New York;
Professor of Psychiatry
Columbia University School of Medicine
New York, New York

Susan Kaplan Jacobs, BSN, MLS, MA
Retired Curator, Health Sciences Librarian
Elmer Holmes Bobst Library
New York University Libraries
New York, New York

Carl A. Kirton, DNP, RN, MBA
Chief Nursing Officer
Patient Care Services
University Hospital
Newark, New Jersey;
Adjunct Faculty-Nursing
New York University
Rory Meyers College of Nursing
New York, New York;
Adjunct Faculty
Business Administration
St. Peter's University
Jersey City, New Jersey

**Melanie McEwen, PhD, RN, CNE, ANEF,
FAAN**
Professor
University of Texas Health Science Center
Cizik School of Nursing
Houston, Texas

Shannon Munro, PhD, APRN, NP
Researcher
Diffusion of Excellence Initiative
Veterans Health Administration
Salem, Virginia

Brennan Parmelee Streck, PhD, RN
Cancer Prevention Fellow
Division of Cancer Prevention
National Cancer Institute, National Institutes
of Health
Bethesda, Maryland

**Susan Sullivan-Bolyai, DNSc, CNS, RN,
FAAN**
Associate Dean for Research & Innovation
Graduate School of Nursing
University of Massachusetts Medical School
Worcester, Massachusetts

Marita Titler, PhD, RN, FAAN
Professor Emerita
University of Michigan School of Nursing
Ann Arbor, Michigan

Geri LoBiondo-Wood, PhD, RN, FAAN
Bette P. Thomas Distinguished Professor for
Innovative Healthcare Delivery
Director, PhD in Nursing Program
University of Texas Health Science Center
Cizik School of Nursing
Houston, Texas

The foundation of the 10th edition of *Nursing Research: Methods and Critical Appraisal for Evidence-Based Practice* continues to be the belief that research is integral to all levels of nursing education and practice. Over the past three decades since the first edition of this textbook, we have seen the depth and breadth of nursing research grow, with more nurses conducting research and using research evidence to shape clinical practice, education, administration, and health policy.

As educators, we are challenged to prepare the next generation of nurses and clinicians at a transformative moment in health care. The COVID-19 pandemic has accelerated a national call to action to advance the integration of public health practices, population health issues, and health disparities related to the social determinants of health. More than ever before, all health professionals are counted on to provide team-based care founded on the best available scientific evidence. This is an exciting challenge. Nurses, as clinicians and interprofessional team members, are using the best available evidence, combined with clinical judgment and patient preferences, to influence the nature and direction of health care delivery and document outcomes related to the quality and cost-effectiveness of patient care.

As editors, we believe that all nurses not only need to understand the research process but also need to know how to critically evaluate research findings and apply them in practice. We realize that understanding research, as a component of evidence-based practice and quality improvement practices, is a challenge, but we believe that the challenge can be accomplished in a stimulating, lively, and learner-friendly manner.

Consistent with this perspective is an ongoing commitment to advancing the implementation of evidence-based health care. Understanding and applying research must be an integral dimension of nursing education, evident not only in a research course but also threaded throughout the curriculum. Graduates need competencies in evidence-based practice and quality improvement; central to these are critical appraisal skills—that is, nurses should be competent research consumers.

Preparing students for this role involves developing their critical thinking skills, thereby enhancing their understanding of the research process and their ability to actually critically appraise, integrate, and apply research findings in clinical practice. Their research course should develop this basic level of competence, an essential requirement if students are to engage in evidence-informed clinical decision making and practice and quality improvement activities.

This book is a valuable resource for all students and clinicians who want a concise presentation of the research process, the critical appraisal process, and the principles and tools for evidence-based practice and quality improvement.

Finally, this text is an important resource for considering how evidence-based practice, quality improvement, and interprofessional collaboration are essential competencies for students and clinicians practicing in a transformed health care system, where nurses and their interprofessional team members are accountable for the quality and cost-effectiveness of care provided to their patient population. Building on the success of the ninth edition, we reaffirm our commitment to evidence-based practice, quality improvement processes, and research principles, thereby providing a cutting-edge, research consumer foundation for clinical practice by doing the following:

- Addressing the essential evidence-based practice and quality improvement role of nurses, thereby embedding evidence-based competencies in clinical practice
- Demystifying research, which is sometimes viewed as a complex process
- Using a user-friendly, evidence-based approach to teach the fundamentals of the research process
- Weaving content and exemplars related to health disparities and the social determinants of health into each chapter
- Including an exciting chapter on the role of theory in research and evidence-based practice
- Featuring an innovative chapter on information literacy, searching, and evidence-based practice competencies that prepare students and nurses to effectively locate and evaluate the best research evidence
- Providing a robust chapter on systematic reviews and clinical guidelines
- Offering two innovative chapters on current strategies and tools for developing an evidence-based practice
- Concluding with an exciting chapter on quality improvement and its application to practice
- Emphasizing the role of evidence-based practice and quality improvement initiatives as the basis for informing clinical decisions that support nursing practice
- Presenting numerous examples of recently published research studies that illustrate and highlight research concepts in a manner that brings abstract ideas to life. These examples are critical links that reinforce evidence-based concepts and competencies.
- Presenting five published articles, including a meta-analysis, in the Appendices, the highlights of which are woven throughout the text as exemplars of research and evidence-based practice
- Showcasing, in four new inspirational **Research Vignettes**, the work of renowned nurse researchers whose careers exemplify the links among research, education, and practice
- Integrating stimulating pedagogical chapter features that reinforce learning, including **Learning Outcomes, Key Terms, Key Points, Clinical Judgment Challenges, Helpful Hints, Evidence-Based Practice Tips, and Critical Thinking Decision Paths,** along with numerous tables, boxes, and figures
- Featuring a section titled **Appraising the Evidence,** accompanied by an updated **Critiquing Criteria** box in each chapter that presents a step of the research process
- Offering a student **Evolve site** with interactive review questions that provide chapter-by-chapter review in a format consistent with that of the NCLEX® Examination
- Offering a **Student Study Guide** that promotes active learning and assimilation of nursing research content
- Presenting **Faculty Evolve Resources** that include a test bank, TEACH lesson plans, PowerPoint slides with integrated audience-response-system questions, and an image collection. Evolve resources for both students and faculty also include a research article library with appraisal exercises for additional practice in reviewing and critiquing, in addition to content updates.

The 10th edition of *Nursing Research: Methods and Critical Appraisal for Evidence-Based Practice* is organized into four parts. Each part is preceded by an introductory section and opens with an engaging Research Vignette by a renowned nurse researcher.

Part I, Overview of Research and Evidence-Based Practice, contains four chapters: Chapter 1, "Integrating Research, Evidence-Based Practice, and Quality Improvement Processes," provides an excellent overview of research and evidence-based practice processes that shape clinical practice. The chapter speaks directly to students and highlights critical appraisal concepts and strategies, facilitating understanding of the research process and its relationship to the critical appraisal process. The chapter introduces a model evidence hierarchy that is used throughout the text. The style and content of this chapter are designed to make subsequent chapters user-friendly. The next two chapters address foundational components of the research process. Chapter 2, "Appraising Research Questions, Hypotheses, and Clinical Questions," focuses on how research questions and hypotheses are derived, operationalized, and critically appraised. Students are also taught how to develop clinical questions that are used to guide evidence-based inquiry, including quality improvement projects. Chapter 3, "Gathering and Appraising the Literature," showcases cutting-edge information literacy content and provides students and nurses with the tools necessary to effectively search for, retrieve, manage, and evaluate research studies and their findings. Chapter 4, "Theoretical Frameworks for Research," is a user-friendly theory chapter that gives students an understanding of how theories provide the foundation of research studies and evidence-based practice projects.

Part II, Processes and Evidence Related to Qualitative Research, contains three interrelated qualitative research chapters. Chapter 5, "Introduction to Qualitative Research," provides an exciting framework for understanding qualitative research and the significant contribution of qualitative research to evidence-based practice. Chapter 6, "Qualitative Approaches to Research," presents, illustrates, and showcases major qualitative methods using examples from the literature as exemplars. This chapter highlights the questions most appropriately answered using qualitative methods. Chapter 7, "Appraising Qualitative Research," synthesizes essential components of and criteria for critiquing qualitative research reports using a published qualitative research study.

Part III, Processes and Evidence Related to Quantitative Research, contains Chapters 8 to 18. This group of chapters delineates the essential steps of the quantitative research process, with published clinical research studies used to illustrate each step. These chapters are streamlined to make the case for linking an evidence-based approach with essential steps of the research process. The steps of the quantitative research process, evidence-based concepts, and critical appraisal criteria are synthesized in Chapter 18 using two published research studies, providing a model for appraising the strengths and weaknesses of studies and determining applicability to practice. Chapter 11, a unique chapter, addresses the use of the types of systematic reviews that support an evidence-based practice and the development and application of clinical guidelines.

Part IV, Application of Research: Evidence-Based Practice, contains three chapters that showcase evidence-based practice models and tools. Chapter 19, "Strategies and Tools for Developing an Evidence-Based Practice," is a revised, vibrant, user-friendly, evidence-based toolkit with exemplars that capture the essence of high-quality, evidence-informed nursing care. It "walks" students and practicing nurses through clinical scenarios and challenges them to consider the relevant evidence-based practice "tools" to develop and answer questions that emerge from clinical situations. Chapter 20, "Developing an Evidence-Based Practice," offers a dynamic presentation of important evidence-based practice models that promote evidence-based decision making. Chapter 21, "Quality Improvement," is an innovative, engaging chapter that outlines the quality improvement process with information from current guidelines. Together, these chapters provide an inspirational conclusion to a text that we hope motivates students and practicing nurses to advance their evidence-based practice and quality improvement knowledge base and clinical competence, positioning them to make important contributions to improving health care outcomes as essential members of interprofessional teams.

The development and refinement of an evidence-based foundation for clinical practice are essential priorities for the future of professional nursing practice. The 10th edition of *Nursing Research: Methods and Critical Appraisal for Evidence-Based Practice* will help students develop a basic level of competence in understanding the research process that will enable them to critically analyze studies, judge their merit, and judiciously apply evidence in clinical practice. To the extent that this goal is accomplished, the next generation of nursing professionals will have a cadre of clinicians who inform their practice using theory, research evidence, and clinical judgment as they strive to provide high-quality, cost-effective, and satisfying health care experiences in partnership with individuals, families, and communities.

Geri LoBiondo-Wood
Geri.L.Wood@uth.tmc.edu

Judith Haber
jh33@nyu.edu

We invite you to join us on an exciting research adventure that begins as you turn the first page of the 10th edition of *Nursing Research: Methods and Critical Appraisal for Evidence-Based Practice*. The adventure is one of discovery! You are preparing to be a nurse or are a practicing clinician at a transformative moment in health care. The COVID-19 pandemic has highlighted the importance of public health practices, population health issues, and the prevalence of health disparities related to the social determinants of health. You will discover that this textbook will prepare you to use research evidence to address these most challenging health care challenges.

As you read the nursing research literature featured throughout this text, you will see that it sparkles with pride, dedication, and excitement about the research dimension of nursing practice. Whether you are a student or a practicing nurse whose goal is to use research evidence as the foundation of your practice, you will discover that nursing research and a commitment to evidence-based practice position our profession at the forefront of change. You will discover that evidence-based practice is integral to being an effective member of an interprofessional team that is prepared to meet the challenge of providing quality, whole-person care in partnership with patients, their families/ significant others, and the communities in which they live. Finally, you will discover the richness in the "who," "what," "where," "when," "why," and "how" of nursing research and evidence-based practice, developing a foundation of knowledge and skills that will prepare you for clinical practice and making a significant contribution to achieving the Triple Aim, that is, contributing to high-quality and cost-effective patient outcomes associated with satisfying patient experiences!

We think you will enjoy reading this text. Your research course will be short but filled with new and challenging learning experiences that will develop your evidence-based practice skills. The 10th edition of *Nursing Research: Methods and Critical Appraisal for Evidence-Based Practice* reflects cutting-edge trends for developing evidence-based nursing practice. The four-part organization and special features in this text are designed to help you develop your critical thinking, information literacy, interprofessional, and evidence-based clinical decision-making skills while providing a user-friendly approach to learning that expands your competence to deal with these new and challenging experiences. The companion Study Guide, with its chapter-by-chapter activities, serves as a self-paced learning tool to reinforce the content of the text. The accompanying Evolve website offers review questions to help you reinforce the concepts discussed throughout the book.

Remember that evidence-based practice skills are used in every clinical setting and can be applied to every patient population or clinical practice issue. Whether your practice involves primary care or critical care or inpatient or outpatient treatment in a hospital, clinic, long-term care facility, school, or home setting, you will be challenged to apply your evidence-based practice skills and use research as the foundation for your evidence-based practice. The 10th edition of *Nursing Research: Methods and Critical Appraisal for Evidence-Based Practice* will guide you through this exciting adventure, where you will discover your ability to play a vital role in contributing to the building of an evidence-based professional nursing practice.

Geri LoBiondo-Wood
Geri.L.Wood@uth.tmc.edu

Judith Haber
jh33@nyu.edu

ACKNOWLEDGMENTS

No major undertaking is accomplished alone; there are those who contribute directly and those who contribute indirectly to the success of a project. We acknowledge, with deep appreciation and our warmest thanks, the help and support of the following people:

- Our students, particularly the students at the University of Texas Health Science Center Cizik School of Nursing and the Rory Meyers College of Nursing at New York University, whose interest, lively curiosity, and challenging questions sparked ideas for revisions in the 10th edition
- Our chapter contributors, whose passion for research and translating evidence into practice, in addition to their expertise, cooperation, commitment, and punctuality, made them a joy to have as colleagues
- Our vignette contributors, whose willingness to share evidence of their research wisdom and leadership made a unique and inspirational contribution to this edition
- Our colleagues, who have taken time out of their busy professional lives to offer feedback and constructive criticism that helped us prepare this 10th edition
- Our editor Lee Henderson for his willingness to listen to yet another creative idea about teaching research in a meaningful way and for their expert help with manuscript preparation and production
- Our families, Rick Scharchburg; Brian Wood; Lenny, Andrew, Abbe, Brett, and Meredith Haber; and Laurie, Bob, Mikey, Benjy, and Noah Goldberg, for their unending love, understanding, and support throughout what is inevitably a consuming, but exciting, experience

Geri LoBiondo-Wood

Judith Haber

CONTENTS

PART I

Overview of Research and Evidence-Based Practice

Research Vignette: Tonda L. Hughes

RESEARCH VIGNETTE

OVERCOMING DISPARITIES TO ACHIEVE GENDER EQUITY

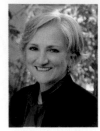

Tonda L. Hughes, PhD, RN, FAAN
Henrik Bendixen Professor of International Nursing
Associate Dean, Global Health
Columbia University School of Nursing
Professor, Psychiatry
Columbia University
New York, New York

Before most health disparities scholars recognized that sexual orientation contributed to inequities in health, I was building a body of work that demonstrated how gender, gender roles, and sexual orientation affect health. My master's and PhD work, completed in the 1980s, focused on alcohol and other drug (AOD) use among women. The scant research on AOD use among lesbian women relied heavily on samples recruited from gay bars. Based on this early research, estimates were that at least one-third of lesbian women were alcoholics or had serious alcohol-related problems. Despite considerable discouragement from well-meaning senior faculty and mentors, I decided it was important to address these biases and gaps in the literature.

Beginning with my doctoral and postdoctoral research, funded by individual fellowships from the National Institutes of Health (NIH), I have examined how gender and culture interact with known risk factors to influence AOD use among vulnerable groups of women. My early work on culture, work roles, and AOD use among nurses was groundbreaking in that it identified barriers to recognition and treatment and clarified standards and policies for employers and treatment providers of nurses addicted to AODs. One example of the impact of this work was my collaboration with the Florida Intervention Project for Nurses, which led to the development or refinement of standards and policies regarding intervention, treatment, and reentry into practice of recovering nurses in Florida. This work was reported in 50 presentations and/or publications, including *Addiction in the Nursing Profession,* winner of the *American Journal of Nursing* Book of the Year Award in 1989.

I also pioneered research related to risk and protective factors associated with hazardous drinking among sexual minority women (SMW) and am internationally known for my work in this area. Compared with heterosexual women, SMW are at higher risk of harmful health behaviors, particularly AOD misuse, and a range of negative health outcomes. My early study on predictors and consequences of hazardous drinking among SMW was the first federally funded study of its kind. This study, the Chicago Health and Life Experiences of Women (CHLEW; K01 AA00266; R01 AA013328-14), is in its 21st year, making it the longest-running study on SMW's health worldwide. Another recent NIH grant (R01 AA027252) will support adding partners of women in the CHLEW to better understand the relationships between hazardous drinking and partner aggression. This work and my collaborative work with leading researchers in the United States and Australia have provided foundational knowledge that has helped to change the field's perspective on the causes and mechanisms underlying sexual-orientation-related health disparities. The result is an improved understanding of the health and well-being of sexual minorities.

Prior to the 1970s and 1980s, nearly all studies were grounded in an illness model that included several implicit assumptions: sexual orientation is a one-dimensional, binary construct that is based on sexual activity (whom one has sex with defines sexual orientation) and exists only in two opposite, discrete forms—heterosexuality or homosexuality. Further, sexual orientation was assumed to form at an early age and to be an enduring, unchanging disposition. My methodological contributions helped to create new paradigms to conceptualize and define sexual orientation, thus raising the standard for rigorous approaches in the study of sexual minority health. For example, the CHLEW and its parent longitudinal study, the National Study of Health and Life Experiences of Women (NSHLEW), were among the first studies to include measures of all three major dimensions of sexual orientation (i.e., identity, behavior, and attraction). Still today, most large-scale surveys assess only one dimension. We developed and pilot-tested these new sexual orientation questions in the mid-1990s, which were added to both the CHLEW and the NSHLEW. These questions also include a broader range of response options. Rather than the typical three-category sexual identity response options of lesbian, bisexual, heterosexual, we included the intermediate responses "mostly lesbian" and "mostly heterosexual," thus providing a more nuanced understanding of sexual identity and related health risks. With data on the three major dimensions of sexual orientation, we found that women whose sexual identity, behavior, and attractions are congruent show higher levels of resilience and lower levels of health-risk behaviors, regardless of whether they identify as lesbian or heterosexual. In contrast, women whose identity does not match their attraction or behavior (e.g., heterosexually identified women who have sex with both men and women) are at elevated risk for a range of AOD and mental health problems.[1]

Using data from large existing population-based samples, my colleagues and I have demonstrated that mental health outcomes differ by sex, dimension of sexual orientation, and sexual minority subgroup. For example, we have conducted pioneering research on women who identify as "mostly heterosexual" when offered the choice of five categories ranging from exclusively heterosexual to exclusively lesbian. Findings from these studies have shown that women who identify as mostly heterosexual differ in important ways from those who identify as exclusively heterosexual,[2-6] including having higher rates of violence and abuse[7-10] and rates of AOD use that are two to four times higher.[5-8] Researchers are increasingly adopting these expanded response options, resulting in more valid assessments of sexual identity in a wide range of studies on health and social behavior.

Because most studies—even large general population surveys—rarely include enough racial/ethnic minority SMW to permit subgroup analyses, very little is known about how health and health care access vary across racial/ethnic groups. Using data from the CHLEW[11-14] and the Youth Risk Behavior Surveys (YRBS),[15,16] my colleagues and I found important racial/ethnic differences. Our findings suggest that SMW of color are more like their White SMW counterparts than their racial/ethnic minority heterosexual counterparts regarding their health risk behaviors. Thus minority race/ethnicity does not appear to confer the same level of protection against health risk behaviors, such as heavy drinking and smoking, among SMW as it does among heterosexual women.[11,17,18]

Perhaps the most important findings of my work are the high rates of lifetime victimization experienced by SMW. Health disparities among sexual minorities most commonly have been explained based on excess stress resulting from their marginalized and stigmatized status. However, my colleagues and my work on victimization drew attention to another critically important and little-recognized factor underlying these health disparities. This work illustrates the disproportionally higher rates of lifetime victimization and highlights the enduring impact of childhood sexual and physical abuse on subsequent victimization and negative mental health and substance use outcomes among SMW.[8,9,19–22] Data from the CHLEW and NSHLEW have shown not only that lesbian and bisexual women are much more likely than heterosexual women to report most forms of interpersonal violence[3,9,23,24] but also that their experiences of violence and abuse are more severe.[25,26] We have replicated findings of higher rates of lifetime victimization among SMW in studies using population-level data from the National Epidemiologic Survey on Alcohol and Related Conditions (NESARC),[8] the National Alcohol Survey,[10] and the Australia Longitudinal Survey on Women's Health.[7,27] For example, we have found that women in the NESARC who identified as lesbian or bisexual were more than twice as likely as those who identified as heterosexual to report any victimization in their lifetime.[8] Furthermore, three times as many lesbian as heterosexual women reported childhood sexual abuse. In addition, among women who reported childhood neglect, lesbian women had more than 30 times the odds of alcohol dependence.[8]

As demonstrated by numerous reports from the Adverse Childhood Events (ACE) study, experiencing more than one adverse event during childhood strongly predicts a plethora of problems in later life. Using data from the CHLEW and NSHLEW, we found that the number of forms of lifetime victimization was significantly associated with hazardous drinking; risk increased by 20% for each additional form of victimization reported.[9] Childhood victimization greatly increased the likelihood of revictimization in adulthood. Given the enormous impact of violence and victimization on health, such findings have major implications for improving the health and quality of life of women—and for progress toward eliminating health disparities based on sexual orientation.

In the third wave of the CHLEW study, we were midway through data collection when Illinois signed into law on January 31, 2011, the Religious Freedom Protection and Civil Union Act, which granted several legal rights (but not legal marriage) to same-sex couples. Participants interviewed after the law's enactment reported lower levels of stigma consciousness, perceived discrimination, depression, and hazardous drinking than those interviewed before enactment.[28] Although these improvements were evident for all SMW, they were most pronounced among African American and Latinx participants and those with lower levels of education. Such findings have important implications regarding other supportive policies, such as employment nondiscrimination, that support the health and well-being of sexual minority people.

Sexual and gender minority (SGM) people are an increasingly open, visible, and accepted part of U.S. society; however, researchers and clinicians continue to grapple with incomplete information about the health behaviors and health needs of these groups. Although research about SGM health has grown over the past 30 years, huge gaps in knowledge remain and are especially glaring regarding SMW's health. For example, less than 0.1% of non-HIV/AIDS–related SGM research funded by the NIH has focused on SMW.[29] Research with sexual minority people has occurred within a complex, changing, and often hostile sociopolitical environment and has been hampered by a variety of challenges, including (1) operationally defining and measuring sexual orientation, (2) overcoming the reluctance of sexual minority people to identify themselves to researchers, and (3) obtaining high-quality samples.[30] Although homosexuality was removed from the *Diagnostic and Statistical Manual of Mental Disorders* in 1973, homophobia still exists within health care professions,[31–34] which likely continues to discourage nurse researchers from studying sexual minority health.

REFERENCES

1. Talley, A. E., Aranda, F., Hughes, T. L., Everett, B., & Johnson, T. P. (2015). Longitudinal associations among discordant sexual orientation dimensions and hazardous drinking in a cohort of sexual minority women. *Journal of Health and Social Behavior, 56*(2), 225–245. http://dx.doi.org/10.1177/0022146515582099.
2. Hughes, T. L., Szalacha, L. A., Johnson, T. P., Kinnison, K. E., Wilsnack, S. C., & Cho, Y. (2010). Sexual victimization and hazardous drinking among heterosexual and sexual minority women. *Addictive Behaviors, 35*(12), 1152–1156. http://dx.doi.org/10.1016/j.addbeh.2010.07.004.
3. Hughes, T., Szalacha, L. A., & McNair, R. (2010). Substance abuse and mental health disparities: Comparisons across sexual identity groups in a national sample of young Australian women. *Social Science & Medicine, 71*(4), 824–831. http://dx.doi.org/10.1016/j.socscimed.2010.05.009.
4. Talley, A. E., Grimaldo, G., Wilsnack, S. C., Hughes, T. L., & Kristjanson, A. F. (2016). Childhood victimization, internalizing symptoms, and substance use among women who identify as mostly heterosexual. *LGBT Health, 3*(4), 266–274. http://dx.doi.org/10.1089/lgbt.2015.0073.
5. Hughes, T. L., Wilsnack, S. C., & Kristjanson, A. F. (2015). Substance use and related problems among U.S. women who identify as mostly heterosexual. *BMC Public Health, 15*(1), 1–8. http://dx.doi.org/10.1186/s12889-015-2143-1.
6. Wilsnack, S. C., Hughes, T. L., Johnson, T. P., Bostwick, W. B., Szalacha, L. A., Benson, P. W., et al. (2008). Drinking and drinking-related problems among heterosexual and sexual minority women. *Journal of Studies on Alcohol and Drugs, 69*(1), 129–139. http://dx.doi.org/10.15288/jsad.2008.69.129.
7. Hughes, T., Szalacha, L. A., & McNair, R. (2010). Substance abuse and mental health disparities: Comparisons across sexual identity groups in a national sample of young Australian women. *Social Science & Medicine, 71*(4), 824–831. http://dx.doi.org/10.1016/j.socscimed.2010.05.009.
8. Hughes, T., McCabe, S. E., Wilsnack, S. C., West, B. T., & Boyd, C. J. (2010). Victimization and substance use disorders in a national sample of heterosexual and sexual minority women and men. *Addiction, 105*(12), 2130–2140. http://dx.doi.org/10.1111/j.1360-0443.2010.03088.x.
9. Hughes, T. L., Johnson, T. P., Steffen, A. D., Wilsnack, S. C., & Everett, B. G. (2014). Lifetime victimization, hazardous drinking, and depression among heterosexual and sexual minority women. *LGBT Health, 1*(3), 192–203. http://dx.doi.org/10.1089/lgbt.2014.0014.
10. Drabble, L., Trocki, K. F., Hughes, T. L., Korcha, R. A., & Lown, A. E. (2013). Sexual orientation differences in the relationship between victimization and hazardous drinking among women in the National Alcohol Survey. *Psychology of Addictive Behaviors, 27*(3), 639–648. http://dx.doi.org/10.1037/a0031486.
11. Hughes, T. L., Wilsnack, S. C., Szalacha, L. A., Johnson, T. P., Bostwick, W. B., Seymour, R., et al. (2006). Age and racial/ethnic differences in drinking and drinking-related problems in a community sample of lesbians. *Journal of Studies on Alcohol, 67*(4), 579–590. http://dx.doi.org/10.15288/jsa.2006.67.579.
12. Aranda, F., Matthews, A. K., Hughes, T. L., Muramatsu, N., Wilsnack, S. C., Johnson, T. P., & Riley, B. B. (2015). Coming out in color: Racial/ethnic differences in the relationship between

level of sexual identity disclosure and depression among lesbians. *Cultural Diversity and Ethnic Minority Psychology, 21*(2), 247–257. http://dx.doi.org/10.1037/a0037644.

13. Jeong, Y. M., Veldhuis, C. B., Aranda, F., & Hughes, T. L. (2016). Racial/ethnic differences in unmet needs for mental health and substance use treatment in a community-based sample of sexual minority women. *Journal of Clinical Nursing, 25*(23-24), 3557–3569. http://dx.doi.org/10.1111/jocn.13477.

14. Parks, C. A., Hughes, T. L., & Matthews, A. K. (2004). Race/ethnicity and sexual orientation: Intersecting identities. *Cultural Diversity and Ethnic Minority Psychology, 10*(3), 241–254. http://dx.doi.org/10.1037/1099-9809.10.3.241.

15. Talley, A. E., Hughes, T. L., Aranda, F., Birkett, M., & Marshal, M. P. (2014). Exploring alcohol-use behaviors among heterosexual and sexual minority adolescents: Intersections with sex, age, and race/ethnicity. *American Journal of Public Health, 104*(2), 295–303. http://dx.doi.org/10.2105/AJPH.2013.301627.

16. Bostwick, W. B., Meyer, I. H., Aranda, F., Russell, S., Hughes, T. L., Birkett, M., & Mustanski, B. (2014). Mental health and suicidality among racially/ethnically diverse sexual minority youths. *American Journal of Public Health, 104*(6), 1129–1136. http://dx.doi.org/10.2105/AJPH.2013.301749.

17. Matthews, A. K., & Hughes, T. L. (2001). Mental health service use by African American women: Exploration of subpopulation differences. *Cultural Diversity and Ethnic Minority Psychology, 7*(1), 75–87. http://dx.doi.org/10.1037//1099-9809.7.1.75.

18. Hughes, T. L., Wilsnack, S. C., & Kantor, L. W. (2016). The influence of gender and sexual orientation on alcohol use and alcohol-related problems: Toward a global perspective. *Alcohol Research Current Reviews, 38*(1), 121–132.

19. Hughes, T. L., Haas, A. P., Razzano, L. A., Cassidy, R., & Matthews, A. K. (2000). Comparing lesbian and heterosexual women's mental health: A multi-site survey. *Journal of Gay & Lesbian Social Services, 11*(1), 57–76.

20. Hughes, T. L., Johnson, T., & Wilsnack, S. C. (2001). Sexual assault and alcohol abuse: A comparison of lesbians and heterosexual women. *Journal of Substance Abuse, 13*, 515–532. https://doi.org/10.1016/S0899-3289(01)00095-5.

21. Gilmore, A. K., Koo, K. H., Nguyen, H. V., Granato, H. F., Hughes, T. L., & Kaysen, D. (2014). Sexual assault, drinking norms, and drinking behavior among a national sample of lesbian and bisexual women. *Addictive Behaviors, 39*(3), 630–636. http://dx.doi.org/10.1016/j.addbeh.2013.11.015.

22. Hughes, T. L., Johnson, T. P., Wilsnack, S. C., & Szalacha, L. A. (2007). Childhood risk factors for alcohol abuse and psychological distress among adult lesbians. *Child Abuse & Neglect, 31*(7), 769–789. http://dx.doi.org/10.1016/j.chiabu.2006.12.014.

23. Andersen, J. P., Hughes, T. L., Zou, C., & Wilsnack, S. C. (2014). Lifetime victimization and physical health outcomes among lesbian and heterosexual women. *PLoS ONE, 9*(7), Article e101939. http://dx.doi.org/10.1371/journal.pone.0101939.

24. Matthews, A. K., Hughes, T. L., Cho, Y. I., Wilsnack, S. C., Aranda, F., & Johnson, T. P. (2018). The effects of sexual orientation on the relationship between victimization experiences and smoking status among US women. *Nicotine and Tobacco Research, 20*(3), 332–339. https://doi.org/10.1093/ntrntx052.

25. Wilsnack, S. C., Kristjanson, A. F., Hughes, T. L., & Benson, P. W. (2012). Characteristics of childhood sexual abuse in lesbians and heterosexual women. *Child Abuse & Neglect, 36*(3), 260–265. http://dx.doi.org/10.1016/j.chiabu.2011.10.008.

26. Alvy, L. M., Hughes, T. L., Kristjanson, A. F., & Wilsnack, S. C. (2013). Sexual identity group differences in child abuse and neglect. *Journal of Interpersonal Violence, 28*(10), 2088–2111. http://dx.doi.org/10.1177/0886260512471081.

27. Szalacha, L. A., Hughes, T. L., & McNair, R. P. (in review). Mental health as predicted by sexual identity and violence: Findings from the Australian Longitudinal Women's Health Study. BMC Women's Health, *17*(1), 94. https://doi.org/10.1186/s12905-017-0452-5.

28. Everett, B. G., Hatzenbuehler, M. L., & Hughes, T. L. (2016). The impact of civil union legislation on minority stress, depression, and hazardous drinking in a diverse sample of sexual-minority women: A quasi-natural experiment. *Social Science & Medicine, 169*, 180–190. http://dx.doi .org/10.1016/j.socscimed.2016.09.036.

29. Coulter, R. W. S., Kenst, K. S., Bowen, D. J., & Scout (2014). Research funded by the national Institutes of Health on the health of lesbian, gay, bisexual, and transgender populations. *American Journal of Public Health, 104*(2), e105–e112. http://dx.doi.org/10.2105/AJPH.2013.301501.

30. Institute of Medicine. (2011). *The health of lesbian, gay, bisexual, and transgender people: Building a foundation for better understanding.* Committee on Lesbian, Gay, Bisexual, and Transgender Health Issues and Research Gaps and Opportunities. Washington (DC): National Academies Press. Available from: https://www.ncbi.nlm.nih.gov/books/NBK64806 / doi: 10.17226/1312.

31. Irwin, L. (2007). Homophobia and heterosexism: Implications for nursing and nursing practice. *Australian Journal of Advanced Nursing, 25*(1), 70–76.

32. Sabin, J. A., Riskind, R. G., & Nosek, B. A. (2015). Health care providers' implicit and explicit attitudes toward lesbian women and gay men. *American Journal of Public Health, 105*(9), 1831–1841. http://dx.doi.org/10.2105/AJPH.2015.302631.

33. Schwinn, S., & Dinkel, S. (2015) Changing the culture of long-term care: Combating heterosexism OJIN: The Online Journal of Issues in Nursing, 20(2). doi: 10.3912/OJIN .Vol20No02PPT03.

34. Chonody, J. M., Woodford, M. R., Brennan, D. J., Newman, B., & Wang, D. (2014). Attitudes toward gay men and lesbian women among heterosexual social work faculty. *Journal of Social Work Education, 50*, 136–152. http://dx.doi.org/10.1080/10437797.2014.856239.

Integrating Research, Evidence-Based Practice, and Quality Improvement Processes

Geri LoBiondo-Wood, Judith Haber

Go to Evolve at **http://evolve.elsevier.com/LoBiondo/** for review questions.

LEARNING OUTCOMES

After reading this chapter, you should be able to do the following:

- State the significance of research, evidence-based practice, and quality improvement (QI).
- Identify the role of the consumer of nursing research.
- Differentiate among research, evidence-based practice, and QI.
- Discuss evidence-based and QI decision making.
- Explain the difference between quantitative and qualitative research.

- Explain the difference between types of systematic reviews.
- Discuss how to use an evidence hierarchy when critically appraising research studies.
- Discuss the format and style of research reports/articles.

KEY TERMS

abstract	evidence-based	levels of evidence	qualitative research
clinical guidelines	guidelines	meta-analysis	quantitative research
consensus guidelines	evidence-based practice	meta-synthesis	research
critical appraisal	integrative review	quality improvement	systematic review

We invite you to join us on an exciting nursing research adventure that begins as you read the first page of this chapter. The adventure is one of discovery! You will discover that the nursing research literature sparkles with pride, dedication, and excitement about this dimension of professional practice. As you progress through your nursing program, you are taught how to ensure quality and safety in clinical practice by acquiring knowledge of the various sciences and health care principles. A critical component of clinical knowledge is understanding research as it applies to practicing from an evidence base.

Whether you are a student or a practicing nurse whose goal is to use research as the foundation of your practice, you will discover that research, evidence-based practice (EBP), and quality improvement (QI) position our profession at the cutting edge of change and improvement in patient outcomes. You will also discover the cutting-edge "who," "what," "where," "when," "why," and "how" of research that help you develop a foundation of EBP knowledge and competencies that will equip you for clinical practice.

Your nursing research adventure will be filled with new and challenging learning experiences that develop your EBP skills. Your critical appraisal skills and clinical decision-making skills will expand as you develop clinical questions, search the research literature, evaluate the research evidence found in the literature, and make clinical decisions about applying the "best available evidence" to your practice. For example, you will be encouraged to ask important clinical questions, such as,

- What makes a telehealth education intervention more effective with one group of patients with a diagnosis of congestive heart failure but not another?
- What is the effect of e-learning health literacy modules on self-management of diabetes in children?
- What research has been conducted to identify barriers to breast cancer screening in African American women?
- What is the quality of studies conducted about the effectiveness of motivational interviewing in promoting behavioral lifestyle changes for populations at high risk for hypertension?
- Which nurse-delivered smoking cessation interventions are most effective?

This book will help you begin your adventure into EBP by developing an appreciation of research as the foundation for EBP and QI.

NURSING RESEARCH, EVIDENCE-BASED PRACTICE, AND QUALITY IMPROVEMENT

Nurses are challenged to stay abreast of new information to provide the highest quality of patient care (Institute of Medicine [IOM], 2011). Nurses are challenged to expand their "comfort zone" by offering creative approaches to old and new health problems and designing new and innovative programs that make a difference in the health status of targeted populations across the life span. These challenges can best be met by integrating rapidly expanding research and evidence-based knowledge about biological, behavioral, and environmental influences on health into the care of patients and their families.

It is important to differentiate among research, EBP, and QI. Research is a systematic, rigorous, critical investigation that aims to answer questions about health-related phenomena. Researchers follow the steps of the scientific process, which are outlined in this chapter and discussed in detail in each chapter of this text. There are two types of research: quantitative and qualitative. The methods used by nurse researchers are the same methods used by other disciplines; the difference is that nurses study questions relevant to nursing practice. Published research studies read and evaluated for applicability to practice are used to inform clinical decisions.

Evidence-based practice is the collection, evaluation, and integration of valid research evidence, combined with clinical expertise and an understanding of patient and family values and preferences, to inform clinical decision making (Sackett et al., 2000). Research studies are gathered from the literature, and the findings are assessed so evidence-based decisions about application to practice can be made. **Example:** ➤ To help you understand the importance of EBP, think about the systematic review and meta-analysis from Facchinetti et al. (2020), which assessed the effectiveness of continuity-of-care interventions in reducing hospital readmission for older adults with chronic disease (see Appendix A). Based on their synthesis of the literature, the researchers put forth several conclusions regarding the implications for practice and the need for further research by nurses working in the field of older adults with chronic disease.

Quality Improvement (QI) is the systematic use of data to monitor the outcomes of care processes and the use of improvement methods to design and test changes in practice for the purpose of continuously improving the quality and safety of health care systems (Cronenwett et al., 2007). Although research supports or generates new knowledge, EBP and QI use currently available evidence to improve health care delivery. When you first read about these three processes, you will notice they have similarities. Each begins with a question. The difference is that in a research study, the question is tested with a design appropriate to the question and specific methodology (i.e., sample, instruments, procedures, and data analysis) used to test the research question and contribute to new, generalizable knowledge. In the EBP and QI processes, a clinical question is used to search the literature for completed research studies to bring about improvements in care.

All nurses share a commitment to the advancement of science by conducting research and using research evidence in practice. Research promotes accountability, one of the hallmarks of the nursing profession and a fundamental concept of the American Nurses Association (ANA) Code of Ethics for Nurses (ANA, 2015). There is a consensus that the research role of the baccalaureate and master's graduate calls for **critical appraisal** skills. That is, nurses must be knowledgeable consumers of research, who can evaluate the strengths and weaknesses of research evidence and use existing criteria to determine the strengths and weaknesses of research and its readiness for use in clinical practice. Therefore to use research for developing an EBP and to practice using the highest-quality evidence, you do not have to conduct research. However, you do need to understand and appraise the steps of the research process to read the research literature critically and use it to inform clinical decisions.

As you venture through this text, you will see the steps of the research, EBP, and QI processes. The steps are systematic and relate to the development of EBP. Understanding the processes that researchers use will help you develop the assessment skills necessary to judge the soundness of research studies.

Throughout the chapters, terminology pertinent to each step of the research process is identified and illustrated with examples. Five published research studies and one QI report are found in the appendices and used as examples to illustrate significant points in each chapter. Judging a study's strengths and weaknesses helps you determine its quality and its applicability to practice. Before you can judge a study, it is important to understand the differences among studies. You will see different study designs throughout this text and the appendices. There are standards or criteria not only for critiquing the soundness of each step of a study but also for judging the strength and quality of evidence provided by a study and determining its applicability to practice.

This chapter provides an overview of research study designs and critical appraisal skills. It introduces the overall format of a research article and provides an overview of the subsequent chapters in the text. It also introduces the QI and EBP processes, a level-of-evidence hierarchy model, and other tools to help you evaluate the strength and quality of research evidence. These topics are designed to help you read research articles more effectively and with greater understanding so you can make evidence-based clinical decisions and contribute to quality and cost-effective patient outcomes.

TYPES OF RESEARCH: QUALITATIVE AND QUANTITATIVE

Research is classified into two major categories: qualitative and quantitative. A researcher chooses between these categories based on the question being asked. That is, a researcher may wish to test a cause-and-effect relationship, assess if variables are related, or discover and understand the meaning of an experience or process. A researcher would choose to conduct a qualitative research study if the question is about understanding the meaning of a human experience such as grief, hope, or loss. The meaning of an experience is based on the view that meaning varies, is subjective, and occurs in a context. That is, the experience of loss as a result of a miscarriage would be different than the experience of losing a parent.

Qualitative research is generally conducted in natural settings and uses data that are words or text rather than numeric to describe the experiences being studied. Qualitative studies are guided by research questions, and data are collected from a small number of subjects, allowing an in-depth study of a phenomenon. **Example:** ➢ Hanna et al. (2020) explored the perceptions that underlie health-related adherence behaviors from the perspective of patients who experienced a heart attack (see Appendix E). Although qualitative research is systematic in its method, it uses a subjective approach. Data from qualitative studies help nurses understand experiences or phenomena that affect patients; these data also assist in generating theories that lead clinicians to develop improved patient care and stimulate further research. Highlights of the general steps of qualitative studies and the journal format for a qualitative article are outlined in Table 1.1. Chapters 5 to 7 provide an in-depth view of qualitative research underpinnings, designs, and methods.

TABLE 1.1   Steps of the Research Process and Journal Format: Qualitative Research

Research Process Steps and/or Format Issues	Usual Location in Journal Heading or Subheading
Identifying the phenomenon	Abstract and/or in introduction
Research question or study purpose	Abstract and/or in beginning or end of introduction
Literature review	Introduction, background and/or discussion
Design	Abstract and/or in introductory section or under method section entitled "Design" or stated in method section
Sample	Method section labeled "Sample" or "Subjects"
Legal-ethical issues	Data collection or procedures section or in sample section
Measurement	Methods section includes instruments used and their reliability and validity
Data collection procedure	Data collection or procedures section
Data analysis	Methods section under subhead "Data Analysis" or "Data Analysis and Interpretation"
Results	Stated in separate heading: "Results" or "Findings"
Discussion and recommendation	Combined in separate section: "Discussion" or "Discussion and Implications"
References	At end of article

Whereas qualitative research looks for meaning, quantitative research encompasses the study of research questions and/or hypotheses that describe phenomena, test relationships, assess differences, seek to explain cause-and-effect relationships between variables, and test for intervention effectiveness. The numeric data in quantitative studies are summarized and analyzed using statistics. Quantitative research designs are systematic, and the methodology is controlled. Appendices B to D illustrate examples of different quantitative approaches to answering research questions or testing hypotheses. Table 1.2 indicates where each step of the research process can usually be located in a quantitative research article and where it is discussed in this text. Chapters 2, 3, and 8 to 18 describe processes related to quantitative research.

TABLE 1.2   Steps of the Research Process and Journal Format: Quantitative Research

Research Process Steps and/or Format Issue	Usual Location in Journal Heading or Subheading	Text Chapter
Introduction or Background	Introductory/background that may or may not be labeled provides information that describes the context and significance of the study.	3
Purpose	Abstract and/or in introduction, or end of literature review or theoretical framework section, or labeled separately: "Purpose"	2
Literature review	At end of heading "Introduction" but not labeled as such, or labeled as separate heading: "Literature Review," "Review of the Literature," "Related Literature," or not labeled, or variables reviewed appear as headings or subheadings	3
Theoretical or conceptual framework	Combined with "Literature Review" or found in separate section as TF or CF; or each concept used in TF or CF may appear as separate subheading	3, 4
Hypothesis/research questions	Stated or implied near end of introduction or literature review; may be labeled or found in separate heading or subheading: "Hypothesis" or "Research Questions"; or reported for first time in "Results"	2
Research design	Stated or implied in abstract or introduction or in "Methods" or "Methodology" section	8–10
Sample: type and size	"Size" may be stated in abstract, in methods section, or as separate subheading under methods section as "Sample," "Sample/Subjects," or "Participants"; "Type" may be implied or stated in any of previous headings described under size	12
Legal-ethical issues	Stated or implied in sections: "Methods," "Procedures," "Sample," or "Subjects"	13
Instruments	Found in sections: "Methods," "Instruments," or "Measures"	14
Validity and reliability	Specifically stated or implied in sections: "Methods," "Instruments," "Measures," or "Procedures"	15
Data collection procedure	In methods section under subheading "Procedure" or "Data Collection," or as separate heading: "Procedure"	14
Data analysis	Under subheading: "Data Analysis"	16
Results	Stated in separate heading: "Results"	16, 17
Discussion of findings and new findings	Combined with results or as separate heading: "Discussion"	17
Implications, limitations, and recommendations	Combined in discussion or as separate major headings	17
References	At end of article	4
Communicating research results	Research articles, poster, and paper presentations	1, 20

CF, Conceptual framework; *TF,* theoretical framework.

The primary difference is that qualitative research seeks to interpret meaning and phenomena, whereas quantitative research seeks to test a hypothesis or answer research questions using statistical methods. Remember as you read research articles that, depending on the research question, a researcher may vary the steps slightly; however, each step should be addressed systematically.

CRITICAL APPRAISAL SKILLS

To develop expertise in EBP, you will need to be able to critically evaluate all types of research articles. As you read a research article, you may be struck by the difference in style or format of a research article versus a clinical article. The terms of a research article are new, and the content is different. You may also be thinking that the research article is hard to read or that it is technical and boring. You may simultaneously wonder, "How will I possibly learn to appraise all of the steps of a research study, the terminology, and the process of EBP? I'm only on Chapter 1. This is not so easy; research is as hard as everyone says."

Learning the research process develops your critical appraisal skills. You will gradually be able to read a research article and determine whether the conclusions are based on the study's findings. Once you have obtained this critical appraisal competency, you will be ready to synthesize the findings of multiple studies to use in developing an EBP.

> **IPE HIGHLIGHT**
>
> Start an interprofessional education journal club with students from other health professions programs on your campus. Select a research study to read, understand, and critically appraise together. It is always helpful to collaborate on deciding whether the findings are applicable to clinical practice.

STRATEGIES FOR APPRAISING RESEARCH STUDIES

Critical appraisal of a study objectively and critically evaluates a study's content for its strengths and weaknesses and overall applicability to practice. It requires some knowledge of the subject matter and knowledge of how to use critical appraisal criteria. In this text, you will find:

- Summarized examples of critical appraisal criteria for qualitative studies and an example of a qualitative critique in Chapter 7
- Summarized critical appraisal criteria and examples of a quantitative critique in Chapter 18
- An in-depth exploration of the criteria for evaluation required in quantitative research in Chapters 8 to 18
- Criteria for qualitative research in Chapters 5 to 7
- Principles for qualitative and quantitative research in Chapters 1 to 4

Critical appraisal criteria are the standards, appraisal guides, or questions used to evaluate an article. When analyzing a research article, you must evaluate each step of the research process and ask questions about whether each step meets the criteria. For instance, the critical appraisal criteria in Chapter 3 ask if "the literature review identifies gaps and inconsistencies in the literature about a subject, concept, or problem," and if "all of the concepts and variables are included in the review." These two questions relate to appraising the research question and the literature review components of the research process. Sometimes beginners confuse critical appraisal with criticism and think they are only being asked to identify the weaknesses of a study. Remember that when critiquing a study, you are pointing out strengths and weaknesses. Hopefully, a research study or group of research studies will have more strengths than weaknesses. Standardized critical appraisal tools such as those from the Centre for Evidence-Based Medicine (CEBM) Critical Appraisal Tools (http://www.cebm.net/critical-appraisal) can be used to systematically appraise the strength and quality of evidence provided in research articles (see Chapters 3 and 20).

Appraising can be thought of as looking at a completed jigsaw puzzle. Does it form a comprehensive picture, or is a piece out of place? What is the level of evidence provided by the study and the findings? What is the balance between the risks and benefits of the findings that contribute to clinical decisions? How can I apply the evidence to my patient, to my patient population, or in my setting? When reading several studies for synthesis, you must assess the overall strength and quality of evidence provided by the group of studies and determine the applicability of their findings to practice. Developing a table of evidence (see Chapter 20) will help you organize appraising one or more studies.

OVERCOMING BARRIERS: USEFUL APPRAISAL STRATEGIES

Throughout the text, you will find features that will help refine the skills essential to understanding and using research in your practice. In each chapter, you will find:
- A Critical-Thinking Decision Path related to each step of the research process that will sharpen your decision-making skills
- IT Resources to enhance your literature search skills
- Helpful Hints designed to reinforce your understanding of key information
- QSEN Evidence-Based Practice Tips to help you apply EBP strategies in your clinical practice
- Interprofessional Education Highlights
- Critical Appraisal Criteria
- Clinical Judgment Challenges at the end of each chapter designed to reinforce your critical reading skills

When you complete your first critique, congratulate yourself; mastering these skills is not easy. As you continue to use and perfect critical appraisal skills by critiquing studies, remember that these skills are an expected competency for delivering evidence-based and quality nursing care.

EVIDENCE-BASED PRACTICE AND RESEARCH

Along with gaining comfort while reading and appraising studies, there is one final step: deciding how, when, and if to apply the studies to your practice so your practice and the clinical care you provide is evidence based. EBP allows you to systematically make clinical decisions using the best available evidence with the integration of clinical expertise and the patient's values and preferences (Sackett et al., 2000). For example, research evidence supports significant disparities in untreated tooth decay for children and adults in the United States. Race/ethnicity, age, family income, education level, and financial and nonfinancial barriers (e.g. insurance, transportation, geographic location) are associated with untreated cavities (Gupta et al., 2018). Determining potential interventions to decrease untreated tooth decay in children for whom dental care is an essential benefit of the Affordable Care

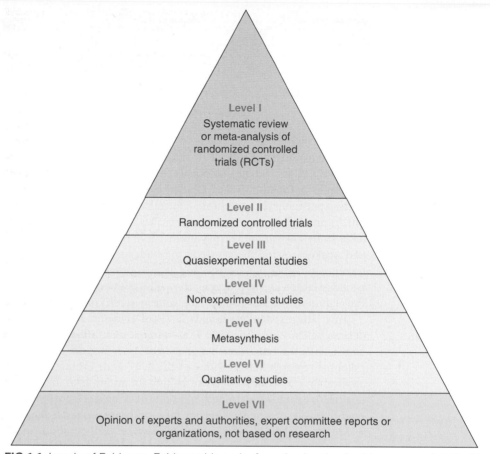

FIG 1.1 Levels of Evidence. Evidence hierarchy for rating levels of evidence associated with a study's design. Evidence is assessed at a level according to its source.

Act (ACA) involves considering interventions that are affordable, accessible, available, and culturally congruent with the targeted community. EBP involves processes and steps, as does the research process. These steps are presented throughout the text. Chapter 19 provides an overview of EBP steps and strategies.

When using EBP strategies, the first step is to be able to read a study with an understanding of how each section is linked to the steps of the research process. The following section introduces you to the research process as presented in published articles. Once you read a study, you must decide which level of evidence the study provides and how well the study was designed and executed. Fig. 1.1 illustrates a model for determining the levels of evidence associated with a study's design, ranging from systematic reviews of randomized controlled trials (RCTs) (see Chapters 9 and 10) to expert opinions. The rating system, or evidence hierarchy model, presented here is just one of many. Many hierarchies for assessing the relative worth of both qualitative and quantitative designs are available. Early in the development of EBP, evidence hierarchies were thought to be very inflexible, with systematic reviews or meta-analyses at the top and qualitative research at the bottom. This is no longer the case. There is no guarantee that a Level II RCT with design flaws will provide stronger evidence than a well-designed Level III cohort study.

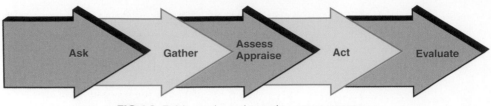

FIG 1.2 Evidence-based practice process steps.

When assessing a research question that tests a cause-and-effect relationship, the meaningfulness of an evidence rating system will become clearer as you read Chapters 8 to 11. **Example:** ➤ The study by De la Fuente Coria et al. (2020) provides Level II evidence because of its experimental, randomized controlled trial design, whereas the study by Hanna et al. (2020) provides Level VI evidence because it is a qualitative study. The level itself does not tell a study's worth; rather it is another tool that helps you think about a study's strengths and weaknesses and the nature of the evidence provided in the findings, conclusions, and recommendations. Chapters 7 and 18 will provide an understanding of how studies can be assessed for use in practice. You will use the evidence hierarchy presented in Fig. 1.1 throughout the text as you develop your research consumer skills.

This rating system represents levels of evidence for judging the strength of a study's design, which is just one level of assessment that influences the confidence one has in the conclusions the researcher has specified. Assessing the strength of scientific evidence or potential research bias provides a vehicle to guide evaluation of research studies for their applicability in clinical decision making. In addition to identifying the level of evidence, one needs to grade the strength of a body of evidence, incorporating the domains of quality, quantity, and consistency (Agency for Healthcare Research and Quality, 2002).

- Quality: Extent to which a study's design, implementation, and analysis minimize bias
- Quantity: Number of studies that have evaluated the research question, including the overall sample size across studies and the strength of the findings from data analyses
- Consistency: Degree to which studies with similar and different designs investigating the same research question report similar findings

The EBP process steps are: ask, gather, assess and appraise, act, and evaluate (Fig. 1.2). These steps of asking clinical questions; identifying and gathering the evidence; critically appraising and synthesizing the evidence or literature; acting to change practice by coupling the best available evidence with your clinical expertise and patient preferences (e.g., values, setting, and resources); and evaluating if the use of the best available research evidence is applicable to your patient or organization will be discussed throughout the text.

To maintain an EBP, studies are evaluated using specific criteria. Studies are evaluated for strength, quality, and consistency of evidence. Before one can proceed with an evidence-based project, it is necessary to understand the steps of the research process.

RESEARCH ARTICLES: FORMAT AND STYLE

Before you begin reading research articles, it is important to understand their organization and format. Many journals publish research, either as the sole type of article or in addition to clinical or theoretical articles. Journals have some common features but also unique characteristics. All journals have guidelines for manuscript preparation and submission. A review of these guidelines, which are found on a journal's website, will give you an idea of the format of articles that appear in specific journals.

Remember that even though each step of the research process is discussed at length in this text, you may find only a short paragraph or a sentence in an article that provides the details of the step. A publication is a shortened version of the researcher(s) completed work. You will also find that some researchers devote more space in an article to the results, whereas others present a longer discussion of the methods and procedures. Decisions about the amount of material presented for each step of the research process are bound by the following:

- The journal's space limitations
- The journal's author guidelines
- The type or nature of the study
- The researcher's decision regarding which component of the study is most important

The following discussion provides a brief overview of each step of the research process and how it may appear in an article. It is important to remember that a quantitative research article will differ from a qualitative research article. The components of qualitative research are discussed in Chapters 5 and 6 and are summarized in Chapter 7.

Abstract

An **abstract** is a short, comprehensive synopsis or summary of a study at the beginning of an article. An abstract quickly focuses the reader on the main points of a study. A well-presented abstract is accurate, self-contained, concise, specific, nonevaluative, coherent, and readable. Abstracts vary in word length. The length and format of an abstract are dictated by the journal's style. Both quantitative and qualitative research studies have abstracts that provide a succinct overview of the study. Examples of abstracts can be found in each of the articles in the appendices.

> **HELPFUL HINT**
>
> An abstract is a concise short overview that provides a reference to the research purpose, research questions, hypotheses, methodology, results, and implications for practice or future research.

Introduction/Study Purpose

Early in a research article, in a section that may or may not be labeled "Introduction," or "Purpose," the researcher presents a background picture of the area researched and its significance to practice (see Chapter 2). The study's purpose may or may not be labeled (see Chapters 2 and 3), or it may be referred to as the study's aim or objective. The studies in Appendices A to E present specific purposes for each study in untitled sections that appear in the beginning of each article and in the article's abstract.

Literature Review and Theoretical Framework

Authors of studies present the literature review and theoretical framework in different ways. Many research articles merge the "Literature Review" and the "Theoretical Framework." This section includes the main concepts investigated and may be called "Review of the Literature," "Literature Review," "Theoretical Framework," "Related Literature," "Background," "Conceptual Framework," or it may not be labeled at all (see Chapters 2 and 3). One style is not better than another; the studies in the appendices contain all of the critical elements but present the elements differently.

> **HELPFUL HINT**
>
> Not all research articles include headings for each step or component of the research process. All steps are presented at some point in the article, but they may be embedded, so you must look for them.

Hypothesis/Research Question

A study's research questions or hypotheses can also be presented in different ways (see Chapter 2 and Appendices B to E). Research articles often do not have separate headings for reporting the "Hypotheses" or "Research Question." They are often embedded in the "Introduction" or "Background" section or at the end of the literature review. Sometimes they are not labeled at all (e.g., as in the studies in the appendices). If a study uses hypotheses, the researcher may report whether the hypotheses were or were not supported toward the end of the article in the "Results" or "Findings" section. Similarly, support for the research questions appear in the same sections. Quantitative research studies have hypotheses or research questions. Qualitative research studies do not have hypotheses, but they have research questions and purposes. The quantitative studies in Appendices A, B, and D have hypotheses.

Research Design

The type of research design can be found in the abstract, the purpose statement, the introduction to the "Procedures" or "Methods" section, or not stated at all (see Chapters 6, 9, and 10). For example, the studies in Appendices A to E identify the design in the abstract and the article.

One of your first objectives is to determine whether the study is qualitative (see Chapters 5 and 6) or quantitative (see Chapters 8, 9, and 10). Although the rigor of the critical appraisal criteria addressed does not substantially change, some of the terminology of the questions differs for qualitative versus quantitative studies. Do not get discouraged if you cannot easily determine the design. One of the best strategies is to review the chapters that address designs. The following tips will help you determine if the study you are reading employs a quantitative design:

- Hypotheses or research questions are stated or implied (see Chapter 2).
- *Fidelity* is an important term that is used to keep conditions constant (see Chapter 8)
- The terms *control group* and *treatment group* are used to identify an *experimental design* (see Chapter 9).
- The terms *survey*, *correlational*, *case control*, or *cohort* are used to identify a nonexperimental design (see Chapter 10).
- The terms *random* or *convenience* are mentioned in relation to the sample (see Chapter 12).
- Variables are measured by instruments or scales (see Chapter 14).
- Reliability and validity of instruments are used to determine their consistency and accuracy (see Chapter 15).
- Statistical analyses are used to determine the study findings (see Chapter 16).

In contrast, qualitative studies generally do not focus on "numbers." Some qualitative studies may use standard quantitative terms (e.g., subjects) rather than qualitative terms (e.g., informants). Deciding on the type of qualitative design can be confusing; one of the best strategies is to review the qualitative chapters (see Chapters 5 to 7).

Begin trying to link the study's design with the level of evidence associated with that design, as illustrated in Fig. 1.1. This will give you a context for evaluating the strength and consistency of the findings and applicability to practice. Chapters 8 to 11 will help you understand how to link the levels of evidence with quantitative designs. A study may not indicate the specific design used; however, all studies inform the reader of the methodology used, which can help you decide the type of design the authors used to guide the study.

Sampling

The population from which the sample was drawn is discussed in the section "Methods" or "Methodology" under the subheadings of "Subjects" or "Sample" (see Chapter 12). Researchers should identify for you the population from which the sample was chosen, the inclusion criteria, the number of subjects who participated in the study, and a description of subjects who dropped out of the study. The authors of the studies in the appendices discuss their samples in enough detail so the reader is clear about who the subjects are and how they were selected.

Reliability and Validity

A discussion of the instruments used to study the variables is usually included in a "Methods" section under the subheading of "Instruments" or "Measures" (see Chapter 14). Usually a discussion of each instrument (or scale) used in the study along with its reliability and validity is included (see Chapter 15). The studies in the appendices discuss each of the measures used in the "Methods" section under the subheading "Measures" or "Instruments," "tools and data collection," and "outcome measures and data collection." The reliability and validity of each measure is not always presented, but references with this information are usually cited.

Procedures and Data Collection Methods

The data collection procedures, or the individual steps taken to gather measurable data (usually with instruments or scales), are generally found in the "Procedures" or "Data Collection" section (see Chapter 14). Notice that the researchers in the studies in the Appendices provided information that the studies were approved by an institutional review board (see Chapter 13), thereby ensuring that each study met ethical standards.

Data Analysis/Results

Data analysis procedures (i.e., the statistical tests used and the results of descriptive and/or inferential tests applied in quantitative studies) are presented in the "Results" or "Findings" section (see Chapters 16 and 17). Although qualitative studies do not use statistical tests, the procedures for analyzing the themes, concepts, and/or observational or print data are usually described in the "Method" or "Data Collection" section and reported in the "Results," "Findings," or "Data Analysis" section (see Appendix E and Chapters 5 and 6).

Discussion

The last section of a research study is the "Discussion" section (see Chapter 17). In this section, the researchers tie together all of the study's components and give a wholistic picture of the study. The researchers return to the literature reviewed and discuss how their study is similar to or different from other studies. Researchers may report the results and discussion in one section but usually report their results in separate "Results" and "Discussion" sections (see Appendices A to E). One particular format is no better than another. Journal and space limitations determine how these sections will be handled. Any new or unexpected findings are usually described in the "Discussion" section.

Recommendations and Implications

In some cases, a researcher reports the limitations and implications, based on the findings, for practice and education. This section captures the overall strengths and weaknesses of the study. Recommendations for future research usually appear in a separate "Conclusions" section; in other cases, this appears in several sections with such titles as "Discussion," "Limitations," "Implications," "Implications for Research and Practice," and "Summary." Again, one approach is not better than the other—only different.

References

All of the references cited are included at the end of the article. The main purpose of the reference list is to support the material presented by identifying the sources in a manner that allows for easy retrieval. Journals use various referencing styles.

Communicating Results

Communicating a study's results can take the form of a published article, poster, or paper presentation. All are valid ways of providing research evidence that have the potential to effect high-quality patient care. Evidence-based nursing care plans and QI practice protocols, guidelines, or standards are outcome measures that effectively indicate communicated research.

HELPFUL HINT

If you have to write a paper on a specific concept or topic that requires you to critique and synthesize the findings from several studies, you might find it useful to create an evidence table of the data (see Chapter 20). Include the following information: author, date, study type, design, level of evidence, sample, data analysis, findings, and implications.

SYSTEMATIC REVIEWS: META-ANALYSES, INTEGRATIVE REVIEWS, AND META-SYNTHESES

Systematic Reviews

Other article types that are important to understand for EBP are review articles. Review articles include systematic reviews, meta-analyses, integrative reviews (sometimes called *narrative reviews* or *scoping reviews*), meta-syntheses, and meta-summaries. A systematic review is a summation and assessment of a group of research studies that test a similar research question. Systematic reviews are based on a clear question, a detailed plan that includes a search strategy, and an appraisal of a group of studies related to the research question. If statistical techniques are used to summarize and assess studies, the systematic review is labeled as a meta-analysis. A meta-analysis is a summary of a number of studies focused on one question or topic, and it uses a specific statistical methodology to synthesize the findings to draw conclusions about the area of focus. An integrative review is a focused review and synthesis of research or theoretical literature in a particular focus area, and it includes specific steps of literature integration and synthesis without statistical analysis; it can include both quantitative and qualitative articles (Cochrane Consumer Network, 2020; Uman, 2011; Whittemore, 2005). At times reviews use the terms systematic review and integrative review interchangeably. Both a meta-synthesis and meta-summary are the synthesis of a number of qualitative research studies on a focused topic using specific qualitative methodology (Kastner et al., 2016; Sandelowski & Barrosos, 2007).

The components of review articles will be discussed in greater detail in Chapters 6, 11, and 20. These articles take a number of studies related to a clinical question and, using a specific set of criteria and methods, evaluate the studies as a whole. Although they may vary somewhat in approach, these reviews all help better inform and develop EBP. The meta-analysis in Appendix E is an example of a systematic review that is a meta-analysis.

CLINICAL GUIDELINES

Clinical guidelines are systematically developed statements or recommendations that serve as a guide for practitioners. Two types of clinical guidelines will be discussed through-out this text: consensus, or expert-developed guidelines, and evidence-based guidelines. Consensus guidelines, or expert-developed guidelines, are developed by an agreement of experts in the field. Evidence-based guidelines are those developed using published research findings. Guidelines are developed to assist in bridging practice and research and are developed by professional organizations, government agencies, institutions, or convened expert panels. Clinical guidelines provide clinicians with an algorithm for clinical management or decision making for specific diseases (e.g., breast cancer) or treatments (e.g., pain management). Not all clinical guidelines are well developed and, like research, must be assessed before implementation. Though they are systematically developed and make explicit recommendations for practice, clinical guidelines may be formatted differently. Guidelines for practice are becoming more important as third-party and government payers are requiring practices to be based on evidence. Guidelines should present the scope and purpose of the practice, detail who the development group included, demonstrate scientific rigor, be clear in its presentation, demonstrate clinical applicability, and demonstrate editorial independence (see Chapter 11).

QUALITY IMPROVEMENT

As a health care provider, you are responsible for continuously improving the quality and safety of health care for your patients and their families through systematic redesign of health care systems in which you work. The IOM (2011) defined quality health care as care that is safe, effective, patient-centered, timely, efficient, and equitable. Therefore the goal of QI is to bring about measurable changes across these six domains by applying specific methodologies within a care setting. Although several QI methods exist, the core steps for improvement commonly include the following:

- Conducting an assessment
- Setting specific goals for improvement
- Identifying ideas for changing current practice
- Deciding how improvements in care will be measured
- Rapidly testing practice changes
- Measuring improvements in care
- Adopting the practice change as a new standard of care

Chapter 21 focuses on building your competence to participate in and lead QI projects by providing an overview of the evolution of QI in health care, including the nurse's role in meeting current regulatory requirements for patient care quality. Chapter 19 discusses QI models and tools, such as cause-and-effect diagrams and process mapping, and skills for effective teamwork and leadership that are essential for successful QI projects.

As you venture through this text, you will be challenged to think not only about reading and understanding research studies but also about applying the findings to your practice. Nursing has a rich legacy of research that has grown in depth and breadth. Producers of research and clinicians must engage in a joint effort to translate findings into practice that will make a difference in the care of patients and families.

KEY POINTS

- Research provides the basis for expanding the unique body of scientific evidence that forms the foundation of evidence-based nursing practice. Research links education, theory, and practice.
- As consumers of research, nurses must have a basic understanding of the research process and critical appraisal skills to evaluate research evidence before applying it to clinical practice.
- Critical appraisal is the process of evaluating the strengths and weaknesses of a research article for scientific merit and application to practice, theory, or education; the need for more research on the topic or clinical problem is also addressed at this stage.
- Critical appraisal criteria are the measures, standards, evaluation guides, or questions used to judge the worth of a research study.
- Critical reading skills will enable you to evaluate the appropriateness of the content of a research article, apply standards or critical appraisal criteria to assess the study's scientific merit for use in practice, or consider alternative ways of handling the same topic.
- A level of evidence model is a tool for evaluating the strength (quality, quantity, and consistency) of a research study and its findings.
- Each article should be evaluated for the study's strength and consistency of evidence as a means of judging the applicability of findings to practice.
- Research articles have different formats and styles depending on journal manuscript requirements and whether they are quantitative or qualitative studies.
- EBP and QI begin with the careful reading and understanding of each article contributing to the practice of nursing, clinical expertise, and an understanding of patient values.
- QI processes are aimed at improving clinical care outcomes for patients and better methods of system performance.

CLINICAL JUDGMENT CHALLENGES

- **IPE** How might nurses discuss the differences between EBP and research with their colleagues in other professions?
- From your clinical practice, discuss several strategies nurses can undertake to promote EBP.
- What are some strategies you can use to develop a more comprehensive critical appraisal of an EBP article?

- A number of different components are usually identified in a research article. Discuss how these sections link with one another to support the researcher's conclusions and recommendations.
- How can QI data be used to improve clinical practice?

REFERENCES

Agency for Healthcare Research and Quality. (2002). Systems to rate the strength of scientific evidence. File inventory, Evidence Report/Technology Assessment No. 47, AHRQ Publication No. 02-E016.

American Nurses Association (ANA). (2015). *Code of ethics for nurses for nurses with interpretive statements*. Washington, DC: The Association.

Cochrane Consumer Network, The Cochrane Library, 2020, retrieved online. www.cochranelibrary.com.

Cronenwett, L., Sherwood, G., Barnsteiner, J., et al. (2007). Quality and safety education for nurses. *Nursing Outlook, 55*(3), 122–131.

De la Fuente Coria, M. C., Cruz-Cobo, C., & Santi-Cano, M. J. (2020). Effectiveness of a primary care nurse delivered educational intervention for patients with a type 2 diabetes mellitus in promoting metabolic control and compliance with long term therapeutic targets: Randomised controlled trial. *International Journal of Nursing Studies, 101*, 1–10. https://doi.org/10.1016/j.ijnurstu.2019.103396. http://dx.doi.org/.

Facchinetti, G., D'Angelo, D., Piredda, M., Petitti, T., Matarese, M., Oliveti, A., & Grazia DeMarinis, M. (2020). Continuity of care interventions for preventing hospital readmission of older people with chronic diseases: A meta-analysis. *International Journal of Nursing Studies*, 1–10. https://doi.org/10.1016/j.ijnurstu.2019.103396.

Gupta, N., Vujicic, M., Yarborough, C., & Harrison, B. (2018). Disparities in untreated caries among children and adults in the U.S., 2011-2014. *BMC Oral Health*, 1–9. https://doi.org/10.1186/s12903-018-0493-7.

Hanna, A., Yael, E-m, Hadassa, L., Iris, E., Eugenia, N., Lior, G., Carmit, S., & Liora, O (2020). It's up to me with a little support" – Adherence after myocardial infraction: A qualitative study. *International Journal of Nursing Studies*. https://doi.org/10.1016/ijnurstu.2019.103416.

Institute of Medicine [IOM]. (2011). *The future of nursing: Leading change, advancing health*. Washington, DC: National Academic Press.

Kastner, M., Antony, J., Soobiah, C., et al. (2016). Conceptual recommendations for selecting the most appropriate knowledge synthesis method to answer research questions related to complex evidence. *Journal of Clinical Epidemiology, 73*, 43–49.

Sackett, D. L., Straus, S., Richardson, S., et al. (2000). *Evidence-based medicine: How to practice and teach EBM* (2nd ed.). London: Churchill Livingstone.

Sandelowski, M., & Barroso, J. (2007). *Handbook of qualitative research*. New York: Springer.

Uman, L. S. (2011). Systematic reviews and meta-analyses. *Journal of the Canadian Academy of Child and Adolescent Psychiatry, 20*(1), 57–59.

Whittemore, R. (2005). Combining evidence in nursing research. *Nursing Research, 54*(1), 56–62.

Go to Evolve at **http://evolve.elsevier.com/LoBiondo/** for review questions, appraisal exercises, and additional research articles for practice in reviewing and appraisal.

2

Appraising Research Questions, Hypotheses, and Clinical Questions

Judith Haber

Go to Evolve at **http://evolve.elsevier.com/LoBiondo/** for review questions.

LEARNING OUTCOMES

After reading this chapter, you should be able to do the following:

- Describe how the research question and hypothesis relate to the other components of the research process.
- Describe the process of identifying and refining a research question or hypothesis.
- Discuss the use of research questions versus hypotheses in a research study.
- Identify the criteria for determining the significance of a research question or hypothesis.

- Discuss how the purpose, research question, and hypothesis suggest the level of evidence to be obtained from the findings of a research study.
- Discuss the purpose of developing a clinical question.
- Discuss the differences between a research question and a clinical question.
- Apply critical appraisal criteria to the evaluation of a research question and hypothesis in a research report.

KEY TERMS

clinical question	independent variable	purpose	testability
dependent variable	nondirectional	research hypothesis	theory
directional hypothesis	hypothesis	research question	variable
hypothesis	population	statistical hypothesis	

As a nurse, you will be a clinical leader who will use research evidence to inform your practice. Evidence-based practice is a key component of the expertise you offer to your patients whether they are individuals, families, or communities. It provides the foundation for learning to critically appraise research questions and hypotheses that guide research studies. It also provides the foundation for developing clinical questions that guide your search for health information that offers the best available evidence to inform your clinical decisions and care planning.

At the beginning of this chapter, you will learn about research questions and hypotheses from the perspective of a researcher. The second part of this chapter will help you generate your own clinical questions to be used to guide the development of quality improvement and evidence-based practice projects. From a clinician's perspective, you must understand the research question and hypothesis as it aligns with the rest of a study. As a practicing nurse, developing clinical questions (see Chapters 19, 20, and 21) is the first step of the evidence-based practice process for quality improvement programs like those that decrease the risk for development of central-line–associated bloodstream infection (CLABSI) (Ferrani and Taylor, 2019; Appendix F).

When nurses ask questions such as, "Why are things done this way?", "I wonder what would happen if . . . ?", "What characteristics are associated with . . .?", or "What is the effect of _____ on patient outcomes?," they are often well on their way to developing a research question or hypothesis. Research questions are usually generated by situations that emerge from practice, leading nurses to wonder about the effectiveness of one intervention versus another for a specific patient population.

The research question or hypothesis is a key preliminary step in the research process. The **research question** tests a measurable relationship to be examined in a research study. The **hypothesis** predicts the outcome of a study.

Hypotheses can be considered intelligent hunches, guesses, or predictions that provide researchers with the direction for the research design and the collection, analysis, and interpretation of data. Hypotheses are a vehicle for testing the validity of the theoretical framework assumptions and provide a bridge between **theory** (a set of interrelated concepts, definitions, and propositions) and the real world (see Chapter 4). The research questions or hypotheses can be found at the beginning of a research article, but they may be embedded or implied in the "Purpose," "Aims," "Goals," or even the "Results" section of the research report.

For a clinician making an evidence-informed decision about a patient care issue, a clinical question, such as whether chlorhexidine or povidone-iodine is more effective in preventing CLABSIs, would guide the nurse in searching and retrieving the best available evidence. This evidence, combined with clinical expertise and patient preferences, would provide an answer on which to base the most effective decision about patient care for this population.

This chapter provides you with a working knowledge of research questions and hypotheses. It also highlights the importance of clinical questions and how to develop them.

DEVELOPING AND REFINING A RESEARCH QUESTION: STUDY PERSPECTIVE

A researcher spends a great deal of time refining a research idea into a testable research question. Research questions or topics are not pulled from thin air. In Table 2.1, you will see that research questions can indicate that practical experience, critical appraisal of the scientific literature, or interest in an untested theory forms the basis for development of a research idea. The research question should reflect a refinement of the researcher's initial thinking. The evaluator of a research study should be able to identify that the researcher has done the following:

- Defined a specific question area
- Reviewed the relevant literature
- Examined the question's potential significance to health care
- Pragmatically examined the feasibility of studying the research question or hypothesis

TABLE 2.1   How Practical Experience, Scientific Literature, and Untested Theory Influence the Development of a Research Idea

Area	Influence	Example
Clinical experience	Clinical practice provides a wealth of experience from which research problems can be derived. The nurse may observe a particular event or pattern and become curious about why it occurs and its relationship to other factors in the patient's environment.	The coronavirus pandemic has decreased access to health care and resulted in an overall hesitancy to keep up with health-promotion visits. Most notable are data from pediatric practice QI retrospective chart reviews that validate the clinical observation about parental hesitancy regarding routine childhood vaccines. A review of literature provides evidence to support that vaccination hesitancy, particularly for influenza vaccine, is prevalent in the United States (Kempe et al., 2020). These data provided the catalyst to develop a health literacy initiative that aimed to improve vaccination outcomes.
Critical appraisal of scientific literature	Critical appraisal of studies in journals may indirectly suggest a clinical problem by stimulating the reader's thinking. The nurse may observe the outcome data from a single study or a group of related studies that provide the basis for developing a pilot study, quality improvement project, or clinical practice guideline to determine the effectiveness of this intervention in his or her setting.	At a staff meeting with members of an interprofessional team at a cancer center, it was noted that the center did not have a standardized clinical practice guideline for mucositis, a painful chemotherapy side effect involving the oral cavity that has a negative impact on nutrition, oral hygiene, and comfort. The team wanted to identify the most effective approaches for treating adults and children experiencing mucositis. Their search for and critical appraisal of existing research studies led the team to develop an interprofessional mucositis guideline that was relevant to their patient population and clinical setting (NYU Langone Medical Center, 2020).
Gaps in the literature	A research idea may also be suggested by a critical appraisal of the literature that identifies gaps and suggests areas for future study. Research ideas also can be generated by research reports that suggest the value of replicating a particular study to extend or refine the existing scientific knowledge base.	Health literacy has been linked to timeliness of breast and cervical cancer screening, with inconsistent findings that may result from the use of nonprobability sampling and a health literacy instrument that only measures a subset of health literacy. The impetus for the cross-sectional, correlational study by Kim and Han (2019) used national-level data from the 2016 Behavioral Risk Factor Surveillance System (BRFSS) for women eligible for breast cancer screening ($n = 44{,}241$) and cervical cancer screening ($n = 38{,}956$) per American Cancer Society guidelines. A health literacy survey consisting of three types of questions: oral (asking for medical advice), listening (understanding the information providers offer), and written (understanding printed health information) literacy. Data were extracted to examine relationships between literacy-related demographic data that reflected the social determinants of health and screening. Oral and listening literacies were significantly related to up-to-date breast cancer ($p = .002$) and cervical cancer ($p < .001$) screenings. The authors concluded that oral and listening literacies are contributing factors to lifetime breast cancer and up-to-date cervical cancer screening. Providers must use strategies that promote effective patient-provider communication that increase these essential health promotion behaviors.

TABLE 2.1 **How Practical Experience, Scientific Literature, and Untested Theory Influence the Development of a Research Idea—cont'd**

Area	Influence	Example
Interest in untested theory	Verification of a theory and its concepts provides a relatively uncharted area from which research problems can be derived. Inasmuch as theories themselves are not tested, a researcher may consider investigating a concept or set of concepts related to a nursing theory or a theory from another discipline. The researcher would pose questions like, "If this theory is correct, what kind of behavior would I expect to observe in particular patients, and under which conditions?" "If this theory is valid, what kind of supporting evidence will I find?"	Adverse childhood experiences (ACE), including abuse, neglect, and household dysfunction, are very common. Almost one-half (45%) have experienced at least one ACE, and the prevalence is higher among Black (61%) and Hispanic (51%) children. ACEs are associated with increased health risks across the life span (Felitti et al., 1998; Hughes et al., 2017). The purpose of this study is to examine risk and protective factors for toxic stress among low-income, multiethnic families that may support the ACE model. This exploratory approach aims to determine effect sizes and generate hypotheses that will form future research studies on the intergenerational transmission of stress and protective factors among vulnerable families (Condon et al., 2019).

IBT, Intensive behavioral therapy.

Defining the Research Question

Brainstorming with faculty or colleagues may provide valuable feedback that helps the researcher focus on a specific research question area. **Example:** ➤ Suppose a researcher tells a colleague that her area of interest is population health problems associated with chronic health conditions like type 2 diabetes (T2D). The colleague may ask, "What is it about the topic that specifically interests you?" The researcher may reply, "Diabetes mellitus has reached global health proportions, with almost 10% of the population worldwide having a diagnosis." This conversation may initiate a chain of thought that results in a decision to explore factors contributing to this population health problem, such as an increase in urbanization, changes in transitions associated with sedentary occupations (e.g., work, food choices), and increased calorie consumption with a dramatic rise in obesity. A search of the literature highlighted the potential benefit of a structured individualized T2D education program provided by a primary care nurse (Coria De la Fuente, 2020) (see Appendix B). Fig. 2.1 illustrates how a broad area of interest (population health, chronic health conditions, evidence-based and cost-effective nursing intervention) was narrowed to a specific research topic (effectiveness of a structured, individualized T2D education program provided by a primary care nurse on glycemic control, fasting blood glucose, cholesterol, triglycerides, and blood pressure).

> **EVIDENCE-BASED PRACTICE TIP**
>
> A well-developed research question guides a focused search for scientific evidence about assessing, diagnosing, treating, or providing patients with information about their prognosis related to a specific health problem.

Beginning the Literature Review

The literature review should reveal a relevant collection of studies and systematic reviews that have been critically examined. Concluding sections in research articles (i.e., the recommendations and implications for practice) often identify remaining gaps in the literature,

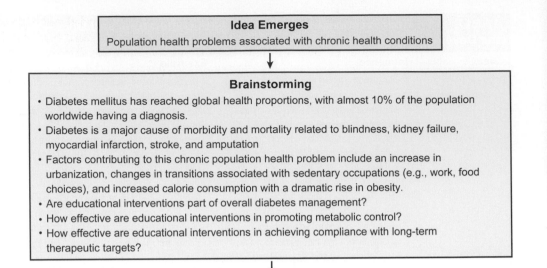

Idea Emerges

Population health problems associated with chronic health conditions

Brainstorming

• Diabetes mellitus has reached global health proportions, with almost 10% of the population worldwide having a diagnosis.
• Diabetes is a major cause of morbidity and mortality related to blindness, kidney failure, myocardial infarction, stroke, and amputation
• Factors contributing to this chronic population health problem include an increase in urbanization, changes in transitions associated with sedentary occupations (e.g., work, food choices), and increased calorie consumption with a dramatic rise in obesity.
• Are educational interventions part of overall diabetes management?
• How effective are educational interventions in promoting metabolic control?
• How effective are educational interventions in achieving compliance with long-term therapeutic targets?

Literature Review

• Evidence-based guidelines consider diabetes education to be one of the keys to managing diabetes.
• The effectiveness of education in terms of improving metabolic control reveals conflicting data.
• The achievement of therapeutic targets of educational programs has been poorly evaluated.
• There is potential benefit on targeted health outcomes of a structured individualized T2D education program provided by a primary care nurse.

Identify Variables

Sociodemographic Variables
• Age
• Gender
• Diabetes Years (DBP)

Health Variables
• Body Mass Index (BMI)
• Systolic Blood Pressure (SBP)
• Diastolic Blood Pressure (DBP)
• Fasting Blood Glucose (FBG)
• Glycated Hemoglobin (Hb A_{1c})
• Total Cholesterol (TC)
• Low-density Lipids (LDL)
• High-density Lipids (HDL)
• Triglycerides (TG)
• Diet/Exercise Treatment
• Oral Antidiabetics (OAD)
• Insulin Treatment

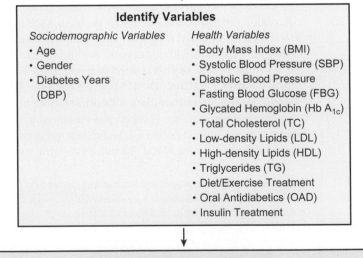

Formulated Research Question

What is the effectiveness of a structured, individualized T2D education program provided by a primary care nurse that featured educational reinforcements and family support to achieve metabolic control and long-term therapeutic targets?

FIG 2.1 Development of a research question.

the need for replication, or the need for additional knowledge about a particular research focus (see Chapter 3). In the previous example, the researcher may have conducted a preliminary review of reports, guidelines, and journals for research studies that provide outcome data about the effectiveness of education in terms of hemoglobin A_{1c} and other cardiovascular parameters. The review revealed conflicting data and that achievement of therapeutic targets following educational programs has been poorly evaluated. These factors, called *variables,* should be potentially relevant, of interest, and measurable.

EVIDENCE-BASED PRACTICE TIP

The answers to questions generated by qualitative data reflect evidence that may provide the first insights about a phenomenon that has not been previously studied.

Other variables, called demographic variables, such as race, ethnicity, gender, geographical location, age, education, and physical and mental health status, are also suggested as essential to consider. **Example:** ➤ A review of the literature revealed that poor oral health of mothers and children (e.g., tooth decay, gum disease, tooth loss) is a predominant health disparity in culturally diverse and economically disadvantaged communities. In a study to determine whether nurse home visitors who received oral health education increased their oral health knowledge and practice behaviors and contributed to positive oral health outcomes in a group of high-risk Medicaid-insured first-time pregnant women, demographic variables like age, zip code, insurance status, and enrollment in the Nurse Family Partnership Program were important to consider (Haber et al., 2020). This information can then be used to further define the research question and continue the search of the literature to identify effective intervention strategies reported in other studies with similar high-risk populations living in different geographical locations and having racial/ethnic backgrounds (e.g., rural) that could be applied to this population. **Example:** ➤ In the study by Coria De la Fuente and colleagues (2020), only two studies are cited that report data about achievement of clinical outcomes of interest to this research team; however, these studies are poorly evaluated. At this point, the research team could write the tentative research question, "What is the effectiveness of using a structured individualized type 2 diabetes education program provided by a primary care nurse to control type 2 diabetes mellitus patients?" You can envision the interrelatedness of the initial definition of the question area, the literature review, and the refined research question.

HELPFUL HINT

Reading the literature review or theoretical framework section of a research article helps you trace the development of the implied research question and/or hypothesis.

Examining Significance

When considering a research question, it is crucial that the researcher examine the question's potential significance for nursing and health care. This is sometimes referred to as the "so what" question, because the research question should have the potential to contribute to and extend the scientific body of nursing knowledge. Guidelines for selecting research questions should meet the following criteria:

- Patients, nurses, the health care community in general, and society will potentially benefit from the knowledge derived from the study.

- Results will be applicable for nursing practice, education, or administration.
- Findings will provide support or lack of support for untested theoretical concepts.
- Findings will extend or challenge existing knowledge by filling a gap or clarifying a conflict in the literature.
- Findings will potentially provide evidence that supports developing, retaining, or revising nursing practices or policies.

If the research question has not met any of these criteria, the researcher would be wise to extensively revise the question or discard it. **Example:** ➤ In the previously cited research question, the significance of the question includes the following facts:

- Diabetes mellitus has reached global epidemic proportions, with a worldwide prevalence of 8.5% in the adult population.
  - In Spain, the prevalence (9.4%) is higher than the worldwide rate.
  - The T2D epidemic has been attributed to urbanization and environmental transitions (e.g., work and diet patterns) that favor sedentary occupations and increased calorie consumption.
  - The increase of T2D in children and young people is attributed to the rise in obesity and physical inactivity and has the potential to become a public health problem.
  - Diabetes is a major cause of morbidity and mortality.
  - The economic costs related to loss of work and income, medications, hospitalization, and ambulatory care are high for patients and health care systems.
- Cost-effective treatments are available to control T2D and prevent or delay complications, but these treatments have been poorly evaluated.
  - This study sought to fill a gap in the related literature by assessing the effectiveness of a structured individualized T2D education program provided by a primary care nurse to achieve the therapeutic targets of long-term control.

> **IPE   HIGHLIGHT**
>
> It is helpful to collaborate with colleagues from other professions to identify an important clinical question that provides data for quality improvement on your unit.

THE FULLY DEVELOPED RESEARCH QUESTION

When a researcher finalizes a research question, the following characteristics should be evident:
- It clearly identifies the variables under consideration.
- It specifies the population being studied.
- It implies the possibility of empirical testing.

Because each element is crucial to developing a satisfactory research question, the criteria will be discussed in greater detail. These elements can often be found in the introduction of the published article; they are not always stated in an explicit manner.

Variables

Researchers call the properties studied "variables." Such properties take on different values. Thus a **variable**, as the name suggests, is something that varies. Properties that differ from each other, such as age, weight, height, religion, and ethnicity, are examples of variables. Researchers attempt to understand how and why differences in one variable relate to differences in another variable. **Example:** ➤ A researcher may be concerned about the variable of hospital-acquired pneumonia (HAP), the leading hospital-acquired bacterial infection. It is a variable because not all hospitalized patients get pneumonia. A researcher may also be interested in which other factors can be linked to HAP. There is clinical evidence to suggest that regular oral hygiene is associated with decreasing risk for HAP. The simple mechanical removal of plaque and bacteria with a toothbrush is a key step in reducing the risk for HAP. You can see that these factors are also variables that must be considered in relation to the development of HAP in hospitalized patients (Munro and Baker, 2019).

When speaking of variables, the researcher is essentially asking, "Is **X** related to **Y**? What is the effect of **X** on **Y**? How are X_1 and X_2 related to **Y**?" The researcher is asking a question about the relationship between one or more independent variables and a dependent variable. (*Note:* In cases in which multiple independent or dependent variables are present, subscripts are used to indicate the number of variables under consideration.)

An **independent variable**, usually symbolized by **X**, is the variable that has the presumed effect on the dependent variable. In experimental research studies, the researcher manipulates the independent variable (see Chapter 9). In nonexperimental research, the independent variable is not manipulated and is assumed to have occurred naturally before or during the study (see Chapter 10).

The **dependent variable**, represented by **Y**, varies with a change in the independent variable. The dependent variable is not manipulated. It is observed and assumed to vary with changes in the independent variable. Predictions are made from the independent variable to the dependent variable. It is the dependent variable that the researcher is interested in understanding, explaining, or predicting. **Example:** ➤ It might be assumed that the perception of pain intensity (the dependent variable) will vary in relation to a person's gender (the independent variable). In this case, we are trying to explain the perception of pain intensity in relation to gender (i.e., male or female). Although variability in the dependent variable is assumed to depend on changes in the independent variable, this does not imply that there is a causal relationship between **X** and **Y**, or that changes in variable **X** cause variable **Y** to change.

Table 2.2 presents a number of examples of research questions. Practice substituting other variables for the examples in Table 2.2. You will be surprised at the skill you develop in writing and critiquing research questions with greater ease.

Although one independent variable and one dependent variable are used in the examples, there is no restriction on the number of variables that can be included in a research question. Research questions that include more than one independent or dependent variable may be broken down into subquestions that are more concise.

Finally, it should be noted that variables are not inherently independent or dependent. A variable that is classified as independent in one study may be considered dependent in another study. **Example**: ➤ A nurse may review an article about depression that identifies depression in older men as predictive of risk for suicide. In this case, depression is the independent variable. When another article about the effectiveness of antidepressant medication alone or in combination with cognitive behavioral therapy (CBT) in decreasing depression in older men is considered, change in depression is the dependent variable. Whether a variable is independent or dependent is a function of the role it plays in a particular study.

Population

The **population** is a well-defined set that has certain characteristics and is either clearly identified or implied in the research question. **Example:** ➤ In a cross-sectional study evaluating whether the stress level of familial caregivers of Parkinson disease patients is related to their

TABLE 2.2	Research Question Format	
Type	**Format**	**Example**
Quantitative		
Correlational	Is there a relationship between **X** (independent variable) and **Y** (dependent variable) in the specified population?	Are there relationships between sociodemographic characteristics (e.g., age, willingness to receive HPV vaccination) and professional characteristics (e.g., education, belief that cervical and oropharyngeal cancer can be prevented by HPV vaccination) and overall knowledge about cervical cancer, HPV, and HPV vaccines?
Comparative	Is there a difference in **Y** (dependent variable) between people who have **X** characteristic (independent variable) versus those who do not have **X** characteristic?	Do female caregivers' appraisals of children's behavior differ by family type (level of hardiness and cohesiveness)?
Experimental	Is there a difference in **Y** (dependent variable) between group A, who received X (independent variable), and group B who did not receive **X**?	What is the effect of pelvic floor muscle training compared with lifestyle advice on the improvement of pelvic floor symptoms after pelvic organ prolapse surgery (Liang et al., 2019).
Qualitative		
Phenomenology	What is your lived experience of **X**?	What are the perceptions and interpretations that underlie health-related adherence behaviors from the perspective of people who have experienced heart attack (Admi et al., 2020; Appendix E)

HBHC, Hospital-based home care.

perception of the need and usefulness of health care education, the study population were older than 18 years of age and were the familial caregiver of Parkinson disease patients at >24" on the Montreal Cognitive Assessment (MoCA) scale. The research question posed was, "Is the stress level of familial caregivers of Parkinson disease patients related to their perception of the need and usefulness of health care education?" (Di Stasio et al., 2020) (Appendix D).

EVIDENCE-BASED PRACTICE TIP

Make sure that the population of interest and the setting have been clearly described so you will know exactly who the study population must be if you want to replicate the study.

Testability

The research question must imply that it is testable (measurable by either qualitative or quantitative methods). **Example:** ➤ The research question "Should postoperative patients control how much pain medication they receive?" is stated incorrectly for a variety of reasons. One reason is that it is not testable; it represents a value statement rather than a research question. A scientific research question must propose a measurable relationship between an independent variable and a dependent variable. A testable research question may be stated the following way: "Is patient-controlled pain medication more effective than nurse-administered pain medication in decreasing postoperative pain?" Many interesting and important clinical questions are not valid research questions because they are not amenable to testing.

TABLE 2.3	**Components of the Research Question and Related Criteria***	
Variables	**Population**	**Testability**
Independent Variable	• High-risk population of HIV-infected racial and ethnic minority adolescents and young adults	• Impact of a peer-led mobile health cognitive behavioral intervention on virologic outcomes and self-reported ART adherence (Navarra et al., 2019)
• Peer-led mobile health cognitive behavioral intervention		
• Age		
• Race/ethnicity		
• Marital and parental status education		
Dependent Variable		
• Antiretroviral therapy (ART) adherence and HIV virologic outcomes		

HELPFUL HINT

Remember that research questions are used to guide all types of research studies but are also used in exploratory, descriptive, qualitative, or hypothesis-generating studies.

The question is: "What is the effectiveness of using an individualized structured T2D education program provided by a primary care nurse to control T2D patients as evaluated by physiological outcomes and achievement of therapeutic targets of long-term control?" Table 2.3 illustrates how this research question is congruent with the three research question criteria.

HELPFUL HINT

- Remember that research questions are often not explicitly stated. The reader must infer the research question from the title of the report, the abstract, the introduction, or the purpose.
- Using your focused question, search the literature for the best available answer to your clinical question.

STUDY PURPOSE, AIMS, OR OBJECTIVES

The **purpose** of the study encompasses the aims or objectives the investigator hopes to achieve with the research. These three terms are synonymous. The researcher selects verbs to use in the purpose statement that suggest the planned approach to be used when studying the research question and the level of evidence to be obtained through the study findings. Verbs such as *explore* or *describe* suggest an investigation of an infrequently researched topic that might appropriately be guided by research questions rather than hypotheses. In contrast, verb statements indicating that the purpose is to test the effectiveness of an intervention or compare two alternative nursing strategies suggest a hypothesis-testing study for which there is an established knowledge base of the topic.

Remember that when the purpose of a study is to test the effectiveness of an intervention or compare the effectiveness of two or more interventions, the level of evidence is likely to have more strength and rigor than a study whose purpose is to explore or describe phenomena. Box 2.1 provides examples of purpose, objective, and aim statements.

BOX 2.1   Examples of Purpose, Objective, and Aim Statements

- The aim of the study was to identify subgroups of Latinas who have distinct symptom profiles when receiving radiation, chemotherapy, and/or hormonal therapy for breast cancer (Crane et al., 2020).
- The purpose of this study was to explore the effect of pelvic floor muscle training on the improvement of pelvic floor symptoms after pelvic organ prolapse surgery to better guide the work of nurse practitioners (Liang et al., 2019).

EVIDENCE-BASED PRACTICE TIP

Purpose, objective, and aim statements often provide the most information about the intent of the research question and hypotheses, and they suggest the level of evidence to be obtained from the findings of the study.

DEVELOPING THE RESEARCH HYPOTHESIS

Like the research question, hypotheses are often not stated explicitly in a research article. You will often find that hypotheses are embedded in the data analysis, results, or discussion section of the research report. Similarly, the population may not be explicitly stated but will have been identified in the background, significance, and literature review. It is then up to you to figure out the hypotheses and population being tested. But sometimes they are explicit. **Example:** ➤ In a study by Kim et al. (2020) predicting smoking abstinence in women with human immunodeficiency virus (HIV) infection, the hypotheses are stated clearly at the end of the "Background" section. The following is an example of one of the three hypotheses: "HIV-infected women who experienced more postquit withdrawal symptoms would be less likely to achieve nicotine-verified smoking abstinence at 3-month follow-up."

Hypotheses flow from the study's purpose, literature review, and theoretical framework. Fig. 2.2 illustrates this flow. A **hypothesis** is a declarative statement about the relationship between two or more variables. A hypothesis predicts an expected outcome of a study.

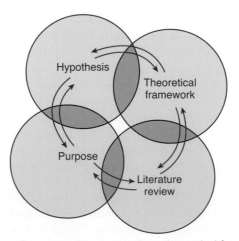

FIG 2.2 Interrelationships of purpose, literature review, theoretical framework, and hypothesis.

Hypotheses are developed before the study is conducted because they provide direction for the collection, analysis, and interpretation of data.

> **HELPFUL HINT**
>
> When hypotheses are not explicitly stated by the author at the end of the "Introduction" section or just before the "Methods" section, they will be embedded or implied in the "Data Analysis," "Results," or "Discussion" section of a research article.

Relationship Statement

The first characteristic of a hypothesis is that it is a declarative statement that identifies the predicted relationship between two or more variables: an independent variable (X) and a dependent variable (Y). The direction of the predicted relationship is also specified in this statement. Phrases such as *greater than, less than, positively, negatively,* or *difference in* suggest the directionality that is proposed in the hypothesis. The following is an example of a directional hypothesis: "HIV-infected women who had higher levels of negative emotional states (i.e., depression and anxiety symptoms) at baseline would report more nicotine withdrawal symptoms during the first 4 weeks after quit day" (Cooley et al., 2020). The dependent and independent variables are explicitly identified, and the relational aspect of the prediction in the hypothesis is contained in the phrase "would report more."

The nature of the relationship, either causal or associative, is also implied by the hypothesis. A causal relationship is one in which the researcher can predict that the independent variable (X) causes a change in the dependent variable (Y). In research, it is rare that one is in a firm enough position to take a definitive stand about a cause-and-effect relationship. **Example:** ➤ In a study investigating disparities in untreated caries (cavities) among children and adults in the United States from 2011 to 2014, the research team identified untreated caries on the crown or enamel surface of a tooth that has not been treated or filled as the independent variable and demographic and socioeconomic characteristics as the dependent variable. The research team hypothesized that improved access to and utilization of dental care post–Affordable Care Act (ACA) are associated with lower odds of untreated caries among children and adults (Gupta et al., 2018). It would be difficult for a researcher to predict a cause-and-effect relationship, however, because of the multiple intervening variables (e.g., race/ethnicity, marital status, gender, education, federal poverty level) related to the social determinants of health (SDOH) that might also influence the subjects' access to and utilization of dental care and contribute to the resultant disparities in this population health issue.

Variables are more commonly related in noncausal ways; that is, the variables are systematically related but in an associative way. This means that the variables change in relation to each other. **Example:** ➤ There is strong evidence that asbestos exposure is related to lung cancer. It is tempting to state that there is a causal relationship between asbestos exposure and lung cancer. Do not overlook the fact, however, that not all of those who have been exposed to asbestos will have lung cancer, and not all of those who have lung cancer have had asbestos exposure. Consequently, it would be scientifically unsound to take a position advocating the presence of a causal relationship between these two variables. Rather, one can say only that there is an associative relationship between the variables of asbestos exposure and lung cancer, a relationship in which there is a strong systematic association between the two phenomena.

Testability

The second characteristic of a hypothesis is its testability. This means that the variables of the study must lend themselves to observation, measurement, and analysis. The hypothesis is either supported or not supported after the data have been collected and analyzed. The predicted outcome proposed by the hypothesis will or will not be congruent with the actual outcome when the hypothesis is tested.

> **HELPFUL HINT**
>
> When a hypothesis contains more than one independent or dependent variable, it is difficult for the findings to indicate unequivocally that the hypothesis is supported or not supported. In such cases, the reader must infer which relationships are significant in the predicted direction from the findings or discussion section.

Theory Base

The third characteristic is that the hypothesis is consistent with an existing body of theory and research findings. Whether a hypothesis is arrived at on the basis of a review of the literature or a clinical observation, it must be based on a sound scientific rationale. You should be able to identify the flow of ideas from the research idea to the literature review, to the theoretical framework, and through the research question(s) or hypotheses. **Example:** ➤ Flanders and colleagues (2020) (see Appendix C) evaluated the impact of a staff resilience program on nursing turnover, employee engagement, and compassion satisfaction among nurses in a PICU. The research team proposed a theoretical framework based on resilience, a "concept that proposes a recurring human need to weather periods of stress and change successfully throughout life" (Resilience, 2009). They further proposed that individuals with high compassion satisfaction and resilience are less likely to suffer from compassion fatigue (CF) and the associated nurse burnout and turnover.

Wording the Hypothesis

As you read the scientific literature and become more familiar with it, you will observe that there are a variety of ways to word a hypothesis that are described in Tables 2.4 and 2.5. Information about hypotheses may be further clarified in the instruments, sample, or methods sections of a research report (see Chapters 12 and 15).

Statistical Versus Research Hypotheses

You may observe that a hypothesis is further categorized as either a research or a statistical hypothesis. A research hypothesis, also known as a scientific hypothesis, consists of a statement about the expected relationship of the variables. A research hypothesis indicates what the outcome of the study is expected to be. A research hypothesis is also either directional or nondirectional. If the researcher obtains statistically significant findings for a research hypothesis, the hypothesis is supported. The examples in Table 2.4 represent research hypotheses.

A statistical hypothesis, also known as a null hypothesis, states that there is no relationship between the independent and dependent variables. The examples in Table 2.5 illustrate statistical hypotheses. If, in the data analysis, a statistically significant relationship emerges between the variables at a specified level of significance, the null hypothesis is rejected. Rejection of the statistical hypothesis is equivalent to acceptance of the research hypothesis.

TABLE 2.4   Examples of How Hypotheses Are Worded

Variables	Hypothesis	Type of Design; Level of Evidence Suggested
1. There are significant differences in self-reported cancer pain, symptoms accompanying pain, and functional status according to self-reported ethnic identity.		
IV: Ethnic identity DV: Self-reported cancer pain DV: Symptoms accompanying pain DV: Functional status	Nondirectional, research	Nonexperimental; level IV
2. Individuals who participate in UC plus BP will have a greater reduction in BP from baseline to 12-month follow-up than individuals who receive UC only.		
IV: TM IV: UC DV: Blood pressure	Directional, research	Experimental; level II
3. There will be a greater decrease in state anxiety scores for patients receiving a structured telehealth health literacy module before abdominal or chest tube removal than for patients receiving standard information.		
IV: Preprocedure structured videotape information IV: Standard information DV: State anxiety	Directional, research	Experimental; level II
4. Participants randomly assigned to the intervention group (dog-walking program) will show a significant increase in physical activity when compared with participants in the control group (no dog-walking program), and these changes will remain 1 year after the start of the intervention.		
IV: Dog-walking intervention among dog owners IV: Control group—usual dog walking DV: Physical activity	Directional, research	Experimental; level II
5. Nurses with high social support from coworkers will have lower perceived job stress.		
IV: Social support DV: Perceived job stress	Directional, research	Nonexperimental; level IV
6. There will be no difference in anesthetic complication rates between hospitals that use CRNAs for obstetrical anesthesia versus those that use anesthesiologists.		
IV: Type of anesthesia provider (CRNA or MD)	Null	Nonexperimental; level IV
7. There will be no significant difference in duration of patency of a 24-gauge intravenous lock in a neonatal patient when flushed with 0.5 mL of heparinized saline (2 u/mL) compared with 0.5 mL of 0.9% of normal saline.		
IV: Heparinized saline IV: Normal saline DV: Duration of patency of intravenous lock	Null	Experimental; level II

BP, Blood pressure; *CRNA,* certified registered nurse anesthetist; *DV,* dependent variable; *IV,* independent variable; *TM,* telemonitoring; *UC,* usual care.

Directional Versus Nondirectional Hypotheses

Hypotheses can be formulated directionally or nondirectionally. A **directional hypothesis** specifies the expected direction of the relationship between the independent and dependent variables. An example of a directional hypothesis is provided in a study by Kim and colleagues (2020) discussed earlier in the chapter, which investigated predictors of smoking abstinence

TABLE 2.5	Examples of Statistical Hypotheses		
Hypothesis	**Variables**	**Type of Hypothesis**	**Type of Design Suggested**
Oxygen inhalation by nasal cannula of up to 6 L/min does not affect oral temperature measurement taken with an electronic thermometer.	IV: Oxygen inhalation by nasal cannula DV: Oral temperature	Statistical; null	Experimental
There will be no difference in the performance accuracy of ANPs and FNPs in formulating accurate diagnoses and acceptable interventions for suspected cases of domestic violence.	IV: Nurse practitioner (ANP or FNP) category DV: Diagnosis and intervention performance accuracy	Statistical; null	Nonexperimental

ANPs, Adult nurse practitioners; *FNPs,* family nurse practitioners; *DV,* dependent variable; *IV,* independent variable.

in women living with HIV infection. The researchers hypothesized that HIV-infected women who received an HIV-tailored smoking cessation intervention would report less nicotine withdrawal symptoms than their counterparts who received an attention-control intervention.

In contrast, a **nondirectional hypothesis** is often implied in the Background or Results section of a study. It indicates the existence of a relationship between the variables but does not specify the anticipated direction of the relationship. **Example:** ➤ Denny and Such (2018) explored the relationship between postoperative pain and subsyndromal delirium (SSD) in older adults after joint replacement surgery. They proposed to determine the relationship between opioid intake and SSD in older adults after joint replacement surgery but did not specify the predicted direction of the relationship. Both the directional and the nondirectional forms of hypothesis statements are acceptable.

RELATIONSHIP BETWEEN THE HYPOTHESIS AND THE RESEARCH DESIGN

Regardless of whether the researcher uses a statistical or a research hypothesis, there is a suggested relationship between the hypothesis, the design of the study, and the level of evidence provided by the results of the study. The type of design, experimental or nonexperimental (see Chapters 9 and 10), will influence the wording of the hypothesis. **Example:** ➤ When an experimental design is used, you would expect to see hypotheses that reflect relationship statements, such as the following:

- X_1 is more effective than X_2 on Y.
- The effect of X_1 on Y is greater than that of X_2 on Y.
- The incidence of Y will not differ in subjects receiving X_1 and X_2 treatments.
- The incidence of Y will be greater in subjects after X_1 than after X_2.

EVIDENCE-BASED PRACTICE TIP

Think about the relationship between the wording of the hypothesis, the type of research design suggested, and the level of evidence provided by the findings of a study using each kind of hypothesis. You may want to consider which type of hypothesis potentially will yield the strongest results applicable to practice.

CRITICAL THINKING DECISION PATH
Determining the Use of a Hypothesis or Research Question

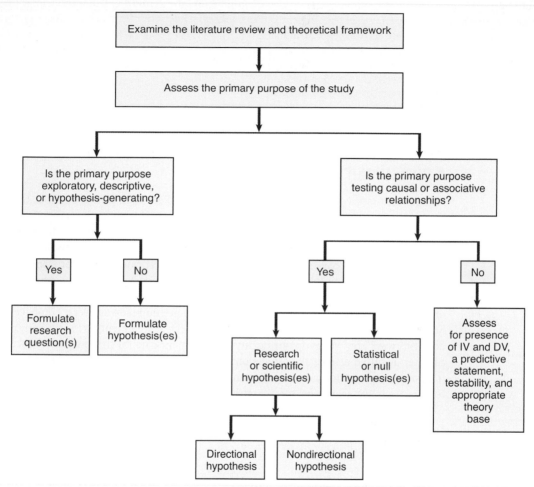

Hypotheses reflecting experimental designs also test the effect of the experimental treatment (i.e., independent variable **X**) on the outcome (i.e., dependent variable **Y**). This suggests that the strength of the evidence provided by the results is level II (experimental design) or level III (quasi-experimental design).

In contrast, hypotheses related to nonexperimental designs reflect associative relationship statements, such as the following:

- **X** will be negatively related to **Y**.
- There will be a positive relationship between **X** and **Y**.

This suggests that the strength of the evidence provided by the results of a study that examined hypotheses with associative relationship statements would be at level IV (nonexperimental design).

Table 2.6 provides an example of this concept. The Critical Thinking Decision Path will help you determine the type of hypothesis or research question presented in a study.

TABLE 2.6   Elements of a Clinical Question

Population	Intervention	Comparison Intervention	Outcome
Older adult patients with hospital-acquired pressure injuries (HAPIs)	The 3T Program (turn, touch, and tidy) was developed to address the areas of concern identified in the root-cause analysis combined with the Lean Six Sigma methodology	HAPI standard of care	Significant decrease in number of HPIs and cost savings to the hospital (Gallo et al., 2019)

HAPI, Hospital-acquired pressure injury.

DEVELOPING AND REFINING A CLINICAL QUESTION: A CONSUMER'S PERSPECTIVE

Practicing nurses as well as students are challenged to keep their practice up to date by searching for, retrieving, and critically appraising research articles that apply to practice issues that are encountered in their clinical setting (see Chapter 20). Practitioners strive to use the current best evidence from research when making clinical and health care decisions. As research consumers, you are not conducting research studies; however, your search for information from and about clinical practice is converted into focused, structured clinical questions that are the foundation of evidence-based practice and quality improvement projects. Clinical questions often arise from clinical situations for which there are no ready answers. You have probably had the experience of asking, "What is the most effective treatment for . . . ?", "Why do we still do it this way?", or "What do our quality improvement data for this quarter reveal about our catheter-acquired urinary tract infection rate."

Using similar criteria related to framing a research question, focused clinical questions form a basis for searching the literature to identify supporting evidence from research. Clinical questions have four components:

- Population
- Intervention
- Comparison
- Outcome

These components, known as *PICO*, provide an effective format for helping nurses develop searchable clinical questions. Box 2.2 presents each component of the clinical question.

BOX 2.2   Components of a Clinical Question Using the PICO Format

Population: The individual patient or group of patients with a particular condition or health care problem (e.g., adolescents 13 to 18 years of age with type 1 insulin-dependent diabetes)

Intervention: The particular aspect of health care that is of interest to the nurse or the health care team (e.g., a therapeutic [inhaler or nebulizer for treatment of asthma], preventive [pneumonia vaccine], diagnostic [measurement of blood pressure], or organizational [implementation of a bar-coding system to reduce medication errors] intervention)

Comparison intervention: Standard care or no intervention (e.g., antibiotic compared with ibuprofen for children with otitis media); a comparison of two treatment settings (e.g., rehabilitation center vs. home care)

Outcome: More effective outcome (e.g., improved glycemic control, decreased hospitalizations, decreased medication errors)

The significance of the clinical question becomes obvious as research evidence from the literature is critically appraised. Research evidence is used together with clinical expertise and the patient's perspective to confirm, develop, or revise nursing standards, protocols, and policies that are used to plan and implement patient care (Cullum, 2000; Sackett et al., 2000; Thompson et al., 2004). Issues or questions can arise from multiple clinical and managerial situations. Using the example of catheter-acquired urinary tract infections (CAUTIs), a team of staff nurses working on a medical unit in an acute care setting were reviewing their unit's quarterly quality improvement data and observed that the number of CAUTIs had increased by 25% over the past 3 months. The nursing staff reviewed the unit's standard of care and noted that although nurses were able to discontinue an indwelling catheter, according to a set of criteria and without a physician order, catheters were remaining in place for what they thought was too long and potentially contributing to an increase in the prevalence of CAUTIs. To focus the nursing staff's search of the literature, they developed the following question: Does the use of daily nurse-led catheter rounds in hospitalized older adults with indwelling urinary catheters lead to a decrease in CAUTIs? Sometimes it is helpful for nurses who develop clinical questions from a quality improvement perspective to consider three elements as they frame their focused question: (1) the situation, (2) the intervention, and (3) the outcome.

- The situation is the patient or problem being addressed. This can be a single patient or a group/population of patients with a particular health problem (e.g., hospitalized adults with indwelling urinary catheters).
- The intervention is the dimension of health care interest that often asks whether a particular intervention is a useful treatment (e.g., daily nurse-led catheter rounds).
- The outcome addresses the effect of the treatment (e.g., intervention) for this patient or patient population in terms of quality and cost (e.g., decreased CAUTIs). It essentially answers whether or not the intervention makes a difference for the patient population.

The individual parts of the question are vital pieces of information to remember when it comes to searching for evidence in the literature. One of the easiest ways to do this is to use a table, as illustrated in Table 2.6. Examples of clinical questions are highlighted in Box 2.3. Chapter 3 provides examples of how to effectively search the literature to find answers to questions posed by researchers and research consumers.

BOX 2.3   Examples of Clinical Questions

- Which factors are associated with patients becoming lost to follow-up at a free transitional and continuing care clinic for patients with uncontrolled diabetes? (Buys et al., 2019)
- Does the Healthy Living with Pain (HeLP) nurse practitioner–led model improve opioid-prescribing practices by family practice residents? (Naimer et al., 2019)
- Can intravenous pentamidine be safely administered to children with cancer who are medically stable outside of the intensive care setting? (Herriage & Hooke, 2020)
- Does the use of telehealth improve symptom awareness and preventive self-care in a community-dwelling population of older adults with heart failure? (Murphy et al., 2019)
- Does a novel live-webinar education program for caregivers improve asthma control in preschoolers? (Sawicki & White, 2020)

≫ APPRAISAL FOR EVIDENCE-BASED PRACTICE
THE RESEARCH QUESTION AND HYPOTHESIS

When you begin to critically appraise a research study, consider the care the researcher takes when developing the research question or hypothesis; it is often representative of the overall conceptualization and design of the study. In a quantitative research study, the remainder of a study revolves around answering the research question or testing the hypothesis. In a qualitative research study, the objective is to answer the research question. Because this text focuses on you as a research consumer, the following sections will primarily pertain to the evaluation of research questions and hypotheses in published research reports.

Critically Appraising the Research Question and Hypothesis

The following Critical Appraisal Criteria box provides several criteria for evaluating the initial phase of the research process—the research question or hypothesis. Because the research question or hypothesis guides the study, it is usually introduced at the beginning of the research report to indicate the focus and direction of the study. You can then evaluate whether the rest of the study logically flows from its foundation—the research question or hypothesis. The author will often begin by identifying the background and significance of the issue that led to crystallizing development of the research question or hypothesis. The clinical and scientific background and/or significance is summarized, and the purpose, aim, or objective of the study is then identified.

Often the research question or hypothesis will be proposed before or after the literature review. Sometimes you will find that the research question or hypothesis is not specifically stated. In some cases, it is only hinted at or is embedded in the purpose statement, and you are challenged to identify the research question or hypothesis. In other cases, the research question is embedded in the findings toward the end of the article. To some extent, this depends on the style of the journal.

Although a hypothesis can legitimately be nondirectional, it is preferable and more common for the researcher to indicate the direction of the relationship between the variables in the hypothesis. Quantifiable words such as *greater than, less than, decrease, increase, positively, negatively,* or *related* convey the idea of objectivity and testability. You will find that when there is a lack of data available for the literature review (i.e., the researcher has chosen to study a relatively undefined area of interest), a nondirectional hypothesis or research question may be appropriate.

You should recognize that how the proposed relationship of the hypothesis or research question is phrased suggests the type of research design that will be appropriate for the study and the level of evidence to be derived from the findings. **Example:** ➤ If a hypothesis proposes that treatment X_1 will have a greater effect on Y than treatment X_2, an experimental design (level II evidence) or quasi-experimental design (level III evidence) is suggested (see Chapter 9). If a research question asks if there will be a positive relationship between variables X and Y, a nonexperimental design (level IV evidence) is suggested (see Chapter 10).

Hypotheses and research questions are never proven beyond the shadow of a doubt. Hypotheses and research questions are only supported or not supported by the findings. Researchers who claim that their data have "proven" the validity of their hypothesis or research question should be regarded with grave reservation. You should realize that, at best, findings that support a hypothesis or the findings of a research question are considered tentative. If repeated replication of a study yields the same results, more confidence can be placed in the conclusions advanced by the researchers.

When critically appraising clinical questions, think about the fact that the clinical question should be focused and specify the patient population or clinical problem being addressed, the intervention, and the outcome for a particular patient population. There should be evidence that the clinical question guided the literature search and that appropriate types of research studies are retrieved in terms of the study design and level of evidence needed to answer the clinical question.

CRITICAL APPRAISAL CRITERIA
Developing Research Questions and Hypotheses

The Research Question
1. Does the research question express a relationship between two or more variables, or at least between an independent variable and a dependent variable, implying empirical testability?
2. How does the research question specify the nature of the population being studied?
3. How has the research question been supported with adequate experiential and scientific background material?
4. How has the research question been placed within the context of an appropriate theoretical framework?
5. How has the significance of the research question been identified?
6. Have pragmatic issues, such as feasibility, been addressed?
7. How have the purpose, aims, or goals of the study been identified?

The Hypothesis
1. Is the hypothesis concisely stated in a declarative form?
2. Are the independent and dependent variables identified in the statement of the hypothesis?
3. Is each hypothesis specific to one relationship so each hypothesis can be either supported or not supported?
4. Is the hypothesis stated in such a way that it is testable?
5. Is the hypothesis stated objectively, without value-laden words?
6. Is the direction of the relationship in each hypothesis clearly stated?
7. How is each hypothesis consistent with the literature review?
8. How is the theoretical rationale for the hypothesis made explicit?
9. Given the level of evidence suggested by the research question, hypothesis, and design, what is the potential applicability to practice?

The Clinical Question
1. Does the clinical question specify the patient population, intervention, comparison intervention, and outcome?
2. Does the clinical question address an outcome applicable to practice?

KEY POINTS

- Developing the research question and stating the hypothesis are key preliminary steps in the research process.
- The research question is refined through a process that proceeds from the identification of a general idea of interest to the definition of a more specific and circumscribed topic.

- A preliminary literature review reveals related factors that appear critical to the research topic of interest and helps further define the research question.
- The significance of the research question must be identified in terms of its potential contribution to patients, nurses, the medical community in general, and society. Applicability of the question for nursing practice and its theoretical relevance must be established. The findings should also have the potential for formulating or altering nursing practices or policies.
- The final research question is a statement about the relationship of two or more variables. It clearly identifies the relationship between the independent variable and the dependent variable, specifies the nature of the population being studied, and implies the possibility of empirical testing.
- Research questions that are nondirectional may be used in exploratory, descriptive, or qualitative research studies.
- Research questions can be directional, depending on the type of study design being used.
- Focused clinical questions arise from clinical practice and guide the literature search for the best available evidence to answer the clinical question.
- A hypothesis is a declarative statement about the relationship between two or more variables that predicts an expected outcome. Characteristics of a hypothesis include a relationship statement, implications regarding testability, and consistency with a defined theory base.
- Hypotheses can be formulated in a directional or a nondirectional manner and be further categorized as either research or statistical hypotheses.
- The purpose, research question, or hypothesis provides information about the intent of the research question and hypothesis and suggests the level of evidence to be obtained from the study findings.
- The interrelationship of the research question or hypothesis and the literature review and the theoretical framework should be apparent.
- The appropriateness of the research design suggested by the research question or hypothesis is also evaluated.

CLINICAL JUDGMENT CHALLENGES

- Discuss how the wording of a research question or hypothesis suggests the type of research design and level of evidence that will be provided.
- Using the study by Di Stasio et al. (2020) (see Appendix D), describe how the background, significance, and purpose of the study are linked to the research questions.
- **IPE** The prevalence of central-line–associated bloodstream infections (CLABSIs) has increased in your critical care unit by 10% in the past quarter. As a member of the quality improvement (QI) committee on your unit, collaborate with your committee colleagues from other professions to develop an interprofessional action plan. Deliberate to develop a clinical question to guide the QI project.
- A nurse is in charge of discharge planning for frail older adults with congestive heart failure. The goal of the program is to promote self-care and prevent rehospitalizations. Using the PICO approach, the nurse wants to develop a clinical question for an evidence-based practice project to evaluate the effectiveness of discharge planning and home telehealth follow-up for this patient population. How can the nurse accomplish that objective?

REFERENCES

Admi, H., Eilon-Moshe, Y., Levy, H., Eisen, I., Nikolsky, E., Gepstein, L., Satran, C., & Ore, L. (2020). "It's up to me with a little support" – adherence after myocardial infarction; A qualitative study. *International Journal of Nursing Studies, 101.* https://doi.org/10.1016/j.inurstu.2019.103416.

Buys, K. C., Selleck, C., & Buys, D. R. (2019). Assessing retention in a free diabetes clinic. *The Journal for Nurse Practitioners, 15*(4), 301–305.

Condon, E. M., Holland, M. L., Slade, A., Redeker, N. S., Mayes, L. C., & Sadler, L. (2019). Maternal adverse childhood experiences, family strengths, and chronic stress in children. *Nursing Research, 68*(3), 189–199.

Coria De la Fuente, M. C., Cruz-Cobo, C., & Santi-Cano, M. J. (2020). Effectiveness of a primary care nurse delivered educational intervention for patients with type 2 diabetes mellitus in promoting metabolic control and compliance with long-term therapeutic targets: A randomized controlled trial. *International Journal of Nursing Studies, 101,* 1–8.

Crane, T. E., Badger, T. A., Sikorski, A., Segrin, C., Hsu, C., & Rosenfeld, A. G. (2020). Symptom profiles of Latina breast cancer survivors. *Nursing Research, 69*(4), 264–271.

Cullum, N. (2000). User's guides to the nursing literature: An introduction. *Evidence-Based Nursing, 3*(2), 71–72.

Denny, D. L., & Such, T. L. (2018). Exploration of relationships between postoperative pain and subsyndromal delirium in older adults. *Nursing Research, 67*(6), 421–429.

Di Stasio, E., Di Simone, E., Galeti, A., Donati, D., Guidotti, C., Tartaglini, D., Massimiliano, C., Marano, M., Di Muzio, M., & Gianfrocca, C. (2020). Stress-related vulnerability and usefulness of healthcare education in Parkinson's disease: The perception of a group of family caregivers, a cross-sectional study. *Applied Nursing Research, 51,* 1–5.

Felitti, V. J., Anda, R. F., Nordenberg, D., Williamson, D. F., Spitz, A. M., Edwards, V., & Marks, J. S. (1998). Relationships of childhood abuse and household dysfunction to many of the leading causes of death in adults: the Adverse Childhood Experiences (ACE) Study. *American Journal of Preventive Medicine, 14,* 245–258. https://doi.org/10.1016/S0749-3797(98)00017-8.

Ferrari, S., & Taylor, K. (2019). Effect of a systemwide approach to a reduction in central line-associated bloodstream infections. *Journal of Nursing Care Quality, 35*(1), 40–44.

Flanders, S., Hampton, D., Missi, P., Ipsan, C., & Gruebbel, C. (2020). Effectiveness of a staff resilience program in a pediatric intensive care unit. *Journal of Pediatric Nursing, 50,* 1–4.

Gallo, A. M., Doyle, R. C., Beckman, J., & Lizarraga, C. G. (2019). Blending evidence-based practice and Lean Six Sigma methodology to reduce hospital-acquired pressure injuries in a progressive care unit. *Journal of Nursing Care Quality, 00*(00), 1–6.

Gupta, N., Vujicic Yarborough, C., & Harrison, B. (2018). Disparities in treated caries among children and adults in the U.S. *BMC Oral Health, 18,* 30. https://doi.org/10.1186/s123903-018-0493-7.

Haber, J., Hartnett, E., Hille, A., & Cipollina, J. (2020). Promoting oral health for mothers and children: A nurse home visitor education program. *Pediatric Nursing, 46*(2), 70–76.

Herriage, T., & Hooke, M. C. (2020). Nursing care of the child with cancer during intravenous pentamidine infusions. *Pediatric Nursing, 46*(2), 61–63.

Hughes, K., Bellis, M. A., Hardcastle, K. A., Seethi, D, Butchart, A., Mikton, C., & Dunne, P. (2017). The effect of multiple adverse childhood experiences on health: a systematic review and meta-analysis. *The Lancet Public Health, 2,* e356–e366. https://doi.org/10.10016/S2368-2667(17)30118-4.

Kempe, A. A. W., Saville, C., Albertin, C., Zimet, G., Breck, A., Helmkamp, L., Vangala, S., Dickinson, M. L., Rand, C., Humiston, S. M., & Szilagyi, P. G. (2020). Parental hesitancy about routine childhood and influenza vaccinations: A national survey. *American Academy of Pediatrics.* https://pediatrics.aappublications.org/node/152121.full.print.

Kim, K., & Han, H. (2019). The association between health literacy and breast and cervical cancer screening behaviors. *Nursing Research, 68*(3), 177–188.

Kim, S. S., Cooley, M. E., Lee, S. A., & DeMarco, R. (2020). Prediction of smoking abstinence in women living with human immunodeficiency virus infection. *Nursing Research, 69*(3), 167.

Liang, Y., Li, X., Wang, J., Liu, Y., Yang, Y., & Dong, M. (2019). Effect of pelvic floor muscle training on improving prolapse-related symptoms after surgery. *Journal for Nurse Practitioners, 15*(8), 600–605.

Munro, S., & Baker, D. (2019). Integrating oral health into patient management to prevent hospital-acquired pneumonia: A team approach. *Journal of the Michigan Dental Association, 20,* 48–57.

Murphy, N., Shanks, M., & Alderman, P. (2019). Management of heart failure with outpatient technology. *The Journal for Nurse Practitioners, 15*(1), 12–18.

Naimer, M. S., Munro, J., Singh, S., & Permaul, J. A. (2019). Improving family Medicine residents' opioid prescribing: A nurse practitioner-led model. *The Journal for Nurse Practitioners, 15*(5), 661–665.

Navarra, A. M. D., Gwadz, M. V., Bakken, S., Whittemore, R., Cleland, C. M., & Melkus, G. M. (2019). Adherence connection for counseling, education, and support: Research protocol for a proof-of-concept study. *Journal of Medical Internet Research, 21*(3). https://doi.org/10.2196/12543.

NYU Langone Medical Center. (2020). *Personal Communication*: New York, NY.

Resilience, (2009). *Mosby's medical dictionary* (8th ed.). Retrieved July 16th, 2019 from https://medical-dictionary.thefreedictionary.com/resilience.

Sackett, D., Straus, S. E., Richardson, W. S., et al. (2000). *Evidence-based medicine: How to practice and teach EBM*. London: Churchill Livingstone.

Sawicki, J. C., & White, K. A. (2020). Controlling asthma in preschoolers: Webinar education for their caregivers. *Pediatric Nursing, 46*(2), 77–82.

Thompson, C., Cullum, N., McCaughan, D., et al. (2004). Nurses, information use, and clinical decision-making: The real world potential for evidence-based decisions in nursing. *Evidence-Based Nursing, 7*(3), 68–72.

Go to Evolve at **http://evolve.elsevier.com/LoBiondo/** for review questions, appraisal exercises, and additional research articles for practice in reviewing and appraisal.

3

Gathering and Appraising the Literature

Brynne A. Campbell, Susan Kaplan Jacobs

Go to **Evolve** at **http://evolve.elsevier.com/LoBiondo/** for review questions.

LEARNING OUTCOMES

After reading this chapter, you should be able to:

- Discuss the purpose of a literature review in a research study.
- Discuss the purpose of reviewing the literature for an evidence-based and quality improvement (QI) project.
- Differentiate between primary and secondary sources.
- Describe how research evidence is hierarchical and based on design, publication type, and peer review.

- Frame background questions, and identify the major sources of background information.
- Identify the core health sciences repositories, recognizing their scope, strengths, and limitations.
- Use the PICO question to guide a systematic search of the literature.
- Use appropriate critical appraisal tools to evaluate both literature reviews and research studies.

KEY TERMS

background questions
Boolean operators
citation management
   software
controlled vocabularies

critical appraisal tools
evidence hierarchy
evidence summaries
grey literature
meta-analysis

metadata
peer review
point-of-care tools
practice guidelines
primary sources

review articles
scholarly journals
search bias
secondary sources
systematic review

Searching for, retrieving, critically appraising, and synthesizing research evidence is essential to supporting an evidence-based practice (EBP). Your ability to locate, retrieve, appraise, and synthesize research articles will help you as both a student and a practicing nurse, enabling you to determine whether you have the best evidence to inform your clinical practice.

EBP is built on the premise that there is an inherent structure and hierarchy to health sciences literature, based on research design and publication practices, such that only the highest-quality evidence should be used in clinical practice. Evidence is often depicted as a pyramid, an evidence hierarchy that distinguishes the strength of the design(s) at each level of evidence (see Chapter 1, Fig. 1.1). The process of identifying, appraising, and synthesizing evidence and then weighing that evidence, in conjunction with patient preference, clinical expertise, and available resources, forms the basis of evidence-based clinical decisions and makes up the heart of EBP/QI projects (Cullum, 2008).

Electronic databases and web-scale search engines have made health information more accessible than ever; a simple Google search can yield thousands of potentially relevant results. However, with this constantly expanding sea of information comes a magnified need for you as students and practicing nurses to be conscious consumers of that information, committed to thoughtfully locating and critically appraising research.

Critical appraisal of research is an organized, systematic approach to evaluating a study or group of studies using standardized critical appraisal criteria. The criteria are used to objectively determine the strength, quality, quantity, and consistency of evidence provided by the literature to determine its applicability to practice, policy, and education (see Chapters 7, 11, and 18).

The purpose of this chapter is to help you understand and navigate the health sciences information landscape to develop the skills necessary to support an EBP. This chapter provides you with the tools to (1) search for, locate, and retrieve studies, systematic reviews/meta-analyses, meta-syntheses (see Chapters 6, 9, 10, and 11), and other documents (e.g., clinical practice guidelines); (2) differentiate between research articles and secondary sources; (3) critically appraise a research study or group of research studies; and (4) organize and synthesize the results of your literature search. You will learn to use discovery and retrieval tools to systematically locate high-quality evidence while maintaining an unbiased and thoughtful approach to gathering, appraising, and synthesizing literature.

REVIEW OF THE LITERATURE

Broadly speaking, a literature review is a synthesis of the completed research on a particular topic, representing the "state of the science" in that area (Card, 2010). The purpose of a literature review differs, depending on the context for the review, specifically whether you are a researcher conducting a review for a study or conducting a QI or EBP project.

The Literature Review: The Researcher's Perspective

Table 3.1 presents the main purposes of a literature review in a research article. In a published study, the literature review generally appears as a short section near the beginning of the report. It may be untitled as a separate section or integrated with the theoretical framework. You may see the literature review section with titles like *background, literature review, review, related literature,* or *conceptual framework.* It provides an abbreviated version of the literature review conducted by the researcher and represents the building blocks, or framework, of the study.

In the literature review, researchers present the relevant primary and secondary sources they have used to establish a foundation and framework for the concepts, hypotheses, or research questions methodologies and analyses that will underpin their quantitative or qualitative research study (see Appendices B–E). Primary sources are research reports or articles in which the researchers themselves describe their original findings ("Primary and Secondary Sources," 2009). In contrast, secondary sources are sources in which the authors have analyzed, interpreted, and synthesized the information presented in primary sources (Table 3.2). The researcher must succinctly present an overview and appraisal of the primary and secondary literature on a topic to generate research questions or hypotheses.

TABLE 3.1 Overall Purposes of a Literature Review

Major Goal

To develop a strong knowledge base to conduct a research study or implement an evidence-based practice/quality improvement project and carry out research

Objectives

A review of the literature supports the following:

For a **research** study...	For an **EBP/QI** project...	For **both** research and EBP/QI...
• Describe theoretical/conceptual frameworks that guide a study.	• Provide information to discuss the findings of a study, draw conclusions, and make recommendations for future research, practice, education, and/or policy changes.	• Determine what is known and unknown about a subject, concept, or problem
• Determine the need for replication or refinement of a study.		• Determine gaps, consistencies, and inconsistencies in the literature about a subject, concept, or problem.
• Generate research questions and hypotheses.	• Uncover a new practice intervention(s) or gain supporting evidence for revising, maintaining current interventions(s), protocols, and policies, or developing new ones.	• Synthesize the strengths and weaknesses of available studies to determine the state of the science on a topic/problem.
• Determine an appropriate research design, methodology, and analysis for a study		• Identify recommendations from the conclusion for future research, practice, education, and/or policy actions.
	• Generate clinical questions that guide development of EBP/QI projects, policies, and protocols	

In some publications, a researcher begins a review of the literature by summarizing the significance, history, and impact of a problem and the need for an intervention. For example, in an article reporting the results of a nurse-led educational intervention for adults with type 2 diabetes (see Appendix B), the introduction section of the article includes citations of global statistics, scientific evidence, references to the economic significance of the disease, and other relevant data supporting the need for the study (De la Fuente Coria et al., 2020). The literature review is a broad, critical evaluation of the literature on the given topic and is essential to inform all steps of the research process.

The Literature Review: The Evidence-based Practice Perspective

In contrast with those *conducting* qualitative or quantitative research, as a clinician who values EBP, you will find yourself as a *consumer* of research. From this perspective, the literature review will focus on the critical appraisal of research studies, systematic reviews, clinical practice guidelines, and other relevant documents. You will seek to comprehensively identify the relevant research evidence on a given clinical topic to inform the development and/or refinement of the clinical question(s) that will guide your EBP or QI project (Box 3.1). After the body of research evidence has been critically appraised, a conclusion about the overall strengths and weaknesses of the body of research evidence can be formulated, allowing you to judge the strength of the evidence available to answer your clinical question and determine its applicability for clinical practice.

Proposing a clear and concise clinical question is essential to conduct a search using one or more electronic databases to find the best available evidence. Clinical questions may sound like research questions, but they are questions used to search the literature for evidence-based answers, not to test research questions or hypotheses. The PICO format is suggested as a framework for developing clear and concise clinical questions:

TABLE 3.2	**Comparing Source Types**	
	Foreground (Primary)	**Background (Secondary)**
Authorship	The researcher(s) who actually conducted the study	Not the original conductor(s) of the research, but a person with some expertise in the field
Examples and Descriptions	Meta-analyses (see example in Appendix A) Nonexperimental studies • Retrospective (see example in Appendix C) • Cross-sectional (see example in Appendix D) • Qualitative research (see example in Appendix E) Experimental studies (e.g., clinical trials, randomized controlled trials) See example in Appendix B: De la Fuente Coria, M. C., Cruz-Cobo, C., & Santi-Cano, M. J. (2020). Effectiveness of a primary care nurse delivered educational intervention for patients with type 2 diabetes mellitus in promoting metabolic control and compliance with long-term therapeutic targets: Randomised controlled trial. *International Journal of Nursing Studies, 101*, 103417.	Articles in abstract journals • Abstract journals contain expert commentary and critical appraisal of published studies (e.g., *Evidence-Based Nursing*) Evidence summaries/syntheses • Aggregation and appraisal of evidence related to clinical topics of interest (e.g., resources from Joanna Briggs Institute EBP Database) Point-of-care (POC) tools • Reference tools designed to help clinicians find evidence-based information at the POC (e.g., Nursing Reference Center, UpToDate) Review articles • Collect, summarize, and sometimes appraise primary evidence on a given research question (e.g., systematic reviews from the Cochrane Database of Systematic Reviews) Practice guidelines • Authored by professional agencies or societies, guidelines often based on systematic reviews (e.g., guidelines recommended by Guideline Central (www.guidelinecentral.com) Government reports and topic summaries • Contain official guidance and overviews from health-related government bodies Example: Centers for Disease Control and Prevention. (2020). *National Diabetes Statistics Report 2020* (CS 314227-A; p. 32). U.S. Department of Health and Human Services. https://stacks.cdc.gov/view/cdc/85309
Uses	• Stay up to date on the most recent emergent information in the field • Provide an evidence base for aggregating, appraising, and synthesizing for an EBP/QI project	Building a knowledge base to understand nuances of clinical questions • Building a capacity to understand and critique primary literature • In a clinical setting, using POC tools, evidence summaries, and practice guidelines to guide decision making

(P) Problem or patient population: Define the specific group, condition, or issue.

(I) Intervention: Identify the intervention or change process that will be used to address the problem or population.

(C) Comparison: Compare how the proposed intervention or process differs from the current standard of care or another intervention.

(O) Outcome: Specify the proposed effect of the intervention or process change.

Box 3.1 provides an example of how the PICO format can be used to frame a clinical question. When working with your student or clinical colleagues to answer the PICO question in Box 3.1, you will work as a team to search the literature using electronic databases to do the following:

> **BOX 3.1 Developing a Clinical Question Using the PICO Format**
>
> In a population of adult patients with type 2 diabetes (P), what is the effectiveness of telehealth educational interventions (I) compared with face-to face care (C) for improving glycemic control by 10% (O)?
> **P** Adult patients with type 2 diabetes with increased glycemic levels
> **I** A telehealth educational intervention delivered by nurses
> **C** Face-to-face counseling
> **O** Improve glycemic control by 10%

- Identify individual research studies, systematic reviews, and clinical practice guidelines to obtain the "best available evidence" related to prevention interventions for type 2 diabetes.
- Critically appraise the evidence gathered using standardized critical appraisal criteria and tools (Table 3.6; Box 3.2).
- Synthesize the overall strengths and weaknesses of the evidence found in the literature.
- Articulate a conclusion about the strength and consistency of the evidence.
- Develop one or more recommendations about the applicability of the evidence to guide the development of an educational intervention to improve glycemic control.

SEARCHING FOR EVIDENCE

Because EBP/QI projects depend heavily on evidence to inform clinical practice, conducting a systematic, reproducible search of the literature is a priority. A body of evidence that is incomplete, of low quality, or biased has the potential to negatively affect your clinical

> **BOX 3.2 Critical Appraisal Criteria for Literature Reviews**
>
> **Content and Source Material**
> 1. Does the literature review have a clear purpose?
>   a. If it is being conducted for EBP, does it answer a clinical question?
> 2. Does the literature review discuss all concepts and variables relevant to the research purpose?
>   a. Does the literature review attempt to identify all relevant studies and source material?
> 3. If it is an evidence synthesis article, does the review include at least one database search strategy? Were multiple databases searched for literature?
> 4. Does the literature review rely on primary sources, including both conceptual and research articles?
> 5. Does the literature review build on earlier studies?
>
> **Critique and Synthesis**
> 6. Does the discussion of each reviewed study reflect the essential components of the study design (e.g., type and size of sample, reliability and validity of instruments, consistency of data collection procedures, appropriate data analysis, identification of limitations)?
> 7. Does the critique of each reviewed study include strengths, weaknesses, or limitations of the design, conflicts, and gaps in information related to the area of interest?
> 8. Does the literature review make connections between the available evidence, synthesizing the results of existing research in a reasonable and logical way?
> 9. Does the literature review uncover gaps or inconsistencies in the available evidence?
>
> **Organization**
> 10. Is the literature review presented in a logical format (e.g., chronologically or grouped by variables), enhancing the reader's ability to evaluate the need for the particular research study or evidence-based practice project?

decision making. Conducting a rigorous search for evidence requires a systematic process, including key steps like framing a researchable question, locating background sources, conducting an initial scoping search, identifying key search terms and subject headings, and testing and revising search strategies. These steps are depicted in the critical thinking decision path and will be covered in greater detail throughout the chapter.

CRITICAL THINKING DECISION PATH: SYSTEMATIC SEARCH PROCESS

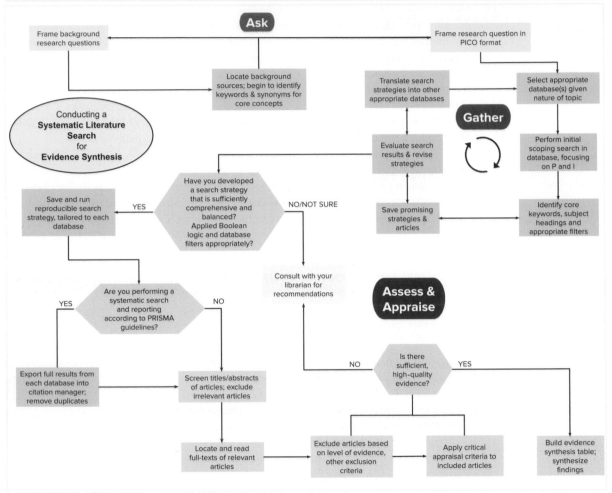

Sources of Literature

All "evidence" in EBP begins with primary research—studies that are designed to answer a clinically relevant question. The ways in which the results of that primary research (the evidence) are disseminated to reach the consumer of the information (often clinicians and students like yourselves) make up the occasionally complex structure of the health sciences information landscape.

The bulk of the evidence that constitutes the basis of your EBP/QI project will take the form of primary sources. After collecting, analyzing, and interpreting research data, researchers write a full report of their findings and submit their paper to scholarly journals, resulting in publications whose purpose is to share their research with other researchers or clinicians in their subject specialty. Scholarly journals are often peer reviewed, meaning that before a study is published, it must have gone through an editorial review process; subject experts appraise the submitted study, offering feedback and suggestions for improvement. Ensuring that a study has been published in a reputable, peer-reviewed journal is a useful first step in quality assessment.

In addition to publishing in scholarly journals, investigators will often present their initial results at discipline-specific conferences. Although these initial research reports have not been peer reviewed, they may be summarized in conference proceedings, which are then made available as part of the published literature. Beyond the body of formally published primary sources, there exists a body of resources known as the grey literature, an umbrella term that refers to information that is produced and distributed outside the traditional bounds of commercial academic publishing, such as reports, policy literature, government documents, preprints, unpublished research studies, white papers, and registrations of in-progress clinical trials (New York Academy of Medicine, 2021).

Once research has been released through these channels, it is read, digested, interpreted, analyzed, appraised, and synthesized into any number of secondary sources. Some secondary sources like evidence summaries/syntheses, clinical practice guidelines, and point-of-care (POC) tools are regularly updated, supported by the highest levels of evidence (see Chapter 1, Fig. 1.1). Other secondary sources, like textbooks, narrative review articles, and critical appraisal commentaries, are useful to provide background and contextualizing information for understanding primary sources. In contrast with primary sources, which contain the original research findings that will be appraised and synthesized as part of an EBP/QI project, secondary sources can offer helpful examples of *how* to digest and analyze original research (see Table 3.2).

Search Bias

It is tempting to think that you can conduct an unbiased, high-quality search using web-scale search tools like Google and Google Scholar. Search bias occurs when a literature search fails to identify all of the highest-quality relevant literature on a particular topic. If the search relies on insufficient selection of databases or incomplete search queries, search results will be biased, representing only an incomplete sample of the existing relevant literature (Opheim et al., 2019; Salvador-Oliván et al., 2019). Because search engines like Google and Google Scholar return results based on keyword relevance, regardless of the nature or validity of the information, they actually retrieve a jumble of resources. The results are likely to be a mixture of scholarly and nonscholarly articles, raw data, editorialized opinions, and user-generated content. The searcher is tempted to "cherry pick" from among the first few results, increasing the likelihood of bias.

Rather than relying on web-scale search tools, it is necessary to use specialized health sciences databases to conduct your literature reviews. These databases offer specific content, filtering capabilities, and the ability to build a structured search query. Using these tools diminishes the likelihood of biased searching and allows the user to develop a more tailored, reliable search strategy that leverages the hierarchical nature of health sciences literature.

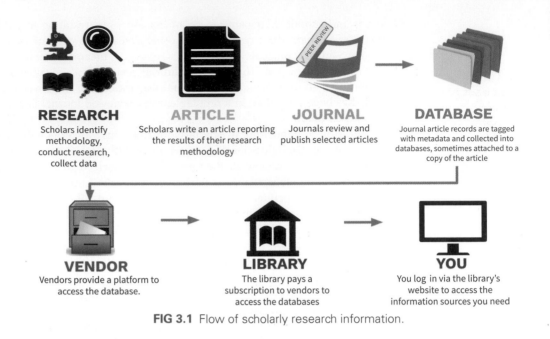

RESEARCH
Scholars identify methodology, conduct research, collect data

ARTICLE
Scholars write an article reporting the results of their research methodology

JOURNAL
Journals review and publish selected articles

DATABASE
Journal article records are tagged with metadata and collected into databases, sometimes attached to a copy of the article

VENDOR
Vendors provide a platform to access the database.

LIBRARY
The library pays a subscription to vendors to access the databases

YOU
You log in via the library's website to access the information sources you need

FIG 3.1 Flow of scholarly research information.

Health Sciences Databases and Digital Repositories

When new issues of scholarly journals are released, the articles are indexed into online databases and described with **metadata**, which are searchable descriptive fields like author, title, abstract, publication date, subject terms, and more. (Fig. 3.2). Databases and indexes are often licensed to institutions like libraries (Fig. 3.1), but some databases have freely discoverable abstracts that are available without an institutional license. These include PubMed, ClinicalTrials.gov, and the Cochrane Library (www.cochranelibrary.com).

Begin your search in databases with a scope and content focus that is concentrated in medical and nursing topics, such as MEDLINE (via PubMed), CINAHL, and PsycINFO (Table 3.3). Records in these databases are tagged with metadata that is particularly useful for refining your search (e.g., article type or methodology, age, sex, and species of the study's subjects). The presence of this metadata allows you to set filters to only retrieve articles that meet particular criteria (see Fig. 3.2).

> **HELPFUL HINT**
>
> Some article databases contain the full text of the article, ready to read and download, but most databases consist only of records with information *about* the articles (metadata). Once you've identified an article of interest via the database, it may be necessary to search the holdings of your institution's library to locate the full text. Only a subset of scholarly articles is open access, or freely available on the Internet; as a seeker of best evidence, you would not want to bias your results by accessing only what is freely available.

Each database has its own areas of strength in content coverage. For instance, MEDLINE via PubMed offers robust coverage of life sciences, biomedical, and pharmaceutical topics. CINAHL has greater coverage of journals related to nursing and allied health sciences, addressing both the biomedical and psychosocial aspects of diseases, conditions, or interventions as well as topics like patient education, health promotion, technology, and administration. Given the diversity in

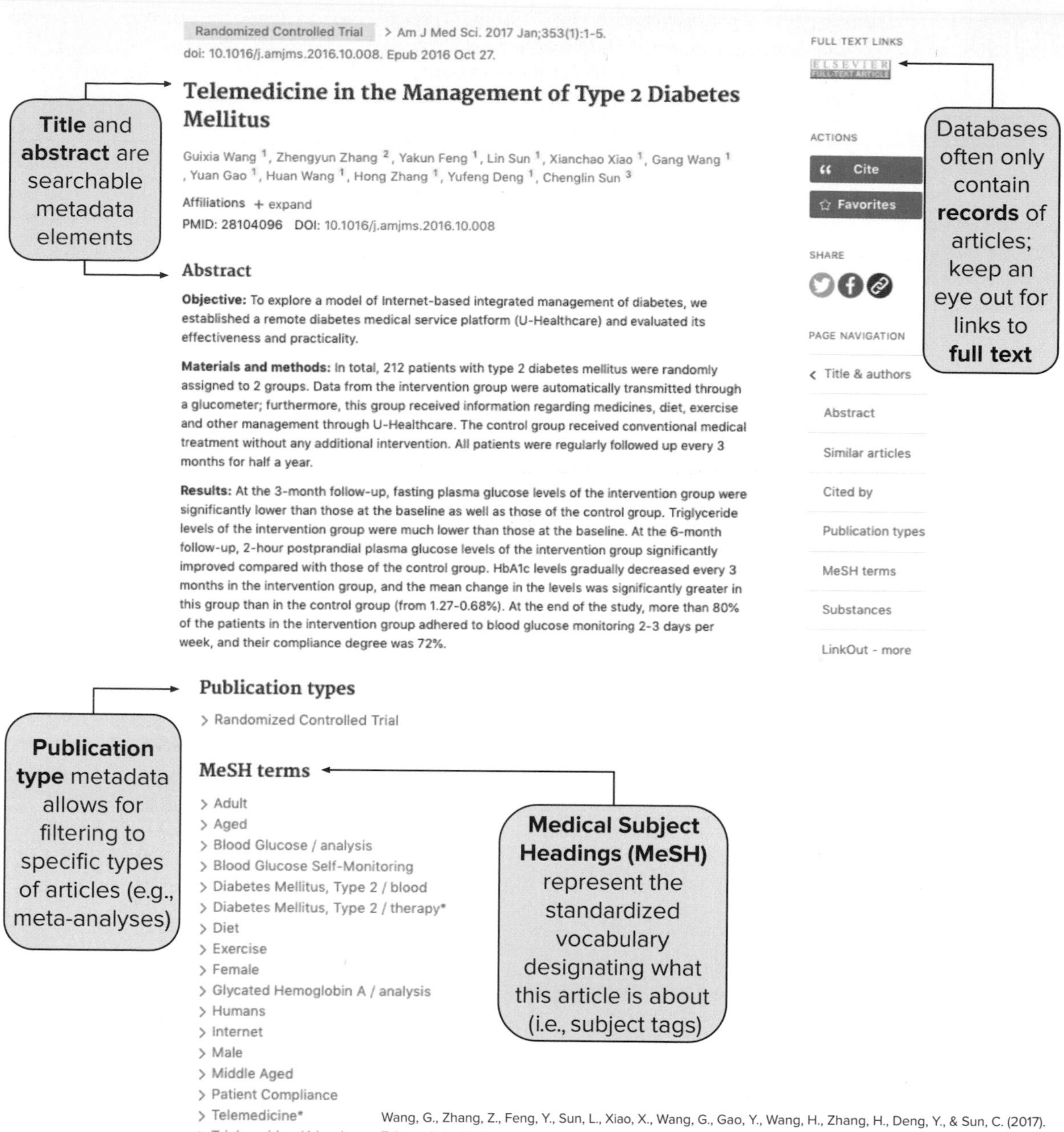

Randomized Controlled Trial   > Am J Med Sci. 2017 Jan;353(1):1-5.
doi: 10.1016/j.amjms.2016.10.008. Epub 2016 Oct 27.

Title and abstract are searchable metadata elements

FULL TEXT LINKS

ELSEVIER
FULL-TEXT ARTICLE

Telemedicine in the Management of Type 2 Diabetes Mellitus

Guixia Wang [1], Zhengyun Zhang [2], Yakun Feng [1], Lin Sun [1], Xianchao Xiao [1], Gang Wang [1], Yuan Gao [1], Huan Wang [1], Hong Zhang [1], Yufeng Deng [1], Chenglin Sun [3]

Affiliations + expand
PMID: 28104096   DOI: 10.1016/j.amjms.2016.10.008

ACTIONS

❝❝ Cite

☆ Favorites

SHARE

🐦 📘 🔗

Databases often only contain records of articles; keep an eye out for links to full text

PAGE NAVIGATION

‹ Title & authors

Abstract

Similar articles

Cited by

Publication types

MeSH terms

Substances

LinkOut - more

Abstract

Objective: To explore a model of Internet-based integrated management of diabetes, we established a remote diabetes medical service platform (U-Healthcare) and evaluated its effectiveness and practicality.

Materials and methods: In total, 212 patients with type 2 diabetes mellitus were randomly assigned to 2 groups. Data from the intervention group were automatically transmitted through a glucometer; furthermore, this group received information regarding medicines, diet, exercise and other management through U-Healthcare. The control group received conventional medical treatment without any additional intervention. All patients were regularly followed up every 3 months for half a year.

Results: At the 3-month follow-up, fasting plasma glucose levels of the intervention group were significantly lower than those at the baseline as well as those of the control group. Triglyceride levels of the intervention group were much lower than those at the baseline. At the 6-month follow-up, 2-hour postprandial plasma glucose levels of the intervention group significantly improved compared with those of the control group. HbA1c levels gradually decreased every 3 months in the intervention group, and the mean change in the levels was significantly greater in this group than in the control group (from 1.27-0.68%). At the end of the study, more than 80% of the patients in the intervention group adhered to blood glucose monitoring 2-3 days per week, and their compliance degree was 72%.

Publication types

> Randomized Controlled Trial

Publication type metadata allows for filtering to specific types of articles (e.g., meta-analyses)

MeSH terms

> Adult
> Aged
> Blood Glucose / analysis
> Blood Glucose Self-Monitoring
> Diabetes Mellitus, Type 2 / blood
> Diabetes Mellitus, Type 2 / therapy*
> Diet
> Exercise
> Female
> Glycated Hemoglobin A / analysis
> Humans
> Internet
> Male
> Middle Aged
> Patient Compliance
> Telemedicine*
> Triglycerides / blood

Medical Subject Headings (MeSH) represent the standardized vocabulary designating what this article is about (i.e., subject tags)

Wang, G., Zhang, Z., Feng, Y., Sun, L., Xiao, X., Wang, G., Gao, Y., Wang, H., Zhang, H., Deng, Y., & Sun, C. (2017). Telemedicine in the management of type 2 diabetes mellitus. *The American Journal of the Medical Sciences*, *353*(1), 1–5. https://doi.org/10.1016/j.amjms.2016.10.008

FIG 3.2 Anatomy of a PubMed database record.

content among different health sciences databases, if you are attempting to complete a comprehensive search on a health care topic, you should expect to look across multiple databases. For example, if your topic pertains to the behavioral aspects of managing type 2 diabetes, you would search a psychology database like PsycINFO in addition to the medical databases.

TABLE 3.3　Recommended Databases (Health Sciences and Multidisciplinary)

Core Health Sciences Databases

List is not meant to be exhaustive; consult your librarian for more institution-specific recommendations

Content Coverage	Types of Materials	Features
CINAHL (Cumulative Index to Nursing and Allied Health Literature) Access via EBSCO (health.ebsco.com/products/the-cinahl-database); requires institutional subscription		
Covers nursing, biomedicine, health sciences librarianship, alternative/complementary medicine, consumer health, and 17 allied health disciplines	Scholarly peer-reviewed journal articles Health care books Nursing dissertations Conference proceedings	Filters for: • Research subject characteristic (age, sex, human), date, publication type, "research" article Preformulated "Clinical Queries" for: • Therapy, Prognosis, Qualitative, Review, Causation Subject Thesaurus: CINAHL Subject Headings
PubMed (with MEDLINE) Free public access to citations and abstracts; links to full-text coverage for some content in PubMed central or open-access journals (pubmed.ncbi.nlm.nih.gov/)		
The premier source for coverage of clinical biomedical topics; also includes coverage of health administration, public health, technology, and other nonclinical aspects of health care	Scholarly, peer-reviewed journal articles A small number of newspapers, magazines, and newsletters	Filters for: • Research subject characteristic (e.g., age, sex, species), date, and article type Preformulated "Clinical Queries" for: • Etiology, Prognosis, Therapy, Clinical Prediction Subject thesaurus: • NLM Medical Subject Headings (MeSH) www.ncbi.nlm.nih.gov/mesh/
PsycINFO Access via Ovid, EBSCO, ProQuest, or directly from APA PsycNET (www.apa.org/pubs/databases/psycinfo); requires subscription		
Coverage centers on psychology and related disciplines, including medicine, psychiatry, nursing, sociology, pharmacology, physiology, and linguistics	Journal articles Books and book chapters Selected dissertations	Filters for: • Population characteristics (e.g., age, sex), methodology, tests and measures, publication type Preformulated "Clinical Queries" for: • Reviews, Therapy, Qualitative Subject Thesaurus *Thesaurus of Psychological Index Terms*®
EMBASE Access via Elsevier (www.elsevier.com/solutions/embase-biomedical-research); requires subscription		
Biomedical and pharmaceutical database indexing journals from more than 90 countries with selective coverage for nursing, psychology, and alternative medicine	Journal articles Conference abstracts (biomedical, drug, and medical device)	Filters for: • Publication type, experimental subjects, subject age and sex (Ovid only) Preformulated "Clinical Queries" for: • Reviews, Therapy, Diagnosis, Prognosis, Causation, Economics, Qualitative Subject Thesaurus • *Emtree*

TABLE 3.3   Recommended Databases (Health Sciences and Multidisciplinary)—cont'd

Recommended Multidisciplinary Databases

Content Coverage	Types of Materials	Features
Web of Science		
Access via Clarivate (clarivate.com/webofsciencegroup/solutions/web-of-science/); requires subscription		
Includes Core Collection, which covers Science Citation, Social Sciences Citation Index, and the Arts and Humanities Citation Index, among others	Scholarly journal articles Conference proceedings	Filters for: • Document types, funding agencies and Web of Science discipline categories, publication date Tools for: • Article and author metrics, cited reference searching
ProQuest Central		
Access via ProQuest (about.proquest.com/products-services/ProQuest_Central.html); requires subscription		
Multidisciplinary source for research across business, health and medical, social sciences, arts and humanities, education, science and technology, and more	Scholarly journal articles Newspaper and magazine articles Dissertations Books	Filters for: • Source and document type, peer-reviewed literature and subject Tools for: • Cited reference search, related articles

---

IPE   HIGHLIGHT

On your EBP/QI team, you may work with colleagues whose expertise and information needs will extend outside the core health sciences resources. Be aware of other subject-specific databases that may be relevant to your work together. For instance, the literature of social work can be found in PsycINFO, but also in Social Services Abstract and/or SocINDEX. A librarian will be able to make database suggestions that are tailored to your team's specific needs.

FRAMING BACKGROUND QUESTIONS AND INITIAL SEARCHING

As you begin your search, it is important to fully understand the context and nuances of a particular clinical topic. You will want to explore background questions, which are questions that seek general knowledge about a condition, disease, or intervention, or a definition of a term. Answers to background questions may be found in secondary sources, like books or topic summaries. For example, imagine you are working in a clinic with an adult patient population with type 2 diabetes whose glycemic control does not meet national guidelines. As a nurse, you are interested in facilitating nonpharmacological behavioral interventions for this population, but you understand the importance of making recommendations that are evidence-based. Before you can do so, it is important to make sure that you have a robust understanding of the topic at hand so you begin to consider background questions about behavioral management of type 2 diabetes. For instance, you may ask:

- What range of blood glucose levels is considered normal for adults?
- What is the state of the science regarding self-management of type 2 diabetes?
- What kinds of nonpharmacological interventions exist for type 2 diabetes?
- What are common barriers to successful blood sugar management?
- What are the current dietary guidelines recommended by the American Diabetes Association for adults with type 2 diabetes?

Background information to address questions like these can be found in a variety of sources, such as textbooks and POC tools. **POC tools** are resources, often mobile apps that provide clinicians with filtered and timely access to high-quality evidence to support patient care decisions in the clinical setting. **Evidence summaries,** like those found in the Joanna Briggs Institute EBP Database, are succinct synopses of available evidence related to selected topics, providing preappraised data and recommendations for research and clinical practice (joannabriggs.org/ebp). **Practice guidelines,** which are often published by health care (e.g., nursing, medicine, dental, pharmacy) organizations, societies, or government agencies, can provide evidence syntheses based on systematic reviews and support clinical decision making by synthesizing evidence related to common clinical problems, diseases, drugs, and therapies (see Table 3.2).

EVIDENCE-BASED PRACTICE TIP

If you are new to a topic, intervention, or disease, start by consulting background sources or POC tools that may synthesize what is known about a disease or intervention in the form of an evidence summary (see Table 3.2). In addition to resources licensed by your library or institution, there are many credible and freely available resources for disease information, data, statistics, and patient education materials. For example:

- WHO website (www.who.int)
- MedlinePlus (patient-facing education materials; medlineplus.gov)
- Clinical practice guidelines available from an association or society website, (e.g., American Diabetes Association www.diabetes.org)

Review articles, which survey the current state of understanding on a topic, can be valuable sources of background information, especially if they are systematic reviews or meta-analyses. A **systematic review** is a specific kind of a review article in which the authors have followed a rigorous, reproducible literature search process, with predefined inclusion and exclusion criteria, to collect all of the studies related to a particular topic or question; they then appraise and synthesize that evidence to present a state-of-the-science conclusion (see Chapter 11). A **meta-analysis** is a type of systematic review that pools the data from multiple studies on a specific topic and then quantitatively analyzes those data in aggregate, presenting a quantitative conclusion about the strength and applicability of the available evidence. Like any source of evidence, both systematic reviews and meta-analyses can vary in quality and should be assessed with the appropriate critical appraisal tools, but they can be valuable resources; not only do they offer an appraisal and synthesis of the available evidence related to a particular topic, but they have extensive reference lists that can serve as a catalyst for further research.

Finally, if your question relates to rapidly changing and current issues in medicine and health care (e.g., recent legislation or emerging public health issues), you will also find it useful to search for news and recent reports in a database whose scope of coverage extends beyond the scholarly health sciences literature (see ProQuest Central in Table 3.3).

IPE HIGHLIGHT

When working with colleagues from other disciplines with varied perspectives, it may be necessary to establish a shared vocabulary and understanding of the concepts at hand. Spending time as a team exploring reference and background sources can help ensure the whole patient care team is on the same page regarding the core components of the research question.

FRAMING CLINICAL QUESTIONS AND SEARCHING FOR PRIMARY EVIDENCE

A robust foundation of background information related to a topic of interest will lead you to developing a narrower clinical question using the PICO format discussed earlier in the chapter (as well as in Chapter 2). The ability to ask a clearly defined clinical question, and acquire evidence to answer that question, is a core competency in EBP (Albarqouni et al., 2018). This practice will require you to locate evidence within recent primary research studies, typically published in peer-reviewed journals that have been indexed in databases like PubMed, CINAHL, EMBASE, and PsycINFO (see Table 3.3). For clinical questions related to more interdisciplinary health care topics like health economics, public policy, ethics, or technology, a health sciences librarian will be able to suggest additional databases.

Translating a Clinical Question into a Database Query

PICO questions are well suited for database searching because they contain clearly defined concepts of interest. For example, consider the question of delivering nonpharmacological interventions for type 2 diabetes. Your background search and information may have revealed that telehealth is an exciting and emerging way to implement behavioral interventions with patients who have type 2 diabetes. You can formulate a more specific PICO question, where you ask:

- In a population of adult patients with type 2 diabetes (P), what is the effectiveness of telehealth educational interventions (I) on blood sugar management compared with face-to-face care (C) for improving glycemic control by 10%? (O)

This PICO question can be used to design a search string to query an article database to retrieve only records that contain these core concepts. An initial search should be structured relatively broadly, just focusing on two or three core concepts (often the *P* and the *I* of the PICO question) (Ho et al., 2016; Higgins et al., 2019). The use of **Boolean operators** (ANDs and ORs) enables you to specify how you would like the search terms to be connected and interpreted by the database search function (Table 3.4b). You can leverage the AND operator to only retrieve records that contain terms for your problem/population *and* intervention together.

As you search, you will begin to generate synonyms and/or alternate spellings for your concepts of interest. To perform a comprehensive search, it is important to keep track of these synonyms. For example, in addition to referring to "type 2 diabetes," some authors use the terms "noninsulin dependent diabetes" or "adult onset diabetes." Synonyms for the problem/population and intervention can be integrated into the search using the Boolean operator "OR," which tells the database to return results that contain *any* one of the given terms. A more comprehensive database search would be: (type 2 diabetes OR "adult onset diabetes" OR "noninsulin dependent diabetes") AND telehealth.

As the search evolves, you will begin to find that some terms are more useful than others; building a concept table is a practical way to track search terms, enabling you to document which terms work well and which terms should be eliminated from the strategy (see Table 3.4a).

Subject Headings and Controlled Vocabularies

Searching for the core concepts as key words or text words is often a good place to start. A text word search will retrieve records where the search term appears *anywhere* in the metadata attached to that record (e.g., the authors' names, the publication title, the abstract). As you become better acquainted with the health sciences databases, you will begin to notice that records are tagged with **controlled vocabularies**, agreed-upon descriptive

TABLE 3.4   Building and Refining a Search for a Problem and Intervention

a. Keep Track of Core Search Concepts

	Concept 1 (Problem/Population) **Type 2 Diabetes**	Concept 2 (Intervention) **Telehealth**
Key words	type 2 diabetes type 2 diabetes diabetes mellitus adult onset diabetes noninsulin dependent diabetes	telehealth mobile app cell phone
MeSH terms *(subject headings for PubMed search)*	"Diabetes Mellitus, Type 2"	Telemedicine "Remote Consultation" Smartphone "Mobile Applications" "Text Messaging"

b. Apply Boolean Operators to Expand or Narrow the Search

Operator	Usage
AND	Retrieve results that include all terms *Tips:* Use AND to narrow a search; the more terms/concept sets connected with AND, the smaller the results pool will be

Example:

Search Query	Results
"Diabetes Mellitus, Type 2"	133,748
"Diabetes Mellitus, Type 2" AND telemedicine	513
"Diabetes Mellitus, Type 2" AND telemedicine AND "glycemic control"	106

Operator	Usage
OR	Retrieve results that include any of linked terms *Tip:* Use OR to expand a search; the more alternate terms/synonyms that are connected with OR, the larger the results pool will be

Example:

Search Query	Results
"Diabetes Mellitus, Type 2"	513
"Diabetes Mellitus, Type 2" AND telemedicine	526
"Diabetes Mellitus, Type 2" AND telemedicine AND "glycemic control"	585

c. Apply Database Filters to Narrow the Search

Search Query	Results
"Diabetes Mellitus, Type 2" AND (telemedicine OR telehealth OR "mobile applications")	585
"Diabetes Mellitus, Type 2" AND (telemedicine OR telehealth OR "mobile applications") *Filters: Randomized Controlled Trials*	194
"Diabetes Mellitus, Type 2" AND (telemedicine OR telehealth OR "mobile applications") *Filters: Randomized Controlled Trials; past 5 years*	119

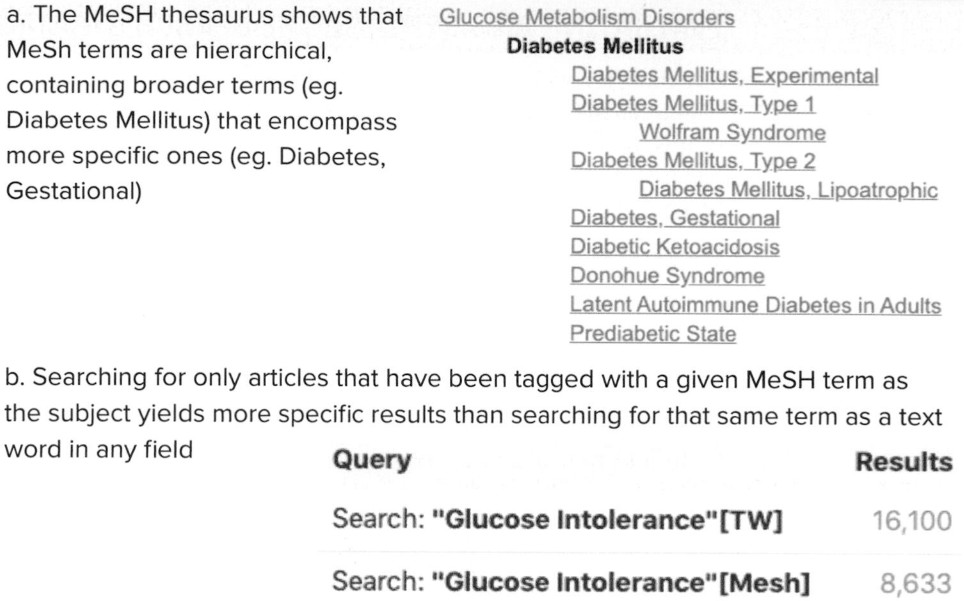

a. The MeSH thesaurus shows that MeSh terms are hierarchical, containing broader terms (eg. Diabetes Mellitus) that encompass more specific ones (eg. Diabetes, Gestational)

Glucose Metabolism Disorders
 Diabetes Mellitus
  Diabetes Mellitus, Experimental
  Diabetes Mellitus, Type 1
   Wolfram Syndrome
  Diabetes Mellitus, Type 2
   Diabetes Mellitus, Lipoatrophic
  Diabetes, Gestational
  Diabetic Ketoacidosis
  Donohue Syndrome
  Latent Autoimmune Diabetes in Adults
  Prediabetic State

b. Searching for only articles that have been tagged with a given MeSH term as the subject yields more specific results than searching for that same term as a text word in any field

Query	Results
Search: **"Glucose Intolerance"[TW]**	16,100
Search: **"Glucose Intolerance"[Mesh]**	8,633

FIG 3.3 Searching using Medical Subject Headings (MeSH).

terms that are assigned to records as they are indexed into the database. These vocabularies are drawn from thesauri that establish definitions and preferred usages; these terms may differ from the natural language text words you initially choose to describe a concept.

For example, indexing in MEDLINE employs metadata known as Medical Subject Headings (MeSH). You may find articles in MEDLINE via PubMed that are written about blood sugar control that have been tagged with the MeSH term "blood glucose/analysis" (see Fig. 3.2). In CINAHL, the subject heading is "glycemic control," indicating that is the preferred term and will return more targeted results. In addition to establishing a shared vocabulary for naming concepts of interest, subject headings are hierarchical, allowing you to select a descriptive term that is more or less specific, depending on how broad or narrow you would like the search to be (Fig. 3.3A).

Most article databases allow you to search specifically for articles that have been tagged with a given subject heading, as opposed to performing a key word or text word search. In contrast with a text word search in which the query returns citations if the term appears *anywhere* in the record, a subject heading search is much more targeted, only returning results in which the search term has been designated as a subject of that article (see Fig. 3.3B). A comprehensive search is usually achieved by searching for a combination of subject headings and text words, so as a strategic searcher you would be well-advised to keep track of both (see Table 3.4a).

HELPFUL HINT

Begin your database search for evidence by just searching for the concepts for the Problem (or Patient or Population) AND the concepts for the Intervention (Higgins et al., 2019). After evaluating the scope and number of results, you may want to add additional refinements for comparator or outcome terms, as suggested in Fig. 3.4.

EVALUATING AND REFINING THE SEARCH STRATEGY

Searching for evidence is a dynamic and exploratory process; the results of an initial scoping search can help you determine whether your search query must be narrowed or broadened, or if your clinical question may need to be refined (Fig. 3.4). Identifying the most relevant records from an initial search allows you to harvest metadata that can help optimize the search to capture additional pertinent records.

Narrowing a Search: Additional Search Concepts and Database Filters

If the initial scoping search retrieves an overwhelming number of results, it may be useful to introduce an additional concept into the search using the Boolean operator AND. If the search is being framed by a PICO question, consider adding a comparison or outcome term as an additional concept to retrieve a smaller, more specific set of results (see Table 3.4b)

In addition to being strategic about search concepts, you can narrow a pool of results by employing filters for date of publication, age group, and/or study methodology and publication type. In searching for the highest level of evidence, it may be helpful to use the database filters to only see studies that have been tagged with the publication type of meta-analysis, systematic review, or randomized controlled trials (see Table 3.4c).

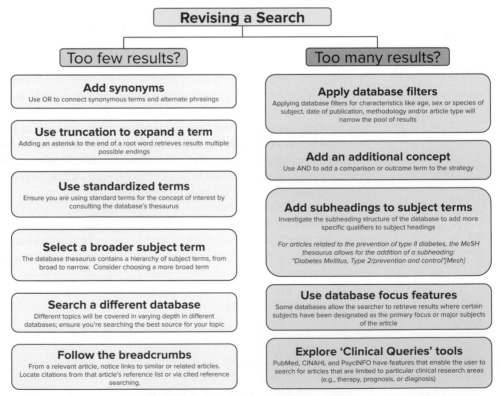

FIG 3.4 Strategies for revising a search.

Remember that you are searching for the highest level of available evidence on *your* question. Different types of clinical questions are suited to different study methodologies; for instance, randomized controlled trials can be used to answer questions regarding the effectiveness of therapies (see Chapter 9), while questions of prognosis are better suited to cohort studies (Roberts and Dicenso, 1999) (see Chapter 10). Moreover, depending on the nature of your question, a strong body of high-level evidence may not yet exist, but experimenting with database filters for publication type can help you develop a sense of what kind of literature has been published.

Expanding a Search: Synonyms and Snowballing

Relevant records from an initial scoping search can be used to harvest additional synonyms and related subject headings for the concepts of interest. These synonyms and related terms can then be integrated into the search string with OR to produce a more flexible query that returns more results. You can use OR to create sets of synonyms, related concepts, and alternate phrases or spellings. Be careful to nest these concepts with parentheses to ensure that the database correctly interprets the logic of the search string (see Table 3.4b).

A promising article can provide a useful trigger for "snowballing," the process of using a germane article as the seed to generate and locate more relevant articles. The references list of that article can be mined for older, classic articles. Cited reference searching, tracing the citation of an article forward in time, is also a useful strategy; certain databases and search tools (Scopus, Web of Science, Google Scholar, and PubMed) have features that allow you to see recent literature that has been cited an older article.

Fine-Tuning a PICO Question

Often, the first version of a PICO question does not result in a fruitful literature search. The question itself may be too broad, so no amount of filtering or revision of the search strategy can lead to a manageable number of results. For example, perhaps you find that your PICO question regarding telehealth interventions for type 2 diabetes is too broad, yielding too many potentially relevant results. This question could be narrowed by identifying a particular kind of telehealth intervention, such as use of a mobile application or a remote consultation program. Additionally, you could choose to narrow only to a particular age group, such as young adults or older adults, or focus your question on a particular population, like African American older adults.

In other cases, the question could be too specific; if research simply does not exist on a topic, even careful expansion of the search will fail to result in a body of relevant literature. In these cases, it may be necessary to refine the PICO question itself. It can be helpful to think about the individual components of the question, especially the problem/population and intervention; consider if one of those concepts can be made more general.

For instance, instead of focusing only on telehealth interventions for type 2 diabetes, perhaps you could expand your search to include any kind of personalized coaching, whether remote or in-person. Additionally, you may find it useful to broaden the search to include all types of patient education for all types of diabetes mellitus rather than just type 2 diabetes. Revisiting your initial results and returning to background sources can guide you toward ways to refine the PICO question.

TABLE 3.5   Tools for Organizing and Citing Literature

Citation Management Software	Citation Formatting Resources	Systematic Review Management Software
Zotero • zotero.org • Free *Mendeley* (Elsevier) • www.mendeley.com • Free and premium versions *RefWorks* (ProQuest) • refworks.proquest.com • Requires institutional subscription *EndNote* (Clarivate) • endnote.com • Requires purchase	APA Style Online (apastyle.apa.org/) • Free ZoteroBib Citation Formatter (zbib.org) • Free Purdue Online Writing Lab— APA (owl.purdue.edu/owl/research_and_citation /apa_style/apa_formatting_and_style _guide/general_format.html) • Free	*Covidence* (www.covidence.org) • Requires subscription *RevMan* (training.cochrane.org/online -learning/core-software-cochrane -reviews/revman) • Free for academic use *DistillerSR* (www.evidencepartners. com/products/distillersr-systematic- review-software/) • Requires subscription

Balancing Sensitivity and Precision

The process of gathering the literature is naturally iterative, meaning the initial results of the search are used to inform and revise the query to improve retrieval of relevant results and minimize the number of irrelevant results (see the critical thinking decision path). Eventually this feedback loop will slow, as tweaks to the search no longer draw in additional useful results and you continue to retrieve the same articles (Higgins et al., 2019). When you reach this point, you know your search is probably concluded. Ideally, a search strategy should attempt to be precise, returning results that are extremely relevant. However, it is important that a search is also sensitive, meaning that it is able to locate all potentially relevant results. A more sensitive search will be less precise (returning some irrelevant articles along with the relevant ones), but it will also be more comprehensive, reducing your risk for missing a key piece of evidence.

Performing a broader, less precise search is preferable because it draws in a large pool of potential articles and puts the power in your hands to make intelligent decisions about what is or is not useful, rather than relying exclusively on the cold logic of a search query. It is typical to have to screen through many titles and abstracts to identify the best-fit articles; there are many tools available to help researchers save and manage database records (Table 3.5).

ORGANIZING AND SCREENING RESULTS

Saving Search Strategies

The practice of experimenting with different search strategies and revising the query based on the results is an important phase in the process of conducting a robust search for research evidence. To facilitate this process, the major databases highlighted in this chapter (see Table 3.3) allow users to create individual accounts to save promising search strategies within the database platform. Moreover, saving search strategies in the database environment and in a separate document or spreadsheet file enables you to develop a search strategy that is reproducible. A reproducible search strategy documents the date when the final search was conducted and includes information about which search terms were used, if

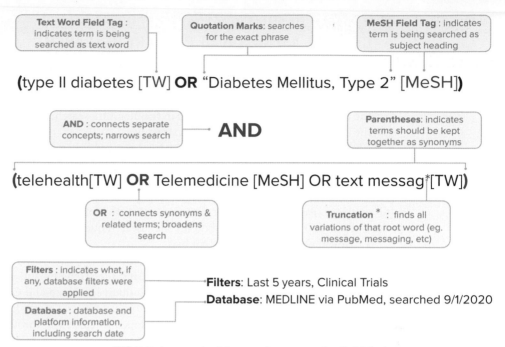

FIG 3.5 A reproducible search strategy for PubMed.

they were searched as text words (appearing anywhere in the record) or specifically designated as subjects, how the terms were connected with Boolean operators, and which (if any) filters were applied (Fig. 3.5).

Screening, Organizing, and Communicating Results

As you begin to sharpen an effective search strategy for your clinical question, you will screen through the titles and abstracts of the articles you locate, setting aside articles that address your PICO question. Within most databases, if you have made a personal account, you can populate a local folder with a collection of records you would like to save for later, a practice that is especially useful in the early stages of search refinement (critical thinking decision path).

In addition to the database features for saving results, you can export selected results to citation management software like *Zotero, EndNote* (Clarivate), *Mendeley* (Elsevier), and *RefWorks* (ProQuest), which allows users to download citation records from article databases, library catalogs, and websites (see Table 3.5). Many of these citation management platforms integrate with popular word processing software to automate the formatting of in-text citations and reference lists.

For more advanced searchers (those who are conducting evidence synthesis projects that demand an exhaustive review of the literature, in accordance with PRISMA guidelines [see Chapter 11]), it is necessary to methodically screen and sort every record that results from the database searches, including tracking the number of duplicate results. To facilitate this process, article databases allow searchers to run their finalized, comprehensive search and perform a bulk export of every resulting record into a citation manager, or specialized systematic review screening software (see Table 3.5).

⟫ APPRAISAL FOR EVIDENCE-BASED PRACTICE
CRITICAL APPRAISAL OF PRIMARY RESEARCH

Once you are confident that you have performed a reasonably exhaustive literature search, it is time to move into the next phase of the process: assessing and appraising the literature you have identified (critical thinking decision path). Even at this stage, reading deeper into the retrieved articles may reveal gaps in the literature search, so do not hesitate to return to the databases and revise your search strategy.

Although identifying research that has been published in peer-reviewed journals is a valuable initial step in identifying high-quality research, not all research evidence is created equal. You will need to critically appraise the pool of studies that address the clinical (PICO) question to determine the quantity, quality, consistency, and strength of the existing evidence. Pay attention to key elements such as the following:

- How well the research method fits the research question
- How the authors controlled for bias
- How the results may be clinically significant

The detailed process of critically appraising the strengths and weaknesses of research evidence is discussed in Chapter 18 for quantitative research and Chapter 7 for qualitative research.

Critical appraisal tools have been developed to guide you through the process of evaluating many types of research (see Table 3.6). These tools are tailored to the specifics of a given research methodology (e.g., clinical trials, cohort studies, qualitative research, systematic reviews). For example, the study in Appendix B (De la Fuente Coria et al., 2020) is a randomized controlled trial and would require a critical appraisal tool designed to assess that specific type of study design. A critical appraisal tool like the Centre for Evidence-Based Medicine's Randomised Controlled Trials (RCT): Critical Appraisal Sheet for assessing randomized controlled trials (see Table 3.6) would be appropriate to use. Identifying the design used in a research article allows you to select and use a critical appraisal tool that is specific to that study design to assess the strength, quality, and consistency of the evidence, including identifying potential sources of bias.

Critical Appraisal of Literature Reviews

As part of your critical appraisal process, it is useful to understand how to read and appraise literature reviews conducted by other researchers. A well-written literature review should establish a sufficient knowledge base to justify the need for a research study or QI/EBP project. Optimistically, the literature review will identify a gap or conflict in the literature or a need to extend the existing knowledge base through further research.

Box 3.2 contains general critical appraisal criteria for literature reviews; the level of scrutiny will depend on the context for the review. If the literature review makes up a portion of a research study (perhaps in the "Background" or "Theoretical Framework" section) or is a nonsystematic narrative review, you may focus on how the review is organized; a thoughtful, well-organized review would be considered of higher quality. Some literature reviews, especially those that are meant to establish a theoretical framework, may be structured chronologically, from the earliest literature to the most recent. Alternatively, you may encounter reviews in which the literature is grouped by concept of interest, by opposing sides of a debate, or to strategically highlight unresolved conflicts in research findings. In all cases, a well-constructed literature review will identify and unpack the key variables

TABLE 3.6	Selected Tools and Checklists for Critical Appraisal
Resource	**Use**
AGREE (Appraisal of Guidelines for Research and Evaluation) www. agreetrust.org	Tool for appraising: • Practice Guidelines
CASP (Critical Appraisal Skills Programme) casp-uk.net	Checklists for appraising: • Systematic Reviews • Qualitative Research • Randomized Controlled Trials • Case Control Studies • Diagnostic Test Studies • Cohort Studies • Economic Evaluations • Clinical Prediction Rules
CEBM (Centre for Evidence-Based Medicine) Critical Appraisal Tools www.cebm.net/2014/06/critical-appraisal/	Worksheets for appraising: • Systematic Reviews • Diagnostic Studies • Prognosis Studies • Randomized Controlled Trials • Qualitative Studies
GRADE (Grading of Recommendations Assessment, Development and Evaluation) gradeworkinggroup.org Handbook: gdt.gradepro.org/app/handbook/handbook.html	System and handbook for rating the quality of a body of evidence
PRISMA (Preferred Reporting Items for Systematic Reviews and Meta-Analyses) www.prisma-statement.org	Checklists for evaluating: • Systematic reviews • Meta-analyses

that underpin the research topic and offer critiques of the strengths and weaknesses of the available literature. Ultimately, an effective literature review will make connections between the cited literature, summarizing and synthesizing the state of research on that topic, which will inform formulation of the research question or hypothesis (see Chapter 2).

When you are evaluating an evidence synthesis project like a systematic review or meta-analysis, critical appraisal of the literature review is much more extensive, rigorous, and transparent. You will pay careful attention to items like the extent to which the review was framed around a well-defined question, the rigor of the search strategy, and how the authors assessed the quality of the studies they included. These appraisal items and more can be found in the appraisal tools that are designed specifically for systematic reviews and meta-analysis (see Table 3.6).

The practice of appraising evidence, whether it is a primary research study or an evidence synthesis article, is a fundamental skill for students and clinicians who are invested in becoming critical consumers of research.

SYNTHESIZING AND COMMUNICATING RESULTS

Evidence Synthesis

Once the studies that you have identified have been critically appraised, you will need to synthesize their overall strengths and weaknesses to establish the state of the science and make an evidence-based conclusion to answer your PICO question and inform clinical practice. To do this, it is helpful to develop an evidence synthesis table in which you extract the key details and variables from each identified study. This table may include information about the study design and methodology, the population/problem, the intervention, the comparison and outcomes that were assessed, and the relative strength of the findings. Ultimately, it is the research question that determines what information is necessary to extract from each study and include in the table (Oh, 2016). For an example of an evidence synthesis table, see Chapter 20.

Presenting the evidence as a table facilitates a holistic assessment of the body of evidence across multiple studies. In particular, you can compare elements like sampling strategy or study design, which affect the quality of the evidence. Using the evidence table, you can identify consistencies as well as potential sources of heterogeneity that may affect the generalizability of the findings.

With the information in the synthesis table as a guide, you will be able to write a descriptive narrative summary that synthesizes the overall quantity, quality, and consistency of the evidence, including potential recommendations for practice. Depending on the overall strength of the evidence you have identified, you may validate current standards of care, suggest changes in practice, or even make recommendations for policy changes.

It is also possible that your synthesis will reveal that the current body of evidence on a question is insufficient to make any recommendations (e.g., there have been too few studies, or only studies of low quality have been conducted). For instance, despite locating 30 studies to synthesize for their meta-analysis on continuity of care interventions, Facchinetti et al. (2020) (Appendix A) determined that the evidence about the effectiveness of these interventions on long-term readmissions was inconclusive, so they could not justify a recommendation, only suggest avenues for further research.

Citing Sources

Proper attribution of the sources you use in your writing is critical. More than just acknowledging the intellectual contribution of previous authors and helping you avoid plagiarism, formatting citations clearly and consistently enables you (and those who read your work) to trace the development of your ideas and more clearly understand your participation in the scholarly conversation around your topic. Although there are a range of standard citation styles, the style of the American Psychological Association (APA) is commonly encountered in nursing publications. The *Publication Manual of the American Psychological Association* (APA, 2019) is available for purchase or may be available in your library; there are also a number of useful citation resources that are freely available on the Internet (see Table 3.5).

CONCLUSION

A targeted, thorough search of the literature is essential for powerful EBP/QI projects. In contrast with literature reviews that are conducted for other reasons (e.g., narrative reviews or as part of research studies), the literature search for an EBP/QI should prioritize the highest level of available evidence as it relates to a specific clinical question (often expressed in PICO format). Conducting background research using secondary sources is a useful practice for establishing a strong contextual understanding of the clinical (PICO) question and a fruitful avenue for refining the question if needed.

The bulk of the primary research that will make up the heart of the EBP/QI project is located in specialized health sciences databases. While these databases are powerful tools for information retrieval, the results are only as good as the search query that generates them. As such, it is up to the searcher to ensure the integrity of the search strategy. Ideally, a search strategy is thoughtful and comprehensive, with targeted database queries that are free from avoidable bias and consider database-specific controlled vocabulary and the platforms' filtering capabilities.

Although there are some elements of quality control built into health sciences databases (e.g., the ability to filter by article type, which may reflect methodology, or filtering for peer-reviewed sources), the onus is on you to critically appraise the quality of the information you encounter, especially given the potential impact that this information could have on clinical practice and patient outcomes. Within the health sciences, frameworks for critical appraisal are designed to help researchers, clinicians, and students to carefully and methodically assess the quality of each element of a research study. With a clear understanding of the strengths and weaknesses of the body of evidence related to a clinical question, it is possible to synthesize that evidence to inform clinical practice.

Finally, although there are many tools designed to help researchers access and organize the networks of information they encounter, it is ultimately up to the researcher to develop the information literacy necessary to intelligently navigate the complex landscape of health care information.

KEY POINTS

- Information in the health sciences takes multiple forms, but synthesizing evidence for EBP/QI projects requires evidence from primary research sources.
- The core health sciences databases offer researchers the necessary content and functionality to perform comprehensive searches that are able to locate high-quality evidence.
- Using the PICO format to ask a clinical question and applying the principles of Boolean logic allow the searcher to build a structured, reproducible search for evidence.
- Acquiring research evidence is an iterative, explorative process; search queries can and should be revised based on the results of initial scoping searches and background research.
- Hands-on database searching and diving into the iterative process of locating evidence is the best way to hone your literature-searching skills.
- Health sciences librarians are skilled professionals who are prepared to help researchers identify sources and design search strategies to locate relevant literature.
- The ability to make EBP recommendations is predicated on the process of locating high-quality evidence; assessing quality requires an integrated understanding of research and publication processes, hierarchies of evidence, and critical appraisal criteria.

CLINICAL JUDGMENT CHALLENGES

- How does locating secondary sources fit into the process of gathering evidence for EBP/QI projects?
- Why is it important and helpful to identify the standard subject headings related to your concepts of interest?

- What are some strategies you could employ to revise a search if it returns too many results?
- When conducting a systematic search, why is it better to design a search that is more sensitive, even if it is less precise?

IPE HIGHLIGHT

Given the importance of communicating clearly with your EBP/QI team colleagues, how can you leverage information resources to ensure that the team has a clear understanding of the core concepts that underpin your project?

REFERENCES

Albarqouni, L., Hoffmann, T., Straus, S., Olsen, N. R., Young, T., Ilic, D., Shaneyfelt, T., Haynes, R. B., Guyatt, G., & Glasziou, P. (2018). Core competencies in evidence-based practice for health professionals: Consensus statement based on a systematic review and Delphi survey. *JAMA Network Open, 1*(2), e180281–e180281. https://doi.org/10.1001/jamanetworkopen.2018.0281.

American Psychological Association (Ed.). (2019). *Publication manual of the American Psychological Association* (Seventh edition). American Psychological Association.

Card, N. A. (2010). Literature review. In N. Salkind (Ed.), *Encyclopedia of research design*. SAGE Publications, Inc. https://doi.org/10.4135/9781412961288.n222.

Cullum, N. (2008). *Evidence-based nursing: An introduction*. Blackwell Pub./BMJ Journals/RCN Pub.

De la Fuente Coria, M. C., Cruz-Cobo, C., & Santi-Cano, M. J. (2020). Effectiveness of a primary care nurse delivered educational intervention for patients with type 2 diabetes mellitus in promoting metabolic control and compliance with long-term therapeutic targets: Randomised controlled trial. *International Journal of Nursing Studies, 101*, 103417. https://doi.org/10.1016/j.ijnurstu.2019.103417.

Facchinetti, G., D'Angelo, D., Piredda, M., Petitti, T., Matarese, M., Oliveti, A., & De Marinis, M. G. (2020). Continuity of care interventions for preventing hospital readmission of older people with chronic diseases: A meta-analysis. *International Journal of Nursing Studies, 101*, 103396. https://doi.org/10.1016/j.ijnurstu.2019.103396.

Higgins, J. P. T., Thomas, J., Chandler, J., Cumpston, M., Li, T., Page, M. J., & Welch, V. A. (2019). *Cochrane handbook for systematic reviews of interventions*. John Wiley & Sons.

Ho, G. J., Liew, S. M., Ng, C. J., Shunmugam, Hisham, R., & Glasziou, P. (2016). Development of a search strategy for an evidence based retrieval service. *PLOS ONE, 11*(12), e0167170. https://doi.org/10.1371/journal.pone.0167170.

New York Academy of Medicine. (2021). What Is grey literature? *Grey Literature Report*. Retrieved June 18, 2020, from https://www.greylit.org/about.

Oh, E. G. (2016). Synthesizing quantitative evidence for evidence-based nursing: Systematic review. *Asian Nursing Research, 10*(2), 89–93. https://doi.org/10.1016/j.anr.2016.05.001.

Opheim, E., Andersen, P. N., Jakobsen, M., Aasen, B., & Kvaal, K. (2019). Poor quality in systematic reviews on PTSD and EMDR: An examination of search methodology and reporting. *Frontiers in Psychology, 10*, 1558. https://doi.org/10.3389/fpsyg.2019.01558.

Primary and secondary sources: Guidelines for authors. (2009). *AJN The American Journal of Nursing, 109*(4), 76–77. https://doi.org/10.1097/01.NAJ.0000348612.62478.db.

Salvador-Oliván, J. A., Marco-Cuenca, G., & Arquero-Avilés, R. (2019). Errors in search strategies used in systematic reviews and their effects on information retrieval. *Journal of the Medical Library Association: JMLA, 107*(2), 210–221. https://doi.org/10.5195/jmla.2019.567.

4

Theoretical Frameworks for Research

Melanie McEwen

Go to Evolve at **http://evolve.elsevier.com/LoBiondo/** for review questions.

LEARNING OUTCOMES

After reading this chapter, you should be able to do the following:

- Describe the relationship among theory, research, and practice.
- Identify the purpose of conceptual and theoretical frameworks for research.
- Differentiate between conceptual and operational definitions.
- Identify the types of theories used in research.
- Describe how a theory or conceptual framework guides research.
- Explain the points of critical appraisal used to evaluate the appropriateness, cohesiveness, and consistency of a framework guiding research.

KEY TERMS

concept	deductive	middle range theory	situation-specific theory
conceptual definition	grand theory	model	theoretical framework
conceptual framework	inductive	operational definition	theory
construct			

To introduce the discussion of the use of theoretical frameworks for research, consider the example of Emily, a novice oncology nurse. From this case study, reflect on how nurses can understand the theoretical underpinnings of both research and evidence-based practice, and reaffirm how nurses should integrate research into practice.

Emily graduated with her bachelor of science in nursing (BSN) a little more than 1 year ago, and she recently changed positions to work on a pediatric oncology unit in a large hospital. She quickly learned that working with very ill and often dying children is tremendously rewarding, even though it is frequently heartbreaking.

One of Emily's first patients was Benny, a 14-year-old boy admitted with a recurrence of leukemia. When she first cared for Benny, he was extremely ill. Benny's oncologist implemented the clinical practice guidelines for cases such as his, but the team was careful to explain to Benny and his family that his prognosis was guarded. In the early days of his hospitalization, Emily cried with his mother when they received his daily laboratory values and there was no apparent improvement. She observed that Benny was growing increasingly fatigued and had little appetite. Despite his worsening condition, however, Benny and his parents were unfailingly positive, making plans for a vacation to the mountains and the upcoming school year.

At the end of her shift one night before several days off, Emily hugged Benny's parents, as she feared that Benny would die before her next scheduled workday. Several days later, when she listened to the report at the start of her shift, Emily was amazed to learn that Benny had been heartily eating a normal diet. He was ambulatory and had been cruising the halls with his baseball coach and playing video games with two of his cousins. When she entered Benny's room for her initial assessment, she saw the much-improved teenager dressed in shorts and a T-shirt, sitting up in bed using his iPad. A half-finished chocolate milkshake was on the table within easy reaching distance. He joked with Emily about Minecraft as she performed her assessment. Benny steadily improved over the ensuing days and eventually went home with his leukemia again in remission.

As Emily became more comfortable in the role of oncology nurse, she continued to notice patterns among the children and adolescents on her unit. Many got better, even though their conditions were often critical. In contrast, some of the children who had better prognoses failed to improve as much or as quickly as anticipated. She realized that the kids who did better than expected seemed to have common attributes or characteristics, including positive attitudes, supportive family and friends, and strong determination to "beat" their cancer. Over lunch one day, Emily talked with her mentor, Marie, about her observations, commenting that on a number of occasions she had seen patients rebound when she thought that death was imminent.

Marie smiled. "Fortunately this is a pattern that we see quite frequently. Many of our kids are amazingly resilient." Marie told Emily about the work of several nurse researchers who studied the phenomenon of resilience and gave her a list of articles reporting on their findings. Emily followed up with Marie's prompting and learned about "psychosocial resilience in adolescents" (Tusaie et al., 2007) and "adolescent resilience" (Ahern, 2006; Ahern et al., 2008). These works led her to a "middle range theory of resilience" (Polk, 1997). Focusing her literature review even more, Emily was able to discover several recent research studies (Ishibashi et al., 2016; Linder et al., 2019; Rosenberg et al., 2018) that examined aspects of resilience among adolescents with cancer, further piquing her interest in the subject.

From her readings, Emily gained insight into resilience, learning to recognize it in her patients. She also identified ways she might encourage and even promote resilience in children and teenagers. Eventually, she decided to enroll in a graduate nursing program to learn how to investigate different phenomena of concern to her patients and discover ways to apply the evidence-based findings to improve nursing care and patient outcomes.

PRACTICE-THEORY-RESEARCH LINKS

Several important aspects of how theory is used in nursing research are embedded in Emily's story. First, it is important to notice the links among practice, theory, and research. Each is inextricably connected with the others to create a knowledge base that can be applied to nursing practice to promote high-quality and cost-effective patient care (Fig. 4.1). In her practice, Emily recognized a pattern of characteristics in some patients that appeared to enhance their recovery. Her mentor directed her to research what other nurses had

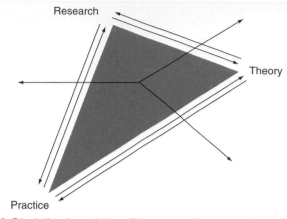

Research

Theory

Practice

FIG 4.1 Discipline knowledge: Theory-practice-research connection.

published on the phenomenon of "resilience." Emily was then able to apply the information on resilience and related research findings as she planned and implemented care. Her goal was to support and enhance each child's resilience as much as possible and thereby improve their outcomes.

Another key message from the case study is the importance of reflecting on an observed phenomenon and discussing it with colleagues. This promotes questioning and collaboration as nurses seek ways to improve practice. Finally, Emily was encouraged to go to the literature to search out what had been published related to the phenomenon she had observed. Reviewing the research led her to a middle range theory of resilience as well as current nursing research that examined its importance in caring for adolescents with cancer. This then challenged her to consider how she might ultimately conduct her own research.

OVERVIEW OF THEORY

Theory is a set of interrelated concepts that provides a systematic view of a phenomenon. A theory allows relationships to be proposed and predictions made, which in turn can suggest potential actions. Beginning with a theory gives the researcher a logical way of collecting data to describe, explain, and predict nursing practice, making it critical in research.

In nursing, science is the result of the interchange between research and theory. The purpose of research is to build knowledge through theory generation and testing the concepts within the theory that can be applied in practice. To build knowledge, research should develop within a theoretical structure or blueprint that facilitates analysis and interpretation of findings. The use of theory provides structure and organization to nursing knowledge. It is important that nurses understand that nursing practice is based on the theories that are generated and validated through research (McEwen & Wills, 2019).

In an integrated, reciprocal manner, theory guides research and practice; practice generates research questions that are tested in research studies or quality improvement projects; research contributes to theory building and establishing practice guidelines (see Fig. 4.1). What is learned through practice, theory, and research interweaves to create the knowledge fabric of nursing. From this perspective, like Emily in the case study, each nurse should be involved in the process of contributing to the knowledge or evidence-based practice.

BOX 4.1   Definitions

Concept

Image or symbolic representation of an abstract idea; the key identified element of a phenomenon that is necessary to understand it. Concept can be concrete or abstract. A concrete concept can be easily identified, quantified, and measured, whereas an abstract concept is more difficult to quantify or measure. For example, weight, blood pressure, and body temperature are concrete concepts. Hope, uncertainty, and spiritual pain are more abstract concepts. In a study, resilience is a relatively abstract concept.

Conceptual Definition

Much like a dictionary definition, a conceptual definition conveys the general meaning of the concept. However, the conceptual definition goes beyond the general language meaning found in the dictionary by defining or explaining the concept as it is rooted in theoretical literature.

Conceptual/Theoretical Framework

A set of interrelated concepts that represents an image of a phenomenon. These two terms are often used interchangeably. The conceptual/theoretical framework refers to a structure that provides guidance for research or practice. The framework identifies the key concepts and describes their relationships to each other and to the phenomena (variables) of concern to nursing. It serves as the foundation on which a study can be developed or as a map to aid in the design of the study.

Construct

Complex concept; constructs usually comprise more than one concept and are built or "constructed" to fit a purpose. Health promotion, maternal-infant bonding, health-seeking behaviors, and health-related quality of life are examples of constructs.

Model

A graphic or symbolic representation of a phenomenon. A graphic model is empirical and can be readily represented. A model of an eye or a heart is an example. A symbolic or theoretical model depicts a phenomenon that is not directly observable and is expressed in language or symbols. Written music or Einstein's theory of relativity are examples of symbolic models. Theories used by nurses or developed by nurses frequently include symbolic models. Models are very helpful in allowing the reader to visualize key concepts/constructs and their identified interrelationships.

Operational Definition

Specifies how the concept will be measured. That is, the operational definition defines what instruments will be used to assess the presence of the concept and will be used to describe the amount or degree to which the concept exists.

Theory

Set of interrelated concepts that provides a systematic view of a phenomenon.

Several key terms are often used when discussing theory. It is necessary to understand these terms when considering how to apply theory in practice and research. They include **concept, conceptual definition, conceptual/theoretical framework, construct, model, operational definition,** and **theory.** Each term is defined and summarized in Box 4.1. Concepts and constructs are the major components of theories and convey the essential ideas or elements of a theory. When a nurse researcher decides to study a concept/construct, the researcher must precisely and explicitly describe and explain the concept, devise a mechanism to identify and confirm the presence of the concept of interest, and determine a method to measure or quantify it. To illustrate, Table 4.1 shows the key concepts and conceptual and operational definitions provided by Flanders and colleagues (2020) in their study of a program to promote resilience among nurses in a pediatric intensive care unit (see Appendix C).

THEORY TYPES

As stated previously, a theory is a set of interrelated concepts that provide a systematic view of a phenomenon. Theory provides a foundation and structure that may be used for the purpose of explaining or predicting another phenomenon. In this way, a theory

TABLE 4.1 Concepts and Variables: Conceptual and Operational Definitions			
Concept	**Conceptual Definition**	**Variable**	**Operational Definition**
Compassion fatigue (Flanders et al., 2020)	Compassion fatigue is seen as the "cost of caring." It is composed of "burnout" and "secondary traumatic stress"	Compassion Fatigue	Burnout + secondary traumatic stress subscales of the Professional Quality of Life Instrument (ProQOL)
Secondary traumatic stress (Flanders et al., 2020)	"The stress one experiences from caring for a person who has suffered from a traumatic event" occurs when health care providers are repeatedly exposed to patients suffering from trauma or devastating illnesses	STS	Subscale of the Professional Quality of Life Instrument (ProQOL)
Burnout (Flanders et al., 2020)	Exhaustion, anger, frustration, and depression	Burnout	Subscale of the Professional Quality of Life Instrument (ProQOL)
Compassion satisfaction (Flanders et al., 2020)	Pleasure derived from doing your job well	Compassion satisfaction	Subscale of the Professional Quality of Life Instrument (ProQOL)
Resilience (Flanders et al., 2020)	A recurrent human need to weather periods of stress and change successfully throughout life	Turnover and employee engagement (outcome of resiliency program)	RN turnover and employee engagement portions of the Press Ganey instrument

is like a blueprint or a guide for building a structure like a house. A blueprint depicts the elements of a structure and the relationships among the elements; similarly, a theory depicts the concepts that compose it and suggests how the concepts are related.

Nurses use a multitude of theories as the foundation for research and practice. Many have been developed by nurses and are explicitly related to practice; others, however, come from other disciplines like psychology, sociology, and anthropology.

Theories From Related Disciplines

Like engineering, architecture, social work, and teaching, nursing is a practice discipline. This means that nurses use concepts, constructs, models, and theories from many disciplines in addition to nursing-specific theories. This is, to a large extent, the rationale for the "liberal arts" education that is required before entering a nursing program. Exposure to knowledge and theories of basic and natural sciences (e.g., mathematics, chemistry, biology) and social sciences (e.g., psychology, sociology, political science) provides a fundamental understanding of these disciplines and allows for application of key principles, concepts, and theories from each, as appropriate.

Likewise, nurses use principles of administration and management and learning theories in patient-centered, holistic practices. Table 4.2 lists a few of the many theories and concepts from other disciplines that are commonly used in practice and research and are part of the foundational framework for nursing.

TABLE 4.2	Theories Used in Nursing Practice and Research
Discipline	**Examples of Theories/Concepts Used by Nurses**
Biomedical sciences	Germ theory (principles of infection), pain theories, immune function, genetics/genomics, pharmacotherapeutics
Sociological sciences	Systems theory (e.g., von Bertalanffy), family theory (e.g., Bowen), role theory (e.g., Merton), critical social theory (e.g., Habermas), cultural diversity (e.g., Leininger)
Behavioral sciences	Developmental theories (e.g., Erikson), human needs theories (e.g., Maslow), personality theories (e.g., Freud), stress theories (e.g., Lazarus & Folkman), health belief model (e.g., Rosenstock)
Learning theories	Behavioral learning theories (e.g., Pavlov, Skinner), cognitive development/interaction theories (e.g., Piaget), adult learning theories (e.g., Knowles)
Leadership/management	Change theory (e.g., Lewin), conflict management (e.g., Rapaport), quality framework (e.g., Donabedian)

Nursing Theories Used in Practice and Research

In addition to the theories from other disciplines, the nursing literature presents a number of theories that were developed by nurses. Typically, nursing theories reflect concepts, relationships, and processes that contribute to the development of a body of knowledge applied to interventions. Understanding these interactions and relationships among the concepts and phenomena is essential to evidence-based care.

HELPFUL HINT

In research and practice, concepts often create descriptions or images that emerge from a conceptual definition. For instance, pain is a concept with different meanings based on the type or aspect of pain being referred to. As such, there are a number of methods and instruments to measure pain. A nurse researching postoperative pain would conceptually define pain based on the patient's perceived discomfort associated with surgery and then select a pain scale/instrument that allows the researcher to operationally define pain as the patient's score on that scale.

Nursing theories are often described based on their scope or degree of abstraction. Typically, these are reported as *grand, middle range,* or *situation-specific* (also called *microrange*) nursing theories. Each is described in this section.

Grand Nursing Theories

Grand nursing theories are sometimes referred to as *conceptual models* and include the theories/models that were developed to describe the discipline of nursing as a whole. This composes the works of nurse theorists such as Florence Nightingale, Virginia Henderson, Martha Rogers, Dorothea Orem, and Betty Neuman. Grand nursing theories/models are all-inclusive conceptual structures that tend to include views on persons, health, and environment to create a perspective about nursing. This most abstract level of theory has established a knowledge base for the discipline. These works are used as the conceptual basis for practice and research, and they are tested in research studies.

One grand theory is not better than another with respect to research. Rather, these varying perspectives allow the researcher to select a framework for research that best depicts the concepts and relationships of interest, and then decide where and how they can be measured as study variables. What is most important about the use of grand nursing theoretical frameworks is the logical connection of the theory to the research

---

BOX 4.2 Grand Theory Example

Kim and Dee (2017) used Orem's self-care deficit nursing theory to examine the factors influencing self-care among Hispanic women at risk for postpartum depression (PPD). The researchers used a descriptive cross-sectional design, collecting data from 223 Hispanic postpartum women in several small towns in California. The key constructs studied were postnatal depression, perceived social support, religiosity, and health practices. Among their findings it was discovered that some 43% of the women surveyed were at risk for PPD. Using Orem's theory as a framework, they determined that social support and spirituality were significantly correlated with positive health practices and healthy living among the women. It was concluded that nurses and other health care professionals should work to provide interventions to assist rural Hispanic women to perform self-care activities during the postpartum period.

---

question and the study design. Nursing literature contains excellent examples of research studies that examine concepts and constructs from grand nursing theories. See Box 4.2 for an example.

Middle Range Nursing Theories

Nurses recognized that grand theories were difficult to apply in research, and considerable attention moved to the development and research of "middle range" nursing theories. In contrast to grand theories, middle range nursing theories contain a limited number of concepts and are focused on a limited aspect of reality. As a result, they are more easily tested through research and more readily used as frameworks for research studies (McEwen & Wills, 2019).

A growing number of middle range nursing theories have been developed, tested through research, and/or used as frameworks for research. Examples are Pender's Health Promotion Model (Murdaugh et al., 2019), the Theory of Uncertainty in Illness (Mishel, 1988, 1990; Clayton, et al., 2018), the Theory of Unpleasant Symptoms (Lenz et al., 1997, 2020), and the Theory of Holistic Comfort (Kolcaba, 1994; Kolcaba & Crawford, 2020).

Examples of development, use, and testing of middle range theories and models are becoming increasingly common in the nursing literature (Box 4.3). The comprehensive health-seeking and coping paradigm (Nyamathi, 1989) is one example. Indeed, Nyamathi's model served as the conceptual framework of a recent research study that examined interventions to improve hepatitis A and B vaccine completion among homeless men (Nyamathi et al., 2015). In this study, the findings were interpreted according to the model. The researchers identified several predictors of vaccine completion and concluded that providers work to recognize factors that promote health-seeking and coping behaviors among high-risk populations.

BOX 4.3 Middle-Range Theory Exemplar

McCutcheon and colleagues (2017) conducted a study of health promotion behaviors specifically related to HPV awareness and vaccination rates in college-age male athletes. This study was based on Pender's health promotion model (Pender et al., 2015). Several variables for the study were operationalized and measured using the Health Promotion Lifestyle Profile II, a survey instrument that was developed to be used in studies that focus on HPM concepts.

HPM, Health Promotion Model.

Situation-Specific Nursing Theories: Microrange, Practice, or Prescriptive Theories

Situation-specific nursing theories are sometimes referred to as *microrange, practice,* or *prescriptive* theories. Situation-specific theories are more specific than middle range theories and are composed of a limited number of concepts. They are narrow in scope, explain a small aspect of phenomena and processes of interest to nurses, and are usually limited to a specific population or field of practice (Chinn & Kramer, 2018; Im, 2014; Peterson, 2020). Im and Chang (2012) observed that as nursing research began to require theoretical bases that are easily operationalized into research, situation-specific theories provided closer links to research and practice. Often what is noted by an author as a middle range theory would more appropriately be termed *situation-specific.* Most commonly, however, a theory is developed from a research study, and no designation (e.g., middle range, situation-specific) is attached to it.

Examples of self-designated, situation-specific theories include the Lee geropalliative caring model, which describes the care of older adults in the last 2 years of life (Lee, 2018), and a situation-specific theory of barriers and facilitators for self-care in patients with heart failure (Kastaun et al., 2019). Increasingly, nurses are using qualitative studies to develop and support theories and models that can and should be expressly identified as situation-specific. This will become progressively more common as more nurses seek graduate study and are involved in research, and increasing attention is given to the importance of evidence-based practice (Im & Chang, 2012; McEwen & Wills, 2019).

Im and Chang (2012) conducted a comprehensive research review that examined how theory has been described in nursing literature for the past decade. They reported a dramatic increase in the number of grounded theory research studies, along with increases in studies using both middle range and situation-specific theories. In contrast, the number and percentage directly dealing with grand nursing theories have fluctuated. Table 4.3 provides examples of grand, middle range, and situation-specific nursing theories used in nursing research.

TABLE 4.3   Levels of Nursing Theory: Examples of Grand, Middle Range, and Situation-Specific Nursing Theories

Grand Nursing Theories	Middle Range Nursing Theories	Situation-Specific (or Micro) Nursing Theories
Florence Nightingale: Notes on Nursing (1860)	Pender's health promotion model (Murdaugh et al., 2019)	Theory of the peaceful end of life (Ruland & Moore, 1998)
Dorothy Johnson: The Behavioral Systems Model for Nursing (1990)	Transitions Theory (Meleis, 2010)	Theory of chronic sorrow (Eakes, 2020; Eakes et al., 1998)
Martha Rogers: Nursing: A Science of Unitary Human Beings (1970, 1990)	Uncertainty in illness theory (Mishel, 1988, 1990; Clayton et al., 2018)	Asian immigrant women's menopausal symptom experience in the United States (Im, 2012)
Betty Neuman: The Neuman Systems Model (2011)	Theory of unpleasant symptoms (Lenz et al., 2020)	Systemic assessment of depressive symptoms among registered nurses (Ross et al., 2020)
Dorothea Orem: The Self Care Deficit Nursing Theory (2001)	Theory of holistic comfort/theory of comfort (Kolcaba, 1994, 2020)	Anticipatory grief (Shore et al., 2016)
Callista Roy: The Roy Adaptation Model (2009)	Theory of resilience (Polk, 1997)	Caregiver contributions to heart failure self-care (Vellone et al., 2019)
	Theory of flight nursing expertise (Reimer & Moore, 2010)	

HOW THEORY IS USED IN RESEARCH

Nursing research is concerned with the study of individuals in interaction with their environments. The intent is to discover interventions that promote optimal functioning and self-care across the life span; the goal is to foster maximum wellness (McEwen & Wills, 2019). In research, theories are used in one of three ways:

- Theory is generated as the outcome of a research study (qualitative designs).
- Theory is used as a research framework, as the context for a study (qualitative or quantitative designs).
- Research is undertaken to test a theory (quantitative designs).

Theory-Generating Nursing Research

When research is undertaken to create or generate theory, the idea is to examine a phenomenon within a particular context and identify and describe its major elements or events. Theory-generating research is focused on "What" and "How," but does not usually attempt to explain "Why." Theory-generating research is **inductive**; that is, it uses a process in which generalizations are developed from specific observations. Research methods used by nurses for theory generation include concept analysis, case studies, phenomenology, grounded theory, ethnography, and historical inquiry. Chapters 5, 6, and 7 describe these research methods. As you review qualitative methods and study examples in the literature, be attuned to the stated purpose(s) or outcomes of the research, and note whether a situation-specific (practice or micro) theory or model or a middle range theory is presented as a finding or outcome.

Theory as Framework for Nursing Research

In nursing research, theory is most commonly used as the conceptual framework, theoretical framework, or conceptual model. Frequently, correlational studies attempt to discover and specify relationships among characteristics of individuals, groups, situations, or events. Correlational research often focuses on one or more concepts, frameworks, or theories to collect data to measure dimensions or characteristics of variables and explain why and the extent to which one variable is related to another. Data are typically gathered by observation or self-report instruments (see Chapter 10 for nonexperimental designs).

HELPFUL HINT

When researchers use conceptual frameworks to guide studies, you can expect to find a system of ideas synthesized for the purpose of organizing, thinking, and providing study direction. Whether the researcher is using a conceptual or theoretical framework, conceptual and then operational definitions will emerge from the framework.

Often in correlational (nonexperimental/quantitative) research, a theory will be used as the study's conceptual/theoretical framework. In these cases, a theory is used as the context for the study and basis for interpretation of the findings. The theory helps guide the study and enhances the value of its findings by setting the findings within the context of the theory, previous works, and describing use of the theory in practice or research. When using a theory as a conceptual framework to guide research, the researcher will do the following:

- Identify an existing theory (or theories), and designate and explain the study's theoretical framework.
- Develop research questions/hypotheses consistent with the framework.

- Provide conceptual definitions taken from the theory/framework.
- Use data collection instrument(s) (and operational definitions) appropriate to the framework.
- Interpret/explain findings based on the framework.
- Determine support for the theory/framework based on the study findings.
- Discuss implications for nursing and recommendations for future research to address the concepts and relationships designated by the framework.

Theory-Testing Research

Finally, nurses may use research to test the concepts of a theory. Theory testing is deductive—that is, hypotheses are derived from theory and tested employing experimental methods. In experimental research such as a randomized controlled trial, the intent is to move beyond explanation to prediction of relationships among characteristics or phenomena within different groups or in various situations. Experimental research requires manipulation of one or more variables to determine how the manipulation affects or changes the dimension or characteristics of other phenomena. In these cases, theoretical statements are posed as research questions or hypotheses. Experimental research requires quantifiable data, and statistical analyses are used to measure differences (see Chapter 9).

In theory-testing research, the researcher (1) chooses a theory and selects a propositional statement to be examined; (2) develops hypotheses that have measurable variables; (3) conducts the study; (4) interprets the findings considering the predictive ability of the theory; and (5) determines whether there are implications for further use of the theory in practice and/or whether further research could be beneficial.

EVIDENCE-BASED PRACTICE TIP

In practice, you can use observation and analysis to consider the nuances of situations that matter to patient health. This process often generates questions that are cogent for improving patient care. In turn, following the observations and questions into the literature can lead to published research that can be applied in practice.

IPE   HIGHLIGHT

When an interprofessional quality improvement team launches a project to develop evidence-based behavior change self-management strategies for a targeted patient population, it may be helpful to think about the Transtheoretical Model of Change and health self-efficacy as an appropriate theoretical framework to guide the project.

APPLICATION TO RESEARCH AND EVIDENCE-BASED PRACTICE

To build knowledge that promotes evidence-based practice, research should develop within a theoretical structure that facilitates analysis and interpretation of findings. When a study is placed within a theoretical context, the theory or theoretical framework guides the research, informs the research questions or hypotheses, and aids in design, analysis, and interpretation. In this regard, a theory, conceptual model, or conceptual framework provides parameters for the research and enables the researcher to weave the facts together.

As you read research, you should know how to recognize the theoretical foundation of a study. Whether evaluating a qualitative or quantitative study, it is essential to understand where and how the research can be integrated within nursing science and applied in evidence-based practice. As a result, it is important to identify whether the intent is to (1) generate a theory, (2) use a theory as the framework that guides the study, or (3) test a theory. This section provides examples that illustrate different types of theories used in nursing research (e.g., non-nursing theories, middle range nursing theories) and examples from the literature highlighting the different ways nurses can use theory in research (e.g., theory-generating study, theory testing, theory as a conceptual framework).

Application of Theory in Qualitative Research

As discussed, in many instances, a theory, framework, or model is the outcome of nursing research. This is often the case in research employing qualitative methods such as grounded theory. From the study's findings, the researcher builds either an implicit or an explicit structure explaining or describing the findings of the research.

Example: ➤ Hanna and colleagues (2020, Appendix E) reported findings from a study examining the perceptions underlying health-related adherence behaviors of patients after they had experienced a heart attack. Using a qualitative approach to data collection, the team interviewed 22 participants recruited from a cardiac rehabilitation program. The researchers discovered two major categories or factors (intrinsic factors and extrinsic factors) and six subfactors (willpower, sense of competency, personal preferences, recurrent event, family and relatives, and health care providers). The research findings were used to develop a model that can be used by health care providers to understand the factors that influence adherence to health promotion therapies and adherence to a healthy lifestyle among patients with long-term health conditions.

Generally, when the researcher is using qualitative methods and inductive reasoning, you will find the framework or theory at the end of the manuscript in the discussion section (see Chapters 5–7). You should be aware that the framework may be implicitly suggested rather than explicitly diagrammed (Box 4.4).

The nursing literature is full of similar examples in which inductive qualitative research methods were used to develop theory. **Example:** ➤ Welch and Carter (2020) used grounded theory methods to conduct interviews with 10 critical care nurses to examine the nurses' perceptions of expertise, expert performance, and transition from novice to expert in clinical practice. They identified three themes describing the performance of the expert critical care nurse. These are: experience, knowledge,

---

BOX 4.4 Research

Martz (2015) used grounded theory research methods to examine actions taken by hospice nurses to alleviate the feelings of guilt often experienced by caregivers. In this study, 16 hospice providers (most were nurses) were interviewed to identify interventions they used to reduce feelings of guilt among family caregivers during the transition from caring for their loved one at home to enlisting their loved one in an assisted living facility. The hospice nurses explained that the family caregivers worked through a five-stage process in their guilt experiences, moving from "feeling guilty" to "resolving their guilt" during the transition period. The actions of the hospice nurses varied based on the stage of the family caregiver's feelings of guilt. These actions included supporting, managing, navigating, negotiating, encouraging, monitoring, and coaching. A situation-specific model was proposed to explain the relationships among these processes and suggest congruent hospice nursing interventions.

and self-actualization. The team concluded that research is needed to understand the processes that result in transformation to expert critical cares nurses and should focus on the interaction among the three themes. In another example, a team led by Markey et al. (2019) used grounded theory methods to develop a theory to explain nurses' behaviors when caring for culturally and linguistically diverse patients. The researchers interviewed 30 nursing students and registered nurses and conducted 10 focus groups to better understand the challenges experienced in caring for patients from diverse backgrounds and gather information. From the interviews, the researchers discussed the observation of "resigned indifference" that resulted in gaps in care. "Masking," "distancing," and "fitting in" were "disengagement strategies" the nurses used to deal with uncertainties of caring for patients from different cultural backgrounds. From their research, it was concluded that nurse managers should work to support and empower ways to address gaps in care by communicating a clearer message of the responsibility to acknowledge and respect cultural differences so as to provide quality, patient-centered care.

Examples of Theory as Research Framework

When the researcher uses quantitative methods, the framework is typically identified and explained at the beginning of the paper, before the discussion of study methods. **Example:** ➤ In their study examining the effectiveness of an individualized structured educational program to promote metabolic control and achievement of long-term therapeutic targets for type 2 diabetes patients, De la Fuente Coria and colleagues (2020) (see Appendix B) indicated that their educational intervention was based on the "model of empowerment" (Asimakopoulou et al., 2012; Inzucchi et al., 2012). The model of empowerment works to promote participation and strengthen autonomy to enhance patient education. In the study, goal setting and motivational interviewing were used to teach the participants basic knowledge of diabetes, including healthy eating, physical activity glucose monitoring, risk reduction, and effective coping. It was determined that the educational intervention had favorable results on fasting blood glucose, total cholesterol, and systolic blood pressure among other indicators. Body mass index was not improved, however. The researchers noted that results might have been improved with group education, particularly with respect to cost-effectiveness and reaching more individuals.

In another example, one of the works read by Emily from the case study dealt with resilience in adolescents (Tusaie et al., 2007). The researchers in this work used Lazarus and Folkman's (1984) theory of stress and coping as part of the theoretical framework, researching factors such as optimism, family support, age, and life events.

Examples of Theory-Testing Research

Although many nursing studies that are experimental and quasi-experimental (see Chapter 9) are frequently conducted to test interventions, examples of research expressly conducted to test a theory are relatively rare in nursing literature. One such work is a quasi-experimental study by Koren (2017) examining the construct of self-care, one of the key constructs of the Theory of Modeling and Role Modeling. The study examined the effectiveness of teaching mindfulness interventions to nursing students. It was concluded that the mindfulness training was somewhat effective in reducing stress and increasing awareness, thereby enhancing self-care among the study cohort.

CRITICAL APPRAISAL CRITERIA

Critiquing Theoretical Framework

1. Is the framework for research clearly identified?
2. Is the framework consistent with a nursing perspective?
3. Is the framework appropriate to guide research on the subject of interest?
4. Are the concepts and variables clearly and appropriately defined?
5. Was sufficient literature presented to support study of the selected concepts?
6. Is there a logical, consistent link between the framework, the concepts being studied, and the methods of measurement?
7. Are the study findings examined in relationship to the framework?

Critiquing the Use of Theory in Nursing Research

It is beneficial to seek out, identify, and follow the theoretical framework or source of the background of a study. The framework for research provides guidance for the researcher as study questions are fine-tuned, methods for measuring variables are selected, and analyses are planned. Once data are collected and analyzed, the framework is used as a base for comparison. Ideally, the research should explain: Did the findings coincide with the framework? Did the findings support or refute findings of other researchers who used the framework? If there were discrepancies, is there a way to explain them using the framework? The reader of research needs to know how to critically appraise a framework for research (see the Critical Appraisal Criteria box).

The first question posed is whether a framework is presented. Sometimes a theory may be guiding the research, but a diagrammed model is not included in the manuscript. You must then look for the theoretical framework in the narrative description of the study concepts. When the framework is identified, it is important to consider its relevance for nursing. The framework does not have to be one created by a nurse, but the importance of its content for nursing should be clear. The question of how the framework depicts a structure congruent with nursing should be addressed. For instance, although the Lazarus Transaction Model of Stress and Coping was not developed by a nurse, it is clearly related to nursing practice when working with people facing stress. Sometimes frameworks from different disciplines, such as physics or art, may be relevant. It is the responsibility of the author to clearly articulate the meaning of the framework for the study and to link the framework to nursing.

Once the meaning and applicability of the theory (if the objective of the research was theory development) or the theoretical framework to nursing are articulated, you will be able to determine whether the framework is appropriate to guide the research. As you critically appraise a study, you would identify a mismatch, for example, in which the researcher presents a study of students' responses to the stress of being in the clinical setting for the first time within a framework of stress related to recovery from chronic illness. You should look closely at the framework to determine whether it is "on target" and the "best fit" for the research question and proposed study design.

Next, the reader should focus on the concepts being studied. Does the researcher clearly describe and explain concepts that are being studied and how they are defined and translated into measurable variables? Is there literature to support the choice of concepts? Concepts should clearly reflect the area of study. **Example:** ➤ Using the concept of "anger," when "incivility" or "hostility" is more appropriate to the research focus creates difficulties in defining variables and determining methods of measurement. These issues are related to the logical consistency among the framework, the concepts being studied, and the methods of measurement.

Throughout the entire critiquing process, from worldview to operational definitions, the reader is evaluating the fit. Finally, the reader will expect to find a discussion of the findings as they relate to the theory or framework. This final point enables evaluation of the framework for use in further research. It may suggest necessary changes to enhance the relevance of the framework for continuing study, and thus serves to let others know where to go from there.

Evaluating frameworks for research requires skills that must be acquired through repeated critique and discussion with others who have critiqued the same work. As with other abilities and skills, you must practice and use the skills to develop them further. With continuing education and a broader knowledge of potential frameworks, you will build a repertoire of knowledge to assess the foundation of a research study and the framework for research and/or to evaluate findings where theory was generated as the outcome of the study.

KEY POINTS

- The interaction among theory, practice, and research is central to knowledge development in the discipline of nursing.
- The use of a framework for research is important as a guide to systematically identify concepts and to link appropriate study variables with each concept.
- Conceptual and operational definitions are critical to the evolution of a study.
- In developing or selecting a framework for research, knowledge may be acquired from other disciplines or directly from nursing. In either case, this knowledge is used to answer specific nursing questions.
- Theory is distinguished by its scope. Grand theories are broadest in scope, and situation-specific theories are the narrowest in scope and at the lowest level of abstraction; middle range theories are in the middle.
- In critiquing a framework for research, it is important to examine the logical, consistent link among the framework, the concepts for study, and the methods of measurement.

CLINICAL JUDGMENT CHALLENGES

- Search recent issues of a prominent nursing journal (e.g., Nursing Research, Research in Nursing & Health) for notations of conceptual frameworks of published studies. How many explicitly discussed the theoretical framework? How many did not mention any theoretical framework? What kinds of theories were mentioned (e.g., grand nursing theories, middle range nursing theories, non-nursing theories)? How many studies were theory generating? How many were theory testing?
- Identify a non-nursing theory that you would like to know more about. How could you find information on its applicability to nursing research and nursing practice? How could you identify if and how it has been used in nursing research?
- Select a nursing theory, concept, or phenomenon (e.g., resilience from the case study) that you are interested in and would like to know more about, and consider: How could you find studies that have used that theory in research and practice? How could you

locate published instruments and tools that reportedly measure concepts and constructs of the theory?

- **IPE** You have just joined an interprofessional primary care quality improvement team focused on developing evidence-based self-management strategies to decrease hospital admissions for the practice's heart failure patients. Which theoretical framework could be used to guide your project?

REFERENCES

Ahern, N. R. (2006). Adolescent resilience: An evolutionary concept analysis. *Journal of Pediatric Nursing, 21*(3), 175–185.

Ahern, N. R., Ark, P., & Byers, J. (2008). Resilience and coping strategies in adolescents. *Pediatric Nursing, 20*(10), 32–36.

Asimakopoulou, K., Gilbert, D., Newton, P., & Scrambler, S. (2012). Back to basics: reexamining the role of patient empowerment in diabetes. *Patient Education, 86*(3), 281–283.

Chinn, P. L., & Kramer, M. K. (2018). *Knowledge development in nursing: Theory and process* (10th ed.). St. Louis, MO: Elsevier.

Clayton, M. F., Dean, M., & Mishel, M. (2018). Theories of uncertainty in illness. In M. J. Smith & P. R. Liehr (Eds.), *Middle range theory for nursing* (4th ed., pp. 49–82). New York, NY: Springer Publishing Co.

De la Fuente Coria, M. C., Cruz-Cobo, Cl., & Santi-Cano, M. J. (2020). Effectiveness of a primary care nurse delivered educational intervention for patients with type 2 diabetes mellitus in promoting metabolic control and compliance with long-term therapeutic targets: Randomised controlled trial. *International Journal of Nursing Studies, 101*, pp.

Eakes, G. (2020). Chronic sorrow. In S. J. Peterson & T. S. Bredow (Eds.), *Middle range theories: Application to nursing research* (5th ed., pp. 1–7). Philadelphia, PA: Wolters Kluwer.

Eakes, G., Burke, M. L., & Hainsworth, M. A. (1998). Middle rang theory of chronic sorrow. *Image: Journal of Nursing Scholarship, 30*(2), 179–185.

Flanders, S., Hampton, D., Missi, P., Ipsan, C., & Greubbl, C. (2020). Effectiveness of a staff resilience program in a pediatric intensive care unit. *Journal of Pediatric Nursing, 50*, 1–4.

Hanna, A., Yael, E. M., Hadassa, L., Iris, E., Eugenia, N., Lior, G., Carmit, S., & Liora, O. (2020). It's up to me with a little support"—Adherence after myocardial infarction: A qualitative study. *International Journal of Nursing Studies, 101*, 1–9.

Im, E. (2014). The status quo of situation-specific theories. *Research and Theory for Nursing Practice: An International Journal, 28*(4), 278–298.

Im, E., & Chang, S. J. (2012). Current trends in nursing theories. *Journal of Nursing Scholarship, 44*(2), 156–164.

Inzucchi, S. E., Bergenstal, R. M., Bruse, J. B., Diamant, M., Ferrannini, E., Nauck, M., Peters, A. L., Tsapas, A, Wender, R., & Matthews, D. R. (2012). Management of hyperglycaemia in Type 2 diabetes: A patient-centered approach: position statement of the American Diabetes Association(ADA) and the European Association for the Study of Diabetes (EASD). *Diabetes Care, 35*(6), 1364–1379.

Ishibashi, A., Okamura, J., Ueda, R., et al. (2016). Psychological strength enhancing resilience in adolescents and young adults with cancer. *Journal of Pediatric Oncology Nursing, 33*(1), 45–54.

Kastaun, S., Wilm, S., Herber, O. R., & Barroso, J. (2019). From qualitative meta-summary to qualitative meta-synthesis: Introducing a new situation-specific theory of barriers and facilitators for self-care in patients with hearth failure. *Qualitative Health Research, 29*(1), 96–106.

Kim, Y., & Dee, V. (2017). Self-care for health in rural Hispanic women at risk for postpartum depression. *Maternal Child Health Journal, 21*, 77–84.

Kolcaba, K. Y. (1994). A theory of holistic comfort for nursing. *Journal of Advanced Nursing, 19*(6), 1178–1184.

Kolcaba, K. Y., & Crawford, C. L. (2020). Comfort. In S. J. Peterson & T. S. Bredow (Eds.), *Middle range theories: Application to nursing research* (5th ed., pp. 189–208). Philadelphia, PA: Wolters Kluwer.

Koren, M. E. (2017). Mindfulness interventions for nursing students: Application of Modelling and Role Modelling Theory. *International Journal of Caring Sciences, 10*(3), 1710–1716.

Lazarus, R. S., & Folkman, S. (1984). *Stress, appraisal and coping.* New York, NY: Springer.

Lee, S. M. (2018). Lee geropalliative caring model: A situation-specific theory for older adults. *Advances in Nursing Science, 41*(2), 161–173.

Lenz, E. R., Pugh, L. C., & Milligan, R. A. (2020). Unpleasant symptoms. In S. J. Peterson & T. S. Bredow (Eds.), *Middle range theories: Application to nursing research* (5th ed.). Philadelphia, PA: Wolters Kluwer.

Lenz, E. R., Pugh, L. C., Miligan, R. A., et al. (1997). The middle range theory of unpleasant symptoms: An update. *Advances in Nursing Science, 19*(3), 14–27.

Linder, L. A, Hooke, M. C., Hockenberry, M., & Landier, W. (2019). Symptoms in children receiving treatment for cancer – Part II: Pain, sadness and symptom clusters. *Journal of Pediatric Oncology Nursing, 36*(4), 262–279.

Markey, K., Tilki, M., & Taylor, G. (2019). Resigned indifference: An explanation of gaps in care for culturally and linguistically diverse patients. *Journal of Nursing Management, 27*(7), 1462–1470.

Martz, K. (2015). Actions of hospice nurses to alleviate guilt in family caregiver during residential care transitions. *Journal of Hospice and Palliative Nursing, 17*(1), 48–55.

McCutcheon, T., Schaar, G., Herline, A., & Hayes, R. (2017). HPV awareness and vaccination rates in college-aged male athletes. *The Nurse Practitioner, 42*(11), 27–34.

McEwen, M., & Wills, E. (2019). *Theoretical basis for nursing* (5th ed.). Philadelphia, PA: Wolters Kluwer.

Meleis, A. I. (2010). *Transitions theory: Middle range and situation specific theories in nursing research and practice.* New York, NY: Springer Publishing.

Mishel, M. H. (1988). Uncertainty in illness. *Journal of Nursing Scholarship, 20*(4), 225–232.

Mishel, M. H. (1990). Reconceptualization of the uncertainty in illness theory. *Image: Journal of Nursing Scholarship, 22*(4), 256–262.

Murdaugh, C., Parsons, M., & Pender, N. J. (2019). *Health promotion in nursing practice* (8th ed.). Upper Saddle River, NJ: Pearson Education.

Nightingale, F. (1969). *Notes on nursing: What it is and what it is not.* New York, NY: Dover Publications (Original work published 1860).

Nyamathi, A. (1989). Comprehensive health seeking and coping paradigm. *Journal of Advanced Nursing, 14*(4), 281–290.

Nyamathi, A., Salem, B. E., Zhang, S., et al. (2015). Nursing case management, peer coaching, and hepatitis A and B vaccine completion among homeless men recently released on parole. *Nursing Research, 64*(3), 177–189.

Orem, D. E. (2001). *Nursing: Concepts of practice* (6th ed.). St Louis, MO: Mosby.

Peterson, S. J. (2020). Introduction to the nature of nursing knowledge. In S. J. Peterson & T. S. Bredow (Eds.), *Middle range theories: Application to nursing research* (5th ed., pp. 1–36). Philadelphia, PA: Wolters Kluwer.

Polk, L. V. (1997). Toward a middle range theory of resilience. *Advances in Nursing Science, 19*(3), 1–13.

Reimer, A. P., & Moore, S. M. (2010). Flight nursing expertise: Towards a middle-range theory. *Journal of Advanced Nursing, 66*(5), 1183–1192.

Rogers, M. E. (1970). *An introduction to the theoretical basis of nursing.* Philadelphia, PA: Davis.

Rogers, M. E. (1990). Nursing: the science of unitary, irreducible, human beings: Update: 1990. In E. A. M. Barrett (Ed.), *Visions of Rogers' science-based nursing* (pp. 5–11). New York, NY: National League for Nursing Press.

Rosenberg, A. R., Bradford, M. C., McCauley, E., Curtis, J. R., Wolfe, J., Baker, K. S., & Yi-Frazier, J. P. (2018). Promoting resilience in adolescents and young adults with cancer: Results from the PRISM randomized controlled trial. *Cancer, 124*(19), 3909–3917.

Ross, R., Letvak, S., Sheppard, F., Jenkins, M., & Almotairy, M. (2020). Systemic assessment of depressive symptoms among registered nurses: A new situation-specific theory. *Nursing Outlook, 68*(2), 207–219.

Roy, C. (2009). *The Roy adaptation model* (3rd ed.). Upper Saddle River, NJ: Pearson.

Ruland, C. M., & Moore, S. M. (1998). Theory construction based on standards of care: A proposed theory of the peaceful end of life. *Nursing Outlook, 46*(4), 169–175.

Shore, J. C., Gelber, M. W., Koch, I. M., & Sower, E. (2016). Anticipatory grief: An evidence-based approach. *Journal of Hospice & Palliative Nursing, 18*(1), 15–19.

Tusaie, K., Puskar, K., & Sereika, S. M. (2007). A predictive and moderating model of psychosocial resilience in adolescents. *Journal of Nursing Scholarship, 39*(1), 54–60.

Vellone, E., Riegel, B., & Alvaro, R. (2019). A situation-specific theory of caregiver contributions to heart failure self-care. *Journal of Cardiovascular Nursing, 34*(2), 166–173.

Welch, T. D., & Carter, M. (2020). Expertise among critical care nurses: A grounded theory study. *Intensive & Critical Care Nursing, 57*, pp. 1–8 (epub).

Go to Evolve at **http://evolve.elsevier.com/LoBiondo/** for review questions, appraisal exercises, and additional research articles for practice in reviewing and appraisal.

PART II

Processes and Evidence Related to Qualitative Research

Research Vignette: Karla M. Abela

RESEARCH VIGNETTE

SELECTING A RESEARCH FOCUS AND STAYING FOCUSED!

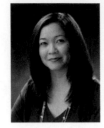

Karla M. Abela, PhD, RN, CCRN-K, CPN
Assistant Professor
University of Texas Health Science Center
Cizik School of Nursing
Houston, Texas

Some nurse scientists begin their doctoral program with a research focus in mind. However, I would venture to say that for most of us, we cycle through several ideas, abandoning many along the way. I think the million-dollar question for those pursuing a doctorate in nursing is, "How does one select a research focus to build a research program?" When I chose to pursue a career in nursing, I did not know I would be developing my own research program more than a decade later.

I was in one of the last classes of diploma-prepared registered nurses in Ontario, Canada. I graduated during a time when hospital-based diploma programs were being closed and community college nursing programs were beginning to partner with larger universities to offer baccalaureate degrees. Evidence-based practice, quality improvement, and research were not part of my undergraduate nursing program. I did not learn about these concepts until I settled into working in a pediatric setting. Although my career began in adult health, I always knew that I wanted to work with children. During nursing school, I often requested to be paired with a pediatric nurse for my clinical rotations and sought volunteer opportunities in local children's centers. However, at that time, novice nurses were encouraged to practice in adult medical-surgical settings before specializing, and most hospitals did not hire new graduate nurses directly into pediatrics. And so, I became a clinical nurse in the adult cardiothoracic surgical unit of a large academic medical center. I resolved to absorb everything from the expert nurses, my role models, while setting my sights on a future that involved working with children.

After several years, I transferred to the pediatric unit, where I cared for children with immune deficiencies, hematological conditions, and oncologic conditions. Many of the children were participants in clinical trials, and in addition to providing nursing care, I also administered investigational drugs and evaluated the children's response to the treatment protocols. After several years, I became the nurse educator for all the pediatric intermediate care units. This experience led me to my first research study and my first interaction with a nurse scientist. A fellow nurse and I worked closely with our nurse scientist to conduct a case-control study of pediatric patients admitted to an intermediate care unit after a post-Fontan procedure, the third and final surgical stage of repair for children with hypoplastic left-heart syndrome. We compared the outcomes of children who participated in an incentive-based ambulation program versus children who received the standard ambulation protocol. Recovery from the Fontan procedure takes weeks, including a lengthy hospitalization in the intensive care unit (ICU). Ambulation was a major component of promoting recovery; the nurses needed to devise a strategy to motivate their patients to get out of bed and walk in the hallways.

At that time, methods to motivate postoperative pediatric patients were limited. We decided to develop a method for the nurses to reward the children with tickets each time they walked in the hallway. Tickets could then be exchanged for developmentally appropriate rewards. Because the operational budget did not include funds for the tickets or prizes, I wrote my first grant application, which was funded to support the rewards. It was such a rewarding experience!

After a few years as an educator, I earned a master's degree in nursing administration and became the nurse manager of the Pediatric ICU (PICU). By this time, I had developed multiple interests in clinical nursing, nursing education, and nursing administration. I experienced the many challenges nurse leaders face daily. Nurse staffing and nursing retention were key issues, and I committed myself to conducting small projects to better understand this problem. With the nurse scientist's guidance, a colleague and I developed a study in response to an unexpected rise in turnover within our organization. We conducted a descriptive qualitative study of registered nurses who had resigned to explore their reasons for leaving, with the hope of using the findings to develop retention strategies. We recruited former staff nurses by mail and conducted interviews by phone. Five main themes emerged from the interview prompts: work environment concerns, emotional and physical distress, distrust of management, lack of support resource use, and reasons for leaving.

When I interviewed for the PhD program a few years later, I was convinced that I would pursue my study of nurse staffing and issues that affect nursing retention. While in the master's program, I was particularly fascinated by the concept of "technostress" and how it applied to the nursing profession. Technostress, or computer anxiety, had not been previously explored in practicing nurses. As an educator and administrator, I was extensively involved in electronic health record implementation at our organization, and I was convinced that many of the challenges we experienced were attributable to technostress and its associated factors. As one of my final assignments, I developed a protocol to examine technostress in practicing nurses and determine its association with personality traits, anxiety, and previous experience using computers. I wanted to continue this work in the doctoral program.

In the first few semesters of my doctoral program, I focused on identifying the specific gap that I would like to address in developing my program of research. As students, we completed several exercises and seminars in which we immersed ourselves in our population of interest, identifying the problems afflicting our specific population. These problems were broken down into concepts that were later explored; I focused on exploring technostress in nurses. Every week, we participated in discussions with faculty and peers to develop our understanding of the research gap and to select the best method to address it. These activities, and those that followed in the subsequent semesters, helped me to shift my focus to a different population in the Pediatric ICU: the patient's family.

Family-centered care (FCC) and its domains were not familiar concepts to me until I became a pediatric nurse. At that time, we had little to no guidance on what FCC was and how to implement best practices such as FCC in subspecialty areas. Visitation restrictions and limitations were slowly easing in hospitals across the country, including ICUs, where visitation rules were stricter. It was not common practice to include the family in rounds, and family conferences were primarily for discussing emergency or end-of-life circumstances. As studies on the impact of critical illness on families started to surface, the attention focused on the parents, who, at the time, were the only ones permitted to visit the hospital. My candidacy committee and I continued the work of Shudy et al. (2006) by conducting a systematic review to examine the impact of pediatric critical illness and injury on families admitted to the PICU. The literature was replete with studies examining the effect on parents, yet siblings of critically ill or injured children were understudied. The review (Abela et al., 2020a) supported that parents experienced stress, anxiety, and worry related to the sights and sounds seen in the PICU environment, the uncertainty of the illness, and changes in family functioning as a result of the hospitalization. However, the experience of siblings of the ill child was still unknown. Given the relatively recent inclusion of siblings at the ill child's bedside, we thought it important to understand their experiences in order to mitigate the stress associated with being in the PICU environment.

Once my focus was established, I was guided by my dissertation committee, composed of my faculty advisor, a nursing faculty member with a mental health background, and a board-certified child psychologist, to develop a research proposal was supported by the American Nurses' Foundation. Because the sibling experience is mostly unknown, we chose to conduct a descriptive qualitative study in which I interviewed school-aged children who were visiting an ill brother or sister in the PICU. Once approved by the institutional review board, I recruited siblings from the PICU. I interviewed 16 siblings from diverse family structures. In addition to what we already knew about parent experiences in the ICU, we discovered that siblings' PICU experiences were influenced by several stressors and coping strategies. Siblings reported being stressed by seeing their parents' physical and emotional suffering and by the uncertainty of the tenuous situation. Siblings coped by distracting themselves with activities unrelated to the illness; reflecting on their relationship with the ill child; and finding support from their friends, family members, and God (Abela et al., 2020b).

Although this study highlighted the experiences of siblings visiting the PICU, many unanswered questions remain. I plan to conduct research to explore the relationships between stressors, coping strategies, and the sibling experience, examining hypothesized relationships between the concepts we identified. I believe that an understanding of the siblings' experiences in the PICU can eventually lead to standardized interventions to support this forgotten population. I also hope that others who wish to conduct studies in PICUs learn from our work. Because siblings have not always been permitted in the ICU setting for prolonged periods of time, we had little knowledge of how to best recruit and study this population. By conducting this study, we gained insight into how parents decided to consent to having their healthy child participate in a study and how to conduct one-to-one interviews with children who are experiencing a profound family crisis. I also experienced the challenges of conducting a study in a clinical setting, such as an ICU, and learned the importance of being patient and nimble.

Now that I have completed the doctoral program, I continue to be guided by faculty mentors in developing my program of research. I have decided to stay in practice for the time being, staying close to my population of interest. For others who wish to do the same, I encourage you to seek an organization that is supportive of nurse scientists who wish to grow their scholarship. With the many competing demands of daily responsibilities and helping others with their own projects, it can be very easy to get distracted from my focus. I also cannot forget that I am a novice researcher with much to learn about developing my program of research, securing funding, and sharing my work with others. Fortunately for me, my relationship with my professors did not end when I graduated. I continue to maintain close ties with the school of nursing faculty, and they help keep me focused on my goals.

My research focus is a product of many years of clinical and leadership experience. The problems I explored in the beginning of the doctoral program were ones I was very passionate about. They were not "bad" ideas, and they all had the potential to have been fruitful. These ideas were not abandoned because I did not see any benefit to pursuing them. Simply put, I had to focus. Focus is what helped me to succeed in the doctoral program. It is what helped me to conduct research and publish while in school and, eventually, earn a grant for my dissertation research. Finally, I highly encourage other doctoral students and novice nurse scientists to heed their faculty advisor's guidance. I am forever indebted to mine for her lessons about pursuing my passions, avoiding distractions, and staying focused.

REFERENCES

Abela, K., Casarez, R., Kaplow, J. B., & LoBiondo-Wood, G. (2020a). Siblings' experience during pediatric intensive care hospitalization. Manuscript submitted for publication.

Abela, K., Wardell, D., Rozmus, C., & LoBiondo-Wood, G. (2020b). Impact of Pediatric Critical Illness and Injury on Families: An Updated Systematic Review. *Journal Of Pediatric Nursing, 51*, 21–31. https://doi.org/10.1016/j.pedn.2019.10.013.

Shudy, M., de Almeida, M., Ly, S., Landon, C., Groft, S., Jenkins, T., & Nicholson, C. (2006). Impact of Pediatric Critical Illness and Injury on Families: A Systematic Literature Review. *PEDIATRICS, 118*(Supplement_3), S203–S218. https://doi.org/10.1542/peds.2006-0951b.

5

Introduction to Qualitative Research

Dalmacio Dennis Flores III, Julie Barroso

Go to Evolve at **http://evolve.elsevier.com/LoBiondo/** for review questions.

LEARNING OUTCOMES

After reading this chapter, you should be able to do the following:

- Describe the components of a qualitative research report.
- Describe the beliefs generally held by qualitative researchers.

- Identify four ways qualitative findings can be used in evidence-based practice.

KEY TERMS

context dependent
data saturation
data collection
   strategies

grand tour question
inclusion and exclusion
   criteria

inductive
naturalistic setting
paradigm

qualitative research
theme

Let's say that you are reading a study that reports findings that highly assimilated young women (e.g., English-speaking second-generation women) from immigrant families with full insurance coverage are reporting more negative sexual health outcomes compared with underinsured newly arrived immigrants. You wonder, "Why is that? Why would US-born young women who have access to reproductive health services have more negative outcomes? Surely it should be the opposite." Or say you are working in a primary care clinic and overhear a patient dismissing the nurse practitioner's suggestion for him to use the new park in the neighborhood for routine walks and regular exercise. You wonder, "What is the process by which patients with weight management issues and high blood pressure decide on which interventions to try and which ones to decline? How do they go about making these decisions?" Like so many other questions we have as nurses, these questions can be best answered through research conducted using qualitative methods. Qualitative research gives us the answers to those difficult "why?" questions. Although qualitative research can be used at many different points in a program of research, you will most often find it answering questions that we have when we understand very little about some phenomenon in nursing.

WHAT IS QUALITATIVE RESEARCH?

Qualitative research is a broad term that encompasses several different methodologies that share many similarities. Qualitative studies help us formulate an understanding of a phenomenon. Nurse scientists who are trained in qualitative methods use these methodological approaches to best answer research questions that require discovery or definition.

Qualitative research is explanatory, descriptive, and **inductive** in nature. It uses words, as opposed to numbers, to explain a phenomenon. Qualitative research lets us see the world through the eyes of another—the young woman who struggles to access sexual health services or the man who quickly dismisses walking in the park near his house as an option for mitigating his obesity and uncontrolled blood pressure. Qualitative researchers assume that we can only understand these things if we consider the context in which they take place, and this is why most qualitative research takes place in naturalistic settings. Qualitative studies make the world of an individual visible to the rest of us; it allows the unique context in which the phenomenon occurs and is experienced to be taken into consideration. Especially in the past few years, qualitative research has moved from a methodology that imposes the perspective of strangers to interpret a phenomenon from the outside to one that centers the perspective of participants and values them as coequals in the research process (Morse, 2020).

WHAT DO QUALITATIVE RESEARCHERS BELIEVE?

Qualitative researchers believe that there are multiple realities that can be understood by carefully studying what people can tell us or what we can observe as we spend time with them. **Example:** ➤ The experience of going to an obstetrician, although it has some shared characteristics, is not the same for any two women, and it is definitely different for a non–English-speaking young woman. Thus qualitative researchers believe that reality is socially constructed and **context dependent**. Even the experience of reading this book is different for any two students; one may be completely engrossed by the content, while another is reading but at the same time worrying about whether or not their financial aid will be approved soon.

Because qualitative researchers believe that the discovery of meaning is the basis for knowledge, their research questions, approaches, and activities are often quite different from quantitative researchers (see the Critical Thinking Decision Path). Qualitative researchers seek to understand the "lived experience" of the research participants. They may use interviews or observations to gather new data and use new data to create narratives about research phenomena. Thus qualitative researchers know that there is a very strong imperative to clearly describe the phenomenon under study. Ideally, the reader of a qualitative research report, if even slightly acquainted with the phenomenon, would have an "aha!" moment of empathetic understanding when reading a well-written qualitative report.

So, you may now be saying, "Wow! This sounds great! Qualitative research is for me!" Many nurses feel very comfortable with this approach because we are educated with regard to how to speak with people about the health issues concerning them; we are used to listening and listening well. Additionally, nurse scientists who employ qualitative research approaches "seek to arouse a perceived mutuality, and an empathic connection" between the participant, scientist, and reader (Gair, 2012, p. 139). Ultimately, this quest "to hear, feel, understand, and value the stories of others, and to convey that felt empathy and understanding back to the client/storyteller/participant" is in the service of positively contributing to health outcomes (Gair, 2012, p. 139). However, the most important consideration for any study is whether or not the methodology fits the question. This means that qualitative researchers must select an approach for exploring phenomena that will actually answer their research questions. Thus, as you read studies and are considering them as evidence on which to base your practice, you should ask yourself, "Does the methodology fit with the research question under study?"

HELPFUL HINT

All research is based on a paradigm, but this is seldom specifically stated in a research report.

DOES THE METHODOLOGY FIT WITH THE RESEARCH QUESTION BEING ASKED?

As we said earlier, qualitative methods are often best for helping us determine the nature of a phenomenon and the meaning of experience. Sometimes authors will state that they are using qualitative methods because little is known about a phenomenon, but this alone is not a good reason for conducting a study. Little may be known about a phenomenon because it does not matter! When researchers ask people to participate in a study, to open themselves and their lives for analysis, they should be asking about things that will help make a difference in people's lives or help us provide more effective nursing care. You should be able to articulate a valid reason for conducting a study beyond "little is known about this topic."

Considering the examples at the start of this chapter, we may want to know why young women born of immigrant parents struggle to use sexual health services that are readily at their disposal, so we can address the unique barriers they face and potentially change clinic processes to overcome those challenges. Similarly, we need to have a comprehension of the decision-making processes older men with hypertension and obesity use to decide whether or not to utilize green spaces and recreational facilities in their neighborhoods for weight loss. To summarize, a qualitative approach "fits" a research question when the researchers seek to understand the nature or experience of phenomena by attending to personal accounts of those with direct experiences related to the phenomena. Keeping in mind the purpose of qualitative research, let's discuss the parts of a qualitative research study.

COMPONENTS OF A QUALITATIVE RESEARCH STUDY

The components of a qualitative study include the literature review, study design, study setting and sample, approaches for data collection and analysis, study findings, and conclusions with implications for practice and research. As we reflect on these parts of qualitative studies, we will see how nurses use the qualitative research process to develop new knowledge for practice (Box 5.1).

> **BOX 5.1 Steps in the Research Process**
>
> - Review of the literature
> - Study design
> - Sample
> - Setting: Recruitment and data collection
>
> - Data collection
> - Data analysis
> - Findings
> - Conclusions

Review of the Literature

When researchers are clear that a qualitative approach is the best way to answer the research question, their first step is to review the relevant literature and describe what is already known about the phenomena of interest. A thorough review is necessary as the same phenomena might have already been investigated and solutions devised in a different part of the country or the world! A review of related published studies is also crucial, as it may inform what "angle" a proposed study will focus on, add research elements you might not have previously considered, and incorporate previous findings to make your investigation more thorough. After a methodical review has been conducted, a researcher may discover that there may not be any published research on the phenomenon in question. In other cases, researchers may identify previous studies on similar subjects, or with the same patient population, or on a closely related concept. **Example:** ➤ Researchers may want to study why English-speaking, second-generation young women with full insurance coverage appear to underutilize sexual health services. Although there may be no other studies in this particular area, there may be some published on the low uptake of HIV and HPV screenings among college-age young adults. There may be literature on the use of sexually transmitted infection prevention services by high school girls at Federally Qualified Health Centers or Planned Parenthood located within ethnic enclaves. These studies would be important in the review of the literature because they identify concepts and relationships that can be used to guide the research process. **Example:** ➤ Findings from the review can show us the precise need for new research, what participants should be in the study sample, and what kinds of questions should be used to collect the data.

Let's consider an example. Say a group of researchers wanted to examine the barriers older men with obesity and uncontrolled hypertension have to using green spaces such as walking paths and recreational parks at urban spaces. If there was no research on this exact topic, the researcher may examine studies on engaging overweight youth with physical activity. They may include studies that examine gender differences in solo or group weight-loss intervention programs. Or they might examine the literature on perceived safety of urban recreational spaces across different generations or look at technology-facilitated smart phone applications and their success rate among different age groups.

The major point is that even though there may be no literature on the exact phenomenon of interest, the review of the literature will identify existing related studies that are useful for exploring the new questions. At the conclusion of an effective review, you should be able to easily identify the strengths and weaknesses in prior research, clearly understand the new research questions, and clearly articulate the significance of the study.

CRITICAL THINKING DECISION PATH

Selecting a Research Process

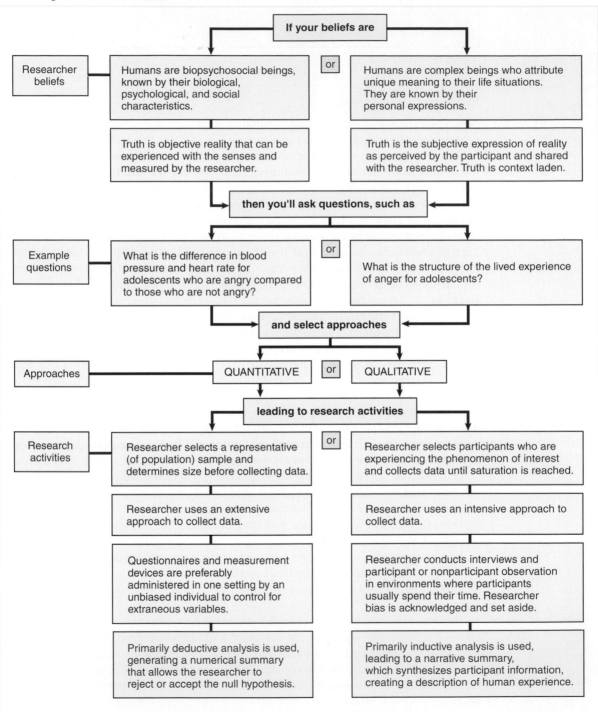

Study Design

The study design is a description of how the qualitative researcher plans to go about answering the research questions. In qualitative research, there may simply be a descriptive or naturalistic design in which the researchers adhere to the general tenets of qualitative research but do not commit to a particular methodology (see Chapter 6). There are many different qualitative methods used to answer the research questions. Some of these methods will be discussed in Chapter 6. What is important, as you read from this point forward, is that the study design must be congruent with the philosophical beliefs that qualitative researchers hold. You would not expect to see a qualitative researcher use methods common to quantitative studies, such as a random sample, a battery of questionnaires administered in a hospital outpatient clinic, or a multiple regression analysis. Rather, you would expect to see a design that includes participant interviews or observations, strategies for inductive analysis, and plans for using data to develop narrative summaries with rich description of the details from participants' experiences. You may also read about a pilot study in the description of a study design; this is work the researchers did before undertaking the main study to make sure that the logistics of the proposed study were reasonable. For example, pilot data may describe if the investigators were able to recruit participants and if the research design led them to the information they needed.

Sample

The study sample refers to the group of people that the researcher will interview or observe in the process of collecting data to answer the research questions. In most qualitative studies, the researchers are looking for a purposeful or purposively selected sample (see Chapter 12). This means that they are searching for a specific person who has firsthand experience or can authoritatively speak about the phenomenon under consideration. **Example:** ➤ The researchers may want to interview Asian American or Latinx young women with recent diagnoses of HPV. There may be other parameters—called inclusion and exclusion criteria—that the researchers impose as well, such as requiring that participants be between 16 and 20 years of age, not under the influence of illicit drugs, or not experiencing a first pregnancy (as opposed to subsequent pregnancies). When researchers are clear about these criteria, they are able to identify and recruit participants with the experiences needed to shed light on the phenomenon in question. Often the researchers make decisions such as determining how to define "recent diagnoses" of HPV. In this case, they must clearly describe why and how they decided who would fit into this category. Is a recent diagnosis limited to ones detected in the past 3, 6, or 12 months? Why is the time of diagnoses relevant? Thus, as a reader of research, you are looking for evidence of sound scientific reasoning behind the sampling plan.

When the researchers have identified the type of person to include in the research sample, the next step is to develop a strategy for recruiting participants, which means locating and engaging them in the research. Recruitment materials are usually very specific. **Example:** ➤ If the researchers want to talk to second-generation young women recently diagnosed with HPV about barriers to accessing sexual health services, they may distribute paper flyers or advertise on social media platforms their interest in recruiting young women who have visited their OBGYNs in the past year and those who have not. Or they may want to talk to young women who fit into only one of these categories. Similarly, the researchers who are examining decision making in older obese men with hypertension would develop recruitment strategies that identify participants with the conditions or characteristics they want to study.

In a research report, the researcher may include a description of the study sample in the findings. (This can also be reported in the description of the sample.) In any event, besides a demographic description of the study participants, a qualitative researcher should also report on key elements in the sample. **Example:** ➤ In a sample of young women with recent HPV diagnoses, there should be information about the length of time since diagnoses, the types of insurance coverage they have, how many sexual partners they have had in the past year, and so on. This information helps you place the findings into a context.

Setting: Recruitment and Data Collection

The study setting refers to the places where participants are recruited from and the data are collected. Settings for recruitment are usually a point of contact for people of common social, medical, or other individual traits. In the example of barriers to sexual health service utilization by second-generation young women, researchers may distribute flyers describing the study at sexual health service organizations, college affinity groups for Asian American or Latinx students, wellness clinics, online support groups, and other places young people frequent. The settings for data collection are another critical area of difference between quantitative and qualitative studies. Data collection in a qualitative study is usually done in a naturalistic setting of the participant's choice, such as someone's home, preferably not in a clinic interview room or researcher's office. This is important in qualitative research because the researcher's observations can inform the data collection. To be in someone else's home is a great advantage, as it helps the researcher understand what the participant values. An entire wall in a participant's living room may contain many pictures their family, so anyone who enters the home would immediately understand the centrality of the family in the participant's life. In the home of someone who is suffering from obesity and uncontrolled hypertension, many household objects may be clustered around a favorite chair: perhaps an oxygen tank, a glass of water, medications, a telephone, and tissues. A qualitative researcher will use clues like these in the study setting to complete the complex, rich drawing that is being rendered in the study.

IPE   HIGHLIGHT

Reading and critically appraising qualitative research studies may be the best way for interprofessional teams to understand the experience of living with a chronic illness so they can provide more effective whole-person care.

Data Collection Strategies

The procedures for data collection differ significantly in qualitative and quantitative studies. Whereas quantitative researchers focus on statistics and numbers, qualitative researchers are concerned with words: what people can tell them and the narratives about meaning or experience. Qualitative researchers have many methods in their research arsenal.

Qualitative researchers commonly interview participants; they may interview an individual or a group of people in what is called a *focus group*. They may also observe individuals as they go about daily tasks, such as sorting medications into a pill minder or caring for a child. Photovoice is another data collection strategy that asks participants to identify, share, and address their experience with a phenomenon by letting them take photographs and engage in a discussion of the images taken afterward with the researchers (Wang & Burris, 1997). Additionally, more qualitative researchers are turning to documentary and other collateral sources such as minutes from important meetings, archived notes, policy papers, and lay autobiographical accounts to glean data about particular topics (Thorne, 2016). Finally, combining several **data collection strategies** is another approach to generate a range of qualitative data that speaks about the same or different facets of a phenomenon. These combined methods may include conducting a focus group with patients, asking nurses who care for them to draw and discuss graphic depictions of a care process, and enlisting parents to create sociograms to map out lines of communication between themselves, the patient, and their providers. And all of these methods may be part of just one study!

Whichever method is used to gather the data, this information as expressed in words is eventually transcribed for analysis. Most qualitative researchers use audio recorders so they can be sure that they have captured what the participant says. This reduces the need to write things down and frees researchers to listen fully. Audio recordings are usually transcribed verbatim and then listened to for accuracy. In a research report, investigators must also describe their procedures for collecting the data, such as obtaining informed consent, the steps from initial contact to the end of the study visit, and how long each interview or focus group lasted or how much time the researcher spent "in the field" collecting data.

A key consideration in qualitative data collection is the researcher's decision that they have a sufficient sample and that data collection is complete. Researchers generally continue to recruit participants until they have reached information redundancy or **data saturation**, which means that nothing new is emerging from the interviews. There usually is not a predetermined number of participants to be selected as there is in quantitative studies; rather, the researcher keeps recruiting until she or he has sufficiently collected and described the depth and richness, and all of the potential configurations of a phenomena under consideration (Thorne, 2016). One important exception to this is if the researcher is very interested in getting different types of people in the study. **Example:** ➤ In the study of second-generation immigrant young women's barriers to accessing sexual health services, the researchers may want to include some young women who initially experienced barriers to care access but then became adept at navigating this care issue, or they may want young women who consistently found sexual health services a challenging health care area to access; alternately, they may want to interview senior students in high school who live with parents and senior college students who no longer live at home. Whatever the specific questions may be, sample sizes tend to be fairly small (fewer than 30 participants) because of the enormous amounts of written text that will need to be analyzed by the researcher.

Researchers use great care to design the interview questions because they must be crafted to help study participants describe their personal experiences and perceptions. Interview questions are different from research questions. Research questions are typically broad, encompassing, and written in scientific language. The interview questions may also be broad, like the overview or **grand tour question** that seeks the "big picture." **Example:** ➤ Researchers may ask, "Tell me about deciding to visit your OBGYN—the things that make it easier and the things that make it harder," or "Tell me what you were thinking about when you heard that young women born in the United States tend to underutilize sexual health services compared with young women born overseas." Along with overview questions, there are usually a series of prompts (additional questions) that were derived from the literature. These are areas that the researcher believes are important to cover (and that the participant will likely cover), but the prompts are there to remind the researcher in case the material is not mentioned. **Example:** ➤ With regard to older men with obesity and uncontrolled hypertension, the researcher may have read in other studies that neighborhood factors can influence openness to weight-loss interventions in two very different ways: safe neighborhoods can become a facilitator for enrollment in weight-loss programs, which would facilitate control of blood pressure, and interventions in public settings make participants self-conscious, leaving them to decline participation where neighbors can see them. Thus a neutrally worded question about the influence of neighborhood factors would be a prompt if the participants do not mention it spontaneously. In a research report, you should expect to find the primary interview questions identified verbatim; without them, it is impossible to know how the data were collected and how the researcher shaped what was discovered in the interviews.

EVIDENCE-BASED PRACTICE TIP

Qualitative researchers use more flexible procedures than quantitative researchers. While collecting data for a project, they consider all of the experiences that may occur.

Data Analysis

Next is the description of data analysis. Here, researchers tell you how they handled the raw data, which, in a qualitative study, are usually transcripts of recorded interviews or focus groups. The goal of qualitative analysis is to find commonalities and differences in the interviews and then group these into broader, more abstract, overarching categories of meaning, sometimes called **themes**, that capture much of the data.

In the example we have been using about underutilization of sexual health services among young women, one participant may talk about the need to keep her parents from finding out that she is sexually active, relaying how her older sister received so much disapproval when her intrauterine device was discovered by their mother years ago. Another woman may talk about how she found the location of the one OBGYN in their community to be a challenge because it was right beside where her family and friends shop for groceries, even though it is right across the local high school. And yet a third young woman may say that the nurse practitioner in the clinic is a local community leader who may disapprove of the fact that she has a longtime boyfriend, and that the young man is not a member of their ethnic group. On a more abstract level, these young women are all talking about sexuality-related shame. So an effective analysis would be one that identifies this pattern of shame and how it interfaces with health care access and, perhaps, goes further by also describing how racial and ethnic considerations for young women's use of sexual health services must be examined to encourage regular and routine health screenings. **Example:** ➤ Consider older men's decision making about a community-based intervention for weight loss. In an ideal situation, written reports about the data will give you an example like the one you just read, but the page limitations of most journals limit the level of detail that researchers can present.

Many qualitative researchers use computer-assisted qualitative data analysis programs to find patterns in the interviews and field notes, which, in many studies, can seem overwhelming because of the sheer quantity of data to be dealt with. With a computer-assisted data analysis program, researchers from multiple sites can simultaneously code and analyze data from hundreds of files without using a single piece of paper. The software is a tool for managing and remembering steps in analysis; however, it does not replace the thoughtful work of the researcher, who must apply the program to guide the analysis of the data. In research reports, you should see a description of the way data were managed and analyzed, and whether the researchers used software or other paper-based approaches such as index cards with handwritten notes.

Findings

At last, we come to the results. Findings in qualitative reports, as we suggested earlier, are words—the findings are patterns of any kind in the data, such as the ways that participants spoke, the things that they spoke about, even their behaviors associated with where the researcher spent time with them. When researchers describe patterns in the data, they may describe a process (such as the way decision making occurs); they may identify a list of things that are functioning in some way (such as a list of barriers and facilitators to accessing sexual health services for second-generation immigrant young women); they may specify a set of conditions that must be present for something to occur (such as what community norms are around sexual activity); or they may describe what it is like to go through some health-related transition (such as what it is like for older obese men to undergo gastric bypass). This is by no means an all-inclusive list; rather, it is a range of examples to help you recognize what types of findings may be possible. It may help if we think of the findings as discoveries. The qualitative researcher has explored a phenomenon, and the findings are a report on what he or she "found" —that is, what was discovered in the interviews and observations.

When researchers describe their results, they usually break down the data into units of meaning that help the data cohere and tell a story. Effective research reports will describe the logic that was used for breaking down the units of data. **Example:** ➤ Are the themes—a means of describing a large quantity of data in a condensed format—identified from the most prevalent to the least prevalent? Are the researchers describing a process in temporal (time-ordered) terms? Are they starting with information that was most important to the subject and then moving to less important items? As a report on the findings unfolds, the researcher should proceed with a thorough description of the phenomenon, defining each of the themes and fleshing out each theme with a thorough explanation of the role that it plays in the question under study. The researcher should also provide quotations that support the themes. Ideally, they will stage the quote, giving you some information about the subject from whom it came. For example, was the college-age participant newly diagnosed with HPV still on her parents' insurance policy? Or was it a high school age woman whose school nurse shared with her information about services offered by the local Planned Parenthood because her family did not have health insurance? The staging of quotes is important because it allows you to put the pieces of information into some understandable social context.

In a well-written report of qualitative research, some of the quotes will indeed give you that "aha!" feeling. You will have a sense that the researcher has done an excellent job of getting to the core of the problem or phenomena. Quotes are as critical to qualitative reports as numbers are to a quantitative study; you would not have a great deal of confidence in a quantitative or qualitative report in which the author asks you to believe the conclusion without also giving concrete, verifiable findings to back it up.

HELPFUL HINT

Values are involved in all research. It is important, however, that they not influence the results of the research.

DISCUSSION OF THE RESULTS AND IMPLICATIONS FOR EVIDENCE-BASED PRACTICE

When the researchers are satisfied that their findings answer the research questions, they should summarize the results for you and compare their findings to the existing literature. Researchers usually explain how these findings are similar to or different from the existing literature. This is one of the great contributions of qualitative research—using findings to open new venues of discovery that were not anticipated when the study was designed. **Example:** ➤ The researchers can use findings to develop new concepts or new conceptual models to explain broader phenomena. The conceptual work also identifies implications for how findings can be used in practice and can direct future research. Another alternative is for researchers to use their findings to extend or refine existing theoretical models. For example, a researcher may learn something new about sexuality and shame that has not been described in the literature, and in writing about these findings, the researcher may refer to an existing shame theory, pointing out how his or her work extends that theory.

Nursing is a practice discipline, and the goal of nursing research is to use research findings to improve patient care. Qualitative methods are the best way to start to answer clinical and research questions that have not been addressed or when a new perspective is needed in practice. The qualitative answers to these questions provide important evidence that offers the first systematic insights into phenomena previously not well understood and often lead to new perspectives in nursing practice and improved patient care outcomes.

Kearney (2001) developed a typology of levels and applications of qualitative research evidence that helps us see how new evidence can be applied to practice (Table 5.1). She described five categories of qualitative findings that are distinguished from one another in their levels of complexity and discovery: those restricted by *a priori* frameworks, descriptive categories, shared pathway or meaning, depiction of experiential variation, and dense explanatory description. She argued that the greater the complexity and discovery within qualitative findings, the stronger the potential for clinical application.

Findings developed with only *a priori* frameworks provide little or no evidence for changing practice because the researchers have prematurely limited what they are able to learn from participants or describe in their analysis. Findings that identify descriptive categories portray a higher level of discovery when a phenomenon is vividly portrayed from a new perspective. For nursing practice, these findings serve as maps of previously uncharted territory in human experience. Findings in Kearney's third category, shared pathway or meaning, are more complex. In this type of finding, there is an integration of concepts or themes that results in a synthesis of a shared process or experience that leads to a logical, complex portrayal of the phenomenon. The researcher's ideas at this level reveal how discrete bits of data come together in a meaningful whole. For nursing practice, this allows us to reflect on the bigger picture and what it means for the human experience (Kearney, 2001). Findings that depict experiential variation describe the essence of an experience and how this experience varies, depending on the individual or context. For nursing practice, this type of finding helps us see a variety of viewpoints, realizations of a human experience, and the contextual sources of that variety. In nursing practice, these findings explain how different variables can produce different consequences in different people or settings. Finally, findings that are presented as a dense explanatory description

TABLE 5.1	Kearney's Categories of Qualitative Findings, From Least to Most Complex	
Category	**Definition**	**Example**
Restricted by *a priori* frameworks	Discovery aborted because researcher obscured the findings with an existing theory	Use of the theory of "intersectionality" to describe women of color's relationships without substantiation in the data, or when there may be an alternative explanation to describe how women exist in relationship to others and their overlapping identities; the data seem to point to an explanation other than "intersectional identities"
Descriptive categories	Phenomenon is vividly portrayed from a new perspective; provides a map into previously uncharted territory in the human experience of health and illness	Same-sex couples' fertility decision-making process when planning for a family
Shared pathway or meaning	Synthesis of a shared experience or process; integration of concepts that provides a complex picture of a phenomenon	Description of recidivism for orphaned youth within the juvenile justice system; each category was fully described, and the conditions for progression were laid out; able to see the origins of a phase in the previous phase
Depiction of experiential variation	Describes the main essence of an experience, but also shows how the experience varies, depending on the individual or context	Description of how pregnant women recovering from opioid abuse may or may not move forward to create a new life, depending on the amount of structure they imposed on their behavior and their desire to give up drugs and change their lives
Dense explanatory description	Rich, situated understanding of a multifaceted and varied human phenomenon in a unique situation; portrays the full range and depth of complex influences; densely woven structure to findings	Unique pandemic conditions and organizational breakdown at the height of COVID-19 resulted in burnout, which led nursing home caregivers in rural settings to stop showing up for work; dedicated and longtime caregivers abandoned their patients to see if anyone else would arrive with supplies and staffing reinforcements; describes trauma and inability to process horrific mortality rates beyond the functional capacity of these isolated nursing homes

are at the highest level of complexity and discovery. They provide a rich, situated understanding of a multifaceted and varied human phenomenon in a unique situation. These types of findings portray the full depth and range of complex influences that propel people to make decisions. Physical and social contexts are fully accounted for. There is a densely woven structure of findings in these studies that provide a rich fund of clinically and theoretically useful information for nursing practice. The layers of detail work together in the findings to increase understanding of human choices and responses in particular contexts (Kearney, 2001).

> **EVIDENCE-BASED PRACTICE TIP**
>
> Qualitative research findings can be used in many ways, including improving ways clinicians communicate with patients and with each other.

So how can we further use qualitative evidence in nursing? The evidence provided by qualitative studies is used conceptually by the nurse: qualitative studies let nurses gain access to the experiences of patients and help nurses expand their ability to understand their patients, which should lead to more helpful approaches to care.

TABLE 5.2 **Kearney's Modes of Clinical Application for Qualitative Research**

Mode of Clinical Application	Example
Insight or empathy: Better understanding our patients and offering more sensitive support	Nurse is better able to understand the behaviors of a woman recovering from depression
Assessment of status or progress: Descriptions of trajectories of illness	Nurse is able to describe the trajectory of recovery from depression and can assess how the patient is moving through this trajectory
Anticipatory guidance: Sharing of qualitative findings with the patient	Nurse is able to explain the phases of recovery from depression to the patient and reassure her that she is not alone and that others have made it through a similar experience
Coaching: Advising patients of steps they can take to reduce distress or improve adjustment to an illness, according to the evidence in the study	Nurse describes the six stages of recovery from depression to the patient, and in ongoing contact, points out how the patient is moving through the stages, coaching her to recognize signs that she is improving and moving through the stages

Kearney (2001) proposed four modes of clinical application: insight or empathy, assessment of status or progress, anticipatory guidance, and coaching (Table 5.2). The simplest mode is to use the information to better understand the experiences of our patients, which in turn helps us offer more sensitive support. Qualitative findings can also help us assess the patient's status or progress through descriptions of trajectories of illness or by offering a different perspective on a health condition. They allow us to consider a range of possible responses from patients. We can then determine the fit of a category to a particular patient or try to locate them on an illness trajectory. Anticipatory guidance includes sharing of qualitative findings directly with patients. The patient can learn about others with a similar condition and can learn what to anticipate. This allows them to better garner resources for what may lie ahead or look for markers of improvement. Anticipatory guidance can also be tremendously comforting in that the sharing of research results can help patients realize they are not alone, that others have been through a similar experience with an illness. Finally, coaching is a way of using qualitative findings; in this instance, nurses can advise patients of steps they can take to reduce distress, improve symptoms, or monitor trajectories of illness (Kearney, 2001).

Unfortunately, qualitative research studies do not fare well in the typical systematic reviews on which evidence-based practice recommendations are based. Randomized controlled trials and other types of intervention studies traditionally have been the major focus of evidence-based practice. Typically, the selection of studies to be included in systematic reviews is guided by levels of evidence models that focus on the effectiveness of interventions according to their strength and consistency of their predictive power. Given that the levels of evidence models are hierarchical in nature and they perpetuate intervention studies as the "gold standard" of research design, the value of qualitative studies and the evidence offered by their results have remained unclear. Qualitative studies historically have been ranked lower in a hierarchy of evidence, as a "weaker" form of research design.

Remember, however, that qualitative research is not designed to test hypotheses or make predictions about causal effects. As we use qualitative methods, these findings become more and more valuable as they help us discover unmet patient needs, entire groups of patients that have been neglected, and new processes for delivering care to a population. Though qualitative research uses different methodologies and has different goals, it is important to explore how and when to use the evidence provided by findings of qualitative studies in practice.

⟫ APPRAISAL FOR EVIDENCE-BASED PRACTICE
FOUNDATION OF QUALITATIVE RESEARCH

A final example illustrates the differences in the methods discussed in this chapter and provides you with the beginning skills of how to critique qualitative research. The information in this chapter, coupled with information presented in Chapter 7, provides the underpinnings of critical appraisal of qualitative research (see the Critical Appraisal Criteria box, Chapter 7). Consider the question of nursing students learning how to conduct research. The empirical analytical approach (quantitative research) may be used in an experiment to see if one teaching method led to better learning outcomes than another. The students' knowledge may be tested with a pretest, the teaching conducted, and then a posttest of knowledge obtained. Scores on these tests would be analyzed statistically to see if the different methods produced a difference in the results.

In contrast, a qualitative researcher may be interested in the process of learning research. The researcher may attend the class to see what occurs and then interview students to ask them to describe how their learning changed over time. They may be asked to describe the experience of becoming researchers or becoming more knowledgeable about research. The goal would be to describe the stages or process of this learning. Alternately, a qualitative researcher may consider the class as a culture and could join to observe and interview students. Questions would be directed at the students' values, behaviors, and beliefs in learning research. The goal would be to understand and describe the group members' shared meanings. Either of these examples are ways of viewing a question with a qualitative perspective. The specific qualitative methodologies are described in Chapter 6.

Many other research methods exist. Although it is important to be aware of the qualitative research method used, it is most important that the method chosen is the one that will provide the best approach to answering the question being asked. One research method does not rank higher than another; rather, a variety of methods based on different **paradigms** are essential for the development of a well-informed and comprehensive approach to evidence-based nursing practice.

KEY POINTS

- All research is based on philosophical beliefs, a worldview, or a paradigm.
- Qualitative research encompasses different methodologies.
- Qualitative researchers believe that reality is socially constructed and is context dependent.
- Values should be acknowledged and examined as influences on the conduct of research.
- Qualitative research follows a process, but the components of the process vary.
- Qualitative research contributes to evidence-based practice.

CLINICAL JUDGMENT CHALLENGES

- Discuss how a researcher's values could influence the results of a study. Include an example in your answer.
- Can the expression, "We do not always get closer to the truth as we slice and homogenize and isolate [it]" be applied to both qualitative and quantitative methods? Justify your answer.
- What is the value of qualitative research in evidence-based practice? Give an example.

- **IPE** Discuss how your interprofessional team could apply the findings of a qualitative study about coping with a diagnosis of multiple sclerosis.

REFERENCES

Gair, S. (2012). Feeling their stories: Contemplating empathy, insider/outsider positionings, and enriching qualitative research. *Qualitative health research, 22*(1), 134–143.

Kearney, M. H. (2001). Levels and applications of qualitative research evidence. *Research in Nursing and Health, 24*, 145–153.

Morse, J. (2020). The Changing Face of Qualitative Inquiry. *International Journal of Qualitative Methods, 19*, 1609406920909938.

Thorne, S. (2016). *Interpretive description: Qualitative research for applied practice.* Routledge.

Wang, C., & Burris, M. A. (1997). Photovoice: Concept, methodology, and use for participatory needs assessment. *Health Education & Behavior, 24*(3), 369–387.

Go to Evolve at **http://evolve.elsevier.com/LoBiondo/** for review questions, appraisal exercises, and additional research articles for practice in reviewing and appraisal.

6

Qualitative Approaches to Research

Dalmacio Dennis Flores III, Julie Barroso

Go to Evolve at **http://evolve.elsevier.com/LoBiondo/** for review questions.

LEARNING OUTCOMES

After reading this chapter, you should be able to do the following:

- Identify the processes of phenomenological, grounded theory, ethnographic, and case study methods.
- Recognize appropriate use of community-based participatory research (CBPR) methods.

- Discuss significant issues that arise in conducting qualitative research in relation to such topics as ethics, criteria for judging scientific rigor, and combination of research methods.
- Apply critical appraisal criteria to evaluate a report of qualitative research.

KEY TERMS

auditability
bracketing
case study method
community-based
   participatory
   research

constant comparative
   method
credibility
data saturation
domains
emic

ethnographic method
etic
fittingness
grounded theory method
key informants
lived experience

meta-summary
meta-synthesis
mixed methods
phenomenological
   method
theoretical sampling

Qualitative research combines the science and art of nursing to enhance understanding of the human health experience. This chapter focuses on four commonly used qualitative research methods: phenomenology, grounded theory, ethnography, and case study. Community-based participatory research (CBPR) is also presented. Each of these methods, although distinct from the others, shares characteristics that identify it as a method within the qualitative research tradition.

Traditional hierarchies of research evaluation and how they categorize evidence from strongest to weakest, with emphasis on support for the effectiveness of interventions, are presented in Chapter 1. This perspective is limited because it does not take into account the ways that qualitative research can support practice, as discussed in Chapter 5. There is no doubt about the merit of qualitative studies; the problem is that no one has developed a satisfactory method for including them in current evidence hierarchies. In addition, qualitative studies can answer the critical "why?" questions that emerge in many evidence-based practice summaries. Such summaries may report the answer to a research question, but they also do not explain how it occurs in the landscape of caring for people.

As a research consumer, you should know that qualitative methods are the best way to start to answer clinical and research questions when little is known or a new perspective is needed for practice. However, this is not the only time qualitative methods are useful; they can be used in any study and at any point in a program of research. Even in a randomized controlled trial, it is very useful to know from participants what worked in terms of the intervention, what did not work, what was cumbersome, and what was easy; this information can be obtained through adding a qualitative component to the study. The very fact that qualitative research studies have increased exponentially in nursing and other social sciences speaks to the urgent need for clinicians to answer these "why?" and "how?" questions and to deepen our understanding of experiences of illness. Thousands of reports of well-conducted qualitative studies exist on topics such as the following:

- Adapting to life transitions, such as childbirth, adolescence, divorce, menopause, and death
- How people view disease, prevention, treatment, and risk, particularly within a cultural context
- Managing the effects of illnesses and their treatments, including the psychological and social effects
- Decision-making experiences at all stages of life from the beginning to the end and assistive and life-extending technological interventions
- How people function within the context of vast health disparities, and how they deal with being at the intersection of multiple disparities
- How people come to value and incorporate health-promotion and disease-prevention self-care into their lives

Findings from qualitative studies provide valuable insights about unique phenomena, patient populations, or clinical situations. In doing so, they provide nurses with the data needed to guide and change practice.

In this chapter, you are invited to look through the lens of human experience to learn about phenomenological, grounded theory, ethnographic, community-based participatory research, and case study methods. You are encouraged to put yourself in the researcher's shoes and imagine how it would be to study an issue of interest from the perspective of each of these methods. No matter which method a researcher uses, there is a focus on the human experience in natural settings.

The researcher using these methods believes that each unique human being attributes meaning to their experience and that experience evolves from one's social and historical context. Thus one person's experience of pain is distinct from another's and can be elucidated by the individual's subjective description of it. **Example:** ➤ Researchers interested in studying the lived experience of pain for the adolescent with sickle cell disease will spend time in the adolescents' natural settings, perhaps in their homes and schools. This allows the researcher to see how the adolescent adapts to their pain in different settings (see Chapter 5). Research efforts will focus on uncovering the meaning of pain as it extends beyond the number of medications

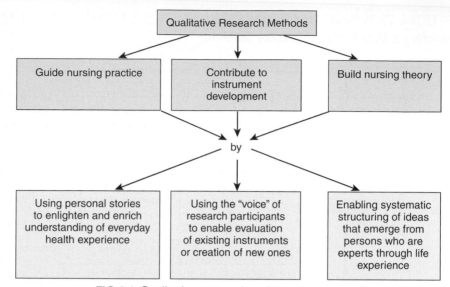

FIG 6.1 Qualitative approach and nursing science.

taken or a rating on a pain scale. Qualitative methods are grounded in the belief that objective data do not capture the whole of the human experience. Rather, the meaning of the adolescent's pain emerges within the context of personal history, current relationships, and future plans as the adolescent lives daily life in dynamic interaction with the environment.

QUALITATIVE APPROACH AND NURSING SCIENCE

The evidence provided by qualitative studies that consider the unique perspectives, concerns, preferences, and expectations each patient brings to a clinical encounter offers in-depth understanding of human experience and the contexts in which they occur. Thus findings in qualitative research often guide nursing practice, contribute to instrument development (see Chapter 15), and contribute to hypothesis generation to inform nursing theory (Fig. 6.1).

QUALITATIVE RESEARCH METHODS

Thus far you have studied an overview of the qualitative research approach (see Chapter 5). Recognizing how the choice to use a qualitative approach reflects one's worldview and the nature of some research questions, you have the necessary foundation for exploring selected qualitative methodologies. Now, as you review the Critical Thinking Decision Path and study the remainder of Chapter 6, note how different qualitative methods are appropriate for distinct areas of interest. Also note how unique research questions may be studied with each qualitative research method. In this chapter, we will explore five qualitative research methods in depth: phenomenological, grounded theory, ethnographic, case study, and CBPR methods.

CRITICAL THINKING DECISION PATH
Selecting a Qualitative Research Method

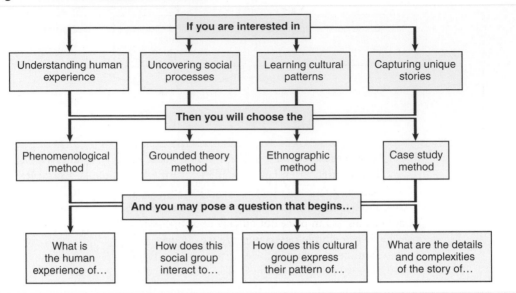

Phenomenological Method

The **phenomenological method** is a process of learning and constructing the meaning of human experience through intensive dialogue with persons who are living the experience. It has strong philosophical underpinnings and rests on the assumption that there is a common meaning for individuals of their lived experiences of a concept or a phenomenon (Creswell & Poth, 2018). The researcher's goal is to understand the meaning of the experience as it is lived by the participant; what do they have in common? The purpose of phenomenology is to reduce individual experiences with a phenomenon to a description of its universal essence, and the end result should be a composite description of the essences of the experience for all of the individuals (Creswell & Poth, 2018). Phenomenological studies usually incorporate data about the lived space, or spatiality; the lived body, or corporeality; lived time, or temporality; and lived human relations, or relationality. Meaning is pursued through a process of dialogue, which extends beyond a simple interview and requires thoughtful presence on the part of the researcher. There are many schools of phenomenological research, and each school of thought uses slight differences in research methods. In all forms of phenomenological research, you will find researchers asking a question about the lived experience and using methods that explore phenomena as they are embedded in people's lives and environments.

Identifying the Phenomenon

Because the focus of the phenomenological method is the **lived experience**, the researcher is likely to choose this method when studying a dimension of day-to-day existence for a particular group of people. An example of this is a study conducted by McKinnon and colleagues (2020) in which they studied the experiences of postanesthesia care unit (PACU) recovery nurses who were facilitating advance directives (ADs) in the immediate postanesthetic period.

Structuring the Study

When thinking about methods, the methodological approach structures the study. This phrase means that the method shapes the way we think about the phenomenon of interest and the way we would go about answering a research question. For the purpose of describing structuring, the following topics are addressed: the research question, the researcher's perspective, and sample selection.

Research Question. The question that guides phenomenological research always asks about some human experience, and it guides the researcher to ask the participant about some past or present experience. In most cases, the research question is not exactly the same as the question used to initiate dialogue with study participants. **Example:** ➤ McKinnon and colleagues (2020) state that the objective of their study was to understand the experiences of PACU nurses when dealing with the uncertainty of what to do when an older adult patient had an AD in place but quickly decompensated physiologically in the PACU. They describe their methodology as interpretive phenomenology. The aims of the project were to develop an understanding of the experience of the PACU nurse when facilitating an AD for a patient to help understand why and how ADs are sometimes carried out successfully and sometimes ignored during the provision of care.

Researcher's Perspective. When using the phenomenological method, the researcher's perspective is bracketed. This means that the researcher identifies their personal thoughts and feelings about the phenomenon of interest to clarify how personal experience and beliefs may color what is heard and reported. Further, the phenomenological researcher is expected to set aside their personal thoughts and feelings—to bracket them—when engaged with the participants. By becoming aware of personal thoughts and feelings, the researcher is more likely to be able to pursue issues of importance as introduced by the participant, rather than leading the participant to issues the researcher deems important (Creswell & Poth, 2018).

IPE HIGHLIGHT

Discuss with your interprofessional quality improvement team why searching for qualitative studies might be most appropriate for understanding about living with hepatitis C and managing the physical, psychological, and social effects of multiple treatments and their effects.

Using phenomenological methods, researchers strive to identify personal experiences with the phenomenon and hold them in abeyance when querying the participant. Readers of phenomenological articles may find it difficult to identify bracketing strategies because they are seldom explicitly identified in a research manuscript. Sometimes a researcher's worldview or assumptions provide insight into biases that have been considered and bracketed.

Sample Selection. As you read a phenomenological study, you will find that the participants were selected purposively (selecting subjects who are considered typical of the population) and that members of the sample either are living the experience the researcher is studying or have lived the experience in their past (Creswell & Poth, 2018). Because phenomenologists believe that each individual's history is a dimension of the present, a past experience exists in the present moment. For the phenomenologist, it is a matter of asking the right questions and listening. Even when a participant is describing a past experience, remembered information is being gathered in the present at the time of the interview.

Data Gathering

Written or oral data may be collected when using the phenomenological method. The researcher may pose the query in writing and ask for a written response, or may schedule a time to interview the participant and record the interaction. In either case, the researcher may return to ask for clarification of written or recorded transcripts. To some extent, the particular data collection procedure is guided by the choice of a specific analysis technique. Different analysis techniques require different numbers of interviews. A concept known as data saturation usually guides decisions regarding how many interviews are enough. Data saturation is the situation of obtaining the full range of themes from the participants so no new data emerge when interviewing additional participants. In phenomenology, the end is reached when the researcher can write a descriptive passage that discusses the essence of an experience for individuals incorporating what they experienced and how they experienced it (Creswell & Poth, 2018).

Data Analysis

Several techniques are available for data analysis when using the phenomenological method. Although the techniques are slightly different from each other, there is a general pattern of moving from the participant's description to the researcher's synthesis of all participants' descriptions. Moustakas (1994) suggests these steps:

1. Generate themes from the analysis of significant statements, read the participants' narratives to acquire a feeling for their ideas to understand them fully. Then highlight significant statements that provide an understanding of how the participants experienced the phenomenon. Then the researcher develops clusters of meaning from these significant statements into themes.
2. Develop textual and structural descriptions. The significant statements and themes are used to write a description of what the participants experienced. The researcher also writes about the context or setting that influenced how the phenomenon was experienced; this is called *structural description*.
3. Report the essence of a phenomenon by using a composite description, focusing on the common experiences of the participants.
4. Present the understanding of the essence of the experience in written form (Moustaskas, 1994).

McKinnon and colleagues (2020) used interpretive phenomenological analysis for their study; the steps closely parallel those of Moustakas. They interviewed and audio-recorded six PACU nurses using a semistructured interview guide, which gives the participant an idea about what the researcher wants them to talk about but is not so prescriptive that it limits the conversation.

It is important to note that giving verbatim transcripts to participants can have unanticipated consequences. It is not unusual for people to deny that they said something in a certain way, or that they said it at all. Even when the actual recording is played for them, they may have difficulty believing it. This is one of the more challenging aspects of any qualitative method: every time a story is told, it changes for the participant. The participant may sincerely feel that the story as it was recorded is not the story as it is when reviewed.

EVIDENCE-BASED PRACTICE TIP

Phenomenological research is an important approach for accumulating evidence when studying a new topic about which little is known.

Describing the Findings

When using the phenomenological method, the researcher provides the subject with a path of information leading from the research question, through samples of participants' words and the researcher's interpretation, to the final detailed description that tells the reader what the participants experienced and how they experienced it. When reading the report of a phenomenological study, the reader should find that detailed descriptive language is used to convey the complex meaning of the lived experience that offers the evidence for this qualitative method. Going back to our example, McKinnon and colleagues (2020) described from the nurses' perspectives an overarching theme of the gray zone, in which the situation in the PACU becomes uncertain and undermines their ability to fulfill a patient's AD. Four themes have emerged that support the gray zone: the trigger of the anesthetic, which could cause the patient's physiological state to deteriorate rapidly and significantly, and which triggered uncertainty about the AD; confusion and frustration as the PACU nurse felt that the anesthetic took away the patient's autonomy to have the AD enacted; consistent paternalism in which the anesthetist sometimes ignored the AD over protests from the nurse; and disempowerment, in which the nurse felt that he or she could not act as an advocate for the patient with an AD. The themes in this phenomenological study describe the need for the operating room team to discuss in advance, preferably with the patient and their loved ones, what exactly the AD meant, especially when in the operating room and in the PACU. By using participant quotes, researchers enable readers to evaluate the connections between what individual nurse participants said and how the researcher labeled or interpreted what they said.

Grounded Theory Method

The **grounded theory method** is an inductive approach involving a systematic set of procedures to arrive at a theory about basic social processes (Charmaz, Thornberg, & Keane, 2018). The emergent theory is based on observations and perceptions of the social scene and evolves during data collection and analysis (Corbin & Strauss, 2015). Grounded theory describes a research approach to construct theory where no theory exists, or in situations in which existing theory fails to provide evidence to explain a set of circumstances.

Developed originally as a sociologist's tool to investigate interactions in social settings (Glaser & Strauss, 1967), the grounded theory method is used in many disciplines. **Example:** ➤ In an area of study such as chronic illness, a nurse may be interested in coping patterns within families, a psychologist may be interested in personal adjustment, and a sociologist may focus on group behavior in health care settings. In grounded theory, the usefulness of the study stems from the transferability of theories; that is, a theory derived from one study is applicable to another.

Identifying the Phenomenon

Researchers typically use the grounded theory method when interested in social processes from the perspective of human interactions or patterns of action and interaction between and among various types of social units (Charmaz, Thornberg, & Keane, 2018; Creswell & Poth, 2018). The basic social process is sometimes expressed in the form of a gerund (i.e., the *-ing* form of a verb when functioning as a noun), which is designed to indicate change occurring over time as individuals negotiate social reality. **Example:** ➤ Zu and Bowers (2020) explored Chinese immigrant women's experiences of postpartum distress, using grounded theory to examine the intersection of cultural and maternal transitions.

Structuring the Study

Research Question. Research questions for the grounded theory method are those that address basic social processes that shape human behavior. In a grounded theory study, the research question can be a statement or a broad question that permits in-depth explanation of the phenomenon. For example, Zu and Bowers (2020) state that the purpose of their study was to develop a conceptual model that describes the experiences of immigrant women's postpartum distress and their social-psychological processes in response to this distress.

Researcher's Perspective. In a grounded theory study, the theory emerges directly from data and reflects the contextual values that are integral to the social processes being studied. Originally it was thought that the researcher should not complete a thorough review of the literature before the study, but this view underestimates the researcher's ability to be reflexive, which is similar to bracketing; the researcher must be aware of the effect of his or her own personal thoughts and feelings when conducting the research so they do not influence the data (Charmaz, Thornberg, & Keane, 2018).

Sample Selection. Sample selection involves choosing participants who are experiencing the circumstance and selecting events and incidents related to the social process under investigation. Zu and Bowers (2020) obtained their purposive sample (initial recruiting) and theoretical sample (second interviews with participants who can help further the development of the theory) (see Chapter 12) through self-referral from flyers and word of mouth.

Data Gathering

In the grounded theory method, data are collected through interviews and skilled observations of individuals interacting in a social setting. Interviews are recorded and transcribed, and observations are recorded as field notes. Open-ended questions are used initially to identify concepts for further focus. At their first data collection point, Zu and Bowers (2020) interviewed 16 women, and 6 were interviewed twice, to further focus the evolving conceptual model. All transcripts were in Chinese and were translated to English by professional translators proficient in both English and Chinese.

Data Analysis

A unique and important feature of the grounded theory method is that data collection and analysis occur simultaneously. The process requires systematic data collection and documentation using field notes and transcribed interviews. Hunches about emerging patterns in the data are noted in memos that the researcher uses to direct activities in fieldwork. This technique, called **theoretical sampling** (referring to theoretical sampling of data, not participants), is used to select experiences that will help the researcher to test hunches and ideas and to gather complete information about developing concepts. The researcher begins by noting indicators or actual events, actions, or words in the data. As data are concurrently collected and analyzed, new concepts, or abstractions, are developed from the indicators (Charmaz, Thornberg, & Keane, 2018; Creswell & Poth, 2018).

The initial analytical process is called *open coding*. Data are examined carefully line by line, broken down into discrete parts, and then compared for similarities and differences (Creswell & Poth, 2018). Coded data are continuously compared with new data as they are acquired during research. This is a process called the **constant comparative method**. When data collection is complete, codes in the data are clustered to form categories. The categories are expanded and developed, or they are collapsed into one another, and relationships among the categories are used to develop a new "grounded" theory. As a result, data collection, analysis, and theory generation have a direct reciprocal relationship that grounds new theory in the perspectives of the research participants (Charmaz, Thornberg, & Keane, 2018; Creswell & Poth, 2018).

> **HELPFUL HINT**
>
> In a report of research using the grounded theory method, you can expect to find a diagrammed model of a theory that synthesizes the researcher's findings in a systematic way.

Describing the Findings

Grounded theory studies are reported in detail, permitting readers to follow the exact steps in the research process. Descriptive language and diagrams of the research process are used as evidence to document the researchers' procedures for moving from the raw data to the new theory. Zu and Bowers (2020) found the basic social processes of transitioning from woman to mother and from native to foreign to be twofold: grayscaling the psychological self (experiencing distress in response to losses) and reviving the psychological self (resolving distress and regaining and/or transforming the psychological self). Grayscaling was described as the extent to which the vibrancy in women's lives was stripped away; women responded to the losses they felt in an immediate response pathway or a delayed response pathway. Reviving the psychological self referred to a gradual process of resolving distress and regaining and/or transforming the psychological self; there were two phases of reviving: preparing and prospecting.

> **EVIDENCE-BASED PRACTICE TIP**
>
> When thinking about the evidence generated by the grounded theory method, consider whether the theory is useful in explaining, interpreting, or predicting the study phenomenon of interest.

Ethnographic Method

Derived from the Greek term *ethnos*, meaning people, race, or cultural group, the **ethnographic method** focuses on scientific description and interpretation of cultural or social groups and systems (Creswell & Poth, 2018). The goal of the ethnographer is to understand the research participants' views of their world, or the emic view. The **emic** view (insiders' view) is contrasted with the **etic** view (outsiders' view), which is obtained when the researcher uses quantitative analyses of behavior. The ethnographic approach requires that the researcher enter the world of the study participants to watch what happens, listen to what is said, ask questions, and collect whatever data are available. It is important to note that the term *ethnography* is used to mean both the research technique and the product of that technique—that is, the study itself (Creswell & Poth, 2018). Ethnography has its roots in the disciplines of sociology and anthropology, as a method borne from the need to understand "other" and "self." Nurses use the method to study cultural variations in health and patient groups as subcultures within larger social contexts.

Identifying the Phenomenon

The phenomenon under investigation in an ethnographic study varies in scope from a long-term study of a very complex culture to a short-term study of a phenomenon within subunits of cultures. The local worlds of patients have cultural, political, economic, institutional, and social-relational dimensions in much the same way as larger complex societies; we only need to look at the coronavirus pandemic as one that touches on all of these dimensions. An example of ethnography is found in Stajduhar and colleagues' (2020) study of people experiencing structural vulnerability (e.g., homelessness, poverty, racism, substance abuse, mental illness) and the barriers they face when trying to access care at the end of life. Family caregivers (including people who are not biologically related) have the potential to play a critical role in providing care to these populations, but we know little about who they are and what their experiences are.

Structuring the Study

Research Question. In ethnographic studies, questions are asked about "lifeways" or particular patterns of behavior within the social context of a culture or subculture. In this type of research, **culture** is viewed as the system of knowledge and linguistic expressions used by social groups, and the researcher looks for patterns of social organization and ideational systems in these groups; the groups must have been intact and interacting long enough to develop social behaviors (Creswell & Poth, 2018). Thus ethnographic nursing studies address questions that concern how cultural knowledge, norms, values, and other contextual variables influence people's health experiences. **Example:** ➤ Stajduhar and colleagues' (2020) research question is implied in their aim statement: To describe family caregiving in the context of providing palliative care to people who are experiencing structural vulnerability; specifically, to understand who these caregivers are and what challenges, burdens, and barriers they face. Remember that ethnographers have a broader definition of culture in which a particular social context is conceptualized as a culture.

Researcher's Perspective. When using the ethnographic method, the researcher's perspective is that of an interpreter entering a different world and attempting to make sense of that world from the insider's point of view (Creswell & Poth, 2018). Like phenomenologists and grounded theorists, ethnographers make their own beliefs explicit and bracket, or set aside, their personal thoughts and feelings as they seek to understand the worldview of others.

Sample Selection. The ethnographer selects a cultural group that is living the phenomenon under investigation. The researcher gathers information from general informants and key informants. **Key informants** are individuals who have special knowledge, status, or communication skills, and who are willing to teach the ethnographer about the phenomenon (Creswell & Poth, 2018). **Example:** ➤ Stajduhar and colleagues' (2020) research took place in an urban area in British Columbia, Canada. They recruited three samples: people experiencing structural vulnerability who were on a palliative care trajectory, their support persons, and their formal service providers (e.g., housing workers and medical professionals).

Data Gathering

Ethnographic data gathering involves immersion in the study setting and the use of participant observation, interviews of informants, and interpretation by the researcher of cultural patterns (Creswell & Poth, 2018). Ethnographic research involves face-to-face interviewing with data collection and analysis taking place in the natural setting. Thus fieldwork is a major focus of the method. Other techniques may include obtaining life histories and collecting material items reflective of the culture. **Example:** ➤ Photographs and films of the informants in their world can be used as data sources. In their study, Stajduhar and colleagues (2020) collected data over 30 months, resulting in about 300 hours of fieldwork. The team observed homes, shelters, transitional housing units, clinics, hospitals, palliative care units, community-based service centers, and streets and parks. They also conducted in-depth interviews with family caregivers.

Data Analysis

Like grounded theory, ethnographic data are collected and analyzed simultaneously. Data analysis proceeds through several levels as the researcher looks for the meaning of cultural symbols in the informant's language and in what they have observed. Analysis begins with a search for domains or symbolic categories that include smaller categories. The researcher moves into a theme analysis of patterns or topics that signifies how the cultural group works and lives. Analysis proceeds through increasing levels of complexity until the data, grounded in the informant's reality, are synthesized by the researcher; a hallmark of ethnography is thick description, a written record of cultural interpretation (Creswell & Poth, 2018). Stajduhar and colleagues (2020) described analysis of data as concurrent with data collection, and beginning with interview transcripts using thematic analysis, with subsequent team meetings to discuss findings and agree on categories. The observation notes were used to substantiate the themes.

Describing the Findings

Ethnographic studies yield large quantities of data that reflect a wide array of evidence amassed as field notes of observations, interview transcriptions, and sometimes other artifacts such as photographs. The first-level description is the description of the scene, the parameters or boundaries of the research group, and the overt characteristics of group members (Creswell & Poth, 2018). Strategies that enhance first-level description include maps and floor plans of the setting, organizational charts, and documents. Researchers may report item-level analysis, followed by pattern- and structure-level of analysis. Ethnographic research articles usually provide examples from data, thorough descriptions of the analytical process, and statements of the hypothetical propositions and their relationship to the ethnographer's frame of reference, which can be rather detailed and lengthy. Stajduhar and colleagues (2020) first tell the reader that many of the caregivers were themselves in structurally vulnerable situations and often recipients of palliative care themselves, which made for complex relationships in which roles often shifted. The researchers identified three core themes related to caregiving in the context of poverty and substance use, housing instability, and challenging relationships. There was incredible stress associated with caregiving, and a constant need for the basics: food, medication, housing. There was also stress associated with the stigma of caring for someone who is structurally vulnerable, and there often was relational tension between the caregiver and the biological family. Policies regarding housing often prevented the caregiver and recipient of care from living together, which complicated caregiving. This study gives us clear direction as to public policies that must change to better help this population.

EVIDENCE-BASED PRACTICE TIP

Evidence generated by ethnographic studies will answer questions about how cultural knowledge, norms, values, and other contextual variables influence the health experience of a particular patient population in a specific setting.

Case Study

Case study research involves the study of a case (or cases) within a real-life contemporary context or setting. A case can be an individual, a group, an organization, a community, or a project. Case study research is not a particular methodology but a choice about what to study (Creswell & Poth, 2018). Thus the case study method is about studying the peculiarities and the commonalities of a specific case, irrespective of the actual strategies for data collection and analysis that are used to explore research questions. Case studies include quantitative and/or qualitative data but are defined by their focus on uncovering an individual case and, in some instances, identifying patterns in variables that are consistent across a set of cases. It is important that the case be a bounded system, that is, bounded by time and place (Creswell & Poth, 2018).

Identifying the Phenomenon

Emerson and colleagues (2020) used a case study design to examine a collaborative program between a local health department and a county jail to offer HPV vaccines to adolescents and young adults. This would offer a preventive health intervention to a vulnerable group that is hard to reach via traditional interventions. A single county municipal jail and a local health department participated. Data collected included phone interviews, focus groups, and site observations.

Structuring the Study

Research Question. Schwandt and Gates (2018) state that there are four uses for case study designs: description; hypothesis generation or theory development; hypothesis and theory testing; and development of normative theory. Although researchers pose questions to begin discussion, the initial questions are never all-inclusive; rather, the researcher uses an iterative process of growing questions in the field. That is, as data are collected to address these questions, it is expected that other questions will emerge and serve as guides to the researcher to untangle the complex, context-laden story within the case. **Example:** ➢ In Emerson and colleagues' (2020) study, they note that even though it has been proven to be effective, uptake of the HPV vaccine has been slow. Women who are incarcerated are diagnosed with abnormal Pap tests and cervical cancer at higher rates than women in the general population. However, jails are not set up to provide preventive health care. When they do get vaccines, they are administered by the county health department. The researchers wanted to learn what it would take to create a collaboration between a county jail and a local health department to implement HPV vaccines, and their research question was about the barriers and facilitators to implementing such a program.

Researcher's Perspective. When the researcher begins with questions developed around suspected issues of importance, they have an **etic** focus, which means the research is focused on the perspective of the researcher. As case study researchers engage the phenomenon of interest in individual cases, the uniqueness of individual stories unfold and shift from an etic (researcher orientation) to an **emic** (participant orientation) focus. Ideally, the case study researcher will develop an insider view that permits narration of the way things happen in the case. **Example:** ➤ In the study by Emerson and colleagues (2020), the etic focus on preventive health care via the HPV vaccine shifted to the emic focus on constrained resources and divergent cultures and priorities between the health department and the jail.

Sample Selection. In case study design, the sample selection is absolutely critical; this is the whole point of case study research. The researcher must think about whether or not they want to study normative cases, extreme cases, or cases that vary on some critical variable; does the study call for the most common cases or the most unusual cases? The convenience of studying the case may even be a factor, especially when case study work often calls for intense interaction with the participant(s). For instance, if there are several patients who have undergone heart transplantation and are willing to participate in the study, practical factors may influence which patient offers the best opportunity for learning. Persons who live in the area and can be easily visited at home or in the medical center may be better choices than those living much farther away (where multiple contacts over time might be impossible). Similarly, the researcher may choose to study a case in which a potential participant has an actively involved family because understanding the family context of transplant patients may shed important new light on their healing. No choice is perfect when selecting a case; however, selecting cases for their contextual features fosters the strength of data that can be learned at the level of the individual case. **Example:** ➤ In Emerson and colleagues' (2020) study, they conducted a 90-minute focus-group session with jail and local health department administrators and staff, and then did individual interviews with administrators at both sites. Nurses working at the jail were not permitted to participate in the study by their employer, a contractor. It is unfortunate that they were not able to obtain data from this critical group, but such is the nature of research.

Data Gathering

Case study data are gathered using interviews, field observations, document reviews, and any other methods that accumulate evidence for describing or explaining the complexity of the case. A data gathering plan should be developed to guide the progress of the study from definition of the case through decisions regarding data collection involving multiple methods, at multiple time points, and sometimes with multiple participants within the case; however, the plan should be flexible enough to accommodate interesting paths that may not have been apparent at the start of the project. In Emerson and colleagues' (2020) study, multiple methods for collecting data were used, including focus groups, individual interviews, field observations, and pulling outcome data on the number of HPV vaccines that were administered.

Data Analysis/Describing Findings

Data analysis is often concurrent with data gathering and description of findings as the narrative in the case develops. A qualitative case study is characterized by researchers spending extended time on site, being personally in contact with activities and operations of the case, and reflecting and revising meanings of what transpires. Reflecting and revising meanings are the work of the case study researcher, who records data, searches for patterns, links data from multiple sources, and develops preliminary thoughts regarding the meaning of collected data. This reflective and iterative process for writing the case narrative produces a unique form of evidence. Many times case study research reports do not list all of the research activities (Creswell & Poth, 2018). **Example:** ➤ Emerson and colleagues (2020) found that administrators and staff in the two agencies were committed to the idea and were willing to work together. However, there were shortages in both agencies of personnel, time, space, and money. It was also complicated because the underage and young adult detainees had to be treated differently from the jail's vantage point. Health department nurses had to be escorted in and out of the jail. At the jail, there was nowhere for the nurses to dispose of the used needles. There were issues with the cost of the vaccine and budget cuts to both agencies. Another issue was the view that each group had of the people who would receive the vaccine: to the jail staff, they were inmates; to the health department staff, they were patients. The jail wanted additional background checks on the nurses, who refused these additional checks. Finally, there was no place at the jail for inmates to receive the vaccine. In the end, only two juveniles were vaccinated, and no adults. This case study enumerated the logistical and structural issues that prohibited successful implementation of the project.

EVIDENCE-BASED PRACTICE TIP

Case studies are a way of providing in-depth evidence-based discussion of clinical topics that can be used to guide practice.

Community-Based Participatory Research

Community-based participatory research (CBPR) is a research method that systematically accesses the voice of a community to plan context-appropriate action and can promote equity between and among academic and community partners (Dickson et al., 2020). CBPR provides an alternative to traditional research approaches that assume a phenomenon may be separated from its context for purposes of study. Investigators who use CBPR recognize that it is crucial to engage members of a study population as active and equal participants in all phases of the research for the research process to be a means of facilitating change (Dickson et al., 2020). Change or action is the intended end product of CBPR, and *action research* is a term related to CBPR. Many scholars consider CBPR to be a type of action research and group this within the tradition of critical science. Most CBPR projects combine qualitative and quantitative methods.

CBPR is based on the assumptions that genuine partnership means colearning (academic and community partners learning from each other); research efforts include capacity building (there is a commitment to training community members in research); findings and knowledge benefit all partners; and CBPR involves a long-term commitment to effectively reduce disparities (Wallerstein & Duran, 2006). Most importantly, the research project itself comes from the community, usually via a needs assessment that is the first step in the research process in CBPR. The researcher may believe that a community needs help with a certain problem, but the community may feel that a different problem is more pressing. In CBPR, what the community believes in and identifies as a priority takes precedence. Once the problem has been determined, the researcher uses a combination of data collection techniques to gather data on the details of the problem in the context of that community to develop interventions to ameliorate it. Interventions are designed with an eye toward capacity building so the interventions endure after the research funding ends. Community members are included as authors on selected publications as well.

Farrales and colleagues (2020) conducted a CBPR study to explore the experiences of grieving parents during their interactions with health care providers during and after a stillbirth. They used four focus groups composed of 27 bereaved parents, who conceptualized the study and participated in all stages of research, including analyses and drafts of articles. Broad-based member checking, which is a method to help ensure rigor in a qualitative study, involved taking the evolving themes back to the parents to ensure fidelity and nuances within themes. The major theme that emerged was provider acknowledgment of the baby as an irreplaceable individual. Subthemes included acknowledgment of parenthood and grief; recognition of the traumatic nature of stillbirth; and acknowledgment of enduring grief coupled with access to support (Farrales et al., 2020). The themes are supported by poignant selections from the interviews to support the data. Interventions for health care providers are clear.

EVIDENCE-BASED PRACTICE TIP

Although qualitative in its approach to research, community-based participatory research leads to an action component in which a nursing intervention is implemented and evaluated for its effectiveness in a specific patient population.

Mixed Methods Research

Mixed methods research is the use of both qualitative and quantitative methods in one study. There are several types of mixed methods designs (Creswell & Plano Clark, 2018). Researchers who choose a mixed methods study choose on the basis of the research question (see Chapter 10 for further information). Although certain questions may be answered effectively by combining qualitative and quantitative methods in a single study, this does not necessarily make the findings and related evidence stronger. In fact, if a researcher inappropriately combines methods in a single study, the findings could be weaker and less credible. As you read research, you will quickly discover that approaches and methods are being combined to best contribute to theory building, guide practice, and facilitate instrument development. **Example:** ➤ Stevens and colleagues (2020) conducted a sequential explanatory mixed methods study to identify the beliefs and behaviors of youth related to substance use by characterizing the content of youths' drug-related tweets. During the quantitative phase, they gathered public tweets from youth 13 to 24 years of age that referenced drug use. The study team then analyzed the content of a subset of the tweets during the subsequent qualitative phase. From their analysis they found functional and relational themes. Functional themes included posts from youth that explicated a function of drugs in one's life, with subthemes of pride, longing, coping, and reminiscing. Relational themes captured substance use as a part of social relationships, with subthemes related to identity and companionship. Across the tweets, the themes of pride and longing were most popular. Most tweets that expressed pride were explicitly related to marijuana. Nearly one-half of the tweets on coping were related to prescription drugs. When both strands of the data were analyzed together, the team found that these tweets normalized drug use for this youth population and, in the absence of any antidrug messages on Twitter, was perceived as justifiable. The study team concluded with a concerted call for public health messaging on social media to provide education and a counternarrative about drug use among youth.

EVIDENCE-BASED PRACTICE TIPS

- Mixed methods research offers an opportunity for researchers to increase the strength and consistency of evidence provided by the use of both qualitative and quantitative research methods.
- The combination of stories with numbers (qualitative and quantitative research approaches) through the use of mixed methods may provide the most complete picture of the phenomenon being studied and, therefore, the best evidence for guiding practice.

SYNTHESIZING QUALITATIVE EVIDENCE: META-SYNTHESIS

The depth and breadth of qualitative research have grown over the years, and it has become important to qualitative researchers to synthesize critical masses of qualitative findings.

The terms most commonly used to describe this activity are *qualitative meta-summary and qualitative meta-synthesis* (Sandelowski & Barroso, 2007). Qualitative meta-summary is a quantitatively oriented aggregation of qualitative findings that are topical or thematic summaries or surveys of data. Meta-summaries are integrations that are approximately equal to the sum of parts, or the sum of findings across reports in a target domain of research. They address the manifest content in findings and reflect a quantitative logic: to discern the frequency of each finding and to find in higher frequency the evidence of replication foundational to validity in most quantitative research. Qualitative meta-summary involves the extraction and further abstraction of findings, and the calculation of manifest frequency effect sizes (Sandelowski & Barroso, 2007). Qualitative meta-synthesis is an integration of qualitative findings that are interpretive syntheses of data, including the phenomenologies, ethnographies, grounded theories, and other integrated and coherent descriptions or explanations of phenomena, events, or cases that are the hallmarks of qualitative research. Meta-syntheses are integrations that are more than the sum of parts in that they offer novel interpretations of findings. These interpretations will not be found in any one research report; rather, they are inferences derived from taking all of the reports in a sample as a whole. Meta-syntheses offer a description or explanation of a target event or experience, instead of a summary view of unlinked features of that event or experience. Such interpretive integrations require researchers to piece the individual syntheses constituting the findings in individual research reports together to craft one or more meta-syntheses. Their validity does not reside in a replication logic, but in an inclusive logic whereby all findings are accommodated, and the accumulative analysis displayed in the final product. Meta-synthesis methods include constant comparison, taxonomic analysis, the reciprocal translation of in vivo concepts, and the use of imported concepts to frame data (Sandelowski & Barroso, 2007). Meta-synthesis integrates qualitative research findings on a topic and is based on comparative analysis and interpretative synthesis of qualitative research findings that seek to retain the essence and unique contribution of each study (Sandelowski & Barroso, 2007). There are a number of meta-synthesis studies conducted by nurse scientists, across a vast array of health and illness experiences and with diverse patient populations.

TABLE 6.1	Characteristics of Qualitative Research Generating Ethical Concerns
Characteristics	**Ethical Concerns**
Naturalistic setting	Some researchers using participant observation methods may believe that consent is not always possible or necessary.
Emergent nature of design	Planning for questioning and observation emerges over the time of the study. Thus it is difficult to inform the participant precisely of all potential threats before he or she agrees to participate.
Researcher-participant interaction	Relationships developed between the researcher and participant may blur the focus of the interaction.
Researcher as instrument	The researcher is the study instrument, collecting data and interpreting the participant's reality.

ISSUES IN QUALITATIVE RESEARCH

Ethics

Protection of human subjects is a critical aspect of all scientific investigation. This demand exists for both quantitative and qualitative research approaches. Protection of human subjects in quantitative approaches is discussed in Chapter 13. These basic tenets hold true for the qualitative approach. However, several characteristics of the qualitative methodologies outlined in Table 6.1 generate unique concerns and require an expanded view of protecting human subjects.

Naturalistic Setting

The central concern that arises when research is conducted in naturalistic settings focuses on the need to gain informed consent. The need to obtain informed consent is a basic researcher responsibility but is not always easy to obtain in naturalistic settings. For instance, when research methods include observing groups of people interacting over time, the complexity of gaining consent becomes apparent: Have all parties consented for all periods of time? Have all parties been consented? What have all parties consented to doing? These complexities generate controversy and debate among qualitative researchers. The balance between respect for human participants and efforts to collect meaningful data must be continuously negotiated. The reader should look for information indicating that the researcher has addressed this issue of balance by recording attention to human participant protection.

Emergent Nature of Design

The emergent nature of the research design in qualitative research underscores the need for ongoing negotiation of consent with participants. In the course of a study, situations change, and what was agreeable at the beginning may become intrusive. Sometimes, as data collection proceeds and new information emerges, the study shifts direction in a way that is not acceptable to participants. For instance, if the researcher were present in a family's home during a time when marital discord arose, the family may choose to renegotiate the consent. The emergent qualitative research process demands ongoing negotiation of researcher-participant relationships, including the consent relationship. The opportunity to renegotiate consent establishes a relationship of trust and respect characteristic of the ethical conduct of research.

Researcher-Participant Interaction

The nature of the researcher-participant interaction over time introduces the possibility that the research experience will become a therapeutic one. It is a case of research becoming practice. It is important to recognize that there are basic differences between the intent of nurses when engaging in practice and when conducting research. In practice, the nurse has caring-healing intentions. In research, the nurse intends to "get the picture" from the perspective of the participant. The process of "getting the picture" may be a therapeutic experience for the participant. When a research participant talks to a caring listener about things that matter, the conversation may promote healing, even though it was not intended. From an ethical perspective, the qualitative researcher is promising only to listen and encourage the other's story. If this experience is therapeutic for the participant, it becomes an unplanned benefit of the research.

Researcher as Instrument

The responsibility to establish rigor in data collection and analysis requires that the researcher acknowledge any personal thoughts and feelings and strive to interpret data in a way that accurately reflects the participant's point of view. This serious ethical obligation may require that researchers return to the subjects at critical interpretive points and ask for clarification or validation. It is also helpful for the researcher to debrief with a trusted colleague who will provide feedback on this matter.

Rigor in Qualitative Research

Quantitative studies are concerned with the reliability and validity of instruments and the internal and external validity criteria as measures of scientific rigor (see the Critical Thinking Decision Path), but these are not appropriate for qualitative work. The rigor of qualitative methodology is judged by criteria appropriate to the research approach; there should be methodological congruence. The criteria for demonstrating rigor in qualitative research are currently in flux, with several scholars advocating for different approaches to determining rigor. All agree, however, that a well-designed study that is true to its stated methodology and that takes all of the appropriate steps at each stage of the research process will have rigor built in to the design. See Table 6.2 for rigor as described by Creswell and Poth (2018).

In summary, the term *qualitative research* is an overriding description of multiple methods with distinct origins and procedures. In spite of distinctions, each method shares a

---

TABLE 6.2   Criteria for Judging Scientific Rigor

Characteristics of rigor in a qualitative study per Creswell and Poth (2018).

The researcher frames the study within the assumptions and characteristics of the qualitative approach to research.

The researcher conducts an ethical study.

The researcher uses a recognized approach to qualitative inquiry.

The researcher begins with a single focus or concept being explored.

The researcher employs rigorous data collection procedures.

The researcher includes detailed methods describing a rigorous approach to data collection, data analysis, and report writing.

The researcher analyzes data using multiple levels of abstraction.

The researcher writes persuasively so the reader experiences "being there."

The researcher situates himself or herself within the study to reflect his or her history, culture, and personal experiences.

common nature that guides data collection from the perspective of the participants to create a story that synthesizes disparate pieces of data into a comprehensible whole that provides evidence and promises direction for building nursing knowledge.

KEY POINTS

- Qualitative research is the investigation of human experiences in naturalistic settings, pursuing meanings that inform theory, practice, instrument development, and further research.
- Qualitative research studies are guided by research questions.
- Data saturation occurs when the information being shared with the researcher becomes repetitive.
- Qualitative research methods include five basic elements: identifying the phenomenon, structuring the study, gathering the data, analyzing the data, and describing the findings.
- The phenomenological method is a process of learning and constructing the meaning of human experience through intensive dialogue with persons who are living the experience.
- The grounded theory method is an inductive approach that implements a systematic set of procedures to arrive at a theory about basic social processes.
- The ethnographic method focuses on scientific descriptions of cultural groups.
- The case study method focuses on a selected phenomenon over a short or long period to provide an in-depth description of its essential dimensions and processes.
- CBPR is a method that systematically accesses the voice of a community to plan context-appropriate action.
- Ethical issues in qualitative research involve issues related to the naturalistic setting, emergent nature of the design, researcher-participant interaction, and researcher as instrument.
- Credibility, auditability, and fittingness are criteria for judging the scientific rigor of a qualitative research study.

CLINICAL JUDGMENT CHALLENGES

- How can mixed methods increase the effectiveness of quantitative or qualitative research alone?
- How can a nurse researcher select a qualitative research method when attempting to accumulate evidence regarding a new topic about which little is known?
- How can the case study approach to research be applied to evidence-based practice?
- Describe characteristics of qualitative research that can generate ethical concerns.
- **IPE** Your interprofessional team is asked to provide a rationale about why they are searching for a meta-synthesis rather than individual qualitative studies to answer their clinical question.

REFERENCES

Charmaz, K., Thornberg, R., & Keane, E. (2018). Evolving grounded theory and social justice inquiry. In N. K. Denzin, & Y. S. Lincoln (Eds.), *The Sage handbook of qualitative research* (5th ed., pp. 411–443). Thousand Oaks, CA: Sage.

Corbin, J., & Strauss, A. (2015). *Basics of qualitative research*. Los Angeles, CA: Sage.

Creswell, J. W., & Plano Clark, V. L. (2018). *Designing and conducting mixed methods research* (3rd ed.). Thousand Oaks, CA: Sage.

Creswell, J. W., & Poth, C. N. (2018). *Qualitative inquiry and research design: Choosing among five approaches* (4th ed.). Thousand Oaks, CA: Sage.

Dickson, E., Magarati, M., Boursaw, B., Oetzel, J., Devia, C., Ortiz, K., & Wallerstein, N. (2020). Characteristics and practices within research partnerships for health and social equity. *Nursing Research, 69,* 51–61.

Emerson, A., Allison, M., Kelly, P. J., & Ramaswamy, M. (2020). Barriers and facilitators of implementing a collaborative HPV vaccine program in an incarcerated population: A case study. *Vaccine.* https://doi.org/ 10.1016/j.vaccine.2020.01.086.

Farrales, L. L., Cacciatore, J., Jonas-Simpson, C., Dharamsi, S., Ascher, J., & Klein, M. C. (2020). What bereaved parents want health care provider to know when their babies are stillborn: A community-based participatory study. *BMC Psychology.* https://doi.org/10.1186/s40359-020 -0385-x .

Glaser, B. G., & Strauss, A. L. (1967). *The discovery of grounded theory: Strategies for qualitative research.* Chicago: Aldine.

McKinnon, M., Donnelly, F., & Perry, J. (2020). Experiences of post anaesthetic unit recovery nurse facilitating advanced directives in the postanaesthetic period: A phenomenological study. *Journal of Advanced Nursing.* https://doi.org/ 10.1111/jan.14357.

Moustakas, C. (1994). *Phenomenological research methods*: Thousand Oaks, CA: Sage.

Sandelowski, M., & Barroso, J. (2007). *Handbook for synthesizing qualitative research.* New York: Springer.

Schwandt, T. A., & Gates, E. F. (2018). Case study methodology. In N. K. Denzin & Y. S. Lincoln (Eds.), *The Sage handbook of qualitative research* (5th ed., pp. 341–358). Thousand Oaks, CA: Sage.

Stajduhar, K. I., Giesbrecht, M., Mollison, A., Dosani, N., & McNeil, R. (2020). Caregiving at the margins: An ethnographic exploration of family caregiver's experiences providing care for structurally vulnerable populations at the end of life. *Palliative Medicine.* https://doi .org/10.1177/0269216320917875.

Stevens, R. C., Brawner, B. M., Kranzler, E., Giorgi, S., Lazarus, E., Abera, M., Huang, S., & Ungar, L. (2020). Exploring substance use tweets of youth in the United States: Mixed methods study. *JMIR Public Health Surveillance.* https://doi.org/10.2196/16191.

Wallerstein, N. B., & Duran, B. (2006). Using community-based participatory research to address health disparities. *Health Promotion Practice, 7,* 312–323.

Zu, Z., & Bowers, B. (2020). "Everything is Greyscaled": Immigrant women's experiences of postpartum distress. *Qualitative Health Research.* https://doi.org/10.1177/10497323209/4868.

Go to Evolve at **http://evolve.elsevier.com/LoBiondo/** for review questions, appraisal exercises, and additional research articles for practice in reviewing and appraisal.

7

Appraising Qualitative Research

Dona Rinaldi Carpenter

Go to Evolve at **http://evolve.elsevier.com/LoBiondo/** for review questions.

LEARNING OUTCOMES

After reading this chapter, you should be able to do the following:

- Discuss the role of critical appraisal in research and evidence-based practice.
- Identify the criteria for critiquing a qualitative research study.
- Identify the stylistic considerations in a qualitative study.
- Apply critical reading skills to the appraisal of qualitative research.
- Evaluate the strengths and weaknesses of a qualitative study.
- Describe applicability of the findings of a qualitative study.
- Construct a written critique of a qualitative study.

KEY TERMS

coding	auditability	phenomena	theme
grounded theory	credibility	saturation	trustworthiness

Qualitative and quantitative research methods vary in terms of purpose, approach, analysis, and conclusions. Therefore the use of each requires an understanding of the traditions on which the methods are based. This chapter aims to provide a set of criteria that can be used to critique qualitative research studies through a process of critical analysis and evaluation.

The critical appraisal of qualitative research continues to be discussed in nursing and related health care professions, providing a framework that includes key concepts for evaluation (Beck, 2009; Sandelowski, 2015; Thorne, 2020; Uma, 2020).

CRITICAL APPRAISAL AND QUALITATIVE RESEARCH CONSIDERATIONS

Qualitative research represents a basic level of inquiry that seeks to discover and understand concepts, phenomena, or cultures. In a qualitative study, you should not expect to find hypotheses; theoretical frameworks; dependent and independent variables; large, random samples; complex statistical procedures; scaled instruments; or definitive conclusions about how to use the findings. A primary reason for conducting a qualitative study is to develop a theory or to discover knowledge about a phenomenon about which little is known. Sample size is expected to be small. This type of research is not generalizable, nor should it be. Findings are presented in a narrative format with raw data used to illustrate identified themes. Thick, rich data are essential to document the rigor of the research, which is called trustworthiness in a qualitative research study. Ensuring trustworthiness in qualitative inquiry is critical, as qualitative researchers seek to have their work recognized in an evidence-driven world (Beck, 2009; Vindrola et al., 2020).

APPLICATION OF QUALITATIVE RESEARCH FINDINGS

The purpose of qualitative research is to describe, understand, or explain phenomena important to nursing. Phenomena are those things that are perceived by our senses. For example, pain and losing a loved one are considered phenomena. In a qualitative study, the researcher gathers narrative data that uses the participants' voices and experiences to describe the phenomenon under investigation. Barbour and Barbour (2003) offer that qualitative research can provide the opportunity to give voice to those who have been disenfranchised and have no history. For example, it may provide an opportunity to learn about the experiences of people in specific communities where the social determinants of health, such as limited access to supermarkets and resultant food scarcity, disproportionately affect the prevalence of health problems like obesity and diabetes. Therefore the application of qualitative findings will necessarily be context-bound.

Qualitative research also has the ability to contribute to evidenced-based practice literature (Ratnapalan, 2019; Thorne, 2020). Describing the lived human experience of patients can contribute to the improvement of care, having those who live it on a day-to-day basis add a dimension of understanding to our work. Fundamentally, principles for evaluating qualitative research are the same. Reviewers are concerned with the plausibility and trustworthiness of the researcher's account of the findings and its potential and/or actual relevance to current or future theory and practice (Sandelowski, 2015; Vindrolla et al., 2020; Williams, 2015). As a framework for understanding how the appraisal of qualitative research can support evidence-based practice, a published research report and critical appraisal criteria follow (Table 7.1). The critical appraisal criteria will be used to demonstrate the process of appraising a qualitative research report. The philosophical underpinnings for appraisal of phenomenology, ethnography, grounded theory, and action research vary. General critiquing guidelines are applied for the purpose of this chapter. For critique guidelines specific to each methodology, see Streubert and Carpenter (2011).

TABLE 7.1	Critical Appraisal of Qualitative Research
Elements of style	1. Was there sufficient detail to enable critical appraisal?
	2. Is there evidence that the researcher has the qualifications, knowledge, and expertise to conduct the research?
	3. Does the abstract give a clear summary of the study, including the research problem, sample, methodology, findings, and recommendations?
	4. Is the title clear, accurate, and reflective of the topic and method?

TABLE 7.1	**Critical Appraisal of Qualitative Research—cont'd**
Statement of the phenomenon of interest	1. Was the title clear, accurate, and related to the research question? 2. What is the phenomenon of interest, and is it clearly stated for the reader? 3. What is the justification for using a qualitative method? 4. What are the philosophical underpinnings of the research method?
Purpose	1. Was the purpose of the study clearly stated? 2. What is the projected significance of the work to nursing?
Ethical considerations	1. Is protection of human participants addressed? 2. Did the author address Institutional Review Board approval? 3. Were the participants fully informed about the nature of the research? 4. Did the researcher address participant autonomy and confidentiality?
Method	1. Is the method used to collect data compatible with the purpose of the research? 2. Is the method adequate to address the phenomenon of interest? 3. If a particular approach is used to guide the inquiry, does the researcher complete the study according to the processes described?
Sampling	1. What type of sampling is used? Is it appropriate, given the particular qualitative method? 2. Are the informants who were chosen appropriate to inform the research? 3. Were the participants and setting adequately described and appropriate for informing the research? 4. Was saturation achieved?
Data collection	1. Is data collection focused on human experience? 2. Does the researcher describe data collection strategies (i.e., interview, observation, field notes)? 3. Were the data gathered of sufficient depth and richness? 4. Were the questions asked and observations made and recorded in an appropriate way? 5. Is saturation of the data described? 6. What are the procedures for collecting data?
Data analysis	1. What strategies are used to analyze the data? 2. Has the researcher remained true to the data? 3. Is there a logical connection between raw data and themes? 4. Does the reader follow the steps described for data analysis?
Authenticity and trustworthiness of data	1. How does the researcher address the credibility, auditability, and transferability of the data? Credibility • Were the study purpose and method clearly described? • Do the participants recognize the experience as their own? • Has adequate time been allowed to fully understand the phenomenon? Auditability • Can the reader follow the researcher's thinking? • Does the researcher document the research process? • Is there a logical connection between data and themes? • Is there a clear description of the findings? • Is there agreement between the findings and conclusions of the study? Transferability • Are the findings applicable outside of the study situation? • Was the selection of participants described? • Did participants fit the context of the study? • Are the results meaningful to individuals not involved in the research? • Is the strategy used for analysis compatible with the purpose of the study?

Continued

TABLE 7.1	**Critical Appraisal of Qualitative Research—cont'd**
Findings	1. Are the findings presented within a context?
	2. Is the reader able to apprehend the essence of the experience from the report of the findings?
	3. Are the researcher's conceptualizations true to the data?
	4. Does the researcher place the report in the context of what is already known about the phenomenon? Was the existing literature on the topic related to the findings?
Conclusions, implications, and recommendations	1. Do the conclusions, implications, and recommendations give the reader a context in which to use the findings?
	2. How do the conclusions reflect the study findings?
	3. What are the recommendations for future study? Do they reflect the findings?
	4. How has the researcher made explicit the significance of the study to nursing theory, research, or practice?

CRITIQUE OF A GROUNDED THEORY RESEARCH STUDY

THE RESEARCH STUDY

The study "Experiences of Care in the Emergency Department Among a Sample of Homeless Male Veterans: A Qualitative Study" by Jillian J. Weber, and colleagues, published in *Journal of Emergency Nursing,* is critiqued. The article is presented in its entirety and followed by the critique.

Experiences of Care in the Emergency Department Among a Sample of Homeless Male Veterans: A Qualitative Study

Jillian J. Weber, PhD, RN, CNL
Rebecca C. Lee, PhD, RN, PHCNS-BC, CTN-A
Donna Martsolf, PhD, RN, CNS, FAAN

Key words

Emergency service

Veterans

Homeless persons

Emergency nursing

Grounded theory

Qualitative research

Department of Veteran's Affairs

Introduction: Homeless populations are historically high users of the emergency department for low-acuity issues that could be treated in more appropriate settings such as primary care. Veterans make up 11% of the homeless adult population and are often seen in community and Veterans Affairs Medical Center (VAMC) emergency departments. The purpose of this study was to describe the experiences of a sample of homeless male veterans as they attempt to access health care in the emergency department. **Methods:** Grounded

Author Affiliations: Member, Greater Cincinnati Emergency Nurses Chapter, is Homeless-PACT RN Care Manager, Community Outreach Division, Cincinnati VA Medical Center, Cincinnati, OH (Dr Webber); Associate Professor, University of Cincinnati, College of Nursing, Cincinnati, OH (Dr Lee); Professor Emerita, University of Cincinnati, College of Nursing, Cincinnati, OH (Dr Martsolf).
The authors have no conflicts of interest to disclose.
Correspondence: Jillian Weber, PhD, RN, CNL, 909 Vine St, Cincinnati, OH 45202 (jillian.weber@va.gov.)
DOI: 10.1016/j.jen.2019.06.009

theory methodology provided the over-arching framework for this research project. Structured interviews were conducted with 34 male homeless veterans, with 25 discussing their ED care. Veterans were recruited and interviewed from one VAMC emergency department, an all-male emergency shelter, and 1 soup kitchen. Text units about ED use were extracted and compared from 25 recorded transcripts to identify categories. **Results:** Three categories defined ED experiences: "no other option," "lack of voice," and "feeling valued." **Discussion:** The sample of homeless veterans in this study provided first-person knowledge about their experiences receiving care in emergency departments. These results are consistent with previous research indicating that homeless populations are high users of ED care; however, they often feel undervalued and lack of empathy from health providers. Emergency nurses are an integral part of the ED health care delivery system for the homeless, providing advocacy and much-needed education about health problems and alternatives to ED care. The insight obtained about the lives and experiences of veterans in the ED is valuable to the practice of emergency nurses.

Introduction

Homelessness is one of the most common characteristics found among people accessing the emergency department for care.[1] These individuals often use emergency departments as their primary source of care because of its ease and accessibility, while contributing to more than 1 million out of 136 million visits to the emergency department every year.[2-5] This overuse by the homeless creates a significant economic, time, and space burden on emergency departments and the overall health care delivery system.[2,3,6] Often, those who use the emergency department frequently represent a small sample of the ED population but make up a significant number of repeat visits.[3] The homeless are at an increased risk for high ED use because of their overall poor health status, including high levels of chronic disease and morbidity,[7] increased exposure to natural elements, high rates of injuries, and unmet physical and mental health needs.[8]

The United States Department of Housing and Urban Development (HUD) and the United States Department of Veterans Affairs (VA) define homelessness as individuals who lack a fixed, regular, and adequate night-time residence or whose primary residence is a place not ordinarily used for routine sleeping accommodations for human beings.[9] Homeless veterans represent 11% of the adult homeless population.[10] The argument can be made that veterans have access to more health-related resources than other homeless subpopulations[11] because of their access to the Veterans Health Administration (VHA). However, only 40% of the nation's 22 million veterans are registered for VHA benefits,[12] and they often choose not to access the VA system.[13-15] Instead, they often opt to receive care in non-VA community settings. Various studies[16-18] indicate that frequent ED use by homeless veterans remains a significant problem both within the VA system and in the community.

Common characteristics and patterns of use of VA emergency departments among veterans has been previously examined.[16-18] The strongest sociodemographic correlation of VA ED use was found to be homelessness, with homeless veterans being 6 times more likely to be among the most frequent ED users.[16] In addition, homelessness has been shown to be 10 times higher among veterans who are treated and released from emergency departments and is a predictor of repeat visits and hospitalizations.[17] Homeless VA ED users are also more likely to use the emergency department repeatedly for nonemergent services and at higher rates than their housed veteran counterparts.[18] The general characteristics of homelessness (food insecurity, exposure to the elements) increases the likelihood of an individual using an emergency department for all health care needs, rather than some other source such as ambulatory care or primary care.[8] In addition to contributing to a crowded and financially burdened environment, the high use of emergency departments by homeless veterans often leads to a lack in continuity of care and poor health outcomes.[2–4,8,16]

In addition, those experiencing homelessness are frequently the subject of negative attitudes and behaviors from other people, including health care personnel.[19] This often leads homeless individuals to report a lack of trust in clinical providers and a further unwillingness to seek care unless deemed necessary.[19–21] Therefore, the purpose of this study was to describe the experiences of a sample of homeless male veterans as they attempt to access health care in the emergency department and make recommendations to emergency nurses and other stakeholders about effective approaches to ED care for this vulnerable population.

Methods

Study Design

Grounded theory methods by Glaser and Strauss were used to answer the research question in this study.[22] This method was chosen for its ability to produce theory that is "grounded" in the research data rather than deduced from a hypothesis and can explain real-world phenomena. Grounded theory requires a close relationship between data collection and data analysis to produce explanatory models of human behavior.[22] To gain a better understanding of the concepts and the main tenets of grounded theory, refer to the Table.[22–26]

The study findings resulted from a larger qualitative study in which the purpose was to explore how homeless veterans manage their chronic health problems. The population of veterans being studied shared the same fundamental problem of being homeless, while also suffering from some chronic disease. The overall focus of the study was to determine how homeless veterans resolve the problem of chronic disease management through a social or psychological process. The specific aim addressed in the present study was to explore the role of the emergency department in how veterans manage these chronic health problems. Participants were included if they were men, United States veterans (self-disclosed), currently homeless as defined by the VA and HUD, and previously diagnosed with at least 1 chronic health problem. Institutional review board and VA Research and Development Committee approval were obtained. Each participant received a $35 gift card to a large chain grocery store as compensation for his time.

Sample and Setting

Purposive or selective sampling followed by theoretical sampling was used to recruit 34 male homeless veterans from 3 locations across 1 large, urban, midwestern city. Detailed flyers were displayed and on-site recruitment occurred at 1 VA emergency department, a soup kitchen, and a large all-male emergency shelter. Informed consent was obtained, and data were collected in a private room at all 3 study sites, with only the participant and the principal investigator present.

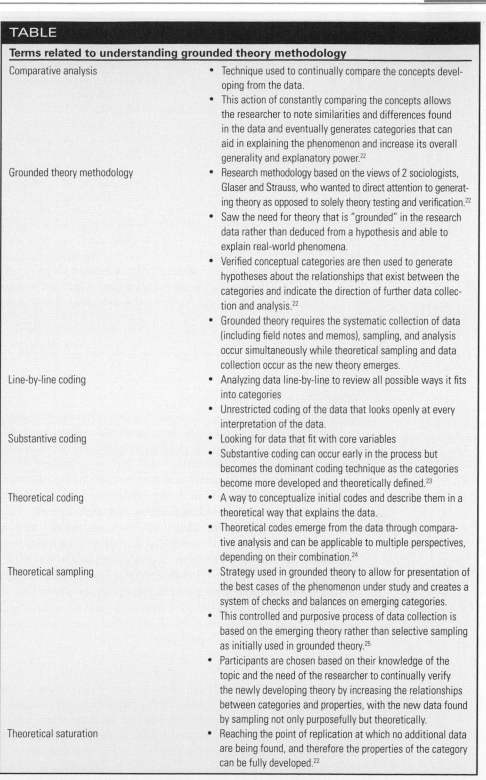

TABLE

Terms related to understanding grounded theory methodology

Comparative analysis	• Technique used to continually compare the concepts developing from the data.
	• This action of constantly comparing the concepts allows the researcher to note similarities and differences found in the data and eventually generates categories that can aid in explaining the phenomenon and increase its overall generality and explanatory power.[22]
Grounded theory methodology	• Research methodology based on the views of 2 sociologists, Glaser and Strauss, who wanted to direct attention to generating theory as opposed to solely theory testing and verification.[22]
	• Saw the need for theory that is "grounded" in the research data rather than deduced from a hypothesis and able to explain real-world phenomena.
	• Verified conceptual categories are then used to generate hypotheses about the relationships that exist between the categories and indicate the direction of further data collection and analysis.[22]
	• Grounded theory requires the systematic collection of data (including field notes and memos), sampling, and analysis occur simultaneously while theoretical sampling and data collection occur as the new theory emerges.
Line-by-line coding	• Analyzing data line-by-line to review all possible ways it fits into categories
	• Unrestricted coding of the data that looks openly at every interpretation of the data.
Substantive coding	• Looking for data that fit with core variables
	• Substantive coding can occur early in the process but becomes the dominant coding technique as the categories become more developed and theoretically defined.[23]
Theoretical coding	• A way to conceptualize initial codes and describe them in a theoretical way that explains the data.
	• Theoretical codes emerge from the data through comparative analysis and can be applicable to multiple perspectives, depending on their combination.[24]
Theoretical sampling	• Strategy used in grounded theory to allow for presentation of the best cases of the phenomenon under study and creates a system of checks and balances on emerging categories.
	• This controlled and purposive process of data collection is based on the emerging theory rather than selective sampling as initially used in grounded theory.[25]
	• Participants are chosen based on their knowledge of the topic and the need of the researcher to continually verify the newly developing theory by increasing the relationships between categories and properties, with the new data found by sampling not only purposefully but theoretically.
Theoretical saturation	• Reaching the point of replication at which no additional data are being found, and therefore the properties of the category can be fully developed.[22]

Continued

Terms related to understanding grounded theory methodology	
	• Complete theoretical saturation fills the various gaps in the theory by maximizing differences among groups and maximizing variations in the data. This is achieved through comparative analysis and theoretical sampling by using "slices of data" to provide alternative views when looking at categories and their properties.[22]
Theoretical sensitivity	• Maintaining theoretical sensitivity throughout the grounded theory process allows the researcher to remain sensitive to the data and allowing the categories and properties to emerge rather than having a priori hypotheses or biases about potential outcomes.[24]
	• Theoretical sensitivity can be increased by professional experience, immersion into the literature, and becoming familiar with common ideas about the phenomenon under study. As grounded theory requires the systematic collection and analyzing of data, categories tend to emerge very quickly.
	• The constant fitting and refitting of data and widespread knowledge of the phenomenon ensures that all the data are explained and best fit in the resulting categories.[26]
	• Preserved throughout the entire grounded theory process to develop a comprehensive formal theory.

Data Collection

Semistructured interviews with participants, lasting between 30 and 60 minutes, were audio-recorded, transcribed, and verified by the principal investigator. Field notes and memos were also used to collect rich data and are consistent with grounded theory methodology.[22] Field notes allowed the researcher to follow up with any clarifying questions and record any general impressions of the environment and/or the participant. Memos were written congruently while data collection and analysis took place to enhance the development of emerging themes. Then, more advanced memos were written as the categories fully developed. Participants were asked 10 interview questions in the larger grounded theory study. Depending on the participants' responses to the guided questions, they were asked additional questions to better understand and capture their experiences in the data. To address the specific aim of this article, the focus was on 2 questions, which included, "Describe a time you needed to seek treatment for your chronic health problems" and "Can you give any advice or recommendations to health care providers working with homeless veterans with chronic health problems?"

Data Analysis Procedures

The transcripts from the 34 participants were analyzed for text units pertaining to self-reported ED visits while homeless. Text units are defined as sentences, phrases, or stories[25] about homeless male veterans' experiences in emergency departments. The grounded theory technique of constant comparative analysis was used to analyze the resulting text units. Line-by-line coding, then substantive coding, and finally theoretical coding were used by the research team, which consisted of the principal investigator, 2 experienced qualitative nurse researchers, and 1 BSN honors student. The principal investigator and 1 nurse researcher met weekly to conduct line-by-line coding on the first 4 transcripts to discuss and establish initial themes. Then, substantive coding and theoretical coding were conducted individually by the entire research team on the remaining 30 transcripts. The research team met weekly to discuss the coded transcripts, analyze the data to reach group consensus and ensure rigor, and review the resulting categories to ensure theoretical saturation was achieved and theoretical sensitivity was maintained. The qualitative software MAXQDA (MAXQDA Analytics Pro, VERBI GmbH, Berlin, Germany)[27] was used to assist with data analysis procedures.

Results

Twenty-five of the 34 study participants discussed care in the emergency department during their interviews when asked to "describe a time you needed to seek treatment for your chronic health problems." The average age of the participants was 56 years. Seventeen participants identified as African American, whereas the remaining 8 identified as Caucasian. More than 80% of the study population had more than 1 diagnosed chronic health problem with substance abuse (drugs and /or alcohol) being the most common; 13 participants used only VA emergency departments, 8 participants used only community emergency departments, and 4 participants used both VA and community emergency departments. Three categories emerged from the data analysis, which represents how veterans described their ED experiences. The categories include "no other option," "lack of voice," and "feeling valued."

No Other Option

This category encompasses homeless veterans feeling that the emergency department is the only place to receive quick and accessible care (20 of 25 participants). They consider their health on a day-to-day basis without future concerns and hope to remain healthy. Participants described feeling how they have no place else to go except the emergency department to be treated immediately for their symptoms. For example, 1 participant described being treated in the emergency department for diabetes:

> I been to the emergency room, in the last 2 months I've been 5 times. They're sick of looking at me, you know what I mean. My sugar was 688, they brought it down to 305 and put me out. I went back; my sugar was 650. They brought it down to 300 and put me out.

Homeless veterans remained concerned about being treated for their health problems at the current time only because they believed the future was beyond their control. They were concerned about receiving follow-up care or making follow-up appointments, as the emergency department was available. One participant described his typical treatment for his health problems:

> I just go to the emergency room, and they give me whatever medication I need, and then when I start to feel better, I leave it alone until another episode. Follow-up after that, me not being stable, I don't even think about that.

Participants described attempting to deal with the problems the best they could because they perceived no other options were available. They were often hopeful that they would remain healthy and not need any health services as 1 participant openly described:

> As far as my health, I just try to take care of myself the best I can, you know there is nothing I can do, you know but deal with the situation.I can't make myself better, so I usually go to the emergency room doctor.

Also, they often lack understanding of how to appropriately navigate the health care system, how to obtain other available resources, and the time needed to access those resources that can be used to manage their care better. Another trend emerging from the data included descriptions associated with the convenience of ED treatment and how this served as a strategy to manage care.

> Well if my back is hurting too bad, I go to the emergency room. Basically, that's what I've been doing, and then after I get the medication I just wait until that episode is over with, and then I won't worry about it until it happens again, or I do something to agitate it, and then I'm running back to the emergency room.

Finally, the lack of health insurance did play a role in homeless veterans accessing the emergency department for care. One participant described using the emergency department for treatment of his chronic obstructive pulmonary disease:

> I have lung disease, and it's not reversible. When I get sick, I normally do go to the emergency room because I don't have any health insurance, and so I can get my treatments by going to the emergency room.

Lack of Voice

This category includes how homeless veterans frequently feel they have no say in their health care situation, which can often lead to a lack of trust in the system and clinical providers (17 of 25 participants). The veteran participants described experiences in which they often felt discounted by the health care system. They wanted to be heard and have a say in their health care and social situations, as 1 participant explained after visiting the emergency department:

> I just would like to be heard sometimes, I don't like to be talked at, I definitely do not like to be talked down to, but I would just like to be heard.if the provider or care source would just maybe listen, he would just know how to treat the person that they're providing service for. We don't need a lot. We may need a little patience but we don't need a lot.

Often, participants described situations that could have been more easily resolved had their health care provider listened to them and tried to better understand their needs and life situations. For instance, 1 participant explained how his needs might be different from another ED patient also experiencing homelessness:

I think health care providers really need to listen to our problems more and really listen and just take each individual case different. We all are different; some people need help with certain things, others need help with other things.

In addition, homeless veterans vividly described experiences of feeling disposable, as 1 participant explained when attempting to interact with ED staff:

Because of my homelessness, I don't think they really take us as being very important people.

Negative perceptions reinforced lack-of-voice experiences and, in our sample, appeared to prevent participants from reaching out for help and establishing relationships with care providers. A participant described not wanting to return for health care services because of his negative ED experience:

The doctor was rude. He came in and told me I had a year; he said "You'll be dead in a year if you don't change your ways."

Feeling Valued

While dealing with their social situation and chronic health problems, participants were still able to provide positive ED experiences that created feelings of value and self-worth (14 of 25 participants). This category incorporates the encouraging words that homeless veterans expressed about those in emergency departments who went out of their way to make a valuable contribution to veterans' health and social situations. Regardless of experiencing both positive and negative situations in the emergency department, many participants were quick to praise those who truly tried to help them. Participants provided encouraging stories in which they either experienced or witnessed other ED staff helping homeless persons:

All these people go beyond their job. I see 1 case worker; she takes a guy across the railroad to pick up stuff that he needs, and the case workers are taking people to their new place.

Much emphasis was placed on feeling that individuals were genuine in their willingness to help and greatly appreciated when there was someone prepared to advocate for them. A veteran with suicidal ideations described how important it was that the ED psychiatric staff stepped in to help him:

I went to the emergency room and told them that I had had it, I was ready to kill myself. Right then, the psychiatric emergency department jumped in and they kept me in the hospital for a while until I felt I was all right. They asked me if I'm ready to go home yet, and I wasn't feeling it, I wasn't ready to go home, so I didn't go home.

Discussion

The study findings indicate that when male homeless veterans required treatment for their chronic health problems they often chose the emergency department as a source for medical care; 75% of study participants noted that they used emergency departments rather than another source, such as primary care, which supports previous research findings.[11,16-18] The theme "no other option" provided some insight regarding why this population are high users of emergency departments.[16-18] The findings suggest that homeless veterans perceive the emergency department as their best option for care rather than primary or ambulatory care services because of convenience, accessibility, and time constraints. Because of their lack of housing and frequent food instability,[8] homeless veterans often described using the emergency department because they had no other options. They are focused on finding food, shelter, and safety[28] rather than seeking appropriate health care services. The emergency department serves as their safety net, and veterans described their attempts to deal with their health issues on their own until symptoms became unavoidable. As a result, they sought out ED care for various reasons such as treatment for diabetes, chronic obstructive pulmonary disease, and medication refills.

Participants describe both positive and negative experiences when encountering emergency health services in both the VA and the community setting. Marginalization of vulnerable populations is not a new concept, and homeless veteran participants in this study describe how they often felt disposable, with no voice in their care, which often created an environment of distrust. The use of ED-integrated social services and/or having a plan to address homelessness—such as emergency shelter access and transitional housing programs—in the emergency department can help increase levels of trust and create positive opportunities for those experiencing homelessness.[20]

Veterans who experience homelessness often have more complex health care needs than the general population.[3,29,30] In addition, they are frequently nomadic and may seek health services across multiple states and health care networks, as participants in this study indicated. Therefore, another way to ensure that homeless veterans are being heard and increase their feelings of value is for ED providers to gain a full understanding of their health and social situations. It is important for providers to be aware, when providing services to our nation's heroes, and allow them the appropriate time, space, and support to adequately explain their health care needs.[21]

Implications for Emergency Nurses

Emergency nurses are likely to encounter homeless populations, including veterans, because of their frequent visits to emergency departments across the United States.[2] Almost half the participants in this study (12 of 25) reported using community emergency departments as opposed to VA emergency departments at some point in time. This puts emergency nurses in the community, along with VA emergency nurses, in a unique position to provide health care, much-needed health education, and advocate for this vulnerable population. Veterans themselves have unique physical and mental health needs, because of their service in the military, to which emergency nurses should be alert. They are often exposed to hazardous materials—such as chemicals, cold injuries, and contaminated water—and experience mental health problems—such as post-traumatic stress disorder, substance abuse, and depression—because of their exposure to combat and other atrocities.[31] It is essential that emergency nurses take the time to ask pertinent health questions related to the veterans' military experience to gain understanding of health needs, increase trust, and create a positive health experience. A VA-developed tool[32] is available to assist nurses and other clinicians in obtaining valuable military and health history information from veterans to best provide for their unique health care needs. This includes asking about military era served; if the veteran experienced combat; talking with the veteran about stress, anxiety, depression, and other mental health issues; and discussing their housing situations.[32]

Findings from this study increase our knowledge and understanding about the experiences of homeless veterans receiving care in emergency departments. Recommendations from the data include emergency nurses working to provide comprehensive care, including evaluating a veteran's military history, while creating a respectful environment to increase trust. In addition, by giving a voice to those homeless individuals who may have been previously ignored through advocacy and health promotion, emergency nurses can create positive health interactions that can lead to open communication and positive health experiences. Ultimately, findings call for more education of emergency nurses and ED staff about homeless veterans and provision of the foundational knowledge for a much-needed educational intervention in the ED setting.

Limitations

One limitation of this study was that participants were interviewed at 1 point in time and may not adequately represent homeless veterans seeking treatment at other VA and non-VA emergency departments across the United States. Another limitation of this study was that the veteran status of participants was self-disclosed. Participants were not asked to provide written proof of military service. However, owing to the nature of the questions asked during the interview process, it would be challenging for a participant to falsify military information and described experiences.

Conclusions

By creating an environment that allows veterans experiencing homelessness to have a voice and feel valued, emergency nurses can generate trust and understanding that opens the door for education about other care options. This study provided a unique first-hand perspective of homeless veterans' experiences seeking care in both VA and community emergency departments. When health care providers listen, support open communication, and convey that they value the patient, these interactions may increase receptivity to learning about other health care options and have a positive impact on follow-up care.[2–4,30] Future research is needed to assess the generalizability of our findings at other sites serving this population. Additional studies may also add to this body of knowledge by devising person-centered strategies that leverage the homeless veteran's experience as an opportunity to provide education about other care-delivery options and help to remove the barriers that perpetuate frequency of ED use.

Author Disclosures

This work was supported by a VISN 10 Research Initiative Program Grant from the United States (U.S.) Department of Veterans Affairs. The contents do not represent the views of the U.S. Department of Veterans Affairs or the United States Government.

REFERENCES

1. Mandelberg, JH, Kuhn, RE, & Kohn, MA. (2000). Epidemiologic analysis of an urban, public emergency department's frequent users. *Acad Emerg Med, 7*, 637–646. https://doi.org/10.1111/j.1553-2712.2000.tb02037.x.

2. Chambers, C, Chiu, S, Katic, M, et al. (2013). High utilizers of emergency health services in a population-based cohort of homeless adults. *Am J Public Health, 103*(suppl 2), 302–310. https://doi.org/10.2105/AJPH.2013.301397.

3. DiPietro, BY, Kindermann, D, & Schenkel, SM. (2012). Ill, itinerant and insured: the top 20 users of the emergency departments in Baltimore city. *Sci World J, 2012*, Article 726568. https://doi.org/10.1100/2012/726568.

4. Kushel, MB, Perry, S, Bangsberg, D, Clark, R, & Moss, AR. (2002). Emergency department use among the homeless and marginally housed: results from a community based study. *Am J Public Health, 92*(5), 778–784. https://doi.org/10.2105/ajph.92.5.778.

5. Centers for Disease Control and Prevention (CDC). *National Hospital Ambulatory Care Survey: 2011 Emergency Department Summary Tables.* http://www.cdc.gov/nchs/data/ahcd/nhamcs_emergency/2011_ed_web_tables.pdf. Accessed February 1, 2016.

6. Chwastiak, L, Tsai, J, & Rosenheck, R. (2012). Impact of health insurance status and a diagnosis of serious mental illness on whether chronically homeless individuals engage in primary care. *Am J Public Health, 102*(12), 83–89. https://doi.org/10.2105/AJPH.2012.301025.

7. Schanzer, B, Dominguez, B, Shrout, PE, & Canton, CLM. (2007). Homelessness, health status, and health care use. *Am J Public Health, 97*(3), 464–469. https://doi.org/10.2105/AJPH.2005.076190.

8. Baggett, TP, O'Connell, JJ, Singer, DE, & Rigotti, NA (2010). The unmet health care needs of homeless adults: a national study. *Am J Public Health, 100*(7), 1326–1333. https://doi.org/10.2105/AJPH.2009.180109.

9. United States Department of Veterans Affairs. Office of Inspector General. *Homeless Incidence and Risk Factors for Becoming Homeless in Veterans.* Retrieved from http://www.va.gov/oig/pubs/VAOIG-11-03428-173.pdf; 2012. Accessed February 21, 2017.

10. United States Department of Housing and Urban Development. *The 2015 Annual Homeless Assessment Report (AHAR) to Congress.* https://www.hudexchange.info/resources/documents/2015-AHAR-Part-1.pdf. Accessed January 5, 2016.

11. Tessler, R, Rosenheck, R, & Gamache, G. (2002). Comparison of homeless veterans with other homeless men in a large clinical outreach program. *Psychiatr Q, 73*(2), 109–119. https://doi.org/10.1023/A:1015051610515.

12. National Center for Veterans Analysis and Statistics. *Department of Veterans Affairs Statistics at a Glance.* http://www.va.gov/vetdata/index.asp; 2014. Accessed January 5, 2016.

13. Agha, Z, Lofgren, RP, VanRuiswyk, JV, & Layde, PM. (2000). Are patients at Veterans Affairs medical centers sicker? A comparative analysis of health status and medical resource use. *Arch Intern Med, 160*, 3252–3257. https://doi.org/10.1001/archinte.160.21.3252.

14. Goldstein G, Luther JF, Jacoby AM, Haas GL. A taxonomy of medical comorbidity for veterans who are homeless. *J Health Care Poor Underserved.* 2008;19(3):991-1005. https://doi.org/10.1353/hpu.0.0040.

15. Goldstein, G, Luther, JF, Haas, GL, Appelt, CJ, & Gordon, AJ. (2010). Factor structure and risk factors for the health status of homeless veterans. *Psychiatr Q, 81*, 311–323. https://doi.org/10.1007/s11126-010-9140-4.

16. Doran, KM, Raven, MC, & Rosenheck, RA. (2013). What drives frequent emergency department use in an integrated health system? National data from the Veterans Health Administration. *Ann Emerg Med, 62*(2), 151–159. https://doi.org/10.1016/j.annemergmed.2013.02.016.

17. Hastings, SN, Smith, VA, Weinberger, M, Schmader, KE, Olsen, MK, & Oddone, EZ. (2011). Emergency department visits in veteran's affairs medical facilities. *Am J Manag Care, 17*(6), e215–e223.

18. Tsai, J, & Rosenheck, RA. (2013). Risk factors for ED use among homeless veterans. *Am J Emerg Med, 31*, 855–858. https://doi.org/10.1016/j.ajem.2013.02.046.

19. Woith, WM, Kerber, C, Astroth, KS, & Jenkins, SH. (2017). Lessons from the homeless: civil and uncivil interactions with nurses, self-care behaviors, and barriers to care. *Nurs Forum, 52*(3), 211–220. https://doi.org/10.1111/nuf.12191.

20. Moore, M, Conrcik, KM, Reddy, A, Allen, A, & Jaffe, C. (2019). From their perspective: the connection between life stressors and health care service use patterns of homeless frequent users of the emergency department. *Health Soc Work, 44*(2), 113–122. https://doi.org/10.1093/hsw/hlz010.

21. Nyamathi, A, Sands, H, Pattatucci-Aragon, A, et al. (2003). Perception of health status by homeless US veterans. *Fam Community Health, 27*(1), 65–74.

22. Glaser, BG, & Strauss, AL. (1967). *The Discovery of Grounded Theory*. Chicago, IL: Aldine.

23. Strauss, AL. (1987). *Qualitative Analysis for Social Scientists*. Cambridge, UK: Cambridge University Press.

24. Glaser, BG. (1978). *Theoretical Sensitivity: Advances in the Methodology of Grounded Theory*. Mill Valley, CA: Sociology Press.

25. Draucker, C, & Martsolf, D. (2010). Life-course typology of adults who experienced sexual violence. *J Interpers Violence, 25*(7), 1155–1182. https://doi.org/10.1177/0886260509340537.

26. Hoare, KJ, Mills, J, & Francis, K. (2012). Dancing with the data: an example of acquiring theoretical sensitivity in a grounded theory study. *Int J Nurs Pract, 18*, 240–245. https://doi.org/10.1111/j.1440-172X.2012.02038.x.

27. MAXQDA. *The art of data analysis*. Berlin, Germany: Version 12; 2015.

28. McCormack, D, & MacIntosh, J. (2001). Research with homeless people uncovers a model of health. *West J Nurs Res, 23*, 679–697. https://doi.org/10.1177/019394590102300704.

29. United States Department of Veterans Affairs. *Ending Veteran Homelessness*. http://www.va.gov/homeless/index.asp. Accessed February 10, 2016.

30. Ku, BS, Scott, KC, Kertesz, SG, & Pitts, SR. (2010). Factors associated with use of urban emergency departments by the US homeless population. *Public Health Rep, 125*, 398–405. https://doi.org/10.1177/003335491012500308.

31. United States Department of Veterans Affairs. *Public Health: Military Exposures*. http://www.publichealth.va.gov/exposures/index.asp. Accessed February 10, 2016.

32. United States Department of Veterans Affairs. *Military Health History Pocket Card for Clinicians*. http://www.va.gov/oaa/archive/Military-Health-History-Card-for-print.pdf; 2015. Accessed February 10, 2016.

CRITICAL APPRAISAL CRITERIA

Qualitative Research Study

As evidenced by published works, Grounded theory is one approach to qualitative research. From a nursing perspective, qualitative research allows caregivers to understand the life experience of patients they care for and, in the case of grounded theory methods, facilitates the development of theory related to a patient care situation that little is known about. Excerpts from "Experiences of Care in the Emergency Department Among a Sample of Homeless Male Veterans: A Qualitative Study" are provided throughout this chapter as examples of grounded theory research. The article was published in *The Journal of Emergency Nursing* in 2020. The primary purpose of this critique is to carefully examine how each step of the research process has been articulated in the study and to examine how this grounded theory study has contributed to nursing knowledge. The article by Weber and colleagues (2020) provides an example of a grounded theory research study true to this qualitative method.

CRITIQUE OF A GROUNDED THEORY RESEARCH STUDY

Grounded theory research creates opportunities for nurse researchers to develop substantive theories regarding phenomena important for nursing practice education and administration. This chapter provides a critique of the study "Experiences of Care in the Emergency Department Among a Sample of Homeless Male Veterans: A Qualitative Study." The authors Jillian J. Weber, PhD, RN, CNL, Rebecca C. Lee, PhD, RN, PHCNS-BC, CTN-A, and Donna Martsolf, PhD, RN, CNS, FAAN, applied grounded theory method to describe specific needs of this vulnerable population in their pursuit of necessary health care. This is a critical appraisal of this grounded theory research study by Weber and colleagues (2020).

Abstract

The purpose of the abstract in any research study is to provide a clear overview of the research and summarize the main features of the findings and recommendations. The abstract must accurately represent the article in its entirety. Weber and colleagues (2020) provide a concise yet detailed abstract of the article that preceded this critique. The authors summarize the research in the following narrative:

> *Homeless populations are historically high users of the emergency department for low-acuity issues with veterans making up 11% of the homeless population. Therefore the purpose of this grounded theory study was to describe the experiences of a sample of homeless male veterans as they attempt to access health care in the emergency department. Grounded theory provided the framework for the study with 34 male homeless veterans, with 25 discussing their Emergency Department Care. Structured interviews were conducted and transcribed verbatim. Three main categories emerged and included "no other option," "lack of voice," and "feeling valued." The findings were consistent with previous research validating the high use of emergency departments by the homeless veteran's population, the lack of empathy from health care providers experienced by this population of patients and the feeling of being undervalued. The insight obtained about the lives and experiences of veterans in the Emergency Department is important to Emergency Department nurses so they are prepared to provide advocacy, education about health problems and alternatives to Emergency Department Care (Weber et al., 2020).*

INTRODUCTION AND REVIEW OF THE LITERATURE

The article provides a clear introduction addressing the focus of the study, and the authors discuss the rationale for a qualitative format. The research presented was a component of a larger grounded theory study, and the authors explicitly noted the purpose for conducting the research. The projected significance to nursing is emphasized throughout the study, noting that homeless veterans primarily seek health care in emergency departments of acute care institutions and often do not receive the long-term care and follow-up that is needed to manage the multitude of chronic health care issues they present with.

This study also helps address the social determinants of health, which include the environments in which people are born, live, learn, work, play, worship, and age that affect a wide range of health, functioning, and quality-of-life outcomes and risks (*Healthy People 2020*). Homeless veterans, unfortunately, have a wide range of acute and chronic health issues as well as a lack of affordable housing, healthy food, and a sense of security and well-being. This research study addresses several aspects of social determinants of health as they apply to the quality of life for homeless veterans.

All research requires the investigator to review the literature. This is the point at which gaps are identified with regard to what is known about a particular topic and what is not known. Unlike with quantitative studies, in qualitative research, only a cursory review of the literature is completed to establish a need for the study. Reviewing the literature a priori has the potential to lead to prejudgments and effect premature closure of ideas or inaccurate interpretation of the raw data. This position is slightly different in grounded theory, as the literature actually may provide one source of data collection.

Selective sampling of the literature is suggested in grounded theory and generally follows or occurs simultaneously with data analysis. The literature review serves to help the researcher become familiar with what has been published about the concepts under study and to fill in the missing pieces in the emerging theory. As theory begins to develop, the existing literature is used as data and woven into a matrix consisting of data, category, and conceptualization. Literature, carefully scrutinized, helps expand the theory and relate it to other theories. Essentially the literature can fill in gaps in the emerging theory and add completeness to the theoretical description (Glaser & Strauss, 1967). The background information provided in the article by Weber and colleagues (2020) provides a concise yet comprehensive review of the literature related to homeless veterans, their health care needs, and the experiences with health care familiar to this very vulnerable population. When critiquing a published study, it is important to note that the literature review will be addressed at the beginning of the article and may appear as though it was completed as a first step in the process. The reader can clarify how the literature was used in the data collection and discussion of the findings. Weber and colleagues (2020) clarified their use of the literature as a component of data collection, which is very appropriate for a grounded theory study. The researchers also use the literature to validate their findings in the discussion section of the article.

The grounded theory method offers an important opportunity to examine clinical practice issues relevant to the discipline of nursing. Weber and colleagues (2020) focused their work on the health care needs of male homeless veterans seeking health care in the emergency departments of hospitals closest to them. The topic is relevant to nurses practicing in the emergency department and to homeless veterans seeking health care that may be related to an acute issue or maintenance of a chronic illness. Weber and colleagues (2020) chose a qualitative approach because "The current literature on homeless veterans' experience using the emergency department for care indicates that, although they use the emergency department for convenience, there is a lack of continuity and follow-up care" (Weber and colleagues 2020, p. 51). Development of theory is critical to understanding and providing for the needs of this vulnerable population.

The researchers further supported the need for the study with a thorough review of the literature. The authors noted that although the topic of homeless veterans has been studied, the voice of the veterans about their experience was missing from the literature. This further substantiated the need for their research study and application of the grounded theory approach. Weber and colleagues (2020) clearly emphasize the significance of the study in relationship to nursing practice and support this with a discussion of the literature that demonstrates a major gap in terms of what is known about homeless veterans and how and where they seek health care.

Philosophical Underpinnings

From a philosophical viewpoint, the study of humans is deeply rooted in descriptive modes of science. Grounded theory methods by Glaser and Strauss (1967) provide a descriptive process to answer the research questions in this study. This method was chosen for its ability to produce theory that is "grounded" in the research data rather than deduced from a hypothesis and can explain real-world phenomena. Grounded theory requires a close relationship between data collection and data analysis to produce explanatory models of human behavior (Glaser 1978; Strauss, 1987). To gain a better understanding of the concepts and the main tenets of grounded theory, the authors provide a comprehensive table (p. 53 of article) addressing the primary tenets of grounded theory methodology. See the reprint of the full article that appears in this chapter before the critique (Weber et al., 2020). The table details steps in grounded theory methodology and further emphasizes the philosophical underpinnings of the method applied in this study (see Chapter 6).

The grounded theory method is specifically aimed at discovering the processes at work in the substantive area of study. Therefore the method is well-suited for uncovering the processes involved in the use of emergency departments for health care by homeless male veterans, their experience of it, and the follow-up care required. Consistent with the approach, the researchers stated the research questions as "Describe a time you needed to seek treatment for your chronic health problems" and "Can you give any advice or recommendations to health care providers working with homeless veterans with chronic health problems?" (Weber et al., 2020). Both questions were broad and open-ended, allowing key issues to emerge, while narrow enough to focus on the specific phenomenon being studied.

Purpose

Weber and colleagues (2020) clearly identified the purpose of the study as "to describe the experiences of a sample of homeless male veterans as they attempt to access health care in the emergency department and make recommendations to emergency nurses and other stakeholders about effective approaches to emergency department care for this vulnerable population." The authors explained why the study was important and the significant contribution the study would make to nursing's body of knowledge. The background information justified the use of a qualitative approach as well as why grounded theory methodology was selected for the study.

Ethical Considerations

The researcher must consider the ethical implications of conducting a grounded theory investigation—or, for that matter, any research study. Informed consent, maintaining confidentiality, and handling of sensitive information are just a few examples of ethical consideration that must be addressed. Because it is impossible to anticipate what sensitive issues may emerge during data collection in a grounded theory investigation, the researcher must be prepared for unexpected concerns.

Addressing the ethical aspects of a research report involves being able to know whether participants were told what the research entailed, how their autonomy and confidentiality will be protected, and what arrangements were made to avoid harm. In qualitative research, the data collection tools generally include interview and participant observation, making anonymity impossible. Because the interviews are open-ended, the possibility of disclosing personal information or uncomfortable information related to the topic may occur. Consent must be a process of continuous negotiation (Oye et al., 2016).

Informed consent was obtained, and data were collected in a private room at all three study sites, with only the participant and the principal investigator present. The sampling technique was appropriate for gathering data relevant to the research questions and is consistent with qualitative research methodology. The sample is appropriate for gathering data relevant to the research questions. Before beginning data collection, the researchers obtained approval from an ethics board. The authors also noted that the participants were assured that they could withdraw from the study at any time (Weber et al., 2020).

Sample

In qualitative research, participants are recruited because of their life experience with the phenomena of interest. This is referred to as *purposive sampling*. The goal is to ensure rich, thick data about the phenomenon of interest. Data are generally collected until no new material is emerging and data saturation has been reached.

Just as it is impossible to finalize the research question before a grounded theory investigation, it is equally impossible to know how many subjects will be involved. The sample size is determined by the data that are generated and the analysis of these data. The grounded theorist continues to collect data until **saturation** is achieved. In terms of grounded theory, *saturation* refers to the completeness of all levels of codes (themes) when no new conceptual information is available to indicate new codes (themes) or the expansion of existing ones (Glaser & Strauss, 1967).

Purposive or selective sampling followed by theoretical sampling was used to recruit 34 male homeless veterans from three locations across one large urban Midwestern city. Flyers were also displayed, and on-site recruitment occurred at one VA emergency department, a soup kitchen, and a large all-male emergency shelter (Weber et al., 2020).

Twenty-five of the 34 study participants discussed care in the emergency department during their interviews when asked to "describe a time you needed to seek treatment for your chronic health problems" (Weber et al., 2020, p. 53). The average age of the participants was 56 years. Seventeen participants identified as African American, whereas the remaining eight identified as Caucasian. More than 80% of the study population had more than 1 diagnosed chronic health problem with substance abuse (drugs and/or alcohol) being the most common; 13 participants used only VA emergency departments, eight participants used only community emergency departments, and four participants used both VA and community emergency departments (Weber et al., 2020, p. 53).

Data Generation

The data generation approach should be sufficiently described so that it is clear to the reader why a particular strategy was selected. Data generation for a grounded theory study may include interviews, observation, documents, or a combination of these sources. Daily journals, participant observation, formal or semistructured interviews, and informal interviewing are valid means of data generation. The choice of data treatment and data collection methods is influenced primarily by the researcher's preference. Interviews are generally recorded and transcribed verbatim. Field notes should be transcribed immediately, and memos should be kept as new interpretations emerge. This is one alternative to data treatment. There are also a variety of computer-based software programs for data treatment/analysis. Weber and colleagues (2020) followed the steps for data generation and used computer programs for data analysis.

Semistructured interviews with participants, lasted between 30 and 60 minutes, were audio-recorded, transcribed verbatim, and verified by the principal investigator. Field notes and Memos were also used to collect rich data and are consistent with grounded theory methodology. Field notes allowed the researcher to follow up with any clarifying questions and record any general impressions of the environment and/or the participant. Memos were written congruently while data collection and analysis took place to enhance the development of emerging themes. Then, more advanced memos were written as the categories fully developed. Depending on the participants' responses to the guided questions, they were asked additional questions to better understand and capture their experiences in the data. Three categories emerged from the data analysis, which represents how veterans described their ED experiences. The categories include "no other option," "lack of voice," and "feeling valued." (Weber et al., 2020)

Data generation was appropriate for this study and was consistent with grounded theory methodology.

Data Analysis

The process of data analysis is fundamental to determining the credibility of qualitative research findings. Data analysis involved the transformation of raw data into a final description or narrative, identifying common thematic elements found in the raw data. The description should enable a reviewer to confirm the processes of concurrent data collection and analysis as well as steps in coding and identifying themes.

The discovery of a core variable is the goal of grounded theory. The researcher undertakes the quest for this essential element of the theory, which illuminates the main theme of the actors in the setting, and explicates what is going on in the data. The core variable serves as the foundational concept for theory generation. The integration and density of the theory are dependent on the discovery of a significant core variable (Glaser & Strauss, 1967).

> *Grounded theory requires that the researcher collect, code and analyze data from the beginning of the study. The method is circular, allowing the researcher to change focus and pursue leads revealed by the ongoing data analysis. The researchers provided a thorough discussion of the application of the findings for educating emergency room nurses, follow-up care for homeless veterans and applicability of the findings to the care of homeless veterans. Further, the findings give voice to this vulnerable population in the determination of health care needs whether chronic or emergent. The study emphasizes the importance of restoring humanity to these individuals and giving them a voice in their care (Weber et al., 2020, p. 54).*

It was clear that follow-up with homeless veterans is at best difficult but critically important. Data analysis was discussed in detail. The table addressing grounded theory language facilitated complete understanding of the method as it was applied to this study.

> *The transcripts from the 34 participants were analyzed for text units pertaining to self-reported ED visits while homeless. Text units are defined as sentences, phrases, or stories about homeless male veterans' experiences in emergency departments. The grounded theory technique of constant comparative analysis was used to analyze the resulting text units. Line-by-line coding, then substantive coding, and finally theoretical coding were used by the research team, which consisted of the principal investigator, two experienced qualitative nurse researchers, and one BSN honors student. The principal investigator and one nurse researcher met weekly to conduct line-by-line coding on the first four transcripts to discuss and establish initial themes. Then, the entire research team on the remaining 30 transcripts conducted substantive coding and theoretical coding individually. The research team met weekly to discuss the coded transcripts, analyze the data to reach group consensus and ensure rigor, and review the resulting categories to ensure theoretical saturation was achieved and theoretical sensitivity was maintained. The qualitative software MAXQDA (MAXQDA Analytics Pro, VERBI GmbH, Berlin, Germany) was used to assist with data analysis procedures (p. 54).*

Coding is a critical element in data analysis. During the conduct of a grounded theory investigation, the processes of data collection, coding, and analysis are occurring simultaneously. As data are collected through interviews, participant observation, field notes, and other data sources, the researcher begins to code the data. Data are examined line by line, processes are identified, and underlying patterns are conceptualized. Weber and colleagues described their process of data analysis in detail as discussed in the previous paragraph. Coding occurred at three levels: Level I coding, Level II coding, and Level III coding (Glaser & Strauss, 1967). Weber and colleagues (2020) refer to this as line-by-line coding, substantive coding, and theoretical coding. Theoretical codes give direction to the process of examining data in the theoretical rather than descriptive modes. Memoing preserves the emerging research question, analytical schemes, hunches, and abstractions. Weber and colleagues (2020) remained faithful to these steps, ensuring that authenticity and trustworthiness of the findings were grounded in the raw data. Authenticity and trustworthiness are determined by the researchers' demonstration of how they remained true to the raw data. As noted earlier, the researchers made every effort to eliminate potential bias. Weekly meetings and individual and group analysis of the raw data facilitated intersubjective agreement, adding to the credibility of the study.

Authenticity and Trustworthiness

Critical to the meaning of the findings is the researcher's ability to demonstrate that the data were authentic and trustworthy or valid. Rigor ensures that there is a correlation between the steps of the research process and the actual study. Procedural rigor relates to accuracy of data collection and analysis. Rigor or trustworthiness is a means of demonstrating the credibility and integrity of the qualitative approach (Cope, 2014; Thorne, 2020). A study's rigor may be established if the reviewer is able to establish an audit trail for the actions and development of the research. It is at this point that the review of literature becomes critical and should be systematically related to the findings. See Table 7.2 for a sampling of raw data the led to the theoretical categories described by the researchers.

TABLE 7.2   Selected Examples of Significant Statements and Their Formulated Meaning

Thematic Element	Raw Data Sample	Formulated Meaning
1 "No other options"	"I been to the emergency department in the past 2 months. I have been five times. They're sick of looking at me, you know what I mean. My sugar was 688; they brought it down to 305 and put me out. I went back. My sugar was 650; they brought it down to 300 and put me out."	The homeless veterans knew of no other way to get health care than to go to the emergency department. Their acute issue would be managed, but with no long-term follow-up, so they come back repeatedly for the same issues.
2 "Lack of voice"	"I just would like to be heard sometimes. I don't like to be talked at. I definitely do not like to be talked down to, but I would just like to be heard. If the provider or care source would just maybe listen, he would just know how to treat the person that they're providing service for. We don't need a lot. We may need a little patience, but we don't need a lot."	Homeless veterans seeking health care in the emergency department feel as though they are not listened to. Assumptions are made because they are homeless, and the triage in the emergency department is one that keeps things moving quickly. This vulnerable population needs a health care facility where they feel their needs are heard and respected.
3 "Feeling valued"	While dealing with their social situation and chronic health problems, participants were still able to provide positive emergency department experiences that created feelings of value and self-worth. "I went to the emergency department and told them that I had had it, I was ready to kill myself. Right then, the psychiatric emergency department jumped in and they kept me in the hospital for a while until I felt I was all right. They asked me if I was ready to go home yet, and I wasn't ready to go home, so I didn't go home."	Homeless veterans need to feel valued when seeking health care, and there are instances where this occurs.

Strauss and Corbin (1998) identified four criteria for judging the applicability of theory to a phenomenon: fit, understanding, generality, and control. If theory is faithful to the everyday reality of the substantive area and is carefully derived from diverse data, then it should fit that substantive area. The emerging theory remained faithful to the substantive area of investigation, mainly homeless veterans who use the emergency department for routine health care. In other words, the grounded theory derived should be immediately recognizable to a practitioner with experience in the area studied, therefore meeting the criteria of understanding. The three main categories described were recognizable to the emergency department nurses, suggesting that the criteria of understanding were met. If the data on which it is based are comprehensive and the interpretations conceptual and broad, then the theory should be abstract enough and include sufficient variation to make it applicable to a variety of contexts related to the phenomenon under study, thus meeting the criteria of generality. The criteria of generality can be interpreted as met given the description provided by the authors related to detailed analysis and intense individual and group reviews to obtain intersubjective agreement. Finally, the theory should provide control with regard to action toward the phenomenon (Strauss & Corbin, 1998). Control in this instance may be assumed by the categories identified in the data.

Although Weber and colleagues (2020) do not discuss in detail authenticity and trustworthiness of the data from a grounded theory perspective, they do however address the limitations of the study, noting:

> One limitation of this study was that participants were interviewed at one point in time and may not adequately represent homeless veterans seeking treatment at other VA and non-VA emergency departments across the United States. Another limitation of this study was that the veteran status of participants was self-disclosed. Participants were not asked to provide written proof of military service. However, owing to the nature of the questions asked during the interview process, it would be challenging a participant to falsify military information and described experiences (p. 57).

Findings, Conclusion, Implications, and Recommendations

Findings from a qualitative study generally are discussed in a narrative format that tells the story of the experience through an exhaustive description and thematic elements. Weber and colleagues (2020) summarized the conclusion, implications, and recommendations from the study.

> Twenty-five of the 34 study participants discussed care in the emergency department during their interviews when asked to "describe a time you needed to seek treatment for your chronic health problems." The average age of the participants was 56 years. Seventeen participants identified as African American, whereas the remaining eight identified as Caucasian. More than 80% of the study population had more than one diagnosed chronic health problem with substance abuse (drugs and/or alcohol) being the most common; 13 participants used only VA emergency departments, 8 participants used only community emergency rooms. Categories emerged from the data analysis, which represents how veterans described their ED experiences. The categories include "no other option," "lack of voice," and "feeling valued" (Weber et al., 2020, p. 56)

The authors did not state a specific core variable but the overarching theme for the participants, a specific vulnerable population, described that their use of the emergency department for health care was clearly related to their feeling that they had *"no other options."*

Findings from this study increase our knowledge and understanding about the experiences of homeless veterans receiving care in emergency departments. Recommendations from the data include emergency nurses working to provide comprehensive care, including evaluating a veteran's military history, while creating a respectful environment to increase trust. In addition, by giving a voice to those homeless individuals who may have been previously ignored through advocacy and health promotion, emergency nurses can create positive health interactions that can lead to open communication and positive health experiences. Ultimately, findings call for more education of emergency nurses and ED staff about homeless veterans and provision of the foundational knowledge for a much-needed educational intervention in the ED setting (Weber et al., 2020, p. 56).

Grounded theory plays a significant role in the conduct of qualitative research. The fundamental characteristics and application of the approach have been reviewed, and this article on health care for homeless veterans makes a significant contribution to the literature in an area about which there was a paucity of information. Applied to the nursing profession, grounded theory can increase development of middle range theory and help explain theoretical gaps between theory, research, and practice.

This study was able to describe the experience of homeless veterans seeking health care through emergency departments. The study, although part of a larger funded study, remained true to grounded theory design. The focus on homeless veterans and how they seek assistance for health care needs has not be studied and is a critically important aspect of care needed in this very vulnerable population. Identifying why the emergency department is used and how homeless veterans are treated can lead to alternative options for care that are more appropriate and provide follow-up for those with chronic health problems.

The critical appraisal of both qualitative and quantitative research is the responsibility of every nurse. This study provides a sound example of grounded theory research and a foundation for the development of critiquing skills.

REFERENCES

Barbour, R. S., & Barbour, M. (2003). Evaluating and synthesizing qualitative research: The need to develop a distinctive approach. *Journal of Evaluation in Clinical Practice, 9*(2), 179–186.

Beck, C. (2009). Critiquing qualitative research. *AORN Journal, 90*(4), 543–554. https://doi .org/10.1016/j.aorn.2008.12.023.

Cleary, M., Escott, P., Horsfall, J., et al. (2014). Qualitative research: The optimal scholarly means of understanding the patient experience. *Issues in Mental Health Nursing, 35*(11), 902–904. https:// doi.org/10.3109/01612840.2014.965619.

Cleary, M., Horsfall, J., & Hayter, M. (2014). Data collection and sampling in qualitative research: Does size matter? *Journal of Advanced Nursing, 70*(3), 473–475. https://doi.org/10.1111/nin.12080.

Cope, D. G. (2014). Methods and meanings: Credibility and trustworthiness of qualitative research. *Oncology Nursing Forum, 41*(1), 89–91. https://doi.org/10.1188/14.ONF.

Glaser, B. G. (1978). *Theoretical sensitivity: Advances in the methodology of grounded theory.* Mill Valley, CA: Sociology Press.

Glaser, B. G, & Strauss, A. (1967). *The Discovery of Grounded Theory*. Chicago, IL: Aldine.

Hegney, D., & Chan, T. W. (2010). Ethical challenges in the conduct of qualitative research. *Nurse Researcher, 18*(1), 4–7.

Oye, C., Sørensen, N. O., & Glasdam, S. (2016). Qualitative research ethics on the spot. *Nursing Ethics, 23*(4), 455–464. https://doi.org/10.1177/0969733014567023.

Ratnapalan, S. (2019). Qualitative approaches: Variations of grounded theory methodology. *Canadian Family Physician, 65*(9), 667–668.

Sandelowski, M. (2015). A matter of taste: Evaluating the quality of qualitative research. *Nursing Inquiry, 22*(2), 86–94. https://doi.org/10.1111/nin.12080.

Strauss, AL. (1987). *Qualitative Analysis for Social Scientists*. Cambridge, UK: Cambridge University Press.

Strauss, A., & Corbin, J. (1998). *Basics of qualitative research: Grounded theory procedures and techniques*. Newbury Park, CA: Sage.

Streubert, H. J., & Carpenter, D. R. (2011). *Qualitative nursing research: Advancing the humanistic imperative*. Philadelphia, PA: Wolters Kluwer Health.

Thorne, S. (2020). Beyond theming: Making qualitative studies matter. *Nursing Inquiry*. https://doi.org/10.1111/nin.12343.

Uma, D., Parameswaran, J., Ozawa-Kirk, L, & Gwen, L. (2020). To live (code) or to not: A new method for coding in qualitative research. *Qualitative Social Work, 19*(2), 169–174. https://doi.org/10.1177/1468794118816618.

Vindrola-Padros, C., & Johnson, G. A. (2020). Rapid techniques in qualitative research: A critical review of the literature. *Qualitative Health Research, 30*(10), 1596–1604. https://doi.org/10.1177/1049732320921835.

Weber, J. J., Lee, R. C., & Martsolf, D. (2020). Experiences of care in the emergency department among a sample of homeless male veterans: A qualitative study. *Journal of Emergency Medicine, 46*(1), 51–56.

Williams, B. (2015). How to evaluate qualitative research. *American Nurse Today, 10*(11), 31–38.

Go to Evolve at **http://evolve.elsevier.com/LoBiondo/** for review questions, appraisal exercises, and additional research articles for practice in reviewing and appraisal.

PART III

Processes and Evidence Related to Quantitative Research

Research Vignette: Abraham A. Brody

RESEARCH VIGNETTE

FOLLOWING YOUR VISION WITH HUMILITY AND PASSION TO IMPACT CARE THROUGH RESEARCH

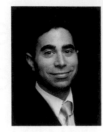

Abraham A. Brody, PhD, RN, FAAN
Associate Professor of Nursing and Medicine
Associate Director, Hartford Institute for Geriatric Nursing
New York University
Rory Meyers College of Nursing
New York, New York

Opportunity can present itself in many ways; the hard part is recognizing the opportunity and taking advantage. As a first-year pre-med biology major at New York University (NYU) who sought to become a pediatric oncologist, I was fortunate to be hired as a student worker at the Hartford Institute for Geriatric Nursing (HIGN). Over the next 4 years, that position would change my life and lead me in a direction I never thought was even possible. I had the good fortune to work for two icons in geriatric nursing, Drs. Mathy Mezey and Terry Fulmer. They, along with many others at HIGN, helped me to see the potential in geriatric nursing research as an avenue for changing the world. By the end of those 4 years, I had helped develop a white paper for the National Institute of Nursing Research on transitions in care at the end of life (Mezey et al., 2002) and moved on to nursing school at the University of California, San Francisco, where I would develop clinical skills as a registered nurse (RN) and gerontological nurse practitioner (GNP) and research skills that I leverage every day.

As a PhD student, I continued to work as a house-call GNP, caring primarily for persons living with dementia (PLWD). In those settings, as I worked with home health and hospice clinicians and emergency rooms, I became frustrated about how little they understood about caring for PLWD. This experience led me to develop a laser-focused vision and passion that I began executing as an assistant professor at the NYU Rory Meyers College of Nursing. My commitment was to translate evidence into practice for PLWD and their caregivers across settings to improve quality and reduce health inequities.

Having never personally practiced as a home health or hospice clinician and only in a limited fashion in emergency departments, I have found it key, to this day, to go into each intervention protocol or new agency/hospital with humility. This humility has helped me and my amazing interdisciplinary team at Aliviado Health within HIGN to further our research into advancing evidence-based care for PLWD and their caregivers and reducing health inequities for older adults.

The primary intervention I have focused on developing is Aliviado Dementia Care, a performance-improvement program that seeks to help interdisciplinary teams provide evidence-based care to PLWD and their caregivers (Bristol et al., 2020; Brody et al., 2016b; Schneider et al., 2020). Aliviado Dementia Care helps home health, hospice, home-based palliative care, hospitals, and other organizations by providing evidence-based online and in-person interactive case-based training, tools (e.g., care plans, caregiver education materials, treatment algorithms), a mobile health point-of-care application, and analytics to improve care for PLWD and their care partners. From its first iteration to today, our team continues to refine Alviado Dementia Care by listening to clinicians in the field and their leadership to ensure we are developing something that is meaningful, useful, and implementable.

Through multiple grant awards, in addition to trial and error, we have been able to refine Aliviado Dementia Care, finally leading to a large-scale semipragmatic clinical trial in home health settings, funded by the National Institute on Aging (NIA). About a year into that grant, a request for applications came along from NIA that seemed tailor-made for me. I could have said, "I had an R01; let me be happy with what I have achieved." Instead, I stuck to my vision and passion and wrote a proposal to translate Aliviado Dementia Care for hospice interdisciplinary teams, leading to the award of a pragmatic stepped-wedge trial in 25 hospices that will touch over 7000 PLWD. It was about following my vision and passion and seizing opportunities, building a team, and running with what seemed like a "big" idea that led to success. A very important component of our preliminary studies and current federally funded studies is the fact that we implemented our research in settings with diverse clinical staff and the PLWD patient population, where health, economic, racial, and other disparities do exist. This purposeful approach allows us to better address the specific needs of diverse populations and ensure substantive recruitment of minority PLWD, which, historically, has been a significant problem in research in general and research into PLWD and their caregivers specifically.

My experience in performing this research with humility and the use of a diverse interdisciplinary-team–based approach also led me to being asked to serve as the pilot core lead of the NIA Imbedded Pragmatic Alzheimer's Disease and Alzheimer's Disease-Related Dementias (AD/ADRD) Clinical Trials (IMPACT) Collaboratory (Brody et al., 2020). I am the only midcareer individual and nurse to serve as a core lead in this significant NIA investment in Alzheimer's disease–focused pragmatic trials. This role provides me the opportunity to lead the development of requests for applications and funding of approximately 40 pilot awards, which has the potential to substantially affect research-driven care for PLWD and their caregivers. This opportunity highlights the nursing leadership role in a major NIA effort.

My research experience and other leadership roles provide an opportunity to "give back" to the nursing profession. In particular, I am committed to guiding the next generation of nurse and interdisciplinary scientists and expanding opportunities to increase the pipeline of diverse researchers, particularly nurses. I consider my success as measured not only by how I affect PLWD and caregivers through my scholarship but also by how I can support others to advance their careers. To this end, I have worked to develop peer-mentoring programs in nursing (Brody et al., 2016a) and strive to highlight the importance of integrating team science principles in nursing programs (Brody et al., 2019).

My aim is to positively affect the care of PWLD, grow the pipeline of nurses with diverse backgrounds not traditionally engaged in academic research roles, and assist them in building their own programs of research. I spend almost as much time mentoring and cultivating emerging scholars as performing my own research. Although I have touched the care of thousands as a clinician and tens of thousands as an implementation scientist, mentoring serves as a force multiplier. Helping diverse nurse researchers to succeed has the potential to affect hundreds of thousands of patients and scholars, if not millions. To me, that is the true mark of success; it is how I live each day. The belief in humble service to others, which advances our profession, helps me to meet my personal vision and passion for improving quality and reducing inequities in care for PLWD and their caregivers.

REFERENCES

Bristol, A. A., Convery, K. A., Sotelo, V., Schneider, C. E., Lin, S. Y., Fletcher, J., & Brody, A. A. (2020). Protocol for an embedded pragmatic clinical trial to test the effectiveness of Aliviado Dementia Care in improving quality of life for persons living with dementia and their informal caregivers. *Contemp Clin Trials, 93*, 106005. https://doi.org/10.1016/j.cct.2020.106005.

Brody, A. A., Barnes, D. E., Chodosh, J., Galvin, J. E., Hepburn, K. W., Troxel, A. B., & Unroe, K. T. (2020). Building a National Program for Pilot Studies of Embedded Pragmatic Clinical Trials in Dementia Care. *Journal of the American Geriatrics Society, 68*(*Suppl 2*), S14–S20. https://doi.org/10.1111/jgs.16618.

Brody, A. A., Bryant, A. L., Perez, G. A., & Bailey, D. E. (2019). Best practices and inclusion of team science principles in appointment promotion and tenure documents in research intensive schools of nursing. *Nurs Outlook, 67*(2), 133–139. https://doi.org/10.1016/j.outlook.2018.11.005.

Brody, A. A., Edelman, L., Siegel, E. O., Foster, V., Bailey, D. E., Jr., Bryant, A. L., & Bond, S. M (2016a). Evaluation of a peer mentoring program for early career gerontological nursing faculty and its potential for application to other fields in nursing and health sciences. *Nurs Outlook, 64*(4), 332–338. https://doi.org/10.1016/j.outlook.2016.03.004.

Brody, A. A., Guan, C., Cortes, T., & Galvin, J. E. (2016b). Development and testing of the Dementia Symptom Management at Home (DSM-H) program: An interprofessional home health care intervention to improve the quality of life for persons with dementia and their caregivers. *Geriatr Nurs, 37*(3), 200–206. https://doi.org/10.1016/j.gerinurse.2016.01.002.

Mezey, M. D., Dubler, N. N., Mitty, E., & Brody, A. A. (2002). What impact do setting and transitions have on the quality of life at the end of life and the quality of the dying process?. *Gerontologist, 42*(Spec No 3), 54–67.

Schneider, C. E., Bristol, A., Ford, A., Lin, S. Y., Palmieri, J., Meier, M. R., & Investigators, H.-Q. T. (2020). The Impact of Aliviado Dementia Care-Hospice Edition Training Program on Hospice Staff's Dementia Symptom Knowledge. *Journal of Pain and Symptom Management*. https://doi.org/10.1016/j.jpainsymman.2020.05.010.

8

Introduction to Quantitative Research

Geri LoBiondo-Wood

Go to Evolve at **http://evolve.elsevier.com/LoBiondo/** for review questions.

LEARNING OUTCOMES

After reading this chapter, you should be able to do the following:

- Define research design.
- Identify the purpose of a research design.
- Define control and fidelity as it affects the outcomes of a study.
- Compare and contrast the elements that affect fidelity and control.
- Begin to evaluate what degree of control should be exercised in a study.
- Define internal validity.
- Identify the threats to internal validity.
- Define external validity.
- Identify the conditions that affect external validity.
- Identify the links between study design and evidence-based practice.
- Evaluate research design using critiquing questions.

KEY TERMS

bias	extraneous or	internal validity	randomization
constancy	mediating variable	intervening variable	reactivity
control	generalizability	intervention fidelity	selection
control group	history	maturation	selection bias
dependent variable	homogeneity	measurement effects	testing
experimental group	independent variable	mortality	
external validity	instrumentation	pilot study	

The word *design* implies the organization of elements into a masterful work of art. In the world of art and fashion, design conjures up images that are used to express a total concept. When an individual creates a structure such as the blueprint for a house, the type of structure depends on the aims of the creator. The same can be said of the research process. The framework that the researcher creates is the design. When reading a study, you should be able to recognize that the literature review, theoretical framework, and research question or hypothesis all interrelate with, complement, and assist in the operationalization of the design (Fig. 8.1).

How a researcher structures, implements, or designs a study affects a study's validity and, ultimately, its application to practice. The implications and usefulness of a study

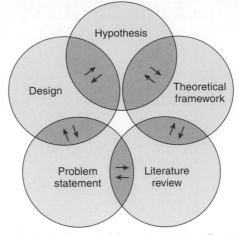

FIG 8.1 Interrelationships of design, problem statement, literature review, theoretical framework, and hypothesis.

for evidence-based practice, the key issues of research design must be understood. This chapter provides an overview of the meaning, purpose, and issues related to quantitative research design, and Chapters 9 and 10 present specific types of quantitative designs.

RESEARCH DESIGN—PURPOSE

Researchers choose from different design types. But the design choice must be consistent with the research question/hypotheses. Quantitative research designs include the following:

- A plan or blueprint
- A vehicle for systematically testing research questions and hypotheses
- Structure for maintaining control in the study

The design, coupled with the methods and analysis, provides control for the study. Control is defined as the measures that the researcher uses to hold the conditions of the study consistent and avoid possible potential of bias or error in the measurement of the dependent variable (outcome variable). Control measures help control threats to the validity of the study.

An example that demonstrates how the design can aid in the solution of a research question and maintain control is illustrated in the study by De la Fuente Coria and colleagues (2020; Appendix B), whose aim was to evaluate the effectiveness of a nurse-delivered intervention for type 2 diabetes. Subjects who met the study's inclusion criteria were randomly assigned to one of the two groups: an interventions group or a control group. The interventions were clearly defined. The authors also discuss how they maintained intervention fidelity or constancy of interventionists, data-collector training, and follow-up throughout the study. By establishing the sample criteria and subject eligibility (see Chapter 12) and by describing the experimental intervention and comparison group, the researchers demonstrated that they had a well-developed plan and were able to consistently maintain the study's conditions. A variety of considerations affect

TABLE 8.1   Pragmatic Considerations in Determining the Feasibility of a Research Question

Factor	Pragmatic Considerations
Time	A question must be one that can be studied within a realistic time period.
Subject availability	A researcher must determine whether a sufficient number of subjects will be available and willing to participate. If one has a captive audience (e.g., students in a classroom), it may be relatively easy to enlist subjects. If a study involves subjects' independent time and effort, they may be unwilling to participate when there is no apparent reward. Potential subjects may have fears about harm and confidentiality and be suspicious of research. Subjects with unusual characteristics may be difficult to locate. Dependent on the design, a researcher may consider enlisting more subjects than needed to prepare for subject attrition. At times, a research report may note how the inclusion criteria were liberalized or the number of subjects altered, as a result of some unforeseen recruitment or attrition consideration.
Facility and equipment availability	Research requires equipment such as questionnaires or computers. Most research requires availability of a facility for data collection (e.g., a hospital unit or laboratory space).
Money	Research requires expenditure of money. Before starting a study, the researcher itemizes expenses and develops a budget. Study costs can include postage, printing, equipment, computer charges, and salaries. Expenses can range from about $1000 for a small study to hundreds of thousands of dollars for a large federally funded project.
Ethics	Research that places unethical demands on subjects is not feasible for study. Ethical considerations affect the design and methodology choice.

a study's successful completion and utility for evidence-based practice. These considerations include the following:

- Objectivity in conceptualizing the research design, question, or hypothesis
- Accuracy
- Feasibility (Table 8.1)
- Control and intervention fidelity
- Validity—internal
- Validity—external

There are statistical principles associated with the mechanisms of control, but it is more important to have a clear conceptual understanding of these mechanisms.

Chapters 9 and 10 present experimental, quasi-experimental, and nonexperimental designs. As you will recall from Chapter 1, a study's type of design is linked to the level of evidence. As you appraise the design, you must also take into account other aspects of how a study is conducted. These aspects are reviewed in this chapter. How they are applied depends on the type of design (see Chapters 9 and 10).

OBJECTIVITY IN THE RESEARCH QUESTION AND DESIGN

Objectivity in the conceptualization of the research question and design is derived from a review of the literature and development of a theoretical framework (see Fig. 8.1). Using the literature, the researcher assesses the depth and breadth of available knowledge about the question (see Chapters 3 and 4), which in turn affects the design chosen. **Example:** ➢ A research question about the length of a breastfeeding teaching program in relation to adherence to breastfeeding may suggest either a correlational or an experimental design (see Chapters 9 and 10), whereas a question related to coping of parents and siblings of adolescent cancer survivors may suggest a survey or correlational study (see Chapter 10).

IPE HIGHLIGHT

There is usually more than one threat to internal and external validity in a study. It is helpful to have a team discussion to summarize specific threats that affect the overall strength and quality of evidence provided by the studies your team are critically appraising.

ACCURACY

Accuracy in determining the appropriate design is aided by a thoughtful theoretical framework and literature review (see Chapters 3 and 4). Accuracy means that all aspects of a study systematically and logically follow from the research question or hypothesis. The simplicity of a research study does not render it useless or of less value. You should feel that the researcher chose a design that was consistent with the research question or hypothesis and offered the maximum amount of control. Issues of control are discussed later in this chapter.

Many research questions have not yet been researched. Therefore a preliminary or **pilot study** is also a wise approach. A pilot study can be thought of as a beginning study conducted to test and refine a study's data collection methods, and it helps to determine the sample size needed for a larger study. **Example:** ➤ Vaughn and colleagues (2020) published a report of a pilot study to (1) explore the feasibility of integrating mobile health (mHealth) technologies to monitor symptom data for pediatric blood and bone marrow transplant patients and (2) evaluate the study design, measures, and procedures. The key is the accuracy, validity, and objectivity used by the researcher in attempting to answer the research question. Accordingly, when conducting research, you should read various types of studies and assess how and if the criteria for each step of the research process was followed.

CONTROL AND INTERVENTION FIDELITY

A researcher chooses a design to maximize the degree of **control**, fidelity, or uniformity of the study methods. Control is maximized by a well-planned study that considers each step of the research process and the potential threats to internal and **external validity**. In a study that tests interventions (randomized controlled trial; see Chapter 9), intervention fidelity (also referred to as *treatment fidelity*) is a key concept. *Fidelity* means trustworthiness or faithfulness. In a study, intervention fidelity means that the researcher standardized the intervention and planned how to administer the intervention to each subject in the same manner under the same conditions. A study designed to address issues related to fidelity maximizes results, decreases bias, and controls preexisting conditions that may affect outcomes. The elements of control and fidelity differ based on the design type. Thus, when research designs are critiqued, the issue of control is always raised but with varying levels of flexibility. The issues discussed here will become clearer as you review the various design types discussed in later chapters (see Chapters 9 and 10).

Control is accomplished by ruling out mediating or intervening variables that compete with the independent variables as an explanation for a study's outcome. An **extraneous, mediating,** or **intervening variable** is one that occurs in between the independent and dependent variable and interferes with interpretation of the dependent variable. An example would be the effect of the stage of cancer and depression during different phases of cancer treatment. Means of controlling mediating variables include the following:

- Use of a homogeneous sample
- Use of consistent data collection procedures
- Training and supervision of data collectors and interventionists
- Manipulation of the independent variable
- Randomization

EVIDENCE-BASED PRACTICE TIP

As you read studies, assess if the study includes an intervention and if there is a clear description of the intervention and how it was controlled. If the details are not clear, it should make you think that the intervention may have been administered differently among the subjects, therefore affecting interpretation of the results.

Homogeneous Sampling

In a smoking cessation study, extraneous variables may affect the dependent variable. The characteristics of a study's subjects are common extraneous variables. Age, gender, length of time smoked, amount smoked, and even smoking rules may affect the outcome in a smoking cessation study. These variables may therefore affect the outcome. As a control for these and other similar problems, the researcher's subjects should demonstrate homogeneity, or similarity, with respect to the extraneous variables relevant to the particular study (see Chapter 12). Extraneous variables are not fixed but must be reviewed and decided on, based on the study's purpose and theoretical base. By using a sample of homogeneous subjects, based on inclusion and exclusion criteria, the researcher has implemented a straightforward method of control.

Example: In the study by De la Fuente Coria and colleagues (2020; see Appendix B), the researchers ensured homogeneity of the sample based on age and history of type 2 diabetes mellitus. This step limits the generalizability or application of the findings to similar populations when discussing the outcomes (see Chapter 17). As you read studies, you will often see the researchers limit the generalizability of the findings to similar samples.

HELPFUL HINT

When critiquing studies, it is better to have a "clean" study with clearly identified controls that enhance generalizability from the sample to the specific population than to have a broad sample from which you can generalize little or nothing.

If a researcher feels that an extraneous variable is important, it may be included in the design. In the smoking cessation example, if individuals are working in an area where smoking is not allowed and this is considered to be important, the researcher could establish a control for it. This can be done by comparing two different work areas: one where smoking is allowed and one where it is not. The key consideration is that before data are collected, the researcher should have identified, planned for, or controlled important extraneous variables.

Constancy in Data Collection

A critical component of control is constancy in data collection. Constancy refers to the notion that the data collection procedures should reflect a step-by-step process of how the researcher controlled the conditions for collecting data. This means that environmental conditions, timing of data collection, data collection instruments, and data collection procedures are the same for each subject (see Chapter 14). Constancy in data collection is also referred to as *intervention fidelity*. The elements of intervention fidelity (Breitstein et al., 2012; Gearing et al., 2011; Preyde & Burnham, 2011) are as follows:

- *Design:* The study is designed to allow adequate testing of the research question(s) or hypothesis (hypotheses) in relation to the underlying theory and clinical processes
- *Training:* Training and supervision of the data collectors and/or interventionists to ensure that the intervention is being delivered as planned and in a similar manner with all subjects
- *Delivery:* Assessing that the intervention is delivered as intended, including that the "dose" (as measured by the number, frequency, and length of contact) is well described for all subjects, the dose is the same in each group, and there is a plan for possible problems
- *Receipt:* Ensuring that the treatment has been received and understood by the subject
- *Enactment:* Assessing that the intervention skills of the subject are enlisted as intended

The study by De la Fuente Coria and colleagues (Appendix B; see the "Interventions" section) is an example of how intervention fidelity was maintained. A review of this study shows that data were collected from each subject in the same manner and under the same conditions by a trained data collector. This type of control aided the investigators' ability to draw conclusions, discuss limitations, and cite the need for further research. When interventions are implemented, researchers will often describe the training of and supervision of interventionists and/or data collectors that took place to ensure constancy. All study designs should demonstrate constancy (fidelity) of data collection, but studies that test an intervention require the highest level of intervention fidelity.

Manipulation of the Independent Variable

A third means of control is manipulation of the independent variable. This refers to the administration of a program, treatment, or intervention to one group in the study and not to the other group in the study. The first group is known as the experimental group or *intervention group,* and the other group is known as the control group. In a control group, the variables under study are held at a constant or comparison level. **Example:** ➤ De la Fuente Coria and colleagues (2020; see Appendix B) implemented a databased intervention and a usual care intervention in two groups of type 2 diabetes mellitus subjects and compared intervention compliance and metabolic outcomes in the groups.

Experimental and quasi-experimental designs are used to test whether a treatment or intervention affects patient outcomes. Nonexperimental designs do not manipulate the independent variable and thus do not have a control group. The use of a control group in an experimental or quasi-experimental design is related to the aim of the study (see Chapter 9).

HELPFUL HINT

The lack of manipulation of the independent variable does not mean a weaker study. The type of question, amount of theoretical development, and the research that has preceded the study affect the researcher's design choice. If the question is amenable to a design that manipulates the independent variable, it increases the power to draw conclusions—that is, if all of the considerations of control are equally addressed.

Randomization

Researchers may also choose other forms of control, such as randomization. Randomization of subjects is used when the required number and type of subjects from a population are obtained in such a manner that each potential subject has an equal chance of being assigned to a treatment group. Randomization, often called *random assignment,* eliminates bias, aids in the attainment of a representative sample, and can be used in various designs (see Chapter 12).

Randomization can also be accomplished with questionnaires. By randomly ordering items on the questionnaires, the investigator can assess if there is a difference in responses related to the order of the items. This may be especially important in longitudinal studies in which bias from completion of the same questionnaire to the same subjects on several occasions can be a problem.

QUANTITATIVE CONTROL AND FLEXIBILITY

The same level of control or elimination of bias *cannot* be exercised equally in all design types. When a researcher wants to explore an area in which little or no research on the concept exists, the researcher may use a qualitative method or a nonexperimental design (see Chapters 5 to 7 and Chapter 10). In these studies, the researcher is interested in describing a phenomenon in a group of individuals.

Control must be exercised as strictly as possible in quantitative research. All studies should be evaluated for potential variables that may affect the outcomes; however, all studies, based on the design, require different levels of control. You should be able to locate in the research report how the researcher maintained control in accordance with its design.

EVIDENCE-BASED PRACTICE TIP

Remember that establishing evidence for practice is determined by assessing the validity of each step of the study, assessing if the evidence assists in planning patient care, and assessing if patients respond to the evidence-based care.

INTERNAL AND EXTERNAL VALIDITY

When reading research, you must be convinced that the results of a study are valid, are obtained with precision, and remain consistent with the aim of the study. For the findings of a study to be applicable to practice and provide the foundation for further research, the study should reflect how the researcher avoided bias. Bias can occur at any step of the research process. Bias can be a result of how research questions are asked (see Chapter 2), which hypotheses are tested (see Chapter 2), how data are collected or observations made (see Chapter 14), the number of subjects and how subjects are recruited and included (see Chapter 12), how subjects are randomly assigned in an experimental study (see Chapter 9), and how data are analyzed (see Chapter 16). There are two important criteria for evaluating bias, credibility, and dependability of the results: internal validity and external validity. An understanding of the threats to internal validity and external validity is necessary for critiquing research and considering applicability to practice. Threats to validity are listed in Box 8.1, and a discussion follows.

BOX 8.1   **Threats to Validity**

Internal Validity
- History
- Maturation
- Testing
- Instrumentation
- Mortality
- Selection bias

External Validity
- Selection effects
- Reactive effects
- Measurement effects

Internal Validity

Internal validity asks whether the *independent variable* really made the difference or the change in the *dependent variable*. To establish internal validity, the researcher rules out other factors or threats as rival explanations of the relationship between the variables—essentially sources of bias. There are a number of threats to internal validity considered by researchers in planning a study and by clinicians before implementing the findings in practice (Campbell & Stanley, 1966). It is important to note that threats to internal validity can compromise outcomes of any study, therefore the overall strength and quality of evidence of a study's findings should be considered in all quantitative designs. How these threats may affect specific designs are addressed in Chapters 9 and 10. Threats to internal validity include history, maturation, testing, instrumentation, mortality, and selection bias. Table 8.2 provides examples of the threats to internal validity. Generally, researchers will note the threats to validity encountered during the conduct of the study in the "Discussion" and/or "Limitations" sections of a research article.

TABLE 8.2   **Examples of Internal Validity Threats**

Threat	Example
History	A study tested an exercise program intervention at one cardiac care rehabilitation center and compared outcomes with those of another center in which usual care was given. During the final months of data collection, the control hospital implemented an e-health physical activity intervention; as a result, data from the control hospital (cohort) were not included in the analysis.
Maturation	Flanders and colleagues (2020, Appendix C) evaluated the effects of staff resilience program in a pediatric intensive care unit. The authors noted that the time frame of the study was a limitation. The program was implemented in 2017 and evaluated in 2018.
Testing	De la Fuente Coria et al. (2020) discussed the limitations of the study noting that no blinding was used regarding group allocation and that changes in medication were not taken into account (see Appendix B).
Instrumentation	DiStasio et al. (2020, Appendix D) discussed how the tools used to assess caregiver vulnerability were not created and based on caregivers of PD patients, but as no tool exists to measure caregiver vulnerability, the researchers adapted the instrument. This issue was acknowledged in the "Limitations" section.
Mortality	Nyamathi and colleagues (2015) noted that more than one-fourth of the subjects (27%) did not complete the vaccine series, despite being informed of their risk for HBV infection.
Selection bias	De la Fuente Coria and colleagues (2020) "noted that due to the type of study there was no blinding was used regarding group allocation" (De la Fuente Coria et al., 2020, Appendix B).

History

In addition to the independent variable, another specific event that can affect the dependent variable may occur either inside or outside the experimental setting; this is referred to as history. An example may be that of an investigator testing the effects of a program aimed at young adults to increase social distancing during the COVID-19 pandemic. During the course of the educational program, an ad featuring a known television figure is released on television and Facebook about the importance of social distancing. The release of this information on social media with a television figure engenders a great deal of media and press attention. In the course of the media attention, medical experts are interviewed widely, and awareness is raised regarding the importance of social distancing. If the researcher finds an increase in the number of young adults who adhere to social distancing in their geographical area, the researcher may not be able to conclude that the change in behavior is the result of the teaching program, as the change may have been influenced by the result of the information on social media and the resultant media coverage. See Table 8.2 for another example.

Maturation

Maturation refers to the developmental, biological, or psychological processes that operate within an individual as a function of time and are external to the events of the study. **Example:** ➤ Suppose one wishes to evaluate the effect of a teaching method on baccalaureate students' achievement on a skills test. The investigator would record the students' abilities before and after the teaching method. Between the pretest and posttest, the students have grown older and wiser. The growth or change is unrelated to the study and may explain the differences between the two testing periods rather than the experimental treatment. It is important to remember that maturation is more than change resulting from an age-related developmental process, but could be related to physical changes as well. **Example:** ➤ In a study of new products to stimulate wound healing, one might ask whether the healing that occurred was related to the product or to the natural occurrence of wound healing. See Table 8.2 for another example.

Testing

Taking the same test repeatedly could influence subjects' responses the next time the test is completed. **Example:** ➤ The effect of taking a pretest on the subject's posttest score is known as testing. The effect of taking a pretest may sensitize an individual and improve the score of the posttest. Individuals generally score higher when they take a test a second time, regardless of the treatment. The differences between posttest and pretest scores may not be a result of the independent variable but rather of the experience gained through the testing. Table 8.2 provides an example.

Instrumentation

Instrumentation threats are changes in the measurement of the variables or observational techniques that may account for changes in the obtained measurement. **Example:** ➤ A researcher may wish to study types of thermometers (e.g., tympanic, oral, infrared) to compare the accuracy of using a digital thermometer with other temperature-taking methods. To prevent instrumentation threat, the researcher must check the calibration of the thermometers according to the manufacturer's specifications before and after data collection.

Another example that fits into this area is related to techniques of observation or data collection. If a researcher has several raters collecting observational data, all raters must be trained in a similar manner so they collect data using a standardized approach, thereby ensuring interrater reliability (see Chapter 13) and intervention fidelity (see Table 8.2). At times, even though the researcher takes steps to prevent instrumentation problems, this threat may still occur and should be evaluated within the total context of the study.

Mortality

Mortality is the loss of study subjects from the first data collection point (pretest) to the second data collection point (posttest). If the subjects who remain in the study are not similar to those who dropped out, the results could be affected. The loss of subjects may be from the sample as a whole, or, in a study that has both an experimental and a control group, there may be a differential loss of subjects. A differential loss of subjects means that more of the subjects in one group dropped out than the other group. See Table 8.2 for an example.

Selection Bias

If precautions are not used to gain a representative sample, selection bias could result from how the subjects were chosen. Suppose an investigator wishes to assess if a new exercise program contributes to weight reduction. If the new program is offered to all, chances are only individuals who are more motivated to exercise will take part in the program. Assessment of the effectiveness of the program is problematic because the investigator cannot be sure if the new program encouraged exercise behaviors or if only highly motivated individuals joined the program. To avoid selection bias, the researcher could randomly assign subjects to groups. In a nonexperimental study, even with clearly defined inclusion and exclusion criteria, selection bias is difficult to avoid completely. See Table 8.2 for an example.

> **HELPFUL HINT**
>
> More than one threat can be found in a study, depending on the type of study design. Finding a threat to internal validity in a study does not invalidate the results and is usually acknowledged by the investigator in the "Results," "Discussion," or "Limitations" section of the study.

> **EVIDENCE-BASED PRACTICE TIP**
>
> Avoiding threats to internal validity can be quite difficult at times. Yet this reality does not render studies that have threats useless. Take them into consideration, and weigh the total evidence of a study for not only its statistical meaningfulness but also its clinical meaningfulness.

External Validity

External validity concerns the generalizability of the findings of one study to additional populations and other environmental conditions. External validity questions under what conditions and with what types of subjects the same results can be expected to occur.

The factors that may affect external validity are related to selection of subjects, study conditions, and type of observations. These factors are termed *selection effects, reactive effects,* and *testing effects.* You will notice the similarity in the names of the factors of selection and testing to those of the threats to internal validity. When considering internal validity threats factors as internal threats, the researcher should assess them as they relate to the testing of *independent* and *dependent* variables within the study. When assessing external validity threats, you should consider them in terms of their *generalizability* or their use outside of the study to other populations and settings. Internal validity threats ask if the independent variable changed or was related to the dependent variable or if it was affected by something else. The Critical Thinking Decision Path for threats to validity displays the way threats to internal and external validity can interact with each other. It is important to remember that this decision path is not exhaustive of the type of threats and their interaction. Problems of internal validity are generally easier to control. Generalizability issues are more difficult to deal with because they indicate that the researcher is assuming that other populations are similar to the one being tested.

CRITICAL THINKING DECISION PATH
Potential Threats to a Study's Validity

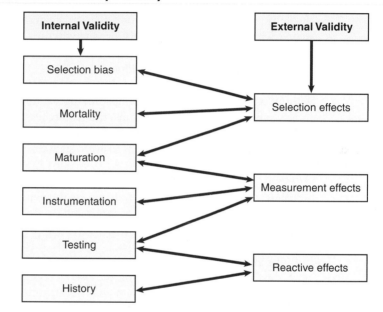

EVIDENCE-BASED PRACTICE TIP

Generalizability depends on who actually participates in a study. Not everyone who is approached actually participates, and not everyone who agrees to participate completes a study. As you review studies, think about how well the subjects represent the population of interest.

Selection Effects

Selection refers to generalizability of the results to other populations. An example of selection effects occurs when the researcher cannot attain the ideal sample. At times, the numbers of available subjects may be low or not accessible (see Chapter 12). Therefore the type of sampling method used and how subjects are assigned to research conditions affect the generalizability to other groups.

Examples of selection effects are reported when researchers note any of the following:

- "This study has some limitations. The first limitation is represented by the small number of the population under study ($n = 69$)" (Enrico et al., 2020, Appendix D).

- "Finally the sample came from a single health center. Therefore the results cannot be generalized for the entire population" (De la Fuente Coria et al., 2020, Appendix B).

These remarks caution you about potentially generalizing beyond the sample in a study, but also point out the usefulness of the findings for practice and future research.

Reactive Effects

Reactivity is defined as the subjects' responses to being studied. Subjects may respond to the investigator not because of the study procedures but merely as an independent response to being studied. This is also known as the *Hawthorne effect,* which is named after Western Electric Corporation's Hawthorne plant, where a study of working conditions was conducted. The researchers developed several different working conditions (e.g., turning up the lights, piping in music loudly or softly, and changing work hours). They found that no matter what was done, the workers' productivity increased. They concluded that production increased as a result of the workers' realization that they were being studied rather than because of the experimental conditions.

In another study that compared daytime physical activity levels in children with and without asthma and the relationships among asthma, physical activity and body mass index, and child report of symptoms, the researchers noted, "Children may change their behaviors due to the Hawthorne effect" (Tsai et al., 2012, p. 258). The researchers made recommendations for future studies to avoid such threats.

Measurement Effects

Administration of a pretest in a study affects the generalizability of the findings to other populations and is known as **measurement effects**. Pretesting can affect the posttest responses within a study (internal validity) and affects the generalizability outside the study (external validity). **Example:** ➤ Suppose a researcher wants to conduct a study with the aim of changing attitudes toward breast cancer screening behaviors. To accomplish this, an education program on the risk factors for breast cancer is incorporated. To test whether the education program changes attitudes toward screening behaviors, tests are given before and after the teaching intervention. The pretest on attitudes allows the subjects to examine their attitudes regarding cancer screening. The subjects' responses on follow-up testing may differ from those of individuals who were given the education program and did not see the pretest. Therefore, when a study is conducted and a pretest is given, it may "prime" the subjects and affect the researcher's ability to generalize to other situations.

> **HELPFUL HINT**
>
> When reviewing a study, be aware of the internal and external validity threats. These threats do not make a study useless—but actually more useful—to you. Recognition of the threats allows researchers to build on data, and allows you to think through what part of the study can be applied to practice. Specific threats to validity depend on the design type.

There are other threats to external validity that depend on the type of design and methods of sampling used by the researcher, but these are beyond the scope of this text. Campbell and Stanley (1966) offer detailed coverage of the issues related to internal and external validity.

⟫ APPRAISAL FOR EVIDENCE-BASED PRACTICE
QUANTITATIVE RESEARCH

Critiquing a study's design requires you to first have knowledge of the overall implications that the choice of a design may have for the study as a whole (see the Critical Appraisal Criteria box). When researchers ask a research question or generate a hypothesis, they design a study and then decide how the data will be collected, what instruments will be used, what the sample's inclusion and exclusion criteria will be, and how large the sample will be to diminish threats to the study's validity. These choices are based on the nature of the research question or hypothesis. Minimizing threats to internal and external validity of a study enhances the strength of evidence. In this chapter, we introduced the meaning, purpose, and important factors of design choice and the vocabulary that accompanies these factors.

Several criteria for evaluating the design related to maximizing control and minimizing threats to internal/external validity and, as a result, sources of bias can be drawn from this chapter. Remember that the criteria are applied differently with various designs (see Chapters 9 and 10). The following discussion pertains to the overall appraisal of a quantitative design.

The research design should reflect that an objective review of the literature and establishment of a theoretical framework guided the development of the hypothesis and the design choice. When reading a study, there may be no explicit statement regarding how the design was chosen, but the literature reviewed will provide clues as to why the researcher chose the study's design. You can evaluate this by critiquing the study's theoretical framework and literature review (see Chapters 3 and 4). Is the question new and not extensively researched? Has a great deal of research been completed on the question, or is it a new or different way of looking at an old question? Depending on the level of the question, the investigators make certain choices.

CRITICAL APPRAISAL CRITERIA
Quantitative Research

1. Is the type of design used appropriate?
2. Are the various concepts of control consistent with the type of design chosen?
3. Does the design used reflect consideration of feasibility issues?
4. Does the design used flow from the proposed research question, theoretical framework, literature review, and hypothesis?
5. What are the threats to internal validity or sources of bias?
6. What are the controls for the threats to internal validity?
7. What are the threats to external validity or generalizability?
8. What are the controls for the threats to external validity?
9. Is the design appropriately linked to the evidence hierarchy?

You should be alert for the means investigators use to maintain control (i.e., homogeneity in the sample, consistent data collection procedures, how or if the independent variable was manipulated, and whether randomization was used). Once it has been established whether or not the necessary control or uniformity of conditions has been maintained, you must determine whether the findings are valid. To assess this aspect, the threats to internal validity should be reviewed. If the investigator's study was systematic, well grounded in theory, and followed the criteria for each step of the research process, you will probably conclude that the study is internally valid. No study is perfect; there is always the potential for bias or threats to validity. This is not because the research was poorly conducted or the researcher did not think through the process completely; rather, it is that there is always some potential for error when conducting research with human subjects. Subjects can drop out of studies, and data collectors can make errors and be inconsistent. Sometimes errors cannot be controlled by the researcher. If there are policy changes during a study, an intervention can be affected. As you read studies, note how each facet of the study was conducted, what potential errors could have arisen, and how the researcher addressed the sources of bias in the "Limitations" section of the study.

Additionally, you must know whether a study has external validity or generalizability to other populations or environmental conditions. For example, the social determinants of health (SDOH), age, education, income, race/ethnicity, and underlying conditions, during the COVID-19 pandemic illustrate how the SDOH have disproportionately affected communities of color, where the population has a higher proportion of underlying conditions like obesity, diabetes, and cardiovascular disease. External validity can be claimed only after internal validity has been established. If the credibility of a study (internal validity) has not been established, a study cannot be generalized (external validity) to other populations. Determination of external validity of the findings goes hand in hand with sampling issues (see Chapter 12). If the study is not representative of any one group or one event of interest, external validity may be limited or not present at all. The issues of internal and external validity and applications for specific designs (see Chapters 9 and 10) provide the remaining knowledge to fully critique the aspects of a study's design.

KEY POINTS

- The purpose of the design is to provide the master plan for a study.
- There are many types of designs.
- You should be able to locate within the study the question that the researcher wished to answer. The question should be proposed with a plan for the accomplishment of the study. Depending on the question, you should be able to recognize the steps taken by the investigator to ensure control, eliminate bias, and increase generalizability.
- The choice of a design depends on the question. The research question and design chosen should reflect the investigator's attempts to maintain objectivity, accuracy, and, most important, control.
- Control affects not only the outcome of a study but also its future use. The design should reflect how the investigator attempted to control both internal and external validity threats.
- Internal validity must be established before external validity can be established.
- The design, literature review, theoretical framework, and hypothesis should all interrelate.
- Pragmatic issues affect the choice of the design. At times, two different designs may be equally valid for the same question.
- The choice of design affects the study's level of evidence.

CLINICAL JUDGMENT CHALLENGES

- How do the three criteria for an experimental design (manipulation, randomization, and control) minimize bias and decrease threats to internal validity?
- Argue your case for supporting or not supporting the following claim: "A study that does not use an experimental design does not decrease the value of the study even though it may influence the applicability of the findings in practice." Include examples to support your rationale.
- **IPE** Have your interprofessional team provide a rationale for why evidence of selection bias and mortality are important sources of bias in research studies. As you critically appraise a study that uses an experimental or quasi-experimental design, why is it important for you to look for evidence of intervention fidelity? How does intervention fidelity increase the strength and quality of the evidence provided by the findings of a study using these types of designs?

REFERENCES

Breitstein, S., Robbins, L., & Cowell, M. (2012). Attention to fidelity: Why is it important? *Journal of School Nursing, 28*(6), 407–408. https://doi.org/10.1186/1748-5908-1-1.

Campbell, D., & Stanley, J. (1966). *Experimental and quasi-experimental designs for research.* Chicago, IL: Rand-McNally.

De la Fuente Coria, M. (2020). Effectiveness of a primary care nurse delivered educational intervention for patients with Type 2 diabetes mellitus in promoting metabolic control and compliance with long term therapeutic targets: Randomised controlled trial. *101*, 1-8, doi.org/10.1016/j.ijnurstu.2019.1034170020-7489.

DiStasio, E., DiSimone, E., Galeti, A., Donati, D., Chiara, G., Tartaglini, D., Massimiliano, C., Massimo, M., & DiMarco, M. (2010). Stress-related vulnerability and usefulness of healthcare education in Parkinson's disease: The perception of a group of family caregivers, a crosssectional study. *Applied Nursing Research.* https://doi.org/10.1016/j.apnr.2019.151186.

Flanders, S., Hampton, D. Missi, P., Ipsan, C., Gruebbel, C. (2020). Effectiveness of a staff resilience. https://doi.org/10.1016/j.pedn.2019.10.007.

Gearing, R. E., El-Bassel, N., Ghesquiere, A., et al. (2011). Major ingredients of fidelity: A review and scientific guide to improving quality of intervention research implementation. *Clinical Psychology Review, 31*, 79–88. https://doi.org/10.1016/jcpr.2010.09.007.

Nyamathi, A., Salem, B., Zhang, S., et al. (2015). Nursing case management, peer coaching, and Hepatitis A and B vaccine completion among homeless men recently released on parole: A randomized trial. *Nursing, 64*(3), 177–189.

Preyde, M., & Burnham, P. V. (2011). Intervention fidelity in psychosocial oncology. *Journal of Evidence-Based Social Work, 8*, 379–396. https://doi.org/10.1080/15433714.2011.54234.

Tsai, S. Y., Ward, T., Lentz, M., & Kieckhefer, G. M. (2012). Daytime physical activity levels in school-age children with and without asthma. *Nursing Research, 61*(4), 159–252.

Turner-Sack, A. M., Menna, R., Setchell, S. R., et al. (2016). Psychological functioning, post traumatic growth, and coping in parent and siblings of adolescent cancer survivors. *Oncology Nursing Forum, 43*(1), 48–56.

Vaughn, J., Gollarahalli, S., Shaw, RJ, Docherty, S., Yang, Q., Malhotra, C., Summers-Goecherma, E., Shah, N. et al. (2020), Mobile Health Technology for Pediatric Symptom Monitoring 69 (2): 142–148.

9

Appraising Experimental and Quasi-Experimental Designs

Susan Sullivan-Bolyai, Carol Bova

Go to **Evolve** at **http://evolve.elsevier.com/LoBiondo/** for review questions.

LEARNING OUTCOMES

After reading this chapter, you should be able to do the following:

- Describe the purpose of experimental and quasi-experimental research.
- Describe the characteristics of experimental and quasi-experimental designs.
- Distinguish between experimental and quasi-experimental designs.
- List the strengths and weaknesses of experimental and quasi-experimental designs.
- Identify the types of experimental and quasi-experimental designs.
- Identify potential internal and external validity issues associated with experimental and quasi-experimental designs.
- Critically evaluate the findings of experimental and quasi-experimental studies.
- Identify the contribution of experimental and quasi-experimental designs to evidence-based practice.

KEY TERMS

after-only design
after-only
   nonequivalent
   control group
   design
antecedent variable
classic experiment
control
dependent variable

design
effect size
experimental design
extraneous variable
independent variable
intervening variable
intervention fidelity
manipulation
mortality

nonequivalent control
   group design
one-group (pretest-
   posttest) design
power analysis
quasi-experimental
   design
randomization (random
   assignment)

randomized controlled
   trial
Solomon four-group
   design
testing
time series design
treatment effect

RESEARCH PROCESS

One purpose of research is to determine cause-and-effect relationships. In nursing practice, we are concerned with identifying interventions to maintain or improve patient outcomes and to base practice on evidence. We test the effectiveness of nursing interventions by using experimental and quasi-experimental designs. These designs differ from nonexperimental designs in one important way: the researcher does not observe behaviors and actions, but actively intervenes by manipulating study variables to bring about a desired effect. By manipulating an independent variable, the researcher can measure a change in behavior(s) or action(s), which is the dependent variable. Experimental and quasi-experimental studies provide the two highest levels of evidence, Level II and Level III, for a single study (see Chapter 1).

Experimental designs are particularly suitable for testing cause-and-effect relationships because they are structured to minimize potential threats to internal validity (see Chapter 8). To infer causality requires that the following three criteria be met:

- The causal (independent) and effect (dependent) variables must be associated with each other.
- The cause must precede the effect.
- The relationship must not be explainable by another variable.

When critiquing experimental and/or quasi-experimental designs, the primary focus is on to what extent the experimental treatment, or independent variable, caused the desired effect on the outcome, the dependent variable. The strength of the conclusion depends on how well other extraneous study variables may have influenced or contributed to the findings.

The purpose of this chapter is to familiarize you with the issues involved in interpreting and applying to practice the findings of studies that use experimental and

CRITICAL THINKING DECISION PATH
Experimental and Quasi-Experimental Designs

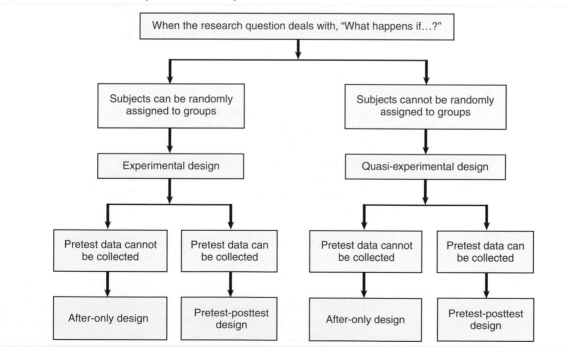

BOX 9.1 **Summary of Experimental and Quasi-Experimental Research Designs**

Experimental Designs
- True experiment (pretest-posttest control group) design
- Solomon four-group design
- After-only design

Quasi-experimental Designs
- Nonequivalent control group design
- After-only nonequivalent control group design
- One group (pretest-posttest) design
- Time series design

---

quasi-experimental designs (Box 9.1). The Critical Thinking Decision Path shows an algorithm that influences the researcher's choice of experimental or quasi-experimental design. In the literature, these types of studies are often referred to as *therapy* or *intervention* studies.

EXPERIMENTAL DESIGN

An **experimental design** has three identifying properties:
- Randomization
- Control
- Manipulation

A study using an experimental design is commonly called a **randomized controlled trial** (RCT). In clinical settings, it may be referred to as a *clinical trial* and is commonly used in drug trials. An RCT is considered the "gold standard" for providing information about cause-and-effect relationships. An RCT generates Level II evidence (see Chapter 1) because randomization, control, and manipulation minimize bias or error. A well-controlled RCT using these properties provides more confidence that the intervention is effective and will produce the same results over time (see Chapters 1 and 8). Box 9.2 shows examples of how these properties were used in the study in Appendix B.

Randomization

Randomization, or **random assignment**, is required for a study to be considered an experimental design with the distribution of subjects to either the experimental or the control group on a random basis. As shown in Box 9.2, each subject has an equal chance of being assigned to one of the two groups. This ensures that other variables that could affect change in the dependent variable will be equally distributed between groups, reducing systematic bias. It also decreases selection bias (see Chapter 8). Randomization may be done individually or by group. Several procedures are used to randomize subjects to groups, such as a table of random numbers or computer-generated number sequences (Suresh, 2011). Note that random assignment to groups is different from random sampling, as discussed in Chapter 12.

Control

Control refers to the process by which the investigator holds conditions constant to limit bias that could influence the dependent variable(s). Control is acquired by manipulating the independent variable, randomly assigning subjects to a group, using a control group, and preparing intervention and data collection protocols that are consistent for all study participants

This study reports specifically on the following:

- The effectiveness of a structured individualized education program for patients with type 2 diabetes, provided by a diabetes nurse, that featured educational reinforcements and family support to achieve metabolic control, and long-term therapeutic targets compared with a control group receiving usual care.
- The intervention group that consisted of individuals with type 1 diabetes including a family member received six one-on-one 30-minute structured, individualized education sessions delivered by a diabetes nurse educator over a period of 6 months and booster sessions at 12 and 18 months.
- The control group received usual medical care at the clinic, which included nurses giving lifestyle advice during routine health care visits (twice a year) without structured diabetes educationaries.
- Fig. 2 in Appendix B: The CONSORT diagram illustrates how $N = 280$ study participants were randomized after excluding 120 who either did not meet inclusion criteria or chose not to participate; 140 were randomized to the experimental arm, and 140 were randomized to the control group.
- The researchers also assessed whether random assignment produced groups that were similar: there were no statistically significant differences observed in the outcome variables between the intervention group and the control group, except for lower body mass index and fewer years with diabetes in the control group. Baseline HgA1c levels in the intervention and control groups

were moderately elevated and similar in both groups. (7.6% vs 7.4, $p = 0.532$).

- Table 1 shows the baseline characteristics of the participants. Over one-half (54.2%) of the participants were male, with mean age for both men and women similar in both study arms (65.1 ± 9.5). The mean number of years living with type 2 diabetes was 8.8 years (±4.4 years) for the intervention group and significantly lower in the control group (M = 6.7 years (±3.6). Thus we would want to consider that randomization did not work for this variable.
- There is no report within this article of **attention-control** (all groups receiving same amount of *attention time*), so we do not know the average amount of time each study arm received. Thus time alone could explain adherence improvement (spending more time teaching/interacting with group members).
- The results include a decrease in HgA1c and systolic blood pressure for the experimental group at 12 months, and at 24 months, other variables significantly improved compared with the control group such as basal glycemia, total cholesterol, low-density lipoprotein cholesterol, and diastolic blood pressure. Very important was that the HgA1c dropped to < 7% in the experimental group compared with the control group (35.2% vs. 24.7%, $p < 0.003$) at 24 months.
- The authors identify several limitations that could have attributed to the findings, such as the sample coming from only one clinic and that medication changes were not measured.

(**intervention fidelity**) (see Chapters 8 and 14). Box 9.2 illustrates how a control group was used by De la Fuente Coria and colleagues (2020; see Appendix B). In an experimental study, the control group receives the usual treatment (in this study, nonstructured diabetes lifestyle advice) or a placebo (an inert pill in drug trials). The experimental group received the intervention by one nurse (interventionist) with diabetes expertise. The nurse did not interact with the control group participants to limit bias by inadvertently offering part of the intervention.

Manipulation

Manipulation is the process of "doing something," a different dose of "something," or comparing different types of treatment by manipulating the independent variable for at least some of the involved subjects (typically those randomly assigned to the experimental group). The independent variable may be a treatment, a teaching plan, or a medication. The effect of this manipulation is measured to determine the result of the experimental treatment on the dependent variable compared with those who did not receive the treatment.

Box 9.2 provides an illustration of how the properties of experimental designs, randomization, control, and manipulation are used in an intervention study and how the researchers ruled out other potential explanations or bias (threats to internal validity) influencing the results. The description in Box 9.2 is also an example of how the researchers used control to minimize bias and its effect on the intervention (De la Fuente Coria et al., 2020). This control helped rule out the following potential internal validity threats:

- *Selection effect:* Bias in the sample contributed to the results versus the intervention.
- *History:* External events may have contributed to the results versus the intervention.
- *Maturation:* Developmental processes that occur and potentially alter the results versus the intervention.

Researchers also tested statistically for differences between the groups and found that there were none, reassuring the reader that the randomization process worked. We have briefly discussed RCTs and how they precisely use control, manipulation, and randomization to test the effectiveness of an intervention.

- RCTs use an experimental and control group, sometimes referred to as *experimental* or *control arms*.
- RCTs have a specific sampling plan, using clear-cut *inclusion* and *exclusion* criteria (see Chapter 12).
- RCTs administer the intervention in a consistent way, called *intervention fidelity*.
- RCTs perform statistical comparisons to determine any baseline and/or postintervention differences between groups.
- RCTs calculate the sample size needed to detect a treatment effect.

It is important that researchers establish a large enough sample size to ensure that there are enough subjects in each study group to statistically detect differences between those who receive the intervention and those who do not. This is called the ability to statistically detect the **treatment effect** or **effect size**—that is, the impact of the independent variable/ intervention on the dependent variable (see Chapter 12). The mathematical procedure to determine the number for each arm (group) needed to test the study's variables is called a **power analysis** (see Chapter 12). You will usually find power analysis information in the "Sample" section of the research article. **Example:** ➤ You will know there was an appropriate plan for an adequate sample size when information like the following is included: that a sample size was calculated at a 95% confidence level with a statistical power of 90%; for HgbA1c a minimum difference of 1% and 4% variance; thus 69 participants were needed for the experimental and 69 for the control arm to obtain an adequate sample size (De la Fuente Coria et al., 2020). This information is critical to assess because with a small sample size, differences may not be statistically evident, thus creating the potential for a *type II error*— that is, acceptance of the null hypothesis when it is false (see Chapter 16). Carefully read the intervention and control group section of an article to see exactly what each group received and what the differences were between groups either at baseline or after the intervention.

In Appendix B, De la Fuente Coria and colleagues (2020) provide a detailed description and illustration of the intervention in the "Methods" section. The "Discussion" section reports that the educational intervention demonstrated improvement in the physiological measures over time. When reviewing RCTs, you also want to assess how well the study incorporates intervention fidelity measures. Fidelity covers several elements of an experimental study (Toomey et al., 2020) that must be evaluated and that can enhance a study's internal validity. These elements are as follows:

1. Well-defined intervention, sampling strategy, and data collection procedures
2. Well-described characteristics of study participants and environment
3. Clearly described protocol for delivering the intervention systematically to all subjects in the intervention group
4. Discussion of threats to internal and *external validity*

Types of Experimental Designs

There are numerous experimental designs (Campbell & Stanley, 1966). Each is based on the classic experimental design called the RCT (Fig. 9.1A). The RCT is conducted as follows:

1. The researcher recruits a sample from the accessible population.
2. Baseline measurements are taken of preintervention demographics, personal characteristics.
3. Baseline measurement is taken of the dependent variable(s).
4. Subjects are randomized to either the intervention or the control group.
5. Each group receives the experimental intervention *or* comparison/control intervention (usual care or standard treatment, or placebo).
6. Both groups complete postintervention measures to see which, if any, changes have occurred in the dependent variables (determining the differential effects of the treatment).
7. Reliability and validity data are clearly described for measurement instruments.

> ### EVIDENCE-BASED PRACTICE TIP
>
> The term *RCT* is often used to refer to an experimental design in health care research and is frequently used in nursing research as the gold-standard design because it minimizes bias or threats to study validity. Because of ethical issues, rarely is "no treatment" acceptable. Typically, either "standard treatment" or another version or dose of "something" is provided to the control group. Only when there is no standard or comparable treatment available is a no-treatment control group appropriate.

The degree of difference between the groups at the end of the study indicates the confidence the researcher has in a causal link (i.e., the intervention caused the difference) between the independent and dependent variables. Because random assignment and control minimizes the effects of many threats to internal validity or bias (see Chapter 8), it is a strong design for testing cause-and-effect relationships. However, the design is not perfect. Some threats to internal validity cannot be controlled in RCTs, including but not limited to:

- Mortality: People tend to drop out of studies, especially those that require participation over an extended period. When reading RCTs, examine the sample and the results carefully to see if excessive dropouts or deaths occurred or if one group had more dropouts than the other, which can affect the study findings.
- Testing: When the same measurement is given twice, subjects tend to score better the second time just by remembering the test items. Researchers can avoid this problem in one of two ways: They may use different or equivalent forms of the same test for the two measurements (see Chapter 15), or they may use a more complex experimental design called the Solomon four-group design.

Solomon Four-Group Design. The Solomon four-group design, shown in Fig. 9.1B, has two groups that are identical to those used in the classic experimental design, plus two additional groups: an experimental after-group and a control after-group. As the diagram shows, subjects are randomly assigned to one of four groups before baseline data are collected. This design results in two groups that receive only a posttest (rather than a pretest and posttest), which provides an opportunity to rule out testing biases that may have occurred because of exposure to the pretest (also called *pretest sensitization*). In other words, pretest sensitization suggests that those who take the pretest learn what to concentrate on during the study and may score higher after the intervention is completed. Although this design

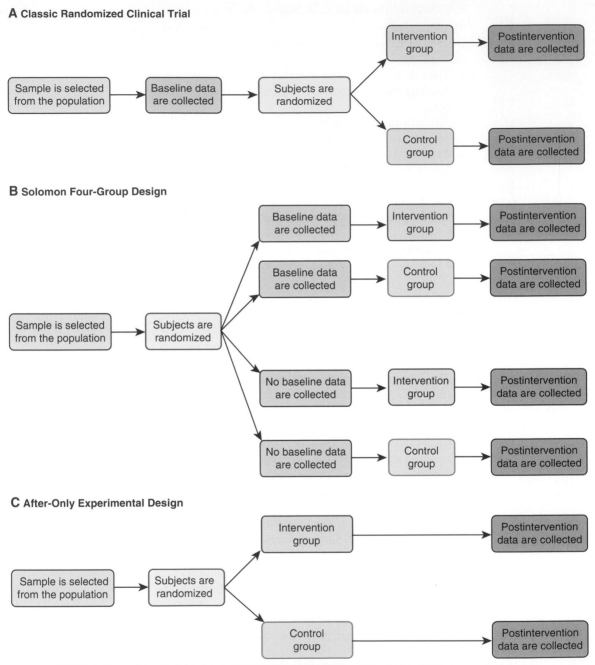

FIG 9.1 Experimental Designs. (A) Classic randomized clinical trial. (B) Solomon four-group design. (C) After-only experimental design.

helps evaluate the effects of testing, the threat of mortality (dropout) is a potential threat to internal validity.

Example: ➤ Barmaki and colleagues (2019) used the Solomon four-group design to test a novel anatomy learning activity (virtual body painting called the REFLECT system) to improve student engagement and learning about the musculoskeletal system. They hypothesized that those who received the virtual body painting exercise would have higher knowledge retention, time on task, and level of engagement compared with those who used a textbook and a virtual mirror.

- The subjects were randomly assigned at the class level (versus individual level) to one of four groups:
  1. Pretest, REFLECT virtual body painting, posttest
  2. Pretest, textbook and virtual mirror, posttest
  3. No pretest, REFLECT virtual body painting, posttest
  4. No pretest, textbook and virtual mirror, posttest
- The study found that classes who used the REFLECT system had greater knowledge retention, increased time on task, and a high level of engagement.

After-Only Design. A less frequently used experimental design is the after-only design (see Fig. 9.1C). This design, which is sometimes called the *posttest-only control group design*, is composed of two randomly assigned groups, but unlike the classic experimental design, neither group is pretested. The independent variable is introduced to the experimental group and not to the control group. The process of randomly assigning the subjects to groups is assumed to be sufficient to ensure lack of bias so the researcher can still determine whether the intervention created significant differences between the two groups. This design is particularly useful when testing effects that are expected to be a major problem, or when outcomes cannot be measured beforehand (e.g., postoperative pain management).

When critiquing research using experimental designs, to help inform your evidence-based decisions, consider which design type was used; how the groups were formed (i.e., if the researchers used randomization); whether the groups were equivalent at baseline; if they were not equivalent, what the possible threats to internal validity were; what kind of manipulation (i.e., intervention) was administered to the experimental group; and what the control group received.

HELPFUL HINT

Look for evidence of preestablished inclusion and exclusion criteria for the study participants.

Strengths and Weaknesses of the Experimental Design

Experimental designs are the most powerful for testing cause-and-effect relationships because of their control, manipulation, and randomization components. Therefore the design offers a better chance of measuring if the intervention caused the change or difference in the two groups. **Example (Appendix B):** ➤ De la Fuente Coria and colleagues (2020) tested structured individualized diabetes education sessions (6 to 30 minutes in person, including a family member) with a nurse diabetes educator over 6 months and booster education follow-up compared with usual care for adults with type 2 diabetes. Those who received the educational intervention had a significant improvement in their HgA1c compared with the control group. If you were working in a clinic caring for this population, you would consider this evidence as a starting point for putting research findings into clinical practice.

Experimental designs have weaknesses as well. They are complicated to design and can be costly to implement. **Example:** ➤ There may not be an adequate number of potential study participants in the accessible population. These studies may be difficult or impractical to carry out in a clinical setting. An example may be trying to randomly assign patients from one hospital unit to different groups because nurses may talk to each other about the different treatments. Experimental procedures also may be disruptive to the setting's usual routine. If several nurses are involved in administering the experimental program, it may be impossible to ensure that the program is administered in the same way with each subject. Another problem is that many important variables that are related to patient care outcomes are not amenable to manipulation for ethical reasons. **Example:** ➤ Cigarette smoking is known to be related to lung cancer, but you cannot randomly assign people to smoking or nonsmoking groups. Health status varies with age and socioeconomic status. No matter how careful a researcher is, no one can assign subjects randomly by age or by a certain income level. Because of these problems in carrying out experimental designs, researchers frequently turn to another type of research design to evaluate cause-and-effect relationships. Such designs, which look like experiments but lack some of the control of the true experimental design, are called *quasi-experimental designs.*

QUASI-EXPERIMENTAL DESIGNS

Quasi-experimental designs also test cause-and-effect relationships. However, in quasi-experimental designs, random assignment or the presence of a control group is lacking. The characteristics of an experimental study may not be possible to include because of the nature of the independent variable or the available subjects.

Without all of the characteristics associated with an experimental study, internal validity may be compromised. Therefore the basic problem with the quasi-experimental approach is a weakened confidence in making causal assertions that the results occurred because of the intervention. Instead, the findings may be a result of other extraneous variables. As a result, quasi-experimental studies provide Level III evidence. **Example (Appendix C):** ➤ Flanders and colleagues (2020) used a quasi-experimental prepost design to evaluate the effect of a staff resilience program in a pediatric intensive care unit on nurse turnover, engagement, compassion satisfaction, and fatigue. This one-group pretest-posttest design was implemented by an interdisciplinary team that included nurse leaders and resulted in improved engagement and decreased turnover. However, it was a convenience sample, and the researchers did not measure the variables over time. In this study, there was no comparison (or control) group to tell if this effect was caused by the staff resilience intervention or something else, such as change over time. We also do not know if this type of program is sustainable as it only had one posttest data point.

> **HELPFUL HINT**
>
> Remember that researchers often make trade-offs and sometimes use a quasi-experimental design instead of an experimental design because it may be impossible to randomly assign subjects to groups. Not using the "purest" design does not decrease the value of the study, even though it may decrease the strength of the findings.

Types of Quasi-experimental Designs

There are many different quasi-experimental designs, but we will limit the discussion to only those most commonly used in nursing research. Refer to the experimental design shown in Fig. 9.1A and compare it with the nonequivalent control group design shown in Fig. 9.2A. Note that this design looks exactly like the true experiment, except that subjects are not randomly assigned to groups. Suppose a researcher is interested in the effects of a new diabetes education program on the physical and psychosocial outcomes of patients newly diagnosed with diabetes. Under certain conditions, the researcher may be able to randomly assign subjects to either the group receiving the new program or the group receiving the usual program, but for any number of reasons, that may not be possible.

- For example, nurses on the unit where patients are admitted may be so excited about the new program that they cannot help but include the new information for all patients.
- The researcher has two choices: to abandon the study or to conduct a quasi-experiment.
- To conduct a quasi-experiment, the researcher can use one unit as the intervention group for the new program, find a similar unit that has not been introduced to the new program, and study the newly diagnosed patients with diabetes who are admitted to that unit as a comparison group. The study would then involve a quasi-experimental design.

Nonequivalent Control Group. The nonequivalent control group design is commonly used in nursing studies conducted in clinical settings. The basic problem with this design is the weakened confidence the researcher can have in assuming that the experimental and comparison groups are similar at the beginning of the study. Threats to internal validity, such as selection effect, maturation, testing, and mortality, are possible. However, the design is relatively strong because by gathering pretest data, the researcher can compare the equivalence of the two groups on important antecedent variables before the independent variable is introduced. Antecedent variables are variables that occur within the subjects before the study, such as in the previous example, where the patients' motivation to learn about their medical condition may be important in determining the effect of the diabetes education program. At the outset of the study, the researcher could include a measure of motivation to learn. Thus differences between the two groups on this variable could be tested, and if significant differences existed, they could be controlled statistically in the analysis.

After-only Nonequivalent Control Group. Sometimes the outcomes simply cannot be measured before the intervention, as with prenatal interventions that are expected to affect birth outcomes. The study that could be conducted would look like the after-only nonequivalent control group design shown in Fig. 9.2B. This design is similar to the after-only experimental design, but randomization is not used to assign subjects to groups and makes the assumption that the two groups are equivalent and comparable before the introduction of the independent variable. The soundness of the design and the confidence that we can put in the findings depend on the soundness of this assumption of preintervention comparability. Often it is difficult to support the assertion that the two nonrandomly assigned groups are comparable at the outset of the study because there is no way of assessing its validity.

One-group (Pretest-Posttest). Another quasi-experimental design is a one-group (pretest-posttest) design (see Fig. 9.2C; Appendix C), such as the Flanders and colleagues (2020) example described earlier. This is used when only one group is available for study. Data are collected before and after an experimental treatment on one group of subjects. In this design, there is no control group and no randomization, which are important characteristics that enhance internal validity. Therefore it becomes important that the evidence

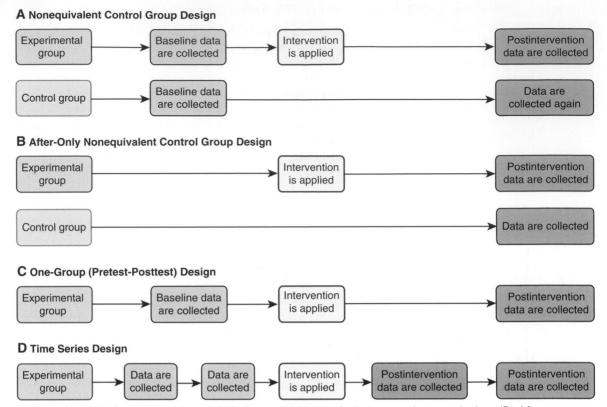

A Nonequivalent Control Group Design

Experimental group → Baseline data are collected → Intervention is applied → Postintervention data are collected

Control group → Baseline data are collected → Data are collected again

B After-Only Nonequivalent Control Group Design

Experimental group → Intervention is applied → Postintervention data are collected

Control group → Data are collected

C One-Group (Pretest-Posttest) Design

Experimental group → Baseline data are collected → Intervention is applied → Postintervention data are collected

D Time Series Design

Experimental group → Data are collected → Data are collected → Intervention is applied → Postintervention data are collected → Postintervention data are collected

FIG 9.2 **Quasi-experimental designs.** (A) Nonequivalent control group design. (B) After-only nonequivalent control group design. (C) One-group (pretest-posttest) design. D, Time series design.

generated by the findings of this type of quasi-experimental design is interpreted with careful consideration of the design limitations.

Time Series. Another quasi-experimental approach used by researchers when only one group is available to study over a longer period is called a **time series design** (see Fig. 9.2D). Time series designs are useful for determining trends over time. Data are collected multiple times before the introduction of the treatment to establish a baseline point of reference on outcomes. The experimental treatment is introduced, and data are collected on multiple occasions to determine a change from baseline. The broad range and number of data collection points help rule out alternative explanations, such as history effects. However, the internal validity of testing is always present because of multiple data collection points. Without a control group, the internal validity threats of selection and maturation cannot be ruled out (see Chapter 8).

IPE HIGHLIGHT

When your team is critically appraising studies that use experimental and quasi-experimental designs, it is important to make sure that your team members understand the difference between random selection and random assignment (randomization).

Strengths and Weaknesses of Quasi-Experimental Designs

Quasi-experimental designs are used frequently because they are practical, less costly, and feasible, with potentially generalizable findings. These designs are more adaptable to the real-world practice setting than the controlled experimental designs. For some research questions and hypotheses, these designs may be the only way to evaluate the effect of the independent variable.

The weaknesses of the quasi-experimental approach involve the inability to make clear cause-and-effect statements.

EVIDENCE-BASED PRACTICE TIP

Experimental designs provide Level II evidence, and quasi-experimental designs provide Level III evidence. Quasi-experimental designs are lower on the evidence hierarchy because of lack of control, which limits the ability to make confident cause-and-effect statements that influence applicability to practice and clinical decision making.

EVIDENCE-BASED PRACTICE

As nursing science expands and as accountability for cost-effective quality clinical outcomes increases, nurses must become more cognizant of what constitutes best practice for their patient population. An understanding of the value of intervention studies that use an experimental or quasi-experimental design is critical for improving clinical outcomes. These study designs provide the strongest evidence for making informed clinical decisions. These designs are those most commonly included in systematic reviews (see Chapter 11).

One cannot assume that because an intervention study has been published that the findings apply to your practice population. When conducting an evidence-based practice project, the clinical question provides a guide for you and your team to collect the strongest, most relevant evidence related to your problem. If your search of the literature reveals experimental and quasi-experimental studies, you will need to evaluate them to determine which studies provide the best available evidence. The likelihood of changing practice based on one study is low, unless it is a large clinical RCT based on prior research evidence.

Key points for evaluating the evidence and whether bias has been minimized in experimental and quasi-experimental designs include the following:

- Random group assignment (experimental or intervention and control or comparison)
- Inclusion and exclusion criteria that are relevant to the clinical problem studied
- Equivalence of groups at baseline on key demographic variables
- Adequate sample size recruitment of a homogeneous sample
- Intervention fidelity and consistent data collection procedures
- Control of antecedent, intervening, or extraneous variables

CRITICAL APPRAISAL CRITERIA
Experimental and Quasi-Experimental Designs

1. Is the design used appropriate to the research question or hypothesis?
2. Is there a detailed description of the intervention?
3. Is there a clear description of the intervention group treatment in comparison with the control group? How is intervention fidelity maintained?
4. Is power analysis used to calculate the appropriate sample size for the study?

Experimental Designs
1. What experimental design is used in the study?
2. How are randomization, control, and manipulation implemented?
3. Are the findings generalizable to the larger population of interest?

Quasi-experimental Designs
1. What quasi-experimental design is used in the study, and is it appropriate?
2. What are the most common threats to internal and external validity of the findings of this design?
3. What does the author say about the limitations of the study?
4. To what extent are the study findings generalizable?

⟫ APPRAISAL FOR EVIDENCE-BASED PRACTICE
EXPERIMENTAL AND QUASI-EXPERIMENTAL DESIGNS

Research designs differ in the amount of control the researcher has over the antecedent and intervening variables that may affect the study's results. Experimental designs, which provide Level II evidence, provide the most possibility for control. Quasi-experimental designs, which provide Level III evidence, provide less control. When conducting an evidence-based practice or quality improvement project, you must always look for studies that provide the highest level of evidence (see Chapter 1). For some PICO questions (see Chapter 2), you will find both Level II and Level III evidence. You will want to determine whether the choice of design, experimental or quasi-experimental, is appropriate to the purpose of the study and can answer the research question or hypotheses.

HELPFUL HINT

When reviewing the experimental and quasi-experimental literature, do not limit your search only to your patient population. For example, it is possible that if you are working with adult caregivers, related parent caregiver intervention studies may provide you with strategies as well. Many times, with some adaptation, interventions used with one sample may be applicable for other populations.

Questions that you should pose when reading studies that test cause-and-effect relationships are listed in the Critical Appraisal Criteria box. These questions should help you judge whether a causal relationship exists.

For studies in which either experimental or quasi-experimental designs are used, you must first try to determine the type of design that was used. Often a statement describing the design of the study appears in the abstract and in the methods section of the article. If such a statement is not present, you should examine the article for evidence of control, randomization, and manipulation. If all are discussed, the design is probably experimental. On the other hand, if the study involves the administration of an experimental treatment but does not involve the random assignment of subjects to groups, the design is quasi-experimental. Next, try to identify which of the experimental and quasi-experimental designs was used. Determining the answer to these questions gives you a head start, because each design has its inherent threats to internal and external validity. This step makes it a bit easier to critically evaluate the study. It is important that the author provide adequate accounts of how the procedures for randomization, control, and manipulation were carried out. The report should include such a clear description of the procedures for random assignment that the reader could determine just how likely it was for any one subject to be assigned to a particular group. The description of the intervention that each group received provides important information about which intervention fidelity strategies were implemented.

The inclusion of this information helps determine whether the intervention group and control group received different treatments that were consistently carried out by trained interventionists and data collectors. The question of threats to internal validity, such as testing and mortality, is even more important to consider when critically evaluating a quasi-experimental study, because quasi-experimental designs cannot possibly feature as much control; there may be a lack of randomization or a control group. A well-written report of a quasi-experimental study systematically reviews potential threats to the internal and external validity of the findings. Your work is to decide if the author's explanations make sense. For either experimental or quasi-experimental studies, you should also check for a reported power analysis that assures you that an appropriate sample size for detecting a treatment effect was planned.

KEY POINTS

- Experimental designs or RCTs provide the strongest evidence (Level II) for a single study that tests whether an intervention or treatment affects patient outcomes.
- Experimental designs are characterized by the ability of the researcher to control extraneous variation, to manipulate the independent variable, and to randomly assign subjects to intervention groups.
- Experimental studies conducted either in clinical settings or in the laboratory provide the best evidence in support of a causal relationship because the following three criteria can be met: (1) the independent and dependent variables are related to each other; (2) the independent variable chronologically precedes the dependent variable; and (3) the relationship cannot be explained by the presence of a third variable.
- Researchers turn to quasi-experimental designs to test cause-and-effect relationships because experimental designs may be impractical or unethical.
- Quasi-experiments may lack the randomization and/or the comparison group characteristics of true experiments. The usefulness of quasi-experiments for studying causal relationships depends on the ability of the researcher to rule out plausible threats to the validity of the findings, such as history, selection, maturation, and testing effects.

CLINICAL JUDGMENT CHALLENGES

- Describe the ethical issues included in a true experimental research design used by a nurse researcher.
- Describe how a true experimental design could be used in a hospital setting with patients.
- How should a nurse go about critically appraising experimental research articles in the research literature so that his or her evidence-based practice is enhanced?
- **IPE** Discuss whether your quality improvement team would use an experimental or quasi-experimental design for a quality improvement project.
- Identify a clinical quality indicator that is a problem on your unit (e.g., falls, ventilator-acquired pneumonia, catheter-acquired urinary tract infection) and consider how a search for studies using experimental or quasi-experimental designs could provide the foundation for a quality improvement project.

REFERENCES

Barmaki, R., Yu, K., Pearlman, R., Shingles, R., Bork, F., Osgood, G. M., & Navab, N. (2019). Enhancement of anatomical education using augmented reality: An empirical study of body painting. *Anatomical Sciences Education, 12*(6), 599–609. https://doi.org/10.1002/ase.1858.

Campbell, D., & Stanley, J. (1966). *Experimental and quasi-experimental designs for research.* Chicago, IL: Rand-McNally.

De la Fuente Coria, Cruz-Cobo, C., & Santi-Cano, M. J. (2020). Effectiveness of a primary care nurse delivered educational intervention for patients with type 2 diabetes mellitus in promoting metabolic control and compliance with long-term therapeutic target. *International Journal of Nursing Studies, 101*, 103417.

Flanders, H., Missi, I., & Gruebbel, C. (2020). Effectiveness of a staff resilience program in a pediatric intensive care unit. *Journal of Pediatric Nursing, 50*, 1–4. https://doi.org/10.1016/j.pedn.2019.10.007. Epub 2019 Oct 25.

Suresh, K. P. (2011). An overview of randomization techniques: An unbiased assessment of outcome in clinical research. Journal of Human Reproductive Science, 4, 8–11.

Toomey, E., Hardeman, W., Hankonen, N., Byrne, M., McSharry, J., Matvienko-Sikar, K., & Lorencatto, F. (2020). Focusing on fidelity: Narrative review and recommendations for improving intervention fidelity within trials of health behaviour change interventions. *Health Psychology and Behavioral Medicine, 8*(1), 132–151. https://doi.org/10.1080/21642850.2020.1738935.

Go to Evolve at **http://evolve.elsevier.com/LoBiondo/** for review questions, appraisal exercises, and additional research articles for practice in reviewing and appraisal.

10

Appraising Nonexperimental Designs

Geri LoBiondo-Wood, Judith Haber

Go to **Evolve** at **http://evolve.elsevier.com/LoBiondo/** for review questions.

LEARNING OUTCOMES

After reading this chapter, you should be able to do the following:

- Describe the purpose of nonexperimental designs.
- Describe the characteristics of nonexperimental designs.
- Define the differences between nonexperimental designs.
- List the advantages and disadvantages of nonexperimental designs.
- Identify the purpose and methods of methodological, secondary analysis, and mixed methods designs.
- Identify the critical appraisal criteria used to critique nonexperimental designs.
- Evaluate the strength and quality of evidence by nonexperimental designs.

KEY TERMS

case control design
cohort design
correlational design
cross-sectional design
developmental design

ex post facto design
longitudinal design
methodological research
mixed methods

prospective design
psychometrics
repeated measures design

retrospective design
secondary analysis
survey design

Many phenomena relevant to nursing do not lend themselves to an experimental design. For example, nurses studying cancer-related fatigue may be interested in the amount of fatigue, variations in fatigue, and patient fatigue in response to chemotherapy. The investigator would not design an experimental study that aims to implement an intervention that could potentially intensify an aspect of a patient's fatigue to study the fatigue experience. Instead, the researcher would examine factors that contribute to the variability in a patient's cancer-related fatigue experience using a nonexperimental design. Nonexperimental designs are used when a researcher wishes to explore events, people, or situations as they occur or test relationships and differences among variables at one point or over a period of time.

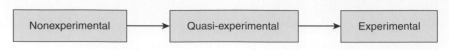

FIG 10.1 Continuum of quantitative research design.

In nonexperimental designs, the independent variables have naturally occurred, so to speak, and the investigator cannot directly control them by manipulation. As the researcher does not actively manipulate the variables, the concepts of control and potential sources of bias (see Chapter 8) should be considered. Nonexperimental designs provide Level IV evidence (see Chapter 1). The information yielded by these designs is critical for developing an evidence-based practice and may represent the best evidence available to answer research or clinical questions.

Researchers are not in agreement on how to classify nonexperimental designs. The types of quantitative research design are presented in Fig. 10.1. Nonexperimental designs explore the relationships or the differences between variables. This chapter divides nonexperimental designs into survey and relationship/difference designs as illustrated in Box 10.1. These categories are somewhat flexible, and other sources may classify nonexperimental designs differently. Some studies fall exclusively within one of these categories, whereas other studies have characteristics of more than one category (Table 10.1). As you read studies, you

---

BOX 10.1 Summary of Nonexperimental Research Designs

I. Survey Designs
  A. Descriptive
  B. Exploratory
  C. Comparative

II. Relationship/Difference Designs
  A. Correlational
  B. Developmental
    1. Cross-sectional
    2. Cohort, longitudinal, and prospective
    3. Case control, retrospective, and ex post facto

TABLE 10.1 Examples of Studies with More Than One Design Label

Design Type	Study's Purpose
Cross-sectional, correlational study	To compare select maternal sleep (sleep quality, caregiver stress, and other sociodemographic variables) and child characteristics (sleep and behavior problems) between mothers with worse mental and physical health and those with better mental and physical health and to determine the contribution of selected characteristics on mental and physical health in mothers of school-age children (6–12) with developmental disabilities (Lee et al., 2018)
Delphi Method/ SURVEY	To identify and agree on a risk assessment and monitoring process for patients at risk of HIV-associated cognitive disorder. Twenty-five experts from four community health centers participated in three rounds of a modified Delphi Survey to reach consensus on the risk assessment tool (Cummins et al., 2019)
Descriptive, secondary analysis of a randomized controlled trial	To identify subgroups of Latina breast cancer survivors who have distinct symptoms profiles while receiving radiation, chemotherapy, and or hormonal therapy. The secondary analysis included intake data from three randomized trials of supportive care psychosocial interventions for Latinas treated for breast cancer ($n = 290$). Prevalence of 12 symptoms, measured using the General Symptom Distress Scale, was entered into the latent class analysis to identify women with different symptom profiles (Crane et al., 2020).
Longitudinal, descriptive	A longitudinal design was used to collect data at three time periods: within 1 month of cancer diagnosis, at 6 months after diagnosis, and at 18 months after diagnosis (Kessler, 2020).

PA, Physical activity; *SEER,* Surveillance, Epidemiology, and End Results.

CRITICAL THINKING DECISION PATH

Nonexperimental Design Choice

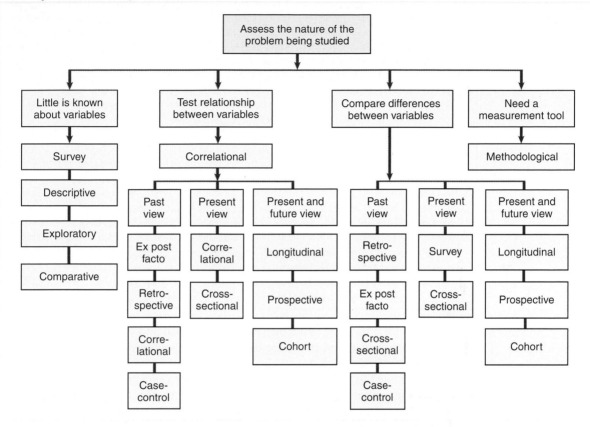

will often find that researchers use several design classifications for one study. This chapter introduces types of nonexperimental designs and discusses their advantages and disadvantages, how nonexperimental designs are used, issues of causality, as well as critical appraisal of nonexperimental designs. The Critical Thinking Decision Path outlines the path to choosing the appropriate nonexperimental design.

EVIDENCE-BASED PRACTICE TIPS

When critically appraising nonexperimental studies, you must be aware of possible sources of bias that can be introduced at any point in the study.

SURVEY DESIGNS

The broadest category of nonexperimental designs is the survey design. Survey designs are further classified as *descriptive, exploratory,* or *comparative.* Surveys collect detailed descriptions of variables and use the data to justify and assess conditions and practices or

---

BOX 10.2   Survey Design Examples

Pontes and colleagues (2020) conducted a secondary analysis of data from a national survey, the Youth Risk Behavior Scale (YRBS), administered to high school students biennially by the Centers for Disease Control and Prevention (CDC) since 1991. The survey assesses depressive symptoms, suicidal ideation, suicide attempts, and suicide attempts that required treatment by a doctor or nurse. This analysis of YRBS survey data for the years 2009 to 2017 investigated additive interactions between female gender in relation to the above symptoms. The findings reveal that during this time frame, suicide attempts increased substantially for female students but not for male students. These survey data support the need for training of nurses and other health professionals about the importance of primary prevention efforts for both males and females from early adolescence through the transition to early adulthood in mental health and primary care settings using evidence-based "gatekeeper" screening such as Applied Suicide Interventions Skills (Bolster, Holliday, Oneal and Shaw, 2015).

   The World Health Organization has designated vaccine hesitancy as 1 of the 10 leading threats to global health, yet there is limited current national data on prevalence of hesitancy among US parents. A survey was conducted using a nationally representative sample of US parents. The survey aimed to (1) assess and compare prevalence of hesitancy and factors driving hesitancy for routine childhood and influenza vaccination and (2) examine associations between sociodemographic characteristics and hesitancy for routine childhood or influenza vaccination. In February 2019, the research team surveyed families with children using the largest online panel generating representative US samples. After weighting, we assessed hesitancy using a modified 5-point Vaccine Hesitancy Scale and labeled parents as hesitant if they scored >3. A total of 2176 of 4445 parents sampled completed the survey (response rate 49%). The survey data revealed that almost 1 in 15 US parents are hesitant about routine childhood vaccination, whereas >1 in 4 are hesitant about influenza vaccination. Furthermore, 1 in 8 parents are concerned about vaccine safety for both routine childhood and influenza vaccines, and only 1 in 4 believe influenza vaccine is effective. Vaccination hesitancy, particularly for influenza vaccine, is prevalent in the United States (Kempe et al., 2020).

---

to make plans for improving health care practices. You will find that the terms *exploratory, descriptive, comparative,* and *survey* are used either alone, interchangeably, or together to describe a survey study (see Table 10.1).

- A survey is used to search for information about the characteristics of particular subjects, groups, populations, institutions, or situations, or about the frequency of a variable's occurrence, particularly when little is known. Box 10.2 provides examples of survey designs.
- Variables can be classified as opinions, attitudes, or facts.
- Fact variables include gender, income level, political and religious affiliations, ethnicity, occupation, and educational level.
- Surveys can provide the basis for the development of intervention studies.
- Surveys are described as comparative when used to determine differences between variables.
- Survey data can be collected with a questionnaire or an interview (see Chapter 14).
- Surveys have small or large samples of subjects drawn from defined populations, can be either broad or narrow, and are composed of people or institutions.
- Surveys relate one variable to another or assess differences between variables, but they do not determine causation.

The advantages of surveys are that a great deal of information can be obtained from a large population in a fairly economical manner, and survey research information can be surprisingly accurate. If a sample is representative of the population (see Chapter 12), even a relatively small number of subjects can provide an accurate picture of the population.

Surveys do have disadvantages. The information obtained in a survey tends to be superficial. The breadth rather than the depth of the information is emphasized.

> **EVIDENCE-BASED PRACTICE TIP**
>
> Evidence gained from a survey may be coupled with clinical expertise and applied to a similar population to develop an educational program to enhance knowledge and skills in a particular clinical area (e.g., a survey designed to measure the nursing staff's knowledge and attitudes about evidence-based practice in which the data are used to develop an evidence-based practice staff development course).

> **HELPFUL HINT**
>
> You should recognize that a well-constructed survey can provide a wealth of data about a particular phenomenon of interest, even though causation is not being examined.

RELATIONSHIP AND DIFFERENCE DESIGNS

Investigators also try to assess the relationships or differences between variables that can provide insight into a phenomenon. The following types of **relationship/difference designs** are discussed: correlational and developmental designs.

Correlational Designs

In a study that uses a **correlational design**, the *relationship* between two or more variables is examined. The researcher does not test whether one variable causes another variable. Rather, the researcher is interested in the following:

- Whether the variables co-vary (i.e., As one variable changes, does a related change occur in another variable?)
- Quantifying the strength of the relationship between variables, or in testing a hypothesis or research question about a specific relationship

The direction of the relationship is important (see Chapter 16 for an explanation of the correlation coefficient). For example, a correlational study by Zhu and colleagues (2019) examined the relationship between fatigue, sleep disturbance, and eating styles in adults with type 2 diabetes (T2D) and found fatigue and sleep disturbance were common in people with T2D, and fatigue accounted for a significant amount of variation in eating style over and above that accounted for by subject characteristics.. Thus the variables were related to (not causal of) outcomes. Each step of this study was consistent with the aims of exploring relationships among variables.

When reviewing a correlational study, remember what relationship the researcher tested and whether the researcher implied a relationship that is consistent with the theoretical framework (see Chapter 4) and research question(s) or hypotheses (see Chapter 2). Correlational designs offer the following advantages:

- An efficient and effective method of collecting a large amount of data about a problem
- A potential for evidence-based application in clinical settings
- A potential foundation for future experimental research studies
- A framework for exploring the relationship between variables that cannot be manipulated
  The following are disadvantages of correlational designs:
- Variables are not manipulated.
- Randomization is not used because the groups are preexisting, and therefore generalizability is decreased.
- A causal relationship cannot be determined between the variables because of a lack of manipulation, control, and randomization.
- The strength and quality of evidence is limited by the associative nature of the relationship between the variables.

Correlational designs may be further labeled as *descriptive correlational* or *predictive correlational*. Based on the literature review and findings, researchers frame the utility of the results in light of previous research that help establish the "best available" evidence that, combined with clinical expertise, informs clinical decisions for a specific patient population. A correlational design is very useful for clinical studies because many of the phenomena of clinical interest are beyond the researcher's ability to manipulate, control, and randomize.

IPE HIGHLIGHT

When your quality improvement team's search for intervention studies reporting evidence-based strategies for preventing ventilator-acquired pneumonia (VAP) yields only studies using nonexperimental designs, your team members should debate whether the evidence is of sufficient quality to be applied to answering your clinical question.

Developmental Designs

There are also nonexperimental designs that use a time perspective. Investigators who use **developmental designs** are concerned not only with the existing status and the relationship and differences among phenomena at one point in time but also with changes that result from elapsed time. The following types of designs are discussed: cross-sectional, cohort/longitudinal/prospective, and case control/retrospective/ex post facto. In the literature, these studies may be designated by more than one design name. This practice is accepted because many studies have elements of several designs. Table 10.1 provides examples of studies classified with more than one design label.

EVIDENCE-BASED PRACTICE TIPS

Replication of significant findings in nonexperimental studies with similar and/or different populations increases your confidence in the conclusions offered by the research and the strength of evidence generated by consistent findings from more than one study that uses a nonexperimental design.

Cross-Sectional Designs

A **cross-sectional design** examines data at one point in time; that is, data are collected on only one occasion with the same subjects rather than with the same subjects at several time points. For example, Enrico et al. (2020) conducted a cross-sectional study (Appendix D) to evaluate whether the stress level of caregivers was related to their perception of the need for health care education in family caregivers of patients with Parkinson disease. The researchers assessed the relationship of various interventions and stress-related vulnerability to assess which interventions were perceived to be more positively associated with usefulness for families of patients with Parkinson disease.

As you review the findings of this study, you will note that the variables studied were related to, not causal of, the outcomes. Each step of this study was consistent with the aims of exploring the relationship among variables in a cross-sectional design. Cross-sectional designs can explore relationships and correlations, or differences and comparisons, or both. Advantages and disadvantages of cross-sectional designs are as follows:

- Cross-sectional designs, compared with longitudinal/cohort/prospective designs are less time-consuming, less expensive, and thus more manageable.

- Large amounts of data can be collected at one point, making results more readily available.
- The confounding variable of maturation, resulting from the elapsed time, is not present.
- The ability to establish an in-depth developmental assessment of the relationships of the variables being studied is lessened. The researcher is unable to determine whether the change that occurred is related to the change that was predicted because the same subjects were not followed over a period of time. In other words, the subjects are unable to serve as their own controls (see Chapter 8).

Cohort/Prospective/Longitudinal/Repeated Measures Designs

In contrast with the cross-sectional design, cohort studies collect data from the same group at different points in time. Cohort designs are also referred to as longitudinal, prospective, and repeated measures designs. These terms are interchangeable. Like cross-sectional studies, cohort studies explore differences and relationships among variables. An example of a longitudinal (cohort) study is found in the study by Cong and colleagues (2020). Over 10 years, this study prospectively collected biomarkers of inflammation, dietary assessment patterns, and depression in childhood. The researchers then assessed the incidence of depression in young adulthood and concluded that higher inflammatory dietary patterns in childhood were associated with higher depression risk in early adulthood.

Cohort designs have advantages and disadvantages. When assessing the appropriateness of a cross-sectional design versus a cohort design, you must first assess the research question or hypothesis: Cohort designs allow clinicians to assess the incidence of a problem over time and potential reasons for changes in the study's variables. However, the disadvantages inherent in a cohort design must be considered. Data collection may be of long duration; therefore subject loss or mortality can be high because of the time it takes for the subjects to progress to each data collection point. The internal validity threat of testing is also present and may be unavoidable in a cohort study. Subject loss to follow-up or attrition may lead to unintended sample bias affecting both the internal validity and external validity of the study (see Chapters 8 and 12).

These realities make a cohort study more costly in terms of time, effort, and money. There is also a chance of confounding variables that could affect interpretation of the results. Subjects may respond in a socially desirable way that they believe is congruent with the investigator's expectations (Hawthorne effect). Advantages of a cohort design are as follows:

- Each subject is followed separately and thereby serves as his or her own control.
- An increased depth of responses can be obtained, and early trends in the data can be analyzed.
- Changes in the variables of interest over time, and both relationships and differences can be explored between variables.

In summary, cohort designs begin in the present and end in the future, and cross-sectional designs look at a broader perspective of a population at a specific point in time.

Retrospective/Case Control/Ex Post Facto Designs

A retrospective design is essentially the same as a case control and an ex post facto design. In these designs, the dependent variable already has been affected by the independent variable, and the investigator attempts to link present events to events that occurred in the past. When researchers wish to explain causality or the factors that determine the occurrence of events or conditions, they prefer to use an experimental design. However, they cannot always manipulate the independent variable, or use random assignments. When experimental designs that test the effect of an intervention or condition cannot be employed,

TABLE 10.2	Paradigm for the Ex Post Facto Design	
Groups (Not Randomly Assigned)	**Independent Variable (Not Manipulated by Investigator)**	**Dependent Variable**
Exposed group: Cigarette smokers	X Cigarette smoking	Y_e Lung cancer
Control group: Nonsmokers	— —	Y_c No lung cancer

retrospective, case control, or ex post facto design may be used. *Ex post facto* literally means "from after the fact." Case control, ex post facto, retrospective, or case control designs also are known as *causal-comparative* designs or *comparative* designs. As we discuss this design further, you will see that many elements of this category are similar to quasi-experimental designs because they explore differences between variables (Campbell & Stanley, 1963).

In case control designs, a researcher hypothesizes, for instance:

- That X (cigarette smoking) is related to and a determinant of Y (lung cancer).
- But X, the presumed cause, is not manipulated, and subjects are not randomly assigned to groups.
- Rather, a group of subjects who have experienced X (cigarette smoking) in a normal situation is located, and a control group of subjects who have not experienced X is chosen.
- The behavior, performance, or condition (lung tissue) of the two groups is compared to determine whether the exposure to X had the effect predicted by the hypothesis.

Table 10.2 illustrates this example. Examination of Table 10.2 reveals that although cigarette smoking appears to be a determinant of lung cancer, the researcher is still not able to conclude that a causal relationship exists between the variables because the independent variable was not manipulated and the subjects were not randomly assigned to groups.

Flanders and colleagues (2020) (Appendix C) conducted a retrospective study to explore the effectiveness of a staff resilience program in a pediatric intensive care unit. The findings indicate that offering a resilience program coupled with interventions designed to promote resilience assisted in the reduction of compassion fatigue for nurses in the pediatric intensive care unit.

EVIDENCE-BASED PRACTICE TIPS

The quality of evidence provided by a cohort/longitudinal/prospective study is stronger than that from other non-experimental designs because the researcher can determine the incidence of a problem and its possible causes.

The advantages of the retrospective/case control/ex post facto design are similar to those of the correlational design. The additional benefit is that it offers an additional level of control not offered by a study using a correlational design, thereby increasing the confidence you would have in the evidence provided by the findings.

Retrospective/case control designs often are used to assess the influence of the social determinants of health on health disparities in relation to targeted population health conditions like diabetes, hypertension, asthma, and other chronic health problems. During the COVID-19 pandemic, retrospective data indicated that race/ethnicity were significant contributors to the disparity in populations at risk for and having the coronavirus. For example, retrospective data about the rate of COVID-19 cases among Black or African

American non-Hispanic persons was 2.6 times higher compared with White non-Hispanic persons. Hospitalizations were 4.7 times higher and 2.1 times higher in comparison with the same population (CDC, 2020). Findings from retrospective/case control studies reveal important population health data that highlight gaps in meeting the public health needs of targeted populations. However, it is important to remember that researchers remain unable to draw a causal linkage between independent and dependent variables. This is the major disadvantage of the retrospective/ex post facto/case control design.

Another disadvantage is the problem of an alternative hypothesis as the reason for the documented relationship. If the researcher obtains data from two existing groups of subjects, such as one that has been exposed to X and one that has not, and the data support the hypothesis that X is related to Y, the researcher cannot be sure whether X or some extraneous variable is the real cause of the occurrence of Y. As such, the impact or effect of the relationship cannot be estimated accurately. Finding naturally occurring groups of subjects who are similar in all respects except for their exposure to the variable of interest is very difficult. There is always the possibility that the groups differ in some other way that can affect the findings of the study and produce spurious or unreliable results. Consequently, you must cautiously evaluate the conclusions drawn by the investigator.

> **HELPFUL HINT**
>
> When reading research reports, you will note that at times researchers classify a study's design with more than one design type label. This is correct because research studies often reflect aspects of more than one design label.

Cohort/longitudinal/prospective designs are considered to be stronger than case control/retrospective designs because of the degree of control that can be imposed on extraneous variables that might confound the data and lead to bias.

> **HELPFUL HINT**
>
> Remember that nonexperimental designs can test relationships, differences, comparisons, or predictions, depending on the purpose of the study.

PREDICTION AND CAUSALITY IN NONEXPERIMENTAL RESEARCH

A concern of researchers and research consumers is the issues of prediction and causality. Researchers are interested in explaining cause-and-effect relationships—that is, estimating the effect of one phenomenon on another without bias. Historically, researchers thought that only findings from experimental research studies could support the concept of causality. For example, if nurses who are interested in discovering what causes anxiety were able to uncover the causes, they could develop interventions that would prevent or decrease the anxiety. Causality makes it necessary to order events chronologically; that is, if we find in a study in which subjects are randomly assigned that event 1 (stress) occurs before event 2 (anxiety) and that those in the stressed group were anxious whereas those in the unstressed group were not, we can say that the hypothesis of stress causing anxiety is supported by empirical data. If these results were found in a nonexperimental study in which some subjects underwent the stress of surgery and were anxious and others did not have surgery and were not anxious, we would say that there is an association or relationship between stress (surgery) and anxiety. But on the basis of the results of a nonexperimental study, we could not say that the stress of surgery caused the anxiety.

EVIDENCE-BASED PRACTICE TIPS

Studies that use nonexperimental designs often precede and provide the data and foundation for building a program of research that leads to experimental designs that test the effectiveness of nursing interventions.

Many variables (e.g., anxiety, vaping, and screening tests) that nurse researchers wish to study cannot be manipulated, nor would it be wise or ethical to manipulate them. Yet there is a need to have studies that can assert a predictive or causal sequence. In light of this need, many nurse researchers are using several analytical techniques that can explain the relationships among variables to establish predictive or causal links. These analytical techniques are called *causal modeling, model testing,* and *associated causal analysis techniques* (Hernan & Robins, 2018, Kline, 2011; Plichta & Kelvin, 2013).

When reading studies, you also will find the terms *path analysis,* LISREL, *analysis of covariance structures, structural equation modeling (SEM),* and *hierarchical linear modeling (HLM)* to describe the statistical techniques (see Chapter 16) used in these studies. These terms do not designate the design of a study, but are statistical tests that are used in many nonexperimental designs to predict how precisely a dependent variable can be predicted based on an independent variable. For example, Moeinslam and colleagues (2020) used SEM to understand quality of life in women with diabetes and health-related quality of life in the whole family. SEM was used to evaluate the network of associations among quality of life, diabetes, and the impact on each family member. This sophisticated design aids understanding how diabetes in women influences their quality of life and affects the quality of life in family members. When developing interventions for either the women or targeted family members, these data will guide structuring of the interventions.

Many studies test models. The statistics used in model-testing studies are advanced, but you should be able to read the article, understand the purpose of the study, and determine whether the model generated was logical and developed and supported by solid evidence from the literature and past research findings.

HELPFUL HINT

Nonexperimental research studies have progressed to the point where prediction models are often used to explore or test relationships between independent and dependent variables.

ADDITIONAL TYPES OF QUANTITATIVE METHODS

Other types of quantitative studies complement the science of research. The additional research methods provide a means of viewing and interpreting phenomena that give further breadth and knowledge to nursing science and practice. The additional types include methodological research, secondary analysis, and mixed methods.

Methodological Research

Methodological research is the development and evaluation of data collection instruments, scales, or strategies. As you will find in Chapters 14 and 15, methodology greatly influences research and the evidence produced.

The most significant and critically important aspect of methodological research addressed in measurement development is called **psychometrics**. Psychometrics focuses on the theory and development of measurement instruments (such as questionnaires) or measurement strategies (such as observational) using the research process. Nurse researchers use psychometric principles to develop and test measurement instruments that focus on nursing phenomena. Many of the phenomena of interest to practice and research are intangible, such as interpersonal conflict, resilience, quality of life, coping, and symptom experience. The intangible nature of various phenomena—yet the recognition of the need to measure them—places methodological research in an important position. Methodological research differs from other research designs in two ways. First, it does not include all steps of the research process as discussed in Chapter 1. Second, to develop a measurement instrument, the researcher must have a sound knowledge of psychometrics or must consult with a researcher knowledgeable about psychometric strategies. The methodological researcher is not interested in the relationship of the independent variable and dependent variable or in the effect of an independent variable on a dependent variable. The methodological researcher is interested in identifying an intangible construct (concept) and making it tangible and measurable with a paper-and-pencil instrument or observation protocol.

A methodological study basically includes the following steps:

- Define the concept or behavior to be measured
- Formulate the instrument's items
- Develop instructions for users and respondents
- Test the instrument's reliability and validity

These steps require a sound, specific, and exhaustive literature review to identify the theories underlying the concept (see Chapter 3). The literature review provides the basis for item formulation. Once the items have been developed, the researcher assesses the tool's reliability and validity (see Chapter 15). As an example of methodological research, Dennis and colleagues (2018) identified that the concept of childcare stress has been shown to predict postpartum depression. A review of the literature identified that there is little research exploring and validating the dimensions of childcare stress instruments so preventive interventions can be developed. Moreover, the literature review revealed inconsistencies in the conceptualization and operationalization of childcare stress. The aim of this methodological study was to develop and psychometrically test a simple childcare stress questionnaire that can be quickly administered with clearly defined dimensions to promote development of preventive interventions. The researchers developed and psychometrically tested The Postpartum Childcare Stress Checklist (PCSC) designed to measure parental perceptions of childcare stress in the early postpartum period (see Chapter 15). Common considerations that researchers incorporate into methodological research are outlined in Table 10.3. Many more examples of methodological research can be found in the research literature. The specific procedures of methodological research are beyond the scope of this book, but you are urged to closely review the instruments used in studies.

Secondary Analysis

Secondary analysis is also not a design but rather a research method in which the researcher takes previously collected and analyzed data from *one* study and reanalyzes the data or a subset of the data for a *secondary* purpose. The original study may be either an experimental or a nonexperimental design. As large data sets become more available, secondary analysis has become more prominent and a useful methodology for answering questions related to

TABLE 10.3 **Common Considerations in the Development of Measurement Tools**	
Consideration	**Example**
A well-constructed scale, test, or interview schedule should consist of an objective, standardized measure of a behavior that has been clearly defined.	Zhang and Ganocy (2020) provided a comprehensive literature review that documented that existing measures do not assess the physical underpinnings of irritability for people with cancer. The literature review supports definitions of the concepts that were operationalized for the Irritability Scale-Initial Version (TISi).
Observations should be made on a small but carefully chosen sampling of the behavior of interest, thus permitting the reader to feel confident that the samples are representative.	Zhang and Ganocy (2020) piloted the instrument for assessing irritability of cancer patients on three dimensions: physical, affective, and behavioral. The authors conducted three pilot studies to develop the 35-item TISi on a 5-point Likert scale. The TISi was tested in 48 early-stage, nonmetastasized breast cancer patients at baseline and 3 months (during chemotherapy) to determine the clarity and sufficiency of the items.
An instrument should be standardized. It should be a set of uniform items and response possibilities, uniformly administered and scored.	Based on the initial pilot test of the instrument. the 35-item scale was developed using a 5-point Likert scale. Ninety-three items were generated and administered to nine consenting cancer patients for testing the appropriateness for wording and the rating scale.
The item types should be limited in the type of variations. Subjects who are expected to shift from one type of item to another may fail to provide a true response as a result of the distraction of making such a change.	Mixing true-or-false items with questions that require a yes-or-no response and items that provide a response format of five possible answers is conducive to a high level of measurement error. The TISi contained only a 5-point Likert scale with responses ranging from never to frequently.
An instrument's diagnostic, predictive, or measurement value depends on the degree to which it serves as an indicator of a relatively broad and significant behavior area, known as the *universe of content* for the behavior. A behavior must be clearly defined before it can be measured. The extent to which test items appear to accomplish this objective is an indication of the instrument's reliability and content and/or construct validity (see Chapter 15).	The TISi demonstrates high internal consistency reliability (Cronbach's alpha = .97), satisfactory test-retest reliability (r = .69). A confirmatory factor analysis yields evidence of construct validity with three factor loadings that align with the conceptualization of the subscales.
An instrument should adequately cover the defined behavior and whether the concept and its multidimensionality are accurately measured.	Zhang and Ganocy (2020) suggest that the findings support the psychometric properties of the TISi and its application for assessing physical, affective, and behavioral manifestations of irritability in people with cancer.
Appropriate discussion of limitations and future instrument development should be identified.	Zhang and Ganocy (2020) clearly identify that future investigations using a large study sample is necessary for improving the construct and criterion validity and reducing item redundancy.

WECS, Women's experience in childbirth survey.

population health issues. Data for secondary analysis may be derived from a large clinical trial and data available through large health care organizations and databases. For example, Bourque and Goldstein (2019) reported on findings of a secondary analysis of communication functions and modalities used in a specific subset of the parent study, minimally verbal preschoolers with severe autism spectrum disorder, from a previous clinical trial by Thiemann-Bourque, Feldmiller Hoffman & Johner (2018). In the parent study, the researchers tested modalities to ensure that others in the environment, such as peers without disabilities, could communicate with the autistic children. Secondary analysis studies have the potential to improve clinical assessment and intervention in specific targeted subpopulations of larger studies.

Mixed Methods

Over the years, studies that use **mixed methods** have been defined in various ways. Historically mixed methods included the use of multimethod research or thought. This means use of a variety of data sources in one study, such as use of different investigators, use of multiple theories in one study, or use of multiple designs and/or methods (Denzin, 1978). The definition and core characteristics that integrate the diverse meaning of mixed methods research are as follows:

In mixed methods, the researcher:

- "Based on the research question collects and analyzes both qualitative and quantitative data
- Mixes the two forms of data concurrently by combining the data
- Gives priority to one or both forms of data in terms of emphasis
- Uses the procedures of both in one study or in multiple phases of a program of study
- Frames the procedures within congruent philosophical worldviews and theoretical lenses
- Combines the procedures into specific research designs that direct the plan for conducting the study" (Creswell & Plano Clark, 2017, pp. 5–6).

The order of data collection in a mixed methods study varies depending on the question that a researcher wishes to answer. In a mixed methods study, the quantitative data may be collected simultaneously with the qualitative data, or one may follow the other. Studying a research question using both methods can contribute to a better understanding of an area of research. An example of a mixed methods study was completed by Jang and colleagues (2019). The aim of the study was to examine the relationships among parental psychological distress, parental feeding practices, child diet, and child body mass index (BMI) in families with young children. The background of the study was based on the concept that parents often play a significant role in establishing the dietary patterns of young children. A gap in the literature revealed that there is no clear understanding about the relationship between parental psychological distress and children's diet and BMI. The quantitative portion was predominant and included well-validated questionnaires completed by parents ($n = 256$ families) that included demographic data, parental general stress, parenting stress, parental sleep quality, parental depressive symptoms, social support for parents, mealtime environment, child feeding practices, child diet, and BMI. For the qualitative component that followed the quantitative data collection, the research team interviewed a subsample of 13 parents. The sequential mixed methods design of this study allowed the research team to understand stressed parents' practices in feeding and food preparation for their preschool children. Among the findings, the data reveal that higher parental psychological distress was associated with higher unhealthy feeding practices ($p < .01$). However, a parental unhealthy feeding practice was not significantly associated with a child's unhealthy diet or BMI. The main theme from the analysis of parent interviews was that parent stress and fatigue influenced their feeding and food preparation. The findings highlight potential foci for intervention programs to address parental psychological distress. Future research may focus on interventions that decrease the risk for parents living in high-stress environments (e.g., neighborhoods with a high rate of food insecurity and unemployment and a lack of safe public transportation) and the impact of those interventions on stress and unhealthy feeding practices.

There is a diversity of opinion on how to evaluate mixed methods designs. Evaluation can include analyzing the quantitative and qualitative designs of the study separately, or, as proposed by Creswell and Plano Clark (2017), there should be a separate set of criteria for mixed methods studies dependent on the designs and methods used.

HELPFUL HINT

As you read the literature, you will find labels such as *outcomes research, needs assessments, evaluation research,* and *quality assurance.* These studies are not designs per se. These studies use either experimental or nonexperimental designs. Studies with these labels are designed to test the effectiveness of health care techniques, programs, or interventions. When reading such a research study, the reader should assess which design was used and if the principles of the design, sampling strategy, and analysis are consistent with the study's purpose.

≫ APPRAISAL FOR EVIDENCE-BASED PRACTICE
NONEXPERIMENTAL DESIGNS

Criteria for appraising nonexperimental designs are presented in the Critical Appraisal Criteria box. When appraising nonexperimental research designs, keep in mind that such designs offer the researcher a lower level of control and an increased risk for bias. The level of evidence provided by nonexperimental designs is not as strong as evidence generated by experimental or quasi-experimental designs. However, there are important clinical research questions that must be answered beyond the testing of interventions and experimental or quasi-experimental designs.

The first step in critiquing nonexperimental designs is to determine which type of design was used in the study. Often a statement describing the design of the study appears in the "Abstract" and in the "Methods" section of the report. If such a statement is not present, you should closely examine the paper for evidence of which type of design was employed. You should be able to discern that either a survey or a relationship design was used. For example, you would expect an investigation of self-concept development in children from birth to 5 years of age to be a relationship study using a cohort/prospective/**longitudinal design**. If a cohort/prospective/longitudinal design was used, you should assess for possible threats to internal validity or bias, such as mortality, testing, and instrumentation. Potential threats to internal or external validity should be recognized by the researchers at the end of a study and, in particular, in the "Limitations" section.

Next, the researcher evaluates the literature review of the study to determine whether a nonexperimental design was the most appropriate approach to the research question or hypothesis. For example, many studies on pain (e.g., intensity, severity, perception) are suggestive of a relationship between pain and any of the independent variables (diagnosis, coping style, and ethnicity) under consideration where the independent variable cannot be manipulated. These studies suggest using a nonexperimental correlational, longitudinal/prospective/cohort, retrospective/ex post facto/case control, or cross-sectional design. Investigators will use one of these designs to examine the relationship between the variables in naturally occurring groups. Sometimes you may think that it would have been more appropriate if the investigators had used an experimental or a quasi-experimental design. However, you must recognize that pragmatic or ethical considerations also may have guided the researchers in their choice of design (see Chapters 8 to 18).

CRITICAL APPRAISAL CRITERIA
Nonexperimental Designs

1. Based on the theoretical framework, is the rationale for the type of design appropriate?
2. How is the design congruent with the purpose of the study?
3. Is the design appropriate for the research question or hypothesis?
4. How do the data collection methods align with the design?
5. How does the researcher present the findings in a manner congruent with the design used?
6. Does the research go beyond the relational parameters of the findings and erroneously infer cause-and-effect relationships between the variables?
7. Where appropriate, how does the researcher discuss the threats to internal validity (bias) and external validity (generalizability)?
8. How does the author identify the limitations of the study?
9. Does the researcher make appropriate recommendations about the applicability based on the strength and quality of evidence provided by the nonexperimental design and the findings?

Finally, the factor or factors that actually influence changes in the dependent variable can be ambiguous in nonexperimental designs. As with all complex phenomena, multiple factors can contribute to variability in the subjects' responses. When an experimental design is not used for controlling some of these extraneous variables that can influence results, the researcher must strive to provide as much control as possible within the context of a nonexperimental design, to decrease bias. For example, when it has not been possible to randomly assign subjects to treatment groups as an approach to controlling an independent variable, the researchers will use strict inclusion and exclusion criteria and calculate an adequate sample size using power analysis that will support valid testing of the research question or hypothesis (see Chapter 12). Threats to internal and external validity or potential sources of bias represent a major influence when interpreting the findings of a nonexperimental study because they impose limitations to the generalizability of the results. It is also important to remember that prediction of patient clinical outcomes is of critical value for clinical researchers. Nonexperimental designs can be used to make predictions if the study is designed with an adequate sample size (see Chapter 12), collects data consistently, and uses reliable and valid instruments (see Chapter 15).

If you are appraising methodological research, you must apply the principles of reliability and validity (see Chapter 15). A secondary analysis must be reviewed from several perspectives. First, you must understand if the researcher followed sound scientific logic in the secondary analysis completed. Second, you must review the original study that the data were extracted from to assess the rigor of the original study. Even though the format and methods vary, it is important to remember that all research has a central goal: to answer questions scientifically and provide the strongest, most consistent evidence possible, while controlling for potential bias. A study using a mixed methods approach should be assessed to determine whether both the quantitative and qualitative components of the study were conducted appropriately. It also is interesting to note whether the researcher indicated which type of design was the predominant one, as was reported in the study by Jang and colleagues (2019) described earlier in this chapter.

KEY POINTS

- Nonexperimental designs are used in studies that construct a picture or make an account of events as they naturally occur.
- Nonexperimental designs can be classified as either survey studies or relationship/difference designs.
- Survey designs and relationship/difference designs are both descriptive and exploratory in nature.
- Survey designs collect detailed descriptions of existing phenomena and use the data either to validate current conditions and practices or to make more informed plans for improvement.
- Correlational designs examine relationships.
- Developmental designs are further broken down into categories of cross-sectional designs, cohort/longitudinal/prospective designs, and case control/retrospective/ex post facto designs.
- Methodological research, secondary analysis, and mixed methods are examples of other means of adding to the body of nursing research. Both the researcher and the reader must consider the advantages and disadvantages of each design.
- Nonexperimental research designs do not enable the investigator to establish cause-and-effect relationships between the variables. Consumers must be wary of nonexperimental studies that make causal claims about the findings unless a causal modeling technique is used.
- Nonexperimental designs also offer the researcher the least amount of control. Threats to validity impose limitations on the generalizability of the results and as such should be fully assessed by the critical reader.
- The critical appraisal process is directed toward evaluating the appropriateness of the selected nonexperimental design in relation to factors, such as the research problem, theoretical framework, hypothesis, methodology, and data analysis and interpretation.
- Though nonexperimental designs do not provide the highest level of evidence (Level IV), they do provide a wealth of data that become useful pieces for formulating both Level I and Level II studies that are aimed at developing and testing nursing interventions.

CLINICAL JUDGMENT CHALLENGES

- **IPE** The mid-term assignment for your interprofessional research course is to critically appraise an assigned study on the relationship of perception of pain severity and quality of life in advanced cancer patients. You and your student nurse colleagues think it is a cross-sectional design, but your medical student colleagues think it is a quasi-experimental design because it has several specific hypotheses. How would each group of students support their argument, and how would they collaborate to resolve their differences?
- You are completing your senior practicum on a surgical unit, and for preconference your student group has just completed a search for studies related to the effectiveness of handwashing in decreasing the incidence of nosocomial infections, but the studies all use an ex post facto/case control design. You want to approach the nurse manager on the unit to present the evidence you have collected and critically appraised, but you are concerned about the strength of the evidence because the studies all use a nonexperimental design. How would you justify that this is the "best available evidence"?

REFERENCES

Bourque, K. S., & Goldstein, H. (2019). Expanding communications modalities expanding communication modalities and functions for preschoolers with autism spectrum disorder: Secondary analysis of a peer partner speech-generating device intervention. *Journal of Speech Hearing Language & Hearing Research, 2019 Dec 19, 63*(1), 190–205. https://doi.org/10.1044/2019_JSLHR-19-00202.

Campbell, D. T., & Stanley, J. C. (1963). *Experimental and quasi-experimental designs for research.* Chicago, IL: Rand-McNally.

Cong, X., Tracy, M., Edmunds, L. S., Hosler, A. S., Appleton, A. A. (2020). The relationship between inflammatory dietary pattern in childhood and depression in early adulthood. *Brain, Behavior & Immunity* – Health. 10.1016/j.bbih.2019.100017. COVID.NET. https://www.cdc.gov/coronavirus/2019-data/covidview/index.html,accessed08/06/20.

Crane, T. E., Badger, T. A., Sikorski, A., Segrin, C., Hsu, C.-H., & Rosenfeld, A. G. (2020). Symptom profiles of Latina breast cancer survivors: A latent class analysis. *Nursing Research, 69*(4), 264–271.

Creswell, J. W., & Plano Clark, V. L. (2017). *Designing and conducting mixed methods research* (3rd ed). Thousand Oaks, CA: Sage Publications.

Cummins, D., Waters, D., Aggar, C., & O'Connor, C. C. (2019). Assessing risk of HIV-associated neurocognitive disorder. *Nursing Research, 68*(1), 22–28.

Dennis, C. L., Brown, H. K., & Brennenstuhl, S. (2018). Development, psychometric assessment and predictive validity of the postpartum childcare stress checklist. *Nursing Research, 67*(6), 439–446.

Denzin, N. K. (1978). *The research act: A theoretical introduction to sociological methods.* New York: McGraw Hill.

Di Stasio, E., Di Simone, E., Galeti, A., Donati, D., Guidotti, C., et al. (2020). Stress-related vulnerability and usefulness of healthcare education in Parkinson's disease: The perception of a group of family caregivers, a cross-sectional study. *Applied Nursing Research, 51*, 1–5.

Flanders, S., Hampton, D., Missi, P., Ipsan, C., & Gruebbel, C. (2020). Effectiveness of a staff resilience program in a pediatric intensive care unit. *Journal of Pediatric Nursing, 50*, 1–4.

Hernán, M. A. (2018). The C-word: Scientific euphemisms do not improve causal inference from observational data (with discussion). *American Journal of Public Health, 108*(5), 616–619.

Jang, M., Brandon, D., & Vorderstrasse, A. (2019). Relationships among parental psychological distress, parental feeding practices, child diet, and child body mass index. *Nursing Research, 68*(4), 296–306.

Kempe, A., Saville, A. W., Albertin, C., Zimet, G., Breck, A., Helmkamp, L., Vangala, S., Dickinson, L. M., Rand, C., Humiston, S., & Szilagyi, P. G. (2020). Parental hesitancy about routine childhood and influenza vaccinations: A national survey. *Pediatrics, 146*(1), e20193852. https://doi.org/10.1542/peds.2019-3852.

Kessler, T. A. (2020). The role of cognitive appraisal in quality of life over time in patients with cancer. *Oncology Nursing Forum, 47*(3), 292–304. https://doi.org/10.1188/20.NF.292-304.

Lee, J., Hayat, M. J., Spratling, R., Sevcik, R. A., & Clark, P. C. (2018). Relationship of mother's mental and physical health to characteristics of mothers and children with developmental disabilities. *Nursing Research, 67*(6), 456–464.

Moeineslam, M., Karmin, M., Jalai-Farahani, S., Shiva, N. & Azizi, F. (2019). Quality of life outcomes 5. doi:101186/s12955-019-1252-4.

Pontes, N. M. H., Ayres, C. G., & Pontes, M. C. F (2020). Trends in depressive symptoms and suicidality: Youth risk behavior survey 2009-2017. *Nursing Research, 69*(3), 176–185.

Zhang, A. Y., & Ganocy, S. J. (2020). Measurement of irritability in cancer patients. *Nursing Research, 69*(2), 91–99.

11

Appraising Systematic Reviews and Clinical Practice Guidelines

Geri LoBiondo-Wood

Go to Evolve at **http://evolve.elsevier.com/LoBiondo/** for review questions.

LEARNING OUTCOMES

After reading this chapter, you should be able to do the following:

- Describe the types of systematic reviews.
- Describe the components of systematic reviews.
- Differentiate between the types of systematic reviews.
- Describe the purpose of clinical guidelines.
- Differentiate between an expert and an evidence-based clinical guideline.
- Critically appraise systematic reviews and clinical practice guidelines.

KEY TERMS

AGREE II
clinical practice
   guidelines
effect size

evidence-based
   practice guidelines
expert-based practice
   guidelines

forest plot
integrative review
meta-analysis
narrative review

rapid review
realist review
scoping review
systematic review

The breadth and depth of clinical research have grown. As the number of studies focused on a similar area conducted by multiple research teams has increased, it has become important to have a means of organizing and assessing the quality, quantity, and consistency among the findings of a group of like studies. The goal of a systematic review is to organize the relevant studies in a focused clinical area. Clinical practice guidelines are informed by the findings of studies, systematic reviews, and expert opinion, and they are used for the development of standards of care, the foundation of the evidence-based practice necessary for the care we provide for individuals, families, and communities.

The previous chapters have introduced the types of qualitative and quantitative designs and how to critically appraise these studies for quality and applicability to practice. The purpose of this chapter is to acquaint you with the types of systematic reviews and clinical practice guidelines that assess multiple studies focused on the same clinical question, and how these reviews and guidelines support evidence-based practice. The terminology used to define systematic reviews and clinical practice guidelines has changed as this area of research and literature assessment has grown. The definitions used in this textbook are consistent with the definitions from the Cochrane Collaboration and the Preferred Reporting for

Systematic Reviews and Meta-Analyses (PRISMA) Group (Cochrane Website, 2020; Higgins & Thomas, 2019; Moher et al., 2009; Stroup et al., 2000). Systematic reviews and clinical guidelines are critical and meaningful for the development of evidence-based practice.

SYSTEMATIC REVIEW COMPONENTS

A systematic review is a review and summary of studies based on a focused clinical question that uses the PICO format discussed in Chapters 2 and 3. It uses a clearly defined search strategy to locate and assess the most current and valid research on intervention effectiveness and clinical knowledge, in an area that will ultimately inform evidence-based decision making. There are various types of reviews, terms, and methods used to systematically review the literature, depending on the review's purpose. Statistical methods may or may not be used to analyze the studies reviewed. If statistical methods are used to synthesize the studies, the review is known as a meta-analysis. A meta-analysis combines the statistical data from all of the included studies to arrive at a more precise estimate of the effect or outcome of the studies. The methods used to systematically review the literature will depend on the review's purpose. Often reviews are categorized under the general category of systematic review but each review type has explicit criteria dependent on its purpose. Basically a systematic review is a summation and assessment of research studies found in the literature. It starts with a clearly focused question called a *PICO question* that uses systematic and explicit criteria and methods to identify, select, critically appraise, and analyze relevant data from the selected studies to summarize the findings as highlighted in Box 11.1 (see Chapters 2 and 3). The components of a PICO question, sometimes identified as a clinical question consists of the following elements:

- Population (P): What is the population of interest?
- Intervention (I): What is the intervention of interest?
- Comparison (C): What will the intervention be compared with? *NB depending on the study design this step may not apply
- Outcome (O): How will you know if the intervention worked? A measurable outcome.

Based on the identified PICO question, the process of conducting a systematic review includes the following:

- Develop an explicit, rigorous reproducible criteria for the studies to be gathered based on the PICO question.
- Locate published and unpublished studies consistent with the PICO question.
- Critically appraise the strength and quality of the evidence in each individual study.
- Synthesize the overall strengths and weaknesses of studies as a group (see Chapter 19 for an example).

Based on the identified PICO question or clinical question, the process of conducting of a systematic review includes the following:

- Identify studies to be included based on rigorous study inclusion and exclusion criteria.
- Develop an explicit reproducible methodology to search for, identify, and collect the studies that meet the eligibility criteria.
- Critically appraise and synthesize of the strength and quality of the evidence in each individual study as well as all the studies as a whole (Moher et al., 2015a).

Systematic reviews may focus on quantitative studies solely, qualitative studies solely, or a mix of both qualitative and qualitative studies. The process for a systematic review of quantitative studies is slightly different than the process for evaluating those that are qualitative. Both quantitative and qualitative reviews begin with a PICO question. The difference

> **BOX 11.1   Systematic Review Components With or Without Meta-Analysis**
>
> **Introduction**
> Review of rationale and a clear clinical question (PICO)
>
> **Methods**
> Information sources, databases used, and search strategy identified: how studies were selected and data extracted as well as the variables extracted and defined
>   Description of methods used to assess risk for bias, summary measures identified (e.g., risk, ratio); identification of how data are combined, if studies are graded, what quality appraisal system was used (see Chapters 1, 17, and 18)
>
> **Results**
> Number of studies screened and characteristics, risk for bias within studies; if a meta-analysis, there will be a synthesis of results including confidence intervals, risk for bias for each study, and all outcomes considered
>
> **Discussion**
> Summary of findings, including the strength, quality, quantity, and consistency of the evidence for each outcome
>   Any limitations of the studies; conclusions and recommendations of findings for practice
>
> **Funding**
> Sources of funding for the systematic review

is how the methodology of the studies are evaluated. The critical appraisal of quantitative studies is presented first followed by the process of evaluating qualitative studies.

Once the studies are gathered, the process of the review should demonstrate that all of the studies related to the PICO (also called a *clinical question*) have been assessed to determine the strength and quality of the evidence for practice provided by the chosen studies in relation to the following:

- Internal validity (bias) threats (Chapter 8)
- External validity (Chapter 8)
- Sampling issues (Chapter 12)
- Variable(s) Measurement (Chapters 14 and 15)
- Data analysis (Chapter 16)
- Applicability of findings to practice (Chapters 17, 19, 20)

Once the studies in a systematic review are gathered from a comprehensive literature search of published and unpublished studies (see Chapter 3), each study is appraised for quality (see Chapters 8 to 10) and synthesized according to quality criteria and/or focus. Practice recommendations are then made and presented. Based on the inclusion criteria, more than one independent judge evaluates the studies to be included or excluded in the review and arrives at an overall quality appraisal for the group of studies. The studies appraised are discussed and presented in table format in the article, which helps you easily identify the studies included in the review and their quality (Moher et al., 2015a).

A systematic review will also include a PRISMA diagram. A PRISMA diagram illustrates the flow of information through the different phases of a systematic review. It maps out the number of records (studies) identified, included and excluded, and the reasons for exclusions (PRISMA website). The most important principle to assess when reading a systematic review is how the author(s) identified the included studies and how the studies were systematically reviewed and appraised to lead to the reviewers' conclusions. The review by Facchinetti et al. (2020) displays a PRISMA diagram in Fig. 1 of their meta-analysis (Appendix A)

The components of a systematic review are the same for a meta-analysis (see Box 11.1), except a meta-analysis quantitatively evaluates the impact of the studies as a whole as noted earlier. Once the studies in a systematic review are **retrieved** from a comprehensive literature search (see Chapter 3), **assessed** for quality, and **synthesized** according to quality or focus, then practice **recommendations** are made and presented in an article.

An example of a systematic review without a meta-analysis was completed by Parmelee Streck and LoBiondo-Wood (2020). The aim of the review was to synthesize the dyadic literature on depression in couples in which one person had breast cancer. The review included the following elements:

- Clinical question
- Background/framework
- Search strategy: inclusion criteria, search terms, study eligibility criteria
- Review and quality assessment
- PRISMA diagram
- Findings/summary and synthesis of studies
- Discussion
- Conclusions
- Table of included studies

All of the sections of a systematic review were presented, except there was no statistical analysis (meta-analysis) of the studies as a whole because the designs used in the studies varied and did not include a homogeneous design type. Based on a set of criteria, each study in this review was considered *individually as well as collectively* for sample size, methodology, and contribution to knowledge in the area. In contrast, a meta-analysis will also feature a statistical analysis of the studies as a whole. Although systematic reviews are highly useful, they also must be reviewed for potential bias and carefully critiqued for scientific rigor.

REVIEW TYPES

There are various types of reviews, terms, and methods used to systematically review the literature. The purpose of the review should be clearly identified. Statistical methods may or may not be used to analyze the studies reviewed. Often reviews are categorized under the general category of systematic review, but each review type has explicit criteria depending on the purpose. Basically a systematic review is a summation and assessment of research studies found in the literature based on a clearly focused question that uses systematic and explicit criteria and methods to identify, select, critically appraise, and analyze relevant data from the selected studies to summarize the findings in a focused area (Cooper, 2020; Liberati et al., 2009; Moher et al., 2015a, 2015b). See Box 11.1 for the components of a systematic review. Some terms are used interchangeably. The terms *systematic review* and *meta-analysis* are often used interchangeably or together, but only a meta-analysis will combine and analyze the studies using statistical methods. Systematic reviews and meta-analyses also grade the level of design or evidence of the studies reviewed. The Critical Thinking Decision Path outlines the path for completing a systematic review. When evaluating a systematic review, it is important to assess how well each of the studies in the review minimized bias or maintained the elements of control (see Chapters 8 and 9).

CRITICAL THINKING DECISION PATH

Completing a Systematic Review

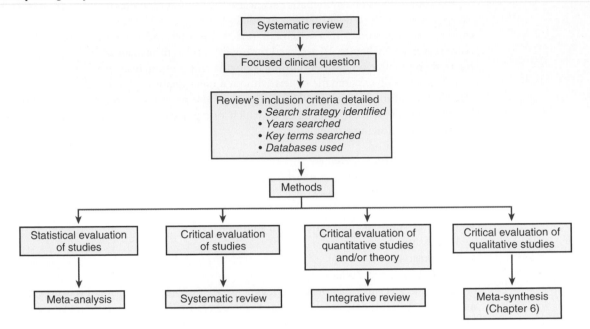

Additional types of reviews have emerged and are discussed later in this chapter. These include integrative reviews, **rapid reviews**, **scoping reviews**, **narrative reviews**, and **realist reviews** (Moher et al., 2015b). Though each review type has a different goal, each type assesses the studies critically for reliability and validity (quality, quantity, and consistency); synthesizes the results of a group of studies in a specific area (see Chapters 1, 8, 17, and 18); and makes recommendations to inform practice, education, or policy. Table 11.1 provides a definition and example for each type of review. Regardless of the type of review you are reading, it is important that the authors have clearly detailed each study's methodology, how well each study in the review minimized bias or maintained the elements of control (see Chapters 8 and 9), and that those methods can be replicated (Moher, et al., 2015b).

META-ANALYSIS

A **meta-analysis** is a systematic summary using *statistical techniques* to assess and combine studies of the same design to obtain a precise estimate of *effect* (impact of an intervention on the dependent variable/outcomes or association between variables). The terms *meta-analysis* and *systematic review* are often used interchangeably. A meta-analysis provides Level I evidence. The unique component of a meta-analysis is that *only* a meta-analysis includes a statistical summary and assessment of the studies reviewed, thereby providing the highest level of evidence. A meta-analysis treats all of the studies reviewed as one large data set to obtain a precise estimate of the effect (impact) of the results (outcomes) of the studies in the review. A well-done meta-analysis assesses for bias in studies and provides clinicians a means of

TABLE 11.1	Review Types, Definitions, and Examples	
Review Type	**Definition**	**Example**
Integrative Review	A critical appraisal of the literature in an area of interest that does not include statistical analysis because of limitations of study designs or heterogeneity of designs and samples. A systematic approach with criteria is used (Whittemore & Knafl, 2005).	Tyo, M. B. & McCurry M. K. (2020). An integrative review measuring caregiver burden in substance abuse disorder. *Nursing Research* 69(5), 391–398. Purpose: To determine what instruments are used to measure caregiver burden in informal caregivers of individuals with substance use disorder.
Narrative Review	A literature review that includes studies that support an authors' perspective and provides a broad background discussion in a focused area of interest. A systematic approach to searching for and appraising papers is often not used (O'Hara, Campbell & Schmidt, 2015).	Shivam, J., Zaki, T., Ostfeld, R.J., & McMacken, M. (2019). Utility of unrefined carbohydrates in type 2 diabetes. Comment on "Reversing type 2 diabetes: A narrative review of the evidence, *Nutrients, 11,* 766. Purpose: To review studies focused on unrefined carbohydrates in patients with type 2 diabetes.
Scoping Review	A preliminary search and assessment of potential size and scope of available research literature, including ongoing research, aimed at determining the value of undertaking a full systematic review (Grant & Booth, 2009).	Pearson, E. J. M., Morris, M. E., di Stefano, M., & McKinstry, C. E. (2018). Interventions for cancer-related fatigue: a scoping review. *European Journal of Cancer Care (Engl). 27*(1). Purpose: This review describes the nature and scope of evidence relating to interventions for cancer-related fatigue.
Rapid Review	A research methodology that uses shorter timeframes than for other evidence-based summaries. Provides a timely, valid view of evidence but sacrifices rigor. As such, rapid reviews are both a review and an assessment, and they respond to urgent clinical and public health–related questions (Khangura, Konnyu, Cushman, Grimshaw & Moher, 2012).	Sipiyaruk, K., Gallagher, J. E., Hatzipanagos, S., Reynolds, P. A. (2018). A rapid review of serious games: From healthcare education to dental education. *European Journal of Dental Education, 22*(4):243–257. Purpose: A rapid review of the literature was undertaken to synthesize available evidence and examine serious games in health care education and dental education.
Realist Review	A review that provides explanatory analysis aimed at discerning what works for whom, in what circumstances, and how. Sources include theoretical, policy, and research that combine theoretical understanding with empirical evidence and focus on the context in which an intervention is applied, the mechanisms by which it works, and outcomes produced. Intended to provide the policy and practice community with rich, yet practical understanding of complex social interventions when planning and implementing programs at a local, regional, or national level (Pawson, Greenhaigh, Harvey & Walshe, 2005).	Mukumbang, F. C., Van Belle, S., Marchal, B., & van Wyk, B. (2017). An exploration of group-based HIV/AIDS treatment and care models in sub-Saharan Africa using a realist evaluation. *Implementation Science*, 12(1), 107–115. Purpose: To examine and explicit how, why, and for whom the adherence club model works at a public health facility in South Africa.

evaluating the merit of a body of clinical research. The Cochrane Library published by the Cochrane Collaboration provides a repository of well-conducted meta-analyses that provide a precise estimate of the effect (impact) of the results (outcomes) of the studies in the review.

Meta-analysis uses a rigorous summary process and determines the impact of a number of studies rather than the impact derived from a single study alone (see Chapter 10). After the clinical question is identified, the search for published and unpublished literature is completed, and studies that meet the eligibility criteria are evaluated. A meta-analysis is conducted in two phases:

Phase I: The data are extracted from each study (i.e., outcome data, sample sizes, quality of the studies, and measures of variability from the identified studies).

Phase II: The decision is made as to whether it is appropriate to calculate what is known as a *pooled average result* (effect) of the studies reviewed.

Effect sizes are calculated using the difference in the average scores between the intervention and control groups (Cochrane Handbook of Systematic Reviews for Interventions, 2019) (see Chapter 12) from each of the studies reviewed to obtain an estimate of the population (or the whole) to create a single effect size of all of the studies. Thus the effect size is an estimate of how large of a difference there is between intervention and control groups in the *summarized* studies. **Example:** ➤ The meta-analysis in Appendix A studied the question: "What is the effectiveness of continuity of care interventions in older people with chronic diseases in reducing short and long term hospital readmission after discharge?" In this meta-analysis, the authors synthesized data from 30 randomized controlled trials (RCTs) on the effectiveness of continuity of care intervention in terms of decreasing hospital readmission (Facchinetti et al., 2020; Appendix A). The studies that focused on this question were reviewed, and each intervention was evaluated for its effect on decreasing short- and long-term hospital readmission. This estimate helps health care providers decide if the interventions reviewed provided supporting evidence that continuity of care interventions decreased hospital readmission. Detailed components of a systematic review with or without meta-analysis (Moher et al., 2009) are listed in Box 11.1.

In addition to calculating effect sizes, meta-analyses use multiple statistical methods to present and depict the data from studies reviewed (see Chapters 19 and 20). One of these methods is a forest plot, sometimes called a *blobbogram*. A forest plot graphically depicts the results of analyzing a number of studies. Fig. 11.1 is an example of a forest plot from the meta-analysis by Facchinetti and colleagues (Facchinetti et al., 2020; Appendix A, Fig. 2).

EVIDENCE-BASED PRACTICE TIP

Evidence-based practice methods such as meta-analysis increase your ability to manage the ever-increasing volume of information produced to develop the best evidence-based practices.

Fig. 11.1 displays a forest plot for the ten studies from the meta-analysis by Facchinetti and colleagues (2020) that assessed readmission rates at 1 month and compared type of care intervention at 1 month. Each study analyzed is listed. To the right of the listed study is a horizontal line that identifies the effect size estimate for each study. The box on the vertical line represents the effect size of each study, and the diamond is the effect or significance of the combined studies. The boxes to the left of the zero line mean that the intervention at 1 month was favored or produced a significant effect. The box to the right of the line indicates studies in which usual care was not favored or significant. The diamond is a more precise estimate of the interventions as it combines the data from all studies. This review identified that the findings suggest that there is evidence to support continuity of care interventions that prevent short-term hospital readmission, but there is inconclusive evidence regarding the effectiveness of continuity interventions aimed at reducing long-term admission.

Returning to the example in Appendix A, you will find that Facchinetti and colleagues (2020) present an introduction, details of the methods used to search the literature (databases, search terms, and years), a PRISMA diagram labeled as Fig. 11.1 – Flow chart of search strategies, data extraction, and analysis. The report also includes an evidence table of the studies

Study or Subgroup	Experimental Events	Total	Control Events	Total	Weight	Risk Ratio M–H, Random, 95% CI	Risk of Bias A B C D E F G
1 month							
Benzo 2016	2	108	10	107	1.3%	0.20 [0.04, 0.88]	+ + ? + + + +
Braun 2009	11	153	12	156	4.6%	0.93 [0.43, 2.05]	+ + ? ? + + +
Chow 2014	14	87	24	98	8.0%	0.66 [0.36, 1.19]	+ + + + + + +
Coleman 2006	31	379	44	371	14.3%	0.69 [0.45, 1.07]	+ + ● + + + +
Dunn 1993	18	102	16	102	7.4%	1.13 [0.61, 2.08]	+ + + + + + +
Jaarsma 1999	11	84	14	95	5.3%	0.89 [0.43, 1.85]	+ + ? ? + + +
Marusic 2012	6	80	5	80	2.2%	1.20 [0.38, 3.77]	+ + ? + + + +
Ritchie 2016	35	233	40	245	15.6%	0.92 [0.61, 1.40]	+ + ● + + + +
Wong 2014	21	196	37	210	11.1%	0.61 [0.37, 1.00]	+ + ? ? + + +
Wong, 2008	58	173	62	181	30.3%	0.98 [0.73, 1.31]	+ + ? + + + +
Total (95% CI)		1595		1645	100.0%	0.84 [0.71, 0.99]	
Total events	207		264				

Heterogeneity: Tau² = 0.00; Chi² = 9.32, df = 9 (P = 0.41); I² = 3%
Test for overall effect: Z = 2.07 (P = 0.04)

0.01 0.1 1 10 100
Favours COC intervention Favours usual care

Study or Subgroup	Experimental Events	Total	Control Events	Total	Weight	Risk Ratio M–H, Random, 95% CI	Risk of Bias A B C D E F G
1–3 months							
Benzo 2016	10	108	22	107	3.2%	0.45 [0.22, 0.91]	+ + ? + + + +
Braun 2009	39	153	55	156	12.2%	0.72 [0.51, 1.02]	+ + ? ? + + +
Chow 2014	32	87	59	98	14.0%	0.61 [0.44, 0.84]	+ + + + + + +
Coleman 2006	63	379	83	371	16.2%	0.74 [0.55, 1.00]	+ + ● + + + +
Dunn 1993	31	102	33	102	9.0%	0.94 [0.63, 1.41]	+ + + + + + +
Harrison 2002	21	92	31	100	6.7%	0.74 [0.46, 1.19]	+ + + ? + + ?
Hermiz 2002	16	67	14	80	3.8%	1.36 [0.72, 2.59]	? ? ? + + + +
Jaarsma 1999	22	84	29	95	6.8%	0.86 [0.54, 1.37]	+ + ? ? + + +
López Cabezas 2006	8	70	16	64	2.6%	0.46 [0.21, 1.00]	+ + ? + + + +
Rich 1995	41	142	59	140	13.7%	0.69 [0.50, 0.95]	+ + + ? + + +
Wong 2014	42	196	54	210	11.7%	0.83 [0.59, 1.19]	+ + ? ? + + +
Total (95% CI)		1480		1523	100.0%	0.74 [0.65, 0.84]	
Total events	325		455				

Heterogeneity: Tau² = 0.00; Chi² = 10.70, df = 10 (P = 0.38); I² = 7%
Test for overall effect: Z = 4.67 (P < 0.00001)

0.01 0.1 1 10 100
Favours COC intervention Favours usual care

Study or Subgroup	Experimental Events	Total	Control Events	Total	Weight	Risk Ratio M–H, Random, 95% CI	Risk of Bias A B C D E F G
3–6 months							
Barker 2011	53	61	39	53	11.3%	1.18 [0.98, 1.43]	+ + ? ? + + +
Benzo 2016	17	108	30	107	5.1%	0.56 [0.33, 0.96]	+ + ? + + + +
Coleman 2006	97	379	114	371	10.4%	0.83 [0.66, 1.05]	+ + ● + + + +
Collinsworth 2018	102	141	105	167	11.9%	1.15 [0.99, 1.34]	+ + ? ? + + +
Courtney 2009	21	58	49	64	7.5%	0.47 [0.33, 0.68]	+ + ? + + + +
Dunn 1993	40	102	43	102	8.2%	0.93 [0.67, 1.30]	+ + + + + + +
Ekman 1998	48	79	45	79	9.7%	1.07 [0.82, 1.38]	+ + ? ? + + +
Hughes 2000	345	981	349	985	12.6%	0.99 [0.88, 1.12]	+ + ? ? + + +
Kwok 2004	53	70	49	79	10.6%	1.22 [0.98, 1.52]	+ + + ? + + +
Kwok 2006	22	49	32	56	7.2%	0.79 [0.54, 1.15]	+ + ● ? + + +
López Cabezas 2006	17	70	27	64	5.4%	0.58 [0.35, 0.95]	+ + + ? + + +
Total (95% CI)		2098		2127	100.0%	0.91 [0.78, 1.06]	
Total events	815		882				

Heterogeneity: Tau² = 0.04; Chi² = 41.22, df = 10 (P < 0.0001); I² = 76%
Test for overall effect: Z = 1.25 (P = 0.21)

0.01 0.1 1 10 100
Favours COC intervention Favours usual care

Study or Subgroup	Experimental Events	Total	Control Events	Total	Weight	Risk Ratio M–H, Random, 95% CI	Risk of Bias A B C D E F G
6–12 months							
Benzo 2016	53	108	73	107	10.8%	0.72 [0.57, 0.91]	+ + ? + + + +
Blue 2001	47	84	49	81	9.9%	0.92 [0.71, 1.20]	+ + ? ? + + +
Cleland 2005	85	170	46	85	10.3%	0.92 [0.72, 1.18]	+ + ? ? + + +
DeBusk 2004	116	228	117	234	12.6%	1.02 [0.85, 1.22]	+ + ● ? + + +
Doughty 2002	64	100	59	97	11.3%	1.05 [0.85, 1.31]	+ + ● ? + + +
Gonzalez–Guerrero 2014	26	59	28	58	6.4%	0.91 [0.62, 1.35]	+ + ? + + + +
Hughes 2000	127	981	196	985	11.7%	0.65 [0.53, 0.80]	+ + ? ? + + +
Jaarsma 1999	31	84	47	95	7.4%	0.75 [0.53, 1.05]	+ + ? ? + + +
Krumholz 2002	16	44	23	44	4.8%	0.70 [0.43, 1.13]	? ? ? + + + +
Leventhal 2011	10	22	6	20	2.1%	1.52 [0.67, 3.41]	+ + ● ? + + +
López Cabezas 2006	23	70	31	64	5.8%	0.68 [0.45, 1.03]	+ + + ? + + +
Rainville 1999	4	17	10	17	1.6%	0.40 [0.16, 1.03]	? ? ? + + + +
Yu 2015	25	90	27	88	5.2%	0.91 [0.57, 1.43]	+ + ? ? + + +
Total (95% CI)		2057		1975	100.0%	0.84 [0.74, 0.95]	
Total events	627		712				

Heterogeneity: Tau² = 0.02; Chi² = 24.63, df = 12 (P = 0.02); I² = 51%
Test for overall effect: Z = 2.71 (P = 0.007)

0.01 0.1 1 10 100
Favours COC intervention Favours usual care

Risk of bias legend
(A) Random sequence generation (selection bias)
(B) Allocation concealment (selection bias)
(C) Blinding of participants and personnel (performance bias)
(D) Blinding of outcome assessment (detection bias)
(E) Incomplete outcome data (attrition bias)
(F) Selective reporting (reporting bias)
(G) Other bias

FIG 11.1 Blobbogram.

reviewed, a description of how the data were summarized, results of the meta-analysis, a forest plot of the reviewed studies (see Chapter 19), conclusions, and implications for practice and research. Meta-analysis is a sophisticated methodology; the exemplar provided in Appendix A is an example of one that includes all of the basic components of a well-designed meta-analysis. For a fuller understanding, several references are provided (Borenstein et al., 2009; da Costa & Juni, 2014; Higgins & Green, 2019); see also Chapters 19 and 20.

An example of how a current meta-analysis termed as a *living review* evaluated a current critical health care question was published in the Cochrane Database of Systematic Reviews. Piechotta et al. (2020) reviewed the literature to assess whether convalescent plasma or hyperimmune immunoglobulin transfusions were effective and safe in the treatment of COVID-19. This review was labeled as a living review as the authors will be adding information from ongoing studies in the area. Reviews such as this assist practitioners in a new critical care area where dependable data are needed.

INTEGRATIVE REVIEW

You will also find critical reviews of an area of research without a statistical analysis or a theory synthesis, termed integrative reviews. An integrative review is the broadest category of review (Whittemore & Knafl, 2005). It can include theoretical literature, research literature, or both. An integrative review can include methodology studies, a theory review, or the results of studies with different designs with wide-ranging clinical implications (Whittemore, 2005). An integrative review can include quantitative or qualitative research, or both. Statistics are not used to summarize and generate conclusions about the studies. Halloway and colleagues (2020) conducted an integrative review of brain-derived neurotropic factor (BDNF) and serious cardiovascular conditions. The purpose of this review was to evaluate BDNF (serum/plasma BDNF levels among humans at risk for or with serious cardiovascular conditions) and to investigate the relationship between BDNF and risk/presence of serious cardiovascular conditions in humans. Additional examples of an integrative review are found in Box 11.2. Recommendations for future research are suggested in each review.

Each study in these reviews was considered *individually as well as collectively* for its sample size, methods, and its contribution to knowledge in the area based on a set of criteria. Although systematic reviews are highly useful, they also must be reviewed for potential bias and carefully critiqued for scientific rigor. Other review types not based on a statistical analysis basically follow the same systematic process but have slightly different foci and can be titled *narrative, scoping, rapid,* and *realist* reviews (see Table 11.1 for definitions and examples).

> **EVIDENCE-BASED PRACTICE TIP**
>
> Evidence-based practice methods such as meta-analysis increase your ability to manage the ever-increasing volume of information produced to develop the best evidence-based practices.

COCHRANE COLLABORATION

In addition to meta-analyses found in journals, the largest repository of meta-analyses is the Cochrane Collaboration/Review. The Cochrane Library published by the Cochrane Collaboration provides a repository of sound meta-analyses. The Cochrane Collaboration prepares and

---

BOX 11.2 Cochrane Review Sections

Review information: Authors and contact person
Abstract
Plain language summary
The review
  Background of the question
  Objectives of the search
  Methods for selecting studies for review
  Type of studies reviewed
Types of participants, types of intervention, types of
  outcomes in the studies
  Search methods for finding studies

Data collection
Analysis of the located studies, including effect
  sizes
Results including description of studies, risk for
  bias, intervention effects
Discussion
Implications for research and practice
References and tables to display the data
  Supplementary information (e.g., appendices, data
  analysis)

---

maintains a body of systematic reviews that focus on health care interventions (Box 11.4). The reviews are found in the Cochrane Database of Systematic Reviews. The Cochrane Collaboration collaborates with a wide range of health care professionals with different skills and backgrounds for developing reviews. These partnerships assist with developing reviews that minimize bias while keeping current with assessment of health care interventions, promoting access to the database, and ensuring the quality of the reviews (Cochrane Handbook for Systematic Reviews, 2019). The steps of a Cochrane Report mirror those of a meta-analysis except for the inclusion of a plain language summary. This useful feature is a straightforward summary of the meta-analysis.

REPORTING GUIDELINES: SYSTEMATIC REVIEWS AND META-ANALYSIS

Systematic reviews and meta-analysis publications are found widely in the research literature. As these resources became more common as a method to present an accumulation of potentially clinically relevant knowledge, a need arose to develop a standard for what information should be included in these reviews. There are several guidelines available for reporting systematic reviews (Table 11.2). These are the PRISMA (Moher et al., 2015a) and MOOSE (Meta-analysis of Observational Studies in Epidemiology) (Stroup et al., 2000) guidelines and the Centre for Evidence Based Medicine (www.cebm.net/category/ebm-resources/tools), who publishes guidelines based on study designs. Tools and checklists for critically appraising the literature are detailed in Chapter 3. A review of these guidelines will help you critically read and interpret if there is any bias in the review.

BOX 11.3 Cochrane Library Databases

- Cochrane Database of Systematic Reviews: Full-text Cochrane reviews
- DARE: Critical assessments and abstracts of other systematic reviews that conform to quality criteria
- CENTRAL: Information of studies published in conference proceedings and other sources not available in other databases
- CMR: Bibliographic information on articles and books on reviewing research and methodological studies

CENTRAL, Cochrane Central Register of Controlled Trials; *CMR,* Cochrane Methodology Register; *DARE,* Database of Abstracts of Review of Effects.

BOX 11.4 Integrative Review Examples

Halloway, S., Jung, M., Yeh, A. Y., Liu, J., McAdams, E., Barley, M., Dorsey, S. G., & Pressler S. J. (2020). An integrative review of brain-derived neurotrophic factor and serious cardiovascular conditions.

There is emerging evidence that suggests a role for brain-derived neurotrophic factor (BDNF) in the risk and presence of serious cardiovascular conditions. This review describes the data related to this relationship.

Lee, M., Ryoo, J. H., Campbell, C., Hollan, P. J., & Williams, I. C. (2019). Exploring the challenges of medical/nursing tasks in home care experienced by caregivers of older adults with dementia: An integrative review.

The purpose of this review was to examine the prevalence, types, challenges and the impact of medical/nursing tasks on caregivers of older adults with dementia.

TABLE 11.2

Evidence Based Resources	Purpose
Centre for Evidenced-Based Medicine (CEBM)	Provides education and dissemination of evidence-based resources for evidence-based health care decision making
Grading of Recommendations Assessment, Development, and Evaluation (GRADE)	Provides consensus resources on rating evidence quality and strength of practice recommendations, system of rating quality, and strength of recommendations in systematic reviews, health technology assessments, and clinical practice guidelines addressing alternative management options.
Critical Appraisal Skills Programme (CASP)	Provides critical appraisal skills training, workshops, and tools used to evaluate research for trustworthiness and relevance. Offers eight appraisal tools designed to be used for assessing research.

CLINICAL PRACTICE GUIDELINES

Clinical practice guidelines are systematically developed statements or recommendations that link research and practice and serve as a guide for practitioners. Guidelines are developed by professional organizations, government agencies, institutions, or convened expert panels. Guidelines provide clinicians with an algorithm for screening, clinical management, or decision making for specific diseases (e.g., colon cancer) or treatments (e.g., pain management). Not all guidelines are well developed, and, like research, they must be assessed before deciding to implement them in clinical practice (see Chapter 9). Guidelines should present the scope and purpose of the practice for a specific population, detail who the development group included, demonstrate scientific rigor, be clear in their presentation, demonstrate clinical applicability, and demonstrate editorial independence. An example is the National Comprehensive Cancer Network, which is an interdisciplinary consortium of 21 cancer centers around the world. Interdisciplinary groups develop practice guidelines for practitioners and education guidelines for oncology patients. These guidelines are accessible at www.nccn.org.

Practice guidelines can be either expert-based or evidence-based. Evidence-based practice guidelines are those developed using a scientific process. This process includes first assembling a multidisciplinary group of experts in a specific field. This group is charged with completing a rigorous search of the literature and completing an evidence table that summarizes the quality and strength of the evidence from which the practice guideline is derived and making recommendations for application to practice (see Chapters 19 and 20). For various reasons, not all areas of clinical practice have a sufficient research base to support a clinical practice guideline. When this is the case, expert-based practice guidelines are developed. Expert-based guidelines depend on having a group of nationally known experts in the field who meet and solely use opinions of experts along with whatever research evidence is developed to date. If limited research is available for such a guideline, a rationale should be presented for the practice recommendations.

Many national organizations develop clinical practice guidelines. It is important to know which one to apply to your patient population. **Example:** ➤ There are numerous evidence-based practice guidelines developed for the management of pain. These guidelines are available from organizations such as the Oncology Nursing Society, American Academy of Pediatrics, National Comprehensive Cancer Network, National Cancer Institute, American College of Physicians, and American Academy of Pain Medicine. You must be able to evaluate each of the guidelines and decide which is the most appropriate for your patient population.

IPE HIGHLIGHT

Recently based on the highest quality of evidence, the American College of Cardiology and the American Heart Association developed a clinical practice guideline for the prevention, detection, evaluation, and management of high blood pressure and prevention of cardiovascular disease in adults (2017). This guideline is widely disseminated and represents a national standard of care for quality cardiovascular care. It is intended to be a resource for the clinical and public health communities. The biggest change reflected in the 2017 guideline is the primary prevention lower target goal for systolic blood pressure of less than 130 systolic/80 diastolic, especially for patients with a history of cardiovascular disease or increased atherosclerotic cardiovascular disease (ASCVD) risk. Based on the 2017 guideline, clinically a normal blood pressure is defined as <120/<80 mm Hg; elevated BP 120 to 129/<80 mm Hg; hypertension stage 1 is 130 to 139 mm Hg/80 to 89 mm Hg, and hypertension stage 2 is ≥140 mm Hg/≥90 mm Hg. These recommendations were based on the results of the SPRINT trial, a large RCT that randomized patients to a target goal of less than 120 systolic or less than 140 systolic (www.acc.org/latest-in-cardiology/ten-points-to-remember/2017/11/09/11/41/2017-guideline-for-high-blood-pressure-in-adults). These types of reviews are key for quality patient care.

The Agency for Healthcare Research and Quality supports the National Guideline Clearinghouse (NGC). The NGC's mission is to provide health care professionals from all disciplines with objective, detailed information on clinical practice guidelines that are disseminated and implemented. The NGC encourages groups to develop guidelines for implementation via their site using the NGC criteria; it is a very useful site for finding well-developed clinical guidelines on a wide range of health- and illness-related topics. Specific guidelines can be found on the AHRQ Effective Health Care Program website (https://www.ahrq.gov/index.html).

IPE HIGHLIGHT

When evaluating a clinical practice guideline (CPG), it is important for an interprofessional team to use an evidence-based critical appraisal tool like **AGREE II** to determine the strength and quality of the CPG for applicability to practice.

EVALUATING CLINICAL PRACTICE GUIDELINES

As evidence-based practice guidelines proliferate, it becomes increasingly important that you critique these guidelines with regard to the rigor of the methods used for guideline formulation and consider how they may be used in practice. The Appraisal of Guidelines Research and Evaluation (Brouwers et al., 2016) is the "gold standard" instrument for critically appraising clinical practice guidelines and is discussed in detail in Chapter 3. Critical areas that should be assessed when critiquing evidence-based practice guidelines include the following:

- Date of publication or release, sponsoring organization(s), and authors
- Endorsement of the guideline
- Clear purpose of what the guideline covers and patient groups for which it was designed
- Types of evidence (research, theoretical) used in guideline formulation
- Types of research included in formulating the guideline (e.g., "We considered only randomized and other prospective controlled trials in determining efficacy of therapeutic interventions.")
- Description of the methods used in grading the evidence
- Search terms and retrieval methods used to acquire evidence used in the guideline
- Well-referenced statements regarding application of the guideline in practice
- Comprehensive reference list
- Review of the guideline by experts
- Whether the guideline has been used or tested in practice and, if so, with which types of patients and in which types of settings

Evidence-based practice guidelines that are formulated using rigorous methods provide a useful starting point for understanding the evidence base for practice. However, because new research becomes available after publication of a guideline, periodic updates and revisions may be needed. Although information in well-developed, national, evidence-based practice guidelines provide a helpful reference, it is usually necessary to localize the guideline using institution-specific evidence-based policies, procedures, or standards before implementing the guideline as a standard of care in a specific clinical setting. Clinical practice guidelines are increasingly being used for quality improvement benchmarks and health care reimbursement.

CRITICAL APPRAISAL CRITERIA

Systematic Reviews

1. Does the PICO question match the studies included in the review?
2. Are the review methods clearly stated and comprehensive?
3. Are the dates of the review's inclusion clear and relevant to the area reviewed?
4. Are the inclusion and exclusion criteria for studies in the review clear and comprehensive?
5. What criteria were used to assess each of the studies in the review for quality and scientific merit?
6. If studies were analyzed individually, were the data clear?
7. Were the methods of study combination clear and appropriate?
8. If the studies were reviewed collectively, how large was the effect?
9. Are the clinical conclusions drawn from the studies relevant and supported by the review?

▶▶ APPRAISAL FOR EVIDENCE-BASED PRACTICE
SYSTEMATIC REVIEWS AND CLINICAL GUIDELINES

For each of the review methods described—systematic, meta-analysis, integrative, and clinical guidelines—think about each method as one that progressively sifts and sorts research studies and the data until the highest quality of evidence is used to arrive at the conclusions. First, the researcher combines the results of all of the studies based on a focused, specific question. The studies that do not meet the inclusion criteria are excluded and the data are assessed for quality. This process is repeated sequentially, excluding studies until only the studies of highest quality available to answer the PICO question are included in the analysis.

The overall results, as an outcome of this sorting and separating process, suggest how sensitive the conclusions are to the quality of studies included (Whittemore, 2005). No matter which type of review is completed, it is important to understand that the included research studies still must be examined through your evidence-based practice lens. This means that evidence you have derived through your critical appraisal and synthesis or through other researchers' reviews must be integrated using your individual clinician's expertise and considering patients' preferences.

CRITICAL APPRAISAL CRITERIA

Critiquing Clinical Guidelines
1. Is the date of publication or release current?
2. Are the authors of the guideline clear and appropriate to the guideline?
3. Is the clinical problem and purpose clear in terms of what the guideline covers and patient groups for which it was designed?
4. What types of evidence were used in formulating the guideline, and are they appropriate to the topic?
5. Is there a description of the methods used to grade the evidence?
6. Were the search terms and retrieval methods used to acquire research and theoretical evidence used in the guideline clear and relevant?
7. Is the guideline well-referenced and comprehensive?
8. Are the recommendations in the guideline sourced according to the level of evidence for its basis?
9. Has the guideline been reviewed and/or endorsed by experts in the appropriate field?
10. Who funded the guideline development?

You should note that a researcher who uses any of the systematic review methods for combining evidence does not conduct the original studies or analyze the data from each study, but rather takes the data from all of the published studies and synthesizes the information by following a set of systematic steps. As such, systematic reviews are considered secondary sources (see Chapter 3). Systematic methods for combining evidence are used to synthesize both nonexperimental and experimental studies.

Finally, evidence-based practice requires that you determine, based on the strength and quality of the evidence provided by the systematic review, coupled with your clinical expertise and patient values, whether or not you would consider implementing a change in practice or conclude that more research is needed.

Systematic reviews that use multiple RCTs to combine study results offer stronger evidence (Level I) in estimating the magnitude of an effect for an intervention (see Chapter 2, Table 2.3). The strength of evidence provided by systematic reviews is a key component for developing a practice based on evidence. The qualitative counterpart to systematic reviews is *meta-synthesis*, which uses qualitative principles to assess qualitative research and is described in Chapter 6.

KEY POINTS

- A systematic review is a summary of a search of quantitative studies that uses similar designs based on a PICO question.
- A meta-analysis is a systematic summary of studies using statistical techniques to assess and combine studies of the same design to obtain a precise estimate of the impact of an intervention.
- The terms *systematic review* and *meta-analysis* are used interchangeably, but only a meta-analysis includes a statistical assessment of the studies reviewed.

- An integrative review is the broadest category of reviews and can include a theoretical literature review or a review of both quantitative and qualitative research literature.
- The Cochrane Collaboration prepares and maintains a body of up-to-date systematic reviews focused on health care interventions.
- There are standardized tools available for evaluating individual studies. An example of such tools are available from the Centre for Evidence Based Medicine.
- Clinical practice guidelines are systematically developed statements or recommendations that link research and practice. There are two types of clinical practice guidelines: evidence-based practice guidelines and expert-based practice guidelines.
- Evidence-based guidelines are practice guidelines developed by experts who assess the research literature for the quality and strength of the evidence for an area of practice.
- Expert-based guidelines are developed typically by a nationally known group of experts in an area using opinions of experts along with whatever research evidence is available to date.
- The Appraisal of Guidelines Research and Evaluation II is a tool for appraising the quality of clinical practice guidelines.

CLINICAL JUDGMENT CHALLENGES

- **IPE** Your interprofessional primary care team is asked to write an evidence-based policy that will introduce depression screening as a required part of the admission protocol in your practice. Debate the pros and cons of considering the evidence to inform your protocol provided by a meta-analysis of 10 RCTs with a combined sample size of $n = 859$ in comparison with 10 individual RCTs, only 2 of which have a sample size of $n = 100$.
- Explain why it is important to have an interprofessional team conducting a systematic review.

REFERENCES

Borenstein, M., Hedges, L. V., Higgins, J. P. T., & Rothstein, H. R (2009). Introduction to meta-analysis. United Kingdom: Wiley.

Brouwers, M. C., Kerkvliet, K., & Spithoff, K. (2016). AGREE Next Steps Consortium. The AGREE Reporting Checklist: a tool to improve reporting of clinical practice guidelines. *BMJ, 352*, i1152. https://doi.org/10.1136/bmj.i1152.

Center for Evidence-Based Medicine Critical Appraisal Tools. http://www.cebm.net/critical-appraisal.

Cochrane Handbook for Systematic Reviews. (2019). http://www.cochrane-handbook.org. Cochrane Website (2020). Retrieved October 29, 2020.

Cooper, H. (2020). *Research synthesis and meta-analysis: A step-by-step approach (applied social research methods)* (5th ed.). ISBN: 9781483331157.

da Costa, B. R., & Juni, P. (2014). Systematic reviews and meta-analyses of randomized trials: Principles and pitfalls. *European Heart Journal, 35*, 3336–3345.

Facchinetti, G., D'Angelo, D., Piredda, M., Petitti, T., Matarese, M., Oliveti, A., & De Mrinis, M. G. (2020). Continuity of care interventions for preventing hospital readmission of older people with chronic diseases: A meta-analysis. *International Journal of Nursing Studies, 101*, 103396. https://doi.org/10.1016/j.ijnurstu.2019.103396.

Grant, M. J., & Booth, B. A. (2009). A typology of reviews: An analysis of 14 review types & associated methodologies. *Health Information & Libraries Journal, 26*, 91–108.

Halloway, S., Jung, M., Yeh, A., Liu, J., McAdams, E., Barley, M., Dorsey, S. G., & Pressler, S. (2020). An integrative review of brain derived neutrotrophic factor and serious cardiovascular conditions. *Nursing Research*, 10/11 69, 5. https://doi.org/10.1009/NNR.0000000000000454.

Higgins, J. P. T., Thomas, J., & Green, S. (2019). Cochrane handbook for systematic reviews of interventions version 6.1.0. http://www.cochrane-handbook.org.

Joshi, S., Zaki, T., Ostfeld, R., & McMacken, M. (2019). Comment on "Reversing Type 2 Diabetes: A Narrative Review of the Evidence. *Nutrients, 11*, 766.

Khangura, S., Konnyu, K., Cushman, R., Grimshaw, J., & Moher, D. (2012). Evidence summaries: The evolution of a rapid review approach. *Systematic Reviews, 1*(10), 1–10.

Lee, M., Ryoo, J. H., Campbell, H. P. J., & Williams, I. C. (2019). Exploring the challenges of medical/nursing tasks in home care experienced by caregivers of older adults with dementia: An integrative review. *Journal of Clinical Nursing, 28*, 23–24.

Liberati, A., Altman, D. G., Tetzlaff, J., et al. (2009). The PRISMA statement for reporting systematic reviews and meta-analyses of studies that evaluate health care interventions: Explanation and elaboration. *Annuals of Internal Medicine, 151*(4), w65–w94.

Martineau, A. R., Cates, C. J., Urashima, M., et al. (2016). Vitamin D for the management of asthma. *Cochrane Database of Systematic Reviews, 9*, CD011511. https://doi.org/10.1002/14651858 .CD011511.pub2.

Moher, D., Liberati, A., Tetzlaff, J., & Altman, D. G. (2009). Preferred reporting items for systematic reviews and meta-analyses: The PRISMA statement. *PLOS Medicine, 62*(10), 1006–1012. https:// doi.org/10.1016/j.jclinepi.2009.06.005.

Moher, D., Shamseer, L., Clarke, M., et al. (2015a). Preferred reporting items for systematic review and meta-analysis protocols (PRISMA—P) 2015 Statement. *Systematic Reviews, 4*(1), 1.

Moher, D., Stewart, L., & Shekelle, P. (2015b). All in the family: Systematic reviews, rapid reviews, scoping reviews, realist reviews and more. *Systematic Reviews, 4*, 183.

Mukumbang, F. C., VanBelle, S., Marchal,B., & Bvanky, B. (2017). An exploration of group based HIV/AIDS treatment and care models in sub-Saharan Africa using a realist evaluation. *Implementation Science, 12*(1),107–115.

O'Hara, C. B., Campbell, I. C., & Schmidt, U. (2015). A reward-centered model of anorexia nervosa: A focused narrative review of the neurological & psychophysiological literature. *Neuroscience & Biobehavioral Reviews*, 52, 131–152.

Parmelee Streck, B., & LoBiondo-Wood, G. (2020). A systematic review of dyadic studies examining depression in couples facing breast cancer. *J Psychosoc Oncol, 38*(4), 463–480. https://doi.org/10 .1080/07347332.2020.1734894.

Pawson, R., Greenhaigh, T., Harvey, G., & Walshe, K. (2005). Realist review – a new method of systematic review designed for complex policy interventions. *Journal of Health Service Research Policy,* 10(Suppl. 1), 21–34.

Pearson, E. J. M., Morris, M. E., diStefano, M., & McKinstry, C. E.(2018). Interventions for cancer-related fatigue: A scoping review. *European Journal of Cancer Care (Engl), 27*, 1.

Piechotta, V., Chai, K. L., Valk, S. J., Monsef, D. C., Wood, E. M., Kimber, L. A., McQuilten, Z., So-Osman, C., Estcourt, L. J., & Skoetz, N. (2020). Convalescent plasma or hyperimmunine immunoglobulin for people with COVID-19: A living systematic review. *Cochrane Database of Systematic Reviews*, Issue 7. Art. No.:CDO13600. https://doi.org/10.1002/14651858.CD013600 .pub2.4, 183.

Shivam, J., Zaki, T., Ostfeld, R. J., & McMacken, M. (2019). Utility of unrefined carbohydrates in type 2 diabetes. *Nutrients, 11*, 766.

Sipiyaruk, K., Gallagher, J. E., Hatzipanagos, S., & Reynolds, P. A. (2018). A rapid review serious games: From healthcare education and to dental health. *European Journal of Dental Education*, 22(4), 243–257.

Stroup, D. F., Berlin, J. A., Morton, S. C., et al. (2000). Meta-analysis of observational studies in epidemiology: A proposal for reporting. Meta-analysis of observational studies in epidemiology (MOOSE) group. *The Journal of the American Medical Association, 283*, 2008–2012.

Tyo, M. B., & McCurry, M. K. (2020). An integrative review measuring caregiver burden in substance abuse disorder. *Nursing Research, 69*(5), 391–398. https://doi.org/10.1097 /NNR.000000000000442.

Whittemore, R. (2005). Combining evidence in nursing research: Methods and implications. *Nursing Research, 54*(1), 56–62. http://www.acc.org/latest-in-cardiology/ten-points-to-remember/2017/11/09/11/41/2017-guideline-for-high-blood-pressure-in-adults.

Whittemore, R., & Knafl, K. (2005). The integrative review: Updated methodology. *Journal of Advanced Nursing, 52*(5), 546–553.

Go to Evolve at **http://evolve.elsevier.com/LoBiondo/** for review questions, appraisal exercises, and additional research articles for practice in reviewing and appraisal.

12

Appraising Sampling

Judith Haber

Go to Evolve at **http://evolve.elsevier.com/LoBiondo/** for review questions.

LEARNING OUTCOMES

After reading this chapter, you should be able to do the following:

- Identify the purpose of sampling.
- Define *population, sample,* and *sampling.*
- Compare a population and a sample.
- Discuss the importance of inclusion and exclusion criteria.
- Define *nonprobability* and *probability sampling.*
- Identify the types of nonprobability and probability sampling strategies.
- Compare the advantages and disadvantages of nonprobability and probability sampling strategies.

- Discuss the contribution of nonprobability and probability sampling strategies to strength of evidence provided by study findings.
- Discuss the factors that influence sample size.
- Discuss potential threats to internal and external validity as sources of sampling bias.
- Use critical appraisal criteria to evaluate the "Sample" section of a research report.

KEY TERMS

accessible population	multistage (cluster) sampling	purposive sampling	simple random sampling
convenience sampling		quota sampling	
data saturation	network sampling	random selection	snowballing
delimitations	nonprobability sampling	representative sample	social determinants of health
element		sample	
eligibility criteria	pilot study	sampling	stratified random sampling
exclusion criteria	population	sampling frame	
inclusion	probability sampling	sampling unit	target population

The sampling section of a study is usually found in the "Methods" section of a research article. You will find it important to understand the sampling process and the elements that contribute to a researcher using the most appropriate sampling strategy for the type of research being conducted. Equally important is knowing how to critically appraise the sampling section of a study to identify how the strengths and weaknesses of the sampling process contributed to the overall strength and quality of evidence provided by the study's findings and applicability to practice. When you are critically appraising the sampling section of a study, it is important to consider the threats to internal and external validity as sources of bias (see Chapter 8).

Sampling is the process of selecting representative units of a population in a study. Many problems in research cannot be solved without employing rigorous sampling procedures. **Example:** ➤ When testing the effectiveness of a medication for patients with type 2 diabetes, the researcher cannot give the drug to every patient with diabetes. Instead, the drug is administered to a sample of the population for whom the drug is potentially appropriate. Because human lives are at stake, the researcher cannot afford to arrive casually at conclusions that are based on the first dozen patients available for study. In this case, the sample must accurately reflect the larger population that has type 2 diabetes.

The impact of arriving at conclusions that are not accurate or making generalizations from a small nonrepresentative sample is much more severe in research than in everyday life. Essentially, researchers sample representative segments of the population because it is rarely feasible or necessary to sample the entire population of interest to obtain relevant information.

This chapter will familiarize you with the basic concepts of sampling as they primarily pertain to the principles of quantitative research design, nonprobability and probability sampling, sample size, and the related critical appraisal process. Sampling issues that relate to qualitative research designs are discussed in Chapters 5 to 7.

SAMPLING CONCEPTS

Population

A **population** is a well-defined set with specified properties. A population can be composed of people, animals, objects, or events. Examples of populations may be all female patients older than 65 years of age admitted to a specific hospital with myocardial infarction during the year 2021, all children diagnosed with COVID-19 in California in 2020, or all men and women with a diagnosis of bipolar disorder in the United States. These examples illustrate that a population may be broadly defined and potentially involve millions of people or narrowly specified to include only several hundred people.

The population criteria establish the **target population**—that is, the entire set of cases about which the researcher would like to make generalizations. A target population may include all undergraduate nursing students enrolled in accelerated baccalaureate programs in the United States. Because of time, money, and personnel, however, it is often not feasible to pursue a study using a target population.

An **accessible population**, one that meets the target population criteria and that is available, is used instead. **Example:** ➤ An accessible population may include all full-time accelerated baccalaureate students attending school in Michigan. Pragmatic factors must also be considered when identifying a potential population of interest.

It is important to know that a population is not restricted to humans. It may consist of hospital records; blood, urine, or other specimens taken from patients at a clinic; historical documents; or laboratory animals. **Example:** ➤ A population may consist of all HgbA1C blood test specimens collected from patients in the City Hospital diabetes clinic or all charts on file for patients who were screened during pregnancy for HIV infection. A population can be defined in a variety of ways. The basic unit of the population must be clearly defined because the generalizability of the findings will be a function of the population criteria.

Inclusion and Exclusion Criteria

When reading a research report, you should consider whether the researcher has identified the population characteristics that form the basis for the inclusion (eligibility) or exclusion (delimitations) criteria used to select the sample—whether people, objects, or events. The terms **inclusion** or **eligibility criteria** and **exclusion criteria** or **delimitations** define characteristics that limit the population to a homogenous group of subjects. The population characteristics that provide the basis for inclusion (eligibility) criteria should be evident in the sample—that is, the characteristics of the population and the sample should be congruent to assess the representativeness of the sample. Examples of inclusion or eligibility criteria and exclusion criteria or delimitations include the following:

- Gender
- Age
- Marital status
- Socioeconomic status
- Geographical location
- Religion
- Race/ethnicity
- Level of education
- Age of children
- Health status
- Diagnosis

These criteria focus on demographic variables frequently associated with the **social determinants of health** (SDOH). The SDOH are conditions in the environment or communities in which people are born, live, work, play, worship, and age that affect their health, functioning, and quality-of-life outcomes (U.S. Department of Health and Human Services, 2020). SDOH are important because often they highlight population-specific health disparities that influence health outcomes. Researchers want to recruit individuals who equitably represent the population of interest. The imperative to recruit underrepresented minorities in research studies, thereby gaining a more accurate understanding of population-specific gaps in health care, has become a national health equity call to action highlighting health disparities related to the SDOH. Inclusion and exclusion criteria are an important research study ingredient for understanding population-specific disparities. Think about the concept of inclusion or eligibility criteria applied to a study in which the subjects are patients. For example, in recent years, the mortality rate for breast cancer among women 60 to 69 years of age decreased 2% per year among white women, but only decreased 1% per year among Black women.

Example: ➤ Findings from a retrospective, cross-sectional population-based study of 177,075 women 40 to 64 years of age who received a diagnosis of stage I to III breast cancer reveal that more women who were either receiving Medicaid or were uninsured received a diagnosis of locally advanced (stage III) cancer compared with women who had health insurance (20% vs 11%). Non-Hispanic Black, American Indian or Alaskan Native, and Hispanic women had a significantly higher risk for locally advanced disease at time of diagnosis than non-Hispanic White women. Nearly one-half of the racial differences were mediated by health insurance coverage (Ko et al., 2020).

Participants had to meet the following inclusion (eligibility) criteria:

1. Age: 40 to 64 years of age
2. Diagnosis: First-time diagnosis of stage I to III breast cancer

3. Race/ethnicity: Non-Hispanic Black, American Indian, Alaskan Native, Hispanic, Non-Hispanic White
4. Insurance status: Commercial, Medicaid, uninsured

Inclusion and exclusion criteria are established to control for extraneous variability or bias that would limit the strength of evidence contributed by the sampling plan in relation to the study's design. Each inclusion or exclusion criterion should have a rationale, presumably related to a potential contaminating effect on the dependent variable. Subjects were excluded from this study if:

- Younger than 40 years of age or older than 64 years of age
- Evidence of metastatic breast cancer (stage IV)

The data analysis, adjusted for SDOH, such as socioeconomic level, education, literacy, and health insurance status, highlights the importance of SDOH, such as race/ethnicity and insurance status, contributing to increased risk for locally advanced breast cancer. Nearly one-half (45% to 47%) of racial differences in the risk for locally advanced disease were mediated by health insurance status (Ko et al., 2020). Careful establishment of sample inclusion or exclusion criteria will increase a study's precision and strength of evidence, thereby contributing to the accuracy and generalizability of the findings (see Chapter 8). The study by De la Fuente Coria and colleagues (2020) provides an example of a flowchart illustrating the progress of individuals in the phases of a randomized controlled trial (RCT) assessing the effectiveness of a primary care nurse–delivered educational intervention for patients with type 2 diabetes (Fig. 1, Appendix B).

HELPFUL HINT

Researchers may not clearly identify the population under study, or the population is not clarified until the "Discussion" section, where the effort is made to discuss the group (population) to which the study findings can be generalized.

Samples and Sampling

Sampling is the selection of a portion or subset of the designated population that represents the entire population. A **sample** is a set of elements that make up the population; an **element** is the most basic unit about which information is collected. The most common element in nursing research is individuals, but other elements (e.g., places, objects) can form the basis of a sample or population. **Example:** ➤ A research team investigated the purported benefits of physical activity (PA), barriers to PA, PA self-efficacy, social support for PA, enjoyment of PA, and motivation (Robbins et al., 2019). The intervention was designed to improve the girls, perceptions of the benefit and enjoyment of physical activity (PA), PA self-efficacy, social support, motivation for PA, and barriers to PA. To account for seasonal variation of moderately vigorous physical activity (MVPA), data collection focused on pairs of schools as sampling units rather than individuals, one intervention school and one control school, at the same time. The purpose of sampling is to increase a study's efficiency. If you think about it, you will realize that it is not feasible to examine every element in the population. When sampling is done properly, the researcher can draw inferences and make generalizations about the population without examining each element in the population. Sampling procedures identify specific selection criteria to ensure that the characteristics of the phenomena of interest will be, or are likely to be, present in all of the units being studied. The researcher's efforts to ensure that the sample is representative of the target population strengthens the evidence generated by the sample, which allows the researcher to draw conclusions that are generalizable to the population and applicable to practice (see Chapter 8).

After having reviewed a number of research studies, you will recognize that samples and sampling procedures vary in terms of merit. The foremost criterion in appraising a sample is its representativeness. A representative sample is one whose key characteristics closely match those of the population. If 70% of the population in a study of child-rearing practices consisted of women and 50% were full-time employees, a representative sample should reflect these characteristics in the same proportions.

EVIDENCE-BASED PRACTICE TIP

Consider whether the choice of participants was biased, thereby influencing the strength of evidence provided by the outcomes of the study.

TYPES OF SAMPLES

Sampling strategies are generally grouped into two categories: nonprobability sampling and probability sampling. In nonprobability sampling, elements are chosen by nonrandom methods. The drawback of this strategy is that there is no way of estimating each element's probability of being included in the total sample. Essentially, there is no way of ensuring that every element has a chance for inclusion in a nonprobability sample.

Probability sampling uses a form of random selection when the sample is chosen. This type of sample enables the researcher to estimate the probability that each element of the population will be included in the sample. Probability sampling is the more rigorous type of sampling strategy and is more likely to result in a representative sample. A summary of sampling strategies appears in Table 12.1 and is discussed in the following sections.

EVIDENCE-BASED PRACTICE TIP

Determining whether the sample is representative of the population being studied will influence your interpretation of the evidence provided by the findings and decision making about their relevance to the patient population and practice setting.

HELPFUL HINT

A research article may not be explicit about the sampling strategy used. If the sampling strategy is not specified, assume that a convenience sample was used for a quantitative study and a purposive sample was used for a qualitative study.

Nonprobability Sampling

Because of lack of random selection, the findings of studies using nonprobability sampling are less generalizable than those using a probability sampling strategy, and they tend to produce less representative samples. When a nonprobability sample is carefully chosen to reflect the target population through the careful use of inclusion and exclusion criteria and adequate sample size, you can have more confidence in the sample's representativeness and the external validity of the findings (see Chapter 8). The three major types of nonprobability sampling are convenience, quota, and purposive sampling strategies.

TABLE 12.1   Summary of Sampling Strategies

Sampling Strategy	Ease of Drawing Sample	Risk for Bias	Representativeness of Sample
Nonprobability			
Convenience	Easy	Greater than any other sampling strategy	Because samples tend to be self-selecting, representativeness is questionable
Quota	Relatively easy	Contains an unknown source of bias that affects external validity	Builds in some representativeness by using knowledge about population of interest
Purposive	Relatively easy	Bias increases with greater heterogeneity of population; conscious bias is also a danger	Very limited ability to generalize because sample is hand-picked
Probability			
Simple random	Time-consuming	Low	Maximized; probability of nonrepresentativeness decreases with increased sample size
Stratified random	Time-consuming	Low	Enhanced
Cluster	Less or more time-consuming depending on the strata	Subject to more sampling errors than simple or stratified	Less representative than simple or stratified

Convenience Sampling

Convenience sampling is the use of the most readily accessible persons or objects as subjects. The subjects may include volunteers, the first 100 patients admitted to hospital X with a particular diagnosis, all people enrolled in program Y during the month of September, or all students enrolled in course Z at a particular university during 2021. The subjects are convenient and accessible to the researcher and are thus called a *convenience sample*.
Example: ➤ A study examining the relationship between two types of social support and self-management of inflammatory bowel disease (IBD) among emerging adults (18 to 29 years of age) used a convenience sample ($n = 61$) of emerging adult IBD individuals (currently prescribed medication to manage IBD) who were recruited through Research Match, Facebook, and word of mouth and met the eligibility criteria (Kamp et al., 2019).

The advantage of a convenience sample is that generally it is easier to obtain subjects. The researcher will still have to be concerned with obtaining a sufficient number of subjects who meet the inclusion criteria. The major disadvantage of a convenience sample is that the risk for bias is greater than in any other type of sample (see Table 12.1). The fact that convenience samples use voluntary participation increases the probability of researchers recruiting those people who feel strongly about the issue being studied, which may favor certain outcomes. In this case, ask yourself the following questions as you think about the strength and quality of evidence contributed by the sampling component of a study:

- What motivated some people to participate and others not to participate (self-selection)?
- What kind of data would have been obtained if nonparticipants had also responded?
- How representative are the people who did participate in relation to the population?
- What kind of confidence can you have in the evidence provided by the findings?

Researchers may recruit subjects in clinic settings; place advertisements in the newspaper; place signs in local churches, community centers, and supermarkets; or post research study information through online platforms indicating that volunteers are needed for a particular study. To assess the degree to which a convenience sample approximates a random sample, the researcher checks for the representativeness of the convenience sample by comparing the sample to population percentages and, in this way, assesses the extent to which bias is or is not evident (Sousa et al., 2004).

Because acquiring research subjects is a problem that confronts many researchers, innovative recruitment strategies may be used. A unique method of accessing and recruiting subjects is the use of online computer networks (e.g., disease-specific chat rooms, blogs, and bulletin boards). **Example:** ➤ In the cross-sectional study by Kamp and colleagues (2019), a convenience sample of subjects with IBD and on medication were recruited through online platforms like Facebook, Research Match, and word of mouth, increasing the likelihood that the sample will reflect bias. When you appraise a study, you should recognize that the convenience sampling strategy, although most common, is the weakest sampling strategy with regard to strength of evidence and generalizability (external validity) unless it is followed by random assignment to groups, as you will find in studies that are RCTs such as the one by De la Fuente Coria and colleagues (2020) in Appendix B (see Chapter 9). When a convenience sample is used, caution should be exercised in interpreting the data and assessing the researcher's comments about the external validity and applicability of the findings (see Chapter 8).

Quota Sampling

Quota sampling refers to a form of nonprobability sampling in which subjects who meet the inclusion criteria are recruited and consecutively enrolled until the target sample size is reached. The study by Wetzstein and colleagues (2020) examining patient activation among community-dwelling persons living with chronic obstructive pulmonary disease (COPD) provides an example of quota sampling. The team conducted a power analysis to identify the number of participants needed to address the study aims. The results showed that 98 participants were needed to detect a treatment effect. Study packets were mailed to 250 eligible individuals who met the eligibility criteria. Subjects were enrolled in the study until the target enrollment was reached.

Sometimes knowledge about the population of interest is used to build some representativeness into the sample (see Table 12.1). A quota sample can identify the strata of the population, and proportionally represents the strata in the sample. **Example:** ➤ The data in Table 12.2 reveal that 40% of the 5000 nurses in city X are associate degree graduates, 30% are 4-year baccalaureate degree graduates, and 30% are accelerated second-degree baccalaureate graduates. Each stratum of the population should be proportionately represented in the sample. In this case, the researcher used a proportional quota sampling strategy and decided to sample 10% of a population of 5000 (i.e., 500 nurses). Based on the proportion of each stratum in the population, 200 associate degree graduates, 150 4-year baccalaureate graduates, and 150 accelerated baccalaureate graduates were the quotas established for the three strata. The researcher recruited subjects who met the study's eligibility criteria until the quota for each stratum was filled. In other words, once the researcher obtained the necessary 200 associate degree graduates, 150 4-year baccalaureate degree graduates, and 150 accelerated baccalaureate degree graduates, the sample was complete.

TABLE 12.2 Numbers and Percentages of Students in Strata of a Quota Sample of 5000 Graduates of Nursing Programs in City X

	Associate Degree Graduates	4-year Baccalaureate Degree Graduates	Accelerated Baccalaureate Degree Graduates
Population	2000 (40%)	1000 (30%)	2000 (30%)
Strata	200	150	150

The characteristics chosen to form the strata are selected according to a researcher's knowledge of the population and the literature review. The criterion for selection should be a variable that reflects important differences in the dependent variables under investigation. Age, gender, religion, ethnicity, medical diagnosis, socioeconomic status, level of completed education, and occupational rank are among the variables that are likely to be important stratifying variables in nursing research studies.

The researcher systematically ensures that proportional segments of the population are included in the sample. The quota sample is not randomly selected (i.e., once the proportional strata have been identified, the researcher recruits and enrolls subjects until the quota for each stratum has been filled) but does increase the sample's representativeness. This sampling strategy addresses the problem of overrepresentation or underrepresentation of certain segments of a population in a sample.

As you critically appraise a study, your aim is to determine whether the sample strata appropriately reflect the population under consideration and whether the stratifying variables are homogeneous enough to ensure a meaningful comparison of differences among strata. Establishment of strict inclusion and exclusion criteria and using power analysis to determine appropriate sample size increase the rigor of a quota sampling strategy by creating homogeneous subject categories that facilitate making meaningful comparisons across strata.

Purposive Sampling

Purposive sampling is a common strategy. The researcher selects subjects who are considered to be typical of the population. Purposive sampling can be found in both quantitative and qualitative studies. When a researcher is considering the sampling strategy for an RCT focusing on a specific diagnosis or patient population, the sampling strategy is often purposive in nature. In such studies, the researcher first purposively selects subjects who are then randomized to groups.

Purposive sampling is commonly used in qualitative research studies. **Example:** ➤ The objective of the qualitative study by Admi and colleagues (2020) was to gain insight into the perceptions that underlie health-related adherence behaviors from the perspective of patients who experienced a heart attack. They selected a purposive sample of 22 participants who were post–myocardial infarction (MI) and recruited from a hospital cardiac rehabilitation unit and from two different communities in northern Israel. Participants were chosen from different cultures to obtain a diversity of experiences from different perspectives. Subjects were selected until the new information obtained did not provide further insight into the themes or no new themes emerged (data saturation; see Chapters 5, 6, and 14). A purposive sample is used also when a highly unusual group is being studied, such as a population with a rare genetic disease (e.g., Huntington chorea). In this case the

> **BOX 12.1   Criteria for Use of a Purposive Sampling Strategy**
>
> - Effective pretesting of newly developed instruments with a purposive sample of divergent types of people
> - Validation of a scale or test with a known-group technique
> - Collection of exploratory data in relation to an unusual or highly specific population, particularly when the total target population remains an unknown to the researcher
> - Collection of descriptive data (e.g., as in qualitative studies) that seek to describe the lived experience of a particular phenomenon (e.g., postpartum depression, caring, hope, surviving childhood sexual abuse)
> - Focus of the study population relates to a specific diagnosis (e.g., type 1 diabetes, ovarian cancer) or condition (e.g., legal blindness, terminal illness) or a demographic characteristic (e.g., same-sex twin pairs)

researcher would describe the sample characteristics precisely to ensure that the reader will have an accurate picture of the subjects in the sample.

Today, computer networks (e.g., online platforms) can be a valuable resource in helping researchers access and recruit subjects for purposive samples. Online support group bulletin boards that facilitate recruitment of subjects for purposive samples exist for people with cancer, rheumatoid arthritis, multiple sclerosis, human immunodeficiency virus/acquired immunodeficiency syndrome (HIV/AIDS), postpartum depression, human papilloma virus (HPV), and many others.

The researcher who uses a purposive sample assumes that errors of judgment in overrepresenting or underrepresenting elements of the population in the sample will tend to balance out. As indicated in Table 12.1, there may be potential bias in the selection of subjects; the ability to generalize from the evidence provided by the findings is very limited. Box 12.1 lists examples of when a purposive sample may be appropriate.

Network Sampling

Network sampling, sometimes referred to as snowballing, is used for locating samples that are difficult or impossible to locate in other ways. This strategy takes advantage of social networks and the fact that friends tend to have characteristics in common. When a few subjects with the necessary eligibility criteria are found, the researcher asks for their assistance in getting in touch with others with similar criteria. **Example:** ➤ Online computer networks and social media platforms, as described earlier in the section on purposive sampling, can be used to assist researchers in acquiring otherwise difficult-to-locate subjects, thereby taking advantage of the networking or snowball effect. A study by Herbel (2019) aimed to diversify recruitment strategies with the use of Facebook to recruit pregnant women into research; an electronic version of the recruitment flyer was created. Herbel developed a Facebook page that displayed the study logo, information about the principal investigator, the study flyer, and contact information. She also created a separate Facebook page for the study so interested participants could refer to the page for more information or invite their friends to "like" the page to generate interest in the study. Herbel also found and then "liked" and "followed" several Facebook groups for mothers and pregnant women to which she gained access. Referrals occurred when a Facebook user "tagged" another user to see the study recruitment flyer. Participants enrolled were the frequency of enrollees who indicated they were recruited into the study because of the study recruitment flyer on Facebook.

> **HELPFUL HINT**
>
> When convenience or purposive sampling is used as the first step in recruiting a sample for an RCT, as illustrated in Fig. 12.1, it is followed by random assignment of subjects to an intervention or control group, which increases the generalizability of the findings.

Probability Sampling

The primary characteristic of probability sampling is the random selection of elements from the population. Random selection occurs when each element of the population has an equal and independent chance of being included in the sample. When probability sampling is used, you have greater confidence that the sample is representative of the population being studied rather than biased. Three commonly used probability sampling strategies are simple random, stratified random, and cluster.

Random selection of sample subjects should not be confused with randomization or random assignment of subjects. The latter, discussed earlier in this chapter and in Chapter 8, refers to the assignment of subjects to either an experimental or a control group on a random basis. Random assignment is most closely associated with RCTs.

Simple Random Sampling

Simple random sampling is a carefully controlled process. The researcher defines the population (a set), lists all units of the population (a sampling frame), and selects a sample of units (a subset) from which the sample will be chosen. **Example:** ➤ If American hospitals specializing in the treatment of cancer were the sampling unit, a list of all such hospitals would be the sampling frame. If certified school nurses constituted the sampling unit, a list of those nurses would be the sampling frame.

Once a list of the population elements has been developed, the best method of selecting a random sample is to use a computer program that generates the order in which the random selection of subjects is to be carried out.

The advantages of simple random sampling are as follows:
- Sample selection is not subject to the conscious biases of the researcher.
- Representativeness of the sample in relation to the population characteristics is maximized.
- Differences in the characteristics of the sample and the population are purely a function of chance.
- The probability of choosing a nonrepresentative sample decreases as the size of the sample increases.

Example: ➤ To increase efficiency and decrease documentation burden, it was thought to be useful for public health nurses engaging in home visiting services for at-risk patients to identify critical data elements most associated with patient care priorities and outcomes that are needed during home visits. Machine learning techniques, an application of artificial intelligence for managing large data sets efficiently, were used with the large home health care data set of the Omaha System (Bose et al., 2019). A sample of 756 patients from a large pool of maternal-child patients who received public health nursing services between 2006 and 2009 were randomly selected from the Omaha System database.

The major disadvantage of simple random sampling is that it can be a time-consuming and inefficient method of obtaining a random sample. **Example:** ➤ Consider the task of listing all baccalaureate nursing students in the United States. With random sampling, it may also be impossible to obtain an accurate or complete listing of every element in the population. **Example:** ➤ Imagine trying to obtain a list of all suicides in New York City for the year 2020. It often is the case that although suicide may have been the cause of death, another cause (e.g., cardiac failure) appears on the death certificate. It would be difficult to estimate how many elements of the target population would be eliminated from consideration. The issue of bias would definitely enter the picture despite the researcher's best efforts. In the final analysis, you, as the evaluator of a research article, must be cautious about generalizing from findings, even when random sampling is the stated strategy or if the target population has been difficult or impossible to list completely.

EVIDENCE-BASED PRACTICE TIP

When thinking about applying study findings to your clinical practice, consider whether the participants making up the sample are similar to your own patients.

Stratified Random Sampling

Stratified random sampling requires that the population be divided into strata or subgroups as illustrated in Fig. 12.1. The subgroups or subsets that the population is divided into are homogeneous. An appropriate number of elements from each subset are randomly selected on the basis of their proportion in the population. The goal of this strategy is to achieve a greater degree of representativeness. Stratified random sampling is similar to the proportional stratified quota sampling strategy discussed earlier in the chapter. The major difference is that stratified random sampling uses a random selection procedure for obtaining sample subjects.

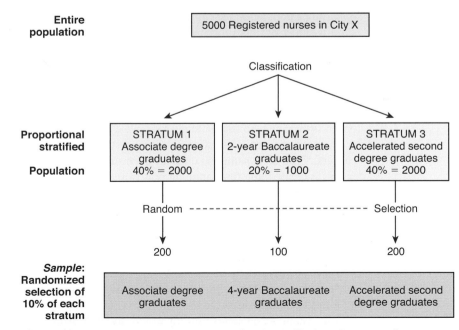

FIG 12.1 Subject selection using a proportional stratified random sampling strategy.

The population is stratified according to any number of attributes, such as age, gender, ethnicity, religion, socioeconomic status, or level of education completed. The variables selected to form the strata should be adaptable to homogeneous subsets with regard to the attributes being studied. **Example:** ➢ The PANDA study (Lewis et al, 2019) investigated the clinical effectiveness of sertraline for patients in primary care with depressive symptoms ranging from mild to severe and tested the role of severity and duration in treatment response.

This study was a pragmatic, multicenter, double-blind, placebo-controlled randomized trial of patients from 179 primary care clinics in four UK cities (Bristol, Liverpool, London, and York). The sample included patients 18 to 74 years of age who had depressive symptoms of any severity or duration in the past 2 years and for whom there was clinical uncertainty about the benefit of an antidepressant. This strategy was designed to improve the generalizability of the sample to current use of antidepressants within primary care. Patients were randomly assigned (1:1) with a remote computer-generated code to sertraline or placebo, and they were stratified by severity, duration, and site with random block length. The primary outcome was depressive symptoms 6 weeks after randomization, measured by Patient Health Questionnaire, 9-item version (PHQ-9) scores. Secondary outcomes at 2, 6, and 12 weeks were depressive symptoms and remission (PHQ-9 and Beck Depression Inventory-II), generalized anxiety symptoms (Generalized Anxiety Disorder Assessment 7-item version), mental and physical health-related quality of life (12-item Short-Form Health Survey), and self-reported improvement.

As illustrated in Table 12.1, several advantages to a stratified random sampling strategy include: (1) representativeness of the sample is enhanced; (2) the researcher has a valid basis for making comparisons among subsets; and (3) the researcher is able to oversample a disproportionately small stratum to adjust for their underrepresentation, statistically weigh the data accordingly, and continue to make legitimate comparisons.

The obstacles encountered by a researcher using this strategy include (1) difficulty of obtaining a population list containing complete critical variable information, (2) time-consuming effort of obtaining multiple enumerated lists, (3) challenge of enrolling proportional strata, and (4) time and money involved in carrying out a large-scale study using a stratified sampling strategy.

Multistage Sampling (Cluster Sampling)

Multistage (cluster) sampling involves a successive random sampling of units (clusters) that progress from large to small and meet sample eligibility criteria. The first-stage sampling unit consists of large units or clusters. The second-stage sampling unit consists of smaller units or clusters. Third-stage sampling units are even smaller. **Example:** ➢ If a sample of critical care nurses is desired, the first sampling unit would be a random sample of hospitals, obtained from an American Hospital Association list, that meet the eligibility criteria (e.g., size, type). The second-stage sampling unit would consist of a list of critical care nurses practicing at each hospital selected in the first stage (i.e., the list obtained from the vice president for nursing at each hospital). The criteria for inclusion in the list of critical care nurses would be as follows:
1. Certified as a Certified Critical Care Registered Nurse (CCRN) with at least 3 years of experience as a critical care nurse
2. Spends at least 75% of the time providing direct patient care in a critical care unit
3. Employed full-time at the hospital

The second-stage sampling unit would obtain a random selection of 10 CCRNs from each hospital who met the previously mentioned eligibility criteria.

When multistage sampling is used in relation to large national surveys, states are used as the first-stage sampling unit, followed by successively smaller units, such as counties, cities, districts, and blocks, as the second-stage sampling unit, and finally households as the third-stage sampling unit. Sampling units or clusters can be selected by simple random or stratified random sampling methods. The main advantage of cluster sampling, as illustrated in Table 12.1, is that it can be more economical in terms of time and money than other types of probability sampling. There are two major disadvantages: (1) more sampling errors tend to occur than with simple random or stratified random sampling, and (2) appropriate handling of the statistical data from cluster samples is very complex. When you are critically appraising a study, it is important to consider whether the use of cluster sampling is justified in light of the research design as well as other pragmatic matters, such as economy.

EVIDENCE-BASED PRACTICE TIP

The sampling strategy, whether probability or nonprobability, must be appropriate to the design and evaluated in relation to the level of evidence provided by the design.

CRITICAL THINKING DECISION PATH
Assessing the Relationship Between the Type of Sampling Strategy and the Appropriate Generalizability

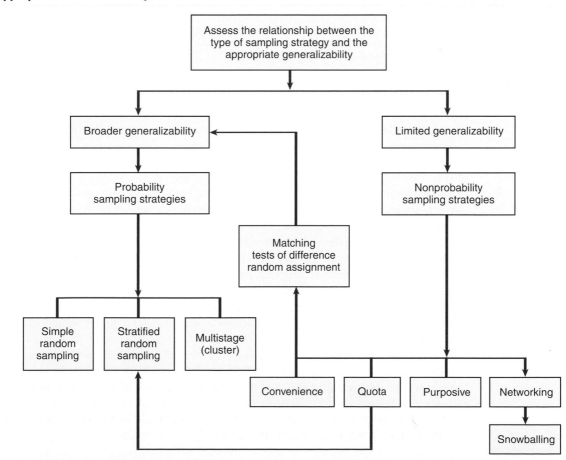

The Critical Thinking Decision Path illustrates the relationship between the type of sampling strategy and the appropriate generalizability.

SAMPLE SIZE

There is no single rule that can be applied to the determination of a sample's size. When arriving at an estimate of sample size, many factors, such as the following, must be considered:

- Type of design
- Type of sampling procedure
- Type of formula used for estimating optimum sample size
- Degree of precision required
- Heterogeneity of the attributes under investigation
- Relative frequency that the phenomenon of interest occurs in the population (i.e., a common versus a rare health problem)
- Projected cost of using a particular sampling strategy

HELPFUL HINT

Look for a brief discussion of a study's sampling strategy in the "Methods" section of a research article. Sometimes there is a separate subsection with the heading "Sample," "Subjects," or "Study Participants." A statistical description of the characteristics of the actual sample often does not appear until the "Results" section of a research article. You may also find a table in the "Results" section that summarizes the sample characteristics using descriptive statistics (see Chapter 14).

The sample size should be determined before a study is conducted. A general rule is always to use the largest sample possible. The larger the sample, the more representative of the population it is likely to be; smaller samples produce less accurate results.

One exception to this principle occurs when using qualitative designs. In this case, sample size is not predetermined. Sample sizes in qualitative research tend to be small because of the large volume of verbal data that must be analyzed, and this type of design tends to emphasize intensive and prolonged contact with subjects (Speziale & Carpenter, 2011). Subjects are added to the sample until data saturation is reached (i.e., new data no longer emerge during the data-collection process). Fittingness of the data is a more important concern than representativeness of subjects (see Chapters 5 to 7).

Another exception is in the case of a pilot study, which is defined as a small sample study conducted as a prelude to a larger-scale study that is often called the *parent study*. The pilot study is typically a smaller scale of the parent study, with similar methods and procedures that yield preliminary data to determine the feasibility of conducting a larger-scale study and establish that sufficient scientific evidence exists to justify subsequent, more extensive research.

The principle of "larger is better" holds true for both probability and nonprobability samples. Results based on small samples (less than 10) tend to be unstable; the values fluctuate from one sample to the next, and it is difficult to apply statistics meaningfully. Small samples tend to increase the probability of obtaining a markedly nonrepresentative sample. As the sample size increases, the mean more closely approximates the population values, thus introducing fewer sampling errors.

It is possible to estimate the sample size needed with the use of a statistical procedure known as *power analysis* (Cohen, 1988). Power analysis is an advanced statistical technique that is commonly used by researchers and is a requirement for external funding. When it is not used, you will have less confidence provided by the findings because the study may be based on a sample that is too small. A researcher may commit a type II error of accepting a null hypothesis when it should have been rejected if the sample is too small (see Chapter 16). No matter how high a research design is located on the evidence hierarchy (e.g., Level II— experimental design consisting of an RCT), the findings of a study and their generalizability are weakened when power analysis is not calculated to ensure an adequate sample size to determine the effect of the intervention.

It is beyond the scope of this chapter to describe this complex procedure in great detail, but a simple example will illustrate its use. De la Fuente Coria and colleagues (2020) evaluated the effectiveness of a structured and individualized education program for type 2 diabetes that was provided by a primary care nurse and featured educational reinforcements and family support to achieve metabolic control and long-term therapeutic targets. They calculated the sample size needed to detect the effect of the intervention by using power analysis to calculate the sample size needed to obtain a confidence level of 95% and a statistical power of 90%. A sample size of 69 participants was needed for both intervention and control groups to detect the difference in glycosylated hemoglobin of 1% and a variance of 4%. The total sample for this study was $n = 280$ and exceeded the minimum number of 69 subjects needed for the intervention and control groups.

HELPFUL HINT

Remember to evaluate the appropriateness of the generalizations made about the study findings in light of the target population, the accessible population, the type of sampling strategy, and the sample size.

When calculating sample size using power analysis, the total sample size needs to consider that attrition, or dropouts, will occur. To address this issue, researchers build in approximately 15% more subjects to make sure that the ability to detect differences between groups or the effect of an intervention remains intact. When expected differences are large, it does not take a very large sample to ensure that differences will be revealed through statistical analysis.

When critically appraising a study, you should evaluate the sample size in terms of the following: (1) how representative the sample is relative to the target population, and (2) to whom the researcher wishes to generalize the study's results. The goal is to have a sample as representative as possible with as little sampling error as possible. Unless representativeness is ensured, all of the data in the world become inconsequential. When an appropriate sample size, including power analysis for calculation of sample size, and sampling strategy have been used, you can feel more confident that the sample is representative of the accessible population rather than biased (Fig. 12.2) and the potential for generalizability of findings is greater (see Chapter 8).

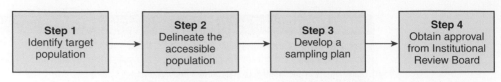

FIG 12.2 Summary of general sampling procedure.

≫ APPRAISAL FOR EVIDENCE-BASED PRACTICE
SAMPLING

The criteria for critical appraisal of a study's sample are presented in the Critical Appraisal Criteria box. As you evaluate the sample section of a study, you must raise two questions:
1. If this study were to be replicated, would there be enough information presented about the nature of the population, the sample, the sampling strategy, and the sample size of another investigator to carry out the study?
2. What are the sampling threats to internal and external validity that are sources of bias?

The answers to these questions highlight the important link of the sample to the findings and the strength of the evidence used to make clinical decisions about the applicability of the findings to clinical practice (see Chapter 8).

In Chapter 8, we talked about how selection effect, as a threat to internal validity, could occur in studies where a convenience, quota, or purposive sampling strategy was used. In these studies, individuals themselves decide whether or not to participate. Subject mortality or attrition is another threat to internal validity related to sampling (see Chapter 8). Mortality is the loss of subjects from the study, usually from the first data-collection point to the second. If the subjects who remain in the study are different from those who drop out, the results can be affected. When more of the subjects in one group drop out than in the other group, the results can also be influenced. It is common for journals to require authors reporting on research results to include a flowchart that diagrams the screening, recruitment, enrollment, random assignment, and attrition process and results (see Fig. 1 flowchart in Appendix B).

Threats to external validity related to sampling are concerned with the generalizability of the results to other populations (see Chapter 8). Generalizability depends on who actually participates in a study. Not everyone who is approached meets the inclusion criteria, agrees to enroll, or completes the study. Bias in sample representativeness and generalizability of findings are important sampling issues that have generated national concern because the presence of these factors decreases confidence in the evidence provided by the findings and limits applicability. Historically, many of the landmark adult health studies (e.g., the Framingham heart study, the Baltimore longitudinal study on aging) excluded women as subjects. Despite the all-male samples, the findings of these studies were generalized from males to all adults, in spite of the lack of female representation in the samples. Similarly, the use of largely European-American subjects in clinical trials limits the identification of variant responses to interventions or drugs in ethnic or racially distinct groups (Ward, 2003). Findings based on European-American data cannot be generalized to African Americans, Asians, Hispanics, or any other cultural group.

CRITICAL APPRAISAL CRITERIA
Sampling

1. Have the sample characteristics been completely described?
2. Can the parameters of the study population be inferred from the description of the sample?
3. To what extent is the sample representative of the population as defined?
4. Are the eligibility/inclusion criteria for the sample clearly identified?
5. Have sample exclusion criteria/delimitations for the sample been established?
6. Would it be possible to replicate the study population?
7. How was the sample selected? Is the method of sample selection appropriate?
8. What kind of bias, if any, is introduced by this sampling method?
9. Is the sample size appropriate? How is it substantiated?
10. Are there indications that rights of subjects have been ensured?
11. Does the researcher identify limitations in generalizability of the findings from the sample to the population? Are they appropriate?
12. Is the sampling strategy appropriate for the design of the study and level of evidence provided by the design?
13. Does the researcher indicate how replication of the study with other samples would provide increased support for the findings?

When appraising the sample of a study, you must remember that despite the use of a carefully controlled sampling procedure that minimizes error, there is no guarantee that the sample will be representative. Factors such as sample heterogeneity and subject dropout may jeopardize the representativeness of the sample despite the most stringent random sampling procedure.

When a purposive sample is used in experimental and quasi-experimental studies, you should determine whether or how the subjects were randomly assigned to groups. If criteria for random assignment have not been followed, you have a valid basis for being cautious about the strength of evidence provided by the proposed conclusions of the study.

Although random selection may be the ideal in establishing the representativeness of a study population, more often realistic barriers (e.g., institutional policy, inaccessibility of subjects, lack of time or money, and current state of knowledge in the field) necessitate the use of nonprobability sampling strategies. Many important research questions that are of interest to nursing do not lend themselves to probability sampling. A well-designed, carefully controlled study using a nonprobability sampling strategy can yield accurate and meaningful evidence that makes a significant contribution to nursing's scientific body of knowledge.

The greatest difficulty in nonprobability sampling stems from the fact that not every element in the population has an equal chance of being represented. Therefore it is likely that some segment of the population will be systematically underrepresented. If the population is homogeneous on critical characteristics, such as age, gender, socioeconomic status, and diagnosis, systematic bias will not be very important. Few of the attributes that researchers are interested in, however, are sufficiently homogeneous to make sampling bias an irrelevant consideration.

Basically you will decide whether the sample size for a quantitative study is appropriate and its size is justifiable. You want to make sure that the researcher indicated how the sample size was determined. The method of arriving at the sample size and the rationale should be briefly mentioned. In a study examining the transition from acute to chronic pain in lower extremity fracture patients (Griffioen et al., 2020) the criterion for detecting a medium treatment effect (95% confidence interval) with a power level set at 0.80, sensitive to the requirements, revealed that a sample size of 158 subjects would be sufficient to detect the effect of the protocol on chronic pain. They anticipated an attrition rate of approximately 15% was accounted for by enrolling 240 subjects. When appraising qualitative research designs, you also apply criteria related to sampling strategies that are relevant for a particular type of qualitative study. In general, sampling strategies for qualitative studies are purposive because the study of specific phenomena in their natural setting is emphasized; any subject belonging to a specified group is considered to represent that group. Keep in mind that qualitative studies will not discuss predetermining sample size or method of arriving at the sample size. Rather, sample size will tend to be small and a function of data saturation. Finally, evidence that the rights of human subjects have been protected should appear in the "Sample" section of the research report and probably consists of no more than one sentence. Remember to evaluate whether permission was obtained from an institutional review board that reviewed the study relative to the maintenance of ethical research standards (see Chapter 13).

KEY POINTS

- Sampling is a process that selects representative units of a population for study. Researchers sample representative segments of the population because it is rarely feasible or necessary to sample entire populations of interest to obtain accurate and meaningful information.
- Researchers establish eligibility criteria; these are descriptors of the population and provide the basis for selection of a sample. Eligibility criteria, which are also referred to as *delimitations,* include age, gender, socioeconomic status, level of education, religion, and ethnicity.
- The researcher must identify the target population (i.e., the entire set of cases about which the researcher would like to make generalizations). Because of the pragmatic constraints, however, the researcher usually uses an accessible population (i.e., one that meets the population criteria and is available).
- A sample is a set of elements that makes up the population.
- A sampling unit is the element or set of elements used for selecting the sample. The foremost criterion in appraising a sample is the representativeness or congruence of characteristics with the population.
- Sampling strategies consist of nonprobability and probability sampling.
- In nonprobability sampling, the elements are chosen by nonrandom methods. Types of nonprobability sampling include convenience, quota, and purposive sampling.
- Probability sampling is characterized by the random selection of elements from the population. In random selection, each element in the population has an equal and independent chance of being included in the sample. Types of probability sampling include simple random, stratified random, and multistage sampling.
- Sample size is a function of the type of sampling procedure being used, the degree of precision required, the type of sample estimation formula being used, the heterogeneity of the study attributes, the relative frequency of occurrence of the phenomena under consideration, and cost.

- Criteria for drawing a sample vary according to the sampling strategy. Systematic organization of the sampling procedure minimizes bias. The target population is identified, the accessible portion of the target population is delineated, permission to conduct the research study is obtained, and a sampling plan is formulated.
- When critically appraising a research report, the sampling plan must be evaluated for its appropriateness in relation to the particular research design and level of evidence generated by the design.
- Completeness of the sampling plan is examined in light of potential replicability of the study. The critiquer appraises whether the sampling strategy is the strongest plan for the particular study under consideration.
- An appropriate systematic sampling plan will maximize the efficiency of a research study. It will increase the strength, accuracy, and meaningfulness of the evidence provided by the findings and enhance the generalizability of the findings from the sample to the population.

CLINICAL JUDGMENT CHALLENGES

- How do inclusion and exclusion criteria contribute to increasing the strength of evidence provided by the sampling strategy of a research study?
- Why is it important for a researcher to use power analysis to calculate sample size? How does adequate sample size affect subject mortality, representativeness of the sample, the researcher's ability to detect a treatment effect, and your ability to generalize from the study findings to your patient population?
- How does a flowchart such as the one in Fig. 1 of the De la Fuente Coria article in Appendix B contribute to the strength and quality of evidence provided by the findings of research study and their potential for applicability to practice?
- **IPE** Your interprofessional team member argues that a random sample is always better, even if it is small and represents *only* one site. Another team member counters that a very large convenience sample with random assignment to groups representing multiple sites can be very significant. Which colleague would you defend, and why? How would each scenario affect the strength and quality of evidence provided by the findings?
- Your research classmate argues that a random sample is always better, even if it is small and represents only one site. Another student counters that a very large convenience sample representing multiple sites can be very significant. Which classmate would you defend, and why? How would each scenario affect the strength and quality of evidence provided by the findings?

REFERENCES

Admi, H., Eilon-Moshe, Y., Levy, H., Eisen, I., Nikolsky, E., Gepstein, L., Satran, C., & Ore, L. (2020). It's up to me with a little support" – Adherence after myocardial infarction: A qualitative study. *International Journal of Nursing Studies, 101*, 1–9.

Bose, E., Maganti, S., Bowles, K. H., & Brueshoff, B. L. (2019). Machine learning methods for identifying critical data elements in nursing documentation. *Nursing Research, 68*(1), 65–72.

Cohen, J. (1988). *Statistical power analysis for the behavioral sciences* (2nd ed.). New York, NY: Academic Press.

De la Fuente Coria, M. C., Cruz-Cobo, C., & Santi-Cano, M. J. (2020). Effectiveness of a primary care nurse delivered educational intervention for patients with type 2 diabetes mellitus in promoting metabolic control and compliance with long-term therapeutic targets: Randomised controlled trial. *International Journal of Nursing Studies, 101*, 1–8.

Griffioen, M. A., Gluttig, J., O'Tolle, R. V., Starkweather, A. R., Lyon, D., Dorsey, S. G., & Renn, C. L. (2020). Transition from acute to chronic pain in lower extremity fracture patients. *Nursing Research, 69*(2), 149–156.

Herbel, K. (2019). Using Facebook to recruit pregnant women for research. *Nursing Research, 68*(3), 242–245.

Kamp, K. J., Luo, Z., Holmstrom, A., Given, B., & Wyatt, G. (2019). Self-management through social support among emerging adults with inflammatory bowel disease. *Nursing Research, 68*(4), 285–295.

Ko, N. Y., Hong, S., Winn, R. A., & Calip, G. S. (2020). Association of insurance status and racial disparities with the detection of early-stage breast cancer. *JAMA Oncology, 6*(3), 385–392.

Lewis, G., Duffy, L., Ades, A., Amos, R., Araya, R., Brabyn, K., Button, K. S., et al. (2019). The clinical effectiveness of sertraline in primary care and the role of depression severity and duration (PANDA): a pragmatic, double-blind, placebo-controlled randomized trial. *The Lancet Psychiatry, 6*(11), 903–914.

Office of Disease Prevention and Health Promotion. *Healthy People 2030.* U.S. Department of Health and Human Services. https://health.gov/healthypeople/objectives-and-data/social-determinants-health.

Robbins, L. B., Wen, F., & Ling, J. (2019). Mediators of physical activity behavior change in the "Girls on the Move" intervention. *Nursing Research, 68*(4), 257–266.

Sousa, V. D., Zauszniewski, J. A., & Musil, C. M. (2004). How to determine whether a convenience sample represents the population. *Applied Nursing Research, 17*(2), 130–133.

Speziale, S., & Carpenter, D. R. (2011). *Qualitative research in nursing* (4th ed.). Philadelphia, PA: Lippincott.

Ward, L. S. (2003). Race as a variable in cross-cultural research. *Nursing Outlook, 51*(3), 120–125.

Wetzstein, M. M., Shanta, L. L., & Chian, L. L. (2020). Patient activation among community-dwelling persons living with chronic obstructive pulmonary disease. *Nursing Research, 69*(5), 347–357.

Go to Evolve at **http://evolve.elsevier.com/LoBiondo/** for review questions, appraisal exercises, and additional research articles for practice in reviewing and appraisal.

13

Appraising Legal & Ethical Issues

Judith Haber, Geri LoBiondo-Wood

Go to Evolve at **http://evolve.elsevier.com/LoBiondo/** for review questions.

LEARNING OUTCOMES

After reading this chapter, you should be able to do the following:

- Describe the historical background that led to the development of ethical guidelines for the use of human subjects in research.
- Identify the essential elements of the informed consent process.
- Evaluate the adequacy of an informed consent.
- Describe the institutional review board's role in the research review process.
- Identify populations of subjects who require special legal and ethical research considerations.
- Describe the nurse's role as a patient advocate.
- Critique the ethical aspects of a research study.

KEY TERMS

anonymity	confidentiality	informed consent	justice
assent	consent	institutional review	respect for persons
beneficence	ethics	boards	risk/benefit ratio

Ethical issues are integral with the conduct of research and implementation of evidence-based practice. Nurses need to remember that research, as well as clinical decision making, is at its core a patient-centered, ethical matter. This is of particular importance when working with underserved and vulnerable populations who often feel less empowered and able to participate in decision making. The focus of this chapter is the legal and ethical considerations that must be addressed before, during, and after the conduct of research. Informed consent, institutional review boards (IRBs), and research involving vulnerable populations—older adults, pregnant women, children, and prisoners—are discussed. The nurse's role as patient advocate, whether functioning as researcher, caregiver, or research consumer, is addressed.

ETHICAL AND LEGAL CONSIDERATIONS IN RESEARCH: A HISTORICAL PERSPECTIVE

Ethical and legal considerations with regard to research first received attention after World War II, when the US Secretary of State and Secretary of War learned that the trials for war criminals would focus on justifying the atrocities committed by Nazi physicians as "medical research." The American Medical Association appointed a group to develop a code of ethics for research that would serve as a standard for judging the medical atrocities committed on concentration camp prisoners.

The resultant Nuremberg Code and its definitions of *voluntary, legal capacity, sufficient understanding,* and *enlightened decision* have been the subject of numerous court cases and presidential commissions involved in setting ethical standards in research (Amdur & Bankert, 2011). The code requires informed consent in all cases but makes no provisions for any special treatment of children, older adults, or the cognitively impaired. In the United States, federal guidelines for the ethical conduct of research were developed in the 1970s. Despite the safeguards provided by the federal guidelines, some of the most atrocious and hence memorable examples of unethical research took place in the United States as recently as 2019. During the COVID pandemic in 2020, many studies of untested therapeutics were called into question. These examples are highlighted in Table 13.1 and are sad reminders of our own tarnished research heritage. They illustrate the human consequences of not adhering to ethical research standards.

TABLE 13.1   Highlights of Unethical Research Studies Conducted in the United States

Research Study	Year(s)	Focus of Study	Ethical Principle Violated
Hyman vs. Jewish Chronic Disease Hospital case	1965	Doctors injected cancer-ridden aged and senile patients with their own cancer cells to study the rejection response.	Informed consent not obtained and no indication that the study was reviewed and approved by an ethics committee. The two physicians claimed they did not wish to evoke emotional reactions or refusals to participate by informing the subjects of the nature of the study (Hershey & Miller, 1976).
Ivory Coast, Africa, AIDS/AZT case	1994	In a study supported by the US government and conducted in the Ivory Coast, Dominican Republic, and Thailand, some pregnant women infected with HIV were given placebo pills rather than AZT, a drug known to prevent mothers from passing on the virus. Babies were in danger of contracting HIV unnecessarily.	Subjects who consented to participate and randomized to the control group were denied access to a medication regimen with a known benefit. This violates a subject's right to fair treatment and protection (French, 1997; Wheeler, 1997).
Midgeville, Georgia, case	1969	Investigational drugs were used on mentally disabled children without first obtaining the opinion of a psychiatrist.	No review of the study protocol or institutional approval of the program before implementation (Levine, 1986).
Tuskegee, Alabama, Syphilis Study	1932–1973	For 40 years, the US Public Health Service conducted a study using two groups of poor black male sharecroppers. One group included those who had untreated syphilis; the other group was judged to be free of the disease. Treatment was withheld from the group having syphilis, even after penicillin became available and accepted as effective treatment. Steps were taken to prevent the subjects from obtaining it. Researchers wanted to study the untreated disease.	Many subjects who consented to participate were not informed about the purpose and procedures of the research. Others were unaware that they were subjects. The degree of risk outweighed the potential benefit. Withholding of known effective treatment violates the subjects' right to fair treatment and protection from harm (Levine, 1986).

TABLE 13.1   Highlights of Unethical Research Studies Conducted in the United States—cont'd

Research Study	Year(s)	Focus of Study	Ethical Principle Violated
San Antonio Contraceptive Study	1969	This study examined side effects of oral contraceptives in 76 impoverished Mexican-American women who were randomly assigned to an experimental group receiving birth control pills or a control group receiving placebos. Subjects were not informed about the placebo and pregnancy risk; 11 subjects became pregnant, 10 of whom were in the placebo control group.	Informed consent principles were violated; full disclosure of potential risk, harm, results, or side effects was not evident in the informed consent document. The potential risk outweighed the benefits of the study. The subjects' right to fair treatment and protection from harm was violated (Levine, 1986).
Willowbrook Hospital Study	1972	Mentally incompetent children ($n = 350$) were not admitted to Willowbrook Hospital, a residential treatment facility, unless parents consented to their children being subjects in a study examining the natural history of infectious hepatitis and the effect of gamma globulin. Children were deliberately infected with the hepatitis virus under various conditions. Some received gamma globulin; others did not.	The principle of voluntary consent was violated. Parents were coerced to consent to their children's participation as research subjects. Subjects or their guardians have a right to self-determination—that is, they should be free from constraint, coercion, or undue influence of any kind.
UCLA Schizophrenia Medication Study	1983	This study examined the effects of withdrawing psychotropic medications of 50 patients being treated for schizophrenia; 23 subjects suffered severe relapses after their medication was stopped. The study's goal was to determine whether some schizophrenics might do better without medications that had deleterious side effects.	Although subjects signed an informed consent, they were not informed how severe their relapses might be or that they could suffer worsening symptoms with each recurrence. Informed consent principles were violated; full disclosure of potential risk, harm, results, or side effects was not evident in the informed consent form. Potential risks outweighed the study's benefits. The subjects' right to fair treatment and protection from harm was violated (Hilts, 1995).

In 1973, the first set of proposed regulations on the protection of human subjects was published. The most important provision was a regulation mandating that an IRB must review and approve all studies. In 1974, the National Commission for the Protection of Human Subjects of Biomedical and Behavioral Research was created. A major change brought forth by the commission was to identify the basic principles that should underlie the conduct of biomedical and behavioral research involving human subjects and to develop guidelines to ensure that research is conducted in accordance with those principles (Amdur & Bankert, 2011). Three ethical principles were identified as relevant to the conduct of research involving human subjects: the principles of respect for persons, beneficence, and justice (Box 13.1). Included in the report, called the Belmont Report, these principles provide the basis for regulations affecting research (National Commission for the Protection of Human Subjects of Biomedical and Behavioral Research, 1978).

BOX 13.1   Basic Ethical Principles Relevant to the Conduct of Research

Respect for Persons

People have the right to self-determination and to treatment as autonomous agents. Thus they have the freedom to participate or not participate in research. Persons with diminished autonomy are entitled to protection.

Beneficence

Beneficence is an obligation to do no harm and maximize possible benefits. Persons are treated in an ethical manner, decisions are respected, they are protected from harm, and efforts are made to secure their well-being.

Justice

Human subjects should be treated fairly. An injustice occurs when a benefit to which a person is entitled is denied without good reason or when a burden is imposed unduly.

The US Department of Health and Human Services (DHHS) also developed a set of regulations that have been revised several times (DHHS, 2020). They include the following:

- Requirements for informed consent
- Documentation of informed consent
- IRB review of research proposals
- Exempt and expedited review procedures for certain kinds of research
- Criteria for IRB approval of research

Protection of Human Rights

Human rights are the claims and demands that have been justified in the eyes of an individual or by a group of individuals. The term refers to the rights outlined in the American Nurses Association guidelines (ANA, 2015):

1. Right to self-determination
2. Right to privacy and dignity
3. Right to anonymity and confidentiality
4. Right to fair treatment
5. Right to protection from discomfort and harm

These rights apply to all involved in research, including research team members who may be involved in data collection, practicing nurses involved in the research setting, and subjects participating in the study. As you read a research article, you must realize that any issues highlighted in Table 13.2 should have been addressed and resolved before a research study is approved for implementation.

Procedures for Protecting Basic Human Rights

Informed Consent

Elements of informed consent illustrated by the ethical principles of respect and related right to self-determination are outlined in Box 13.2 and Table 13.2. It is critical to note that informed consent is not just giving a potential subject a consent form, but is a *process* that the researcher completes with each subject. Informed consent is documented by a consent form that is given to prospective subjects and contains standard elements.

Informed consent is a legal principle that means that potential subjects understand the implications of participating in research and they knowingly agree to participate

TABLE 13.2 Protection of Human Rights

Definition	Violation of Basic Human Right	Example
Right to Self-Determination		
Based on the principle of respect for persons, people should be treated as autonomous with the freedom to choose without external controls. An autonomous agent is one who is informed about a proposed study and allowed to choose to participate or not; subjects have the right to withdraw from a study without penalty. Subjects with diminished autonomy are entitled to protection. They are more vulnerable because of age, legal or mental incompetence, terminal illness, or confinement to an institution. Justification for use of vulnerable subjects must be provided.	A subject's right to self-determination is violated through use of coercion, covert data collection, and deception. • Coercion occurs when an overt threat of harm or excessive reward is presented to ensure compliance. • Covert data collection occurs when people become subjects and are exposed to research treatments without their knowledge. • Deception occurs when subjects are actually misinformed about the research's purpose. • Potential for violation of the right to self-determination is greater for subjects with diminished autonomy; they have decreased ability to give informed consent and are vulnerable.	Subjects may feel that their care will be adversely affected if they refuse to participate in research. The Jewish Chronic Disease Hospital Study (see Table 13.1) is an example in which patients and their doctors did not know that cancer cells were being injected. In another study, subjects were deceived when asked to administer electric shocks to another person; the person was really an actor who pretended to feel the shocks. Subjects administering the shocks were very stressed by participating in this study, although they were not administering shocks at all. The Willowbrook Study (see Table 13.1) is an example of how coercion was used to obtain parental consent of vulnerable mentally retarded children who would not be admitted to the institution unless the children participated in a study in which they were deliberately injected with the hepatitis virus.
Right to Privacy and Dignity		
Based on the principle of respect, privacy is the freedom of a person to determine the time, extent, and circumstances under which private information is shared or withheld from others.	The Privacy Act (1974) was instituted to protect subjects from such violations. These occur most frequently during data collection when invasive questions are asked that may result in loss of job or dignity, or may create embarrassment and mental distress. It also may occur when subjects are unaware that information is being shared with others.	Subjects may be asked personal questions such as the following: "Were you sexually abused as a child?" "Do you use drugs?" "What are your sexual preferences?" When questions are asked using hidden microphones or hidden tape recorders, the subjects' privacy is invaded because they have no knowledge that the data are being shared with others. Subjects also have a right to control access of others to their records.
Right to Anonymity and Confidentiality		
Based on the principle of respect, **anonymity** exists when a subject's identity cannot be linked, even by the researcher, with their individual responses.	Anonymity is violated when the subjects' responses can be linked with their identity.	Subjects are given a code number instead of using names for identification purposes. Subjects' names are never used when reporting findings.
Confidentiality means that individual identities of subjects will not be linked to the information they provide and will not be publicly divulged.	Confidentiality is breached when a researcher, either by accident or by direct action, allows an unauthorized person to gain access to study data that contains subjects' identity information or responses that create a potentially harmful situation for subjects.	Breaches of confidentiality with regard to sexual preference, income, drug use, prejudice, or personality variables can be harmful to subjects. Data are analyzed as group data so individuals cannot be identified by their responses.

Continued

TABLE 13.2   Protection of Human Rights—cont'd

Definition	Violation of Basic Human Right	Example
Right to Self-Determination		
Based on the principle of justice, people should be treated fairly and receive what they are due or owed. Fair treatment is equitable subject selection and treatment during a study, including selection of subjects for reasons directly related to the problem studied versus convenience, compromised position, or vulnerability. Also included is fair treatment of subjects during a study, including fair distribution of risks and benefits regardless of age, race, or socioeconomic status.	Injustices with regard to subject selection have occurred as a result of social, cultural, racial, and gender biases in society. Historically, research subjects often have been obtained from groups of people who were regarded as having less "social value," such as the poor, prisoners, slaves, the mentally incompetent, and the dying. Often subjects were treated carelessly, without consideration of physical or psychological harm.	The Tuskegee Syphilis Study (1973), the Jewish Chronic Disease Hospital Study (1965), the San Antonio Contraceptive Study (1969), and the Willowbrook Study (1972) (see Table 13.1) all provide examples related to unfair subject selection. Investigators should not be late for data collection appointments, should terminate data collection on time, should not change agreed-on procedures or activities without consent, and should provide agreed-on benefits such as a copy of the study findings or a participation fee.
Right to Protection From Discomfort and Harm		
Based on the principle of beneficence, people must take an active role in promoting good and preventing harm in the world around them, as well as in research studies. Discomfort and harm can be physical, psychological, social, or economic in nature. There are five categories of studies based on levels of harm and discomfort: 1. No anticipated effects 2. Temporary discomfort 3. Unusual level of temporary discomfort 4. Risk for permanent damage 5. Certainty of permanent damage	Subjects' right to be protected is violated when researchers know in advance that harm, death, or disabling injury will occur and thus the benefits do not outweigh the risk.	Temporary physical discomfort involving minimal risk includes fatigue or headache, and emotional discomfort including travel expenses incurred to and from the data collection site. Studies examining sensitive issues, such as rape, incest, or spouse abuse, may cause unusual levels of temporary discomfort by opening up current and/or past traumatic experiences. In these situations, researchers assess distress levels and provide debriefing sessions during which the subject may express feelings and ask questions. The researcher makes referrals for professional intervention. Studies having the potential to cause permanent damage are more likely to be medical rather than nursing in nature. A recent clinical trial of a new drug, a recombinant activated protein C (rAPC) (Zovan) for treatment of sepsis, was halted when interim findings from the Phase III clinical trials revealed a reduced mortality rate for the treatment group versus the placebo group. Evaluation of the data led to termination of the trial to make available a known beneficial treatment to all patients. In some research, such as the Tuskegee Syphilis Study or the Nazi medical experiments, subjects experienced permanent damage or death.

BOX 13.2   Elements of Informed Consent

1. Title of protocol
2. Invitation to participate
3. Basis for subject selection
4. Overall purpose of study
5. Explanation of procedures
6. Description of risks and discomforts
7. Potential benefits
8. Alternatives to participation
9. Financial obligations
10. Assurance of confidentiality
11. In case of injury compensation
12. HIPAA disclosure
13. Subject withdrawal
14. Offer to answer questions
15. Concluding consent statement
16. Identification of investigators

(Amdur & Bankert, 2011). Informed consent (DHHS, 2020; US Food and Drug Administration [FDA], 2020a) is defined as follows:

The knowing consent of an individual or his/her legally authorized representative, under circumstances that provide the prospective subject or representative sufficient opportunity to consider whether or not to participate without undue inducement or any element of force, fraud, deceit, duress, or other forms of constraint or coercion.

No investigator may involve a person as a research subject before obtaining the legally effective informed consent of a subject or legally authorized representative. The study must be explained to all potential subjects, including the study's purpose; procedures; risks, discomforts, and benefits; and expected duration of participation (i.e., when the study's procedures will be implemented, how many times, and in what setting). Potential subjects must also be informed about any appropriate alternative procedures or treatments, if any, that might be advantageous to the subject. For example, in the Tuskegee Syphilis Study, the researchers should have disclosed that penicillin was an effective available treatment for syphilis. Any compensation for subjects' participation must be delineated when there is more than minimal risk through disclosure about medical treatments and/or compensation that is available if injury occurs.

IPE HIGHLIGHT

It is important to remember that the right to personal privacy may be more difficult to protect when researchers are carrying out qualitative studies because of the small sample size, and the subjects' verbatim quotes are often used in the findings/results section of the research article to highlight the findings.

Prospective subjects must have time to decide whether or not to participate in a study. The researcher must not coerce the subject into participating or collect data on subjects who have explicitly refused to participate in a study. An ethical violation of this principle is illustrated by the halting of eight experiments by the FDA at the University of Pennsylvania's Institute for Human Gene Therapy 4 months after the death of an 18-year-old man, Jesse Gelsinger, who received experimental treatment as part of the institute's research. The institute could not document that all patients had been informed of the risks and benefits of the procedures. Furthermore, some patients who received the therapy should have been considered ineligible, as their illnesses were more severe than allowed by the clinical protocols. Mr. Gelsinger had a non–life-threatening genetic disorder that permits toxic amounts of ammonia to build up in the liver. Nevertheless, he volunteered for an experimental treatment in which normal genes were implanted directly into his liver, and he subsequently died of multiple organ failure. The institute failed to report to the FDA that two patients in the same trial as Mr. Gelsinger had suffered severe side effects, including inflammation of the liver, as a result of the treatment. This should have triggered a halt to the trial (Brainard & Miller, 2000). Of course, subjects may discontinue participation or withdraw from a study at any time without penalty or loss of benefits.

It is important to recognize that the principles of informed consent are not stagnant. For example, ethics related to genomic specimens has led to changes in the Common Rule (DHHS, 2018b). Often researchers gather specimens during the course of a study for a specific study and wish to bank or save the specimen (s) for later study. Thus a new type of consent was identified called *broad consent*. Broad consent asks the participant for permission to store or bank specimens for future studies. These specimens are de-identified when stored, but the researcher may retain a code number.

HELPFUL HINT

Research reports rarely provide detailed information regarding the degree to which the researcher adhered to ethical principles, such as informed consent, because of space limitations in journals that make it impossible to describe all aspects of a study. Failure to mention procedures to safeguard subjects' rights does not necessarily mean that such precautions were not taken.

The language of the consent form must be understandable and in the language of the potential subject. The reading level should be no higher than eighth grade for adults, it should be presented in lay language, and avoidance of technical terms should be observed (DHHS, 2009). If necessary, translators must be made available. Subjects should not be asked to waive their rights or release the investigator from liability for negligence. The elements for an informed consent form are listed in Box 13.2.

Investigators obtain **consent** through personal discussion with potential subjects. This process allows the person to obtain immediate answers to questions. Discussion coupled with consent forms that are written in narrative or outline form will highlight elements that both inform and remind subjects of the nature of the study and their participation (Amdur & Nakert, 2011). For low-risk online or mail-returned questionnaire studies in which responses are anonymous and questionnaires require low-risk responses, researchers may use implied consent only. Implied consent means that completion and submission of the study document(s) is considered consent to participate.

Assurance of anonymity and confidentiality (defined in Table 13.2) is conveyed in writing and describes how subjects' confidentiality will be maintained. The right to privacy is also protected through protection of individually identifiable health information (IIHI). The DHHS developed the following guidelines to help researchers, health care organizations, health care providers, and academic institutions determine when they can use and disclose IIHI:

- IIHI is "de-identified" under the HIPAA Privacy Rule.
- Data are part of a limited data set, and a data use agreement with the researcher is in place.
- A potential subject provides authorization for the researcher to use and disclose protected health information (PHI).
- A waiver or alteration of the authorization requirement is obtained from the IRB.

- The consent form is signed and dated by the subject. The presence of witnesses is not always necessary but does constitute evidence that the subject actually signed the form. If the subject is a minor or is physically or mentally incapable of signing the consent, the legal guardian or representative must sign. The investigator also signs the form to indicate commitment to the agreement.

A copy of the signed informed consent is given or sent to the subject. The researcher maintains the original for their records. Some research, such as a retrospective chart audit, may not require informed consent—only institutional approval. In some cases, when minimal risk is involved, the investigator may have to provide the subject only with an information sheet and verbal explanation. In other cases, such as a volunteer convenience sample, completion and return of research instruments provide evidence of consent. The IRB advises on exceptions to these guidelines, and there are cases in which the IRB may grant waivers or amend its guidelines in other ways. The IRB makes the final determination regarding the most appropriate documentation format. You should note whether and what kind of evidence of informed consent has been provided in a research article.

> **HELPFUL HINT**
>
> Researchers may not obtain written informed consent when the major means of data collection is through self-administered questionnaires. The researcher usually assumes implied consent in such cases—that is, the return of the completed questionnaire reflects the respondent's voluntary consent to participate.

Institutional Review Boards

IRBs review studies to assess that ethical standards are met in relation to the protection of the rights of human subjects. The National Research Act (1974) requires that agencies such as universities, hospitals, and other health care organizations (e.g., managed care companies) where biomedical or behavioral research involving human subjects is conducted must submit an application with assurances that they have an IRB, sometimes called a *human subjects' committee,* that reviews the research projects and protects the rights of the human subjects (FDA, 2012b). At agencies where no federal grants or contracts are awarded, there is usually a review mechanism similar to an IRB process, such as a research advisory committee. The National Research Act requires that the IRBs have at least five members of various research backgrounds to promote complete and adequate study reviews. The members must be qualified by virtue of their expertise and experience and reflect professional, gender, racial, and cultural diversity. Membership must include one member whose concerns are primarily nonscientific (lawyer, clergy, ethicist) and at least one member from outside the agency. IRB members have mandatory training in scientific integrity and prevention of scientific misconduct, as do the principal investigators of a study and their research team members. In an effort to protect research subjects, the HIPAA Privacy Rule has made IRB requirements much more stringent for researchers (Code of Federal Regulations, Part 46, 2009). The revised Department of Health and Human Services Common Rule put forth in 2018 details the needed expertise and experience of IRB members.

The IRB is responsible for protecting subjects from undue risk and loss of personal rights and dignity. The **risk/benefit ratio**, the extent to which a study's benefits are maximized and the risks are minimized such that the subjects are protected from harm, is always a major consideration. For a research proposal to be eligible for consideration by an IRB, it must already have been approved by a departmental review group, such as a nursing research

> **BOX 13.3 Code of Federal Regulations for International Review Board Approval of Research Studies**
>
> To approve research, the IRB must determine that the following has been satisfied:
> 1. Risks to subjects are minimized.
> 2. Risks to subjects are reasonable in relation to anticipated benefits.
> 3. Selection of the subjects is equitable.
> 4. Informed consent must be and will be sought from each prospective subject or the subject's legally authorized representative.
> 5. Informed consent form must be properly documented.
> 6. Where appropriate, the research plan makes adequate provision for monitoring the data collected to ensure subject safety.
> 7. There are adequate provisions to protect subjects' privacy and the confidentiality of data.
> 8. Where some or all of the subjects are likely to be vulnerable to coercion or undue influence, additional safeguards are included.

committee that attests to the proposal's scientific merit and congruence with institutional policies, procedures, and mission. The IRB reviews the study's protocol to ensure that it meets the requirements of ethical research that appear in Box 13.3.

IRBs provide guidelines that include steps to be taken to receive IRB approval. For example, guidelines for writing a standard consent form or criteria for qualifying for an expedited rather than a full IRB review may be made available. The IRB has the authority to approve research, require modifications, or disapprove a study. A researcher must receive IRB approval before beginning to conduct research. IRBs have the authority to audit, suspend, or terminate approval of research that is not conducted in accordance with IRB requirements or that has been associated with unexpected serious harm to subjects.

IRBs also have mechanisms for reviewing research in an expedited manner when the risk to research subjects is minimal (DHHS, 2018b). Keep in mind that although a researcher may determine that a project involves minimal risk, the IRB makes the final determination, and the research may not be undertaken until approved. A full list of research categories eligible for expedited review is available from any IRB office. Examples include the following:

- Prospective collection of specimens by noninvasive procedure (e.g., buccal swab, deciduous teeth, hair/nail clippings)
- Research conducted in established educational settings in which subjects are de-identified
- Research involving materials collected for clinical purposes
- Research on taste, food quality, and consumer acceptance
- Collection of excreta and external secretions, including sweat
- Recording of data on subjects 18 years of age or older, using noninvasive procedures routinely employed in clinical practice
- Voice recordings
- Study of existing data, documents, records, pathological specimens, or diagnostic data

An expedited review does not automatically exempt the researcher from obtaining informed consent, and most importantly, the department or agency mechanisms retains the final judgment as to whether or not a study may be exempt.

When critiquing research, it is important to be conversant with current regulations to determine whether ethical standards have been met. The Critical Thinking Decision Path illustrates the ethical decision-making process an IRB might use in evaluating the risk/benefit ratio of a research study.

CRITICAL THINKING DECISION PATH

Evaluating the Risk/Benefit Ratio of a Research Study

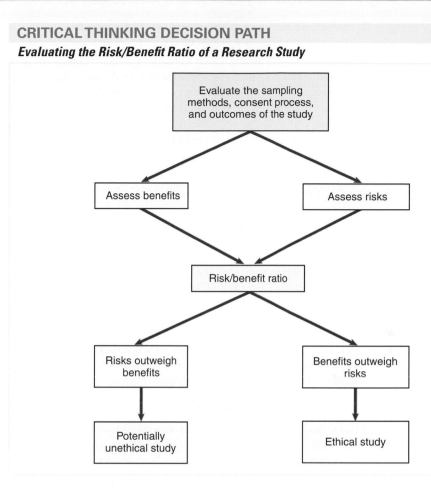

Protecting Basic Human Rights of Vulnerable Groups

Researchers are advised to consult their agency's IRB for the most recent federal and state rules and guidelines when considering research involving vulnerable groups who may have diminished autonomy, such as older adults, children, pregnant women, the unborn, those who are emotionally or physically disabled, prisoners, the deceased, students, and persons with AIDS. In addition, researchers should consult the IRB before planning research that potentially involves an oversubscribed research population, such as individuals experiencing COVID 19, or "captive" and convenient populations, such as prisoners. It should be emphasized that use of special populations does not preclude undertaking research; extra precautions must be taken to protect their rights.

Research with Children. The age of majority differs from state to state, but there are some general rules for including children as subjects (Title 45, CFR46, Subpart D; DHHS, 2018b). Usually a child can assent between 7 and 18 years of age. Research in children requires parental permission and child assent. Assent contains the following fundamental elements:

1. A basic understanding of what the child will be expected to do and what will be done to the child

2. A comprehension of the basic purpose of the research
3. An ability to express a preference regarding participation

In contrast with assent, consent requires a relatively advanced level of cognitive ability. Informed consent reflects competency standards requiring abstract appreciation and reasoning regarding the information provided. Federal guidelines have specific criteria and standards that must be met for children to participate in research. If the research involves more than minimal risk and does not offer direct benefit to the individual child, both parents must give permission. When individuals reach maturity, usually at 18 years of age, they may render their own consent. They may do so at a younger age if they have been legally declared emancipated minors. Questions regarding this are addressed by the IRB and/or research administration office and not left to the discretion of the researcher to answer.

Research With Pregnant Women, Fetuses, and Neonates. Research with pregnant women, fetuses, and neonates requires additional protection but may be conducted if specific criteria are met (Title 45, CFR 46, Subpart B; DHHS, 2018b). Decisions are made relative to the direct or indirect benefit or lack of benefit to the pregnant woman and the fetus. For example, pregnant women may be involved in research if the research suggests the prospect of direct benefit to the pregnant women and fetus by providing data for assessing risks to pregnant women and fetuses. If the research suggests the prospect of direct benefit to the fetus solely, then both the mother and father must provide consent.

Research With Prisoners. The federal guidelines also provide guidance to IRBs regarding research with prisoners. These guidelines address the issues of allowable research, understandable language, adequate assurances that participation does not affect parole decisions, and risks and benefits (Code of Federal Regulations, Title 45, Part 46, Subpart C; DHHS, 2018b).

Research With Older Adults. Older adults have been historically and are potentially vulnerable to abuse and as such require special consideration. There is no issue if the potential subject can supply legally effective informed consent. Competence is not a clear issue. The complexity of the study may affect one's ability to consent to participate. The capacity to obtain informed consent should be assessed in each individual for each research protocol being considered. For example, an older person may be able to consent to participate in a simple observational study but not in a clinical drug trial. The issue of the necessity of requiring an older adult to provide consent often arises, and each situation must be evaluated for its potential to preserve the rights of this population.

No vulnerable population may be singled out for study because it is convenient. For example, neither people with mental illness nor prisoners may be studied because they are an available and convenient group. Prisoners may be studied if the studies pertain to them—that is, studies concerning the effects and processes of incarceration. Similarly, people with mental illness may participate in studies that focus on expanding knowledge about psychiatric disorders and treatments. Students also are often a convenient group. They must not be singled out as research subjects because of convenience; the research questions must have some bearing on their status as students. In all cases, the burden is on the investigator to show the IRB that it is appropriate to involve vulnerable subjects in research. The Office of Clinical Research provides guidance for organizations for the protection of vulnerable research subjects including minority groups, and non–English-speaking individuals. Researchers must provide potential subjects a fair opportunity to understand key information for the consent to be considered valid (https://www.hhs.gov/ohrp/sites/default/files/meeting-new-challenges).

APPRAISAL FOR EVIDENCE-BASED PRACTICE
LEGAL AND ETHICAL ASPECTS OF A RESEARCH STUDY

Published research articles and reports do not contain detailed information regarding the ways in which the investigator adhered to the legal and ethical principles presented in this chapter. Lack of written evidence regarding the protection of human rights does not imply that appropriate steps were not taken.

The Critical Appraisal Criteria box provides guidelines for evaluating the legal and ethical aspects of a study. When reading a study, you will not see all areas explicitly addressed in the article because of space constraints. Box 13.4 provides examples of statements in research articles that illustrate the brevity with which the legal and ethical component of a study is reported.

Information about the legal and ethical considerations of a study is usually presented in the "Methods" section of an article. The subsection on the sample or data-collection methods is the most likely place for this information. The author most often indicates in a sentence that informed consent was obtained and that approval from an IRB was granted. To protect subject and institutional privacy, the locale of the study frequently is described in general terms in the sample subsection of the report. For example, the article may state that data were collected at a 1000-bed tertiary care center in the southwest, without mentioning its name. Protection of subject privacy may be explicitly addressed by statements indicating that anonymity or confidentiality of data was maintained or that grouped data were used in the data analysis.

CRITICAL APPRAISAL CRITERIA

Legal and Ethical Issues

1. Was the study approved by an IRB or other agency committees?
2. Is there evidence that informed consent was obtained from all subjects or their representatives? How was it obtained?
3. Were the subjects protected from physical or emotional harm?
4. Were the subjects or their representatives informed about the purpose and nature of the study?
5. Were the subjects or their representatives informed about any potential risks that may result from participation in the study?
6. How was the research study designed to maximize the benefit(s) to human subjects and minimize the risks?
7. Were subjects coerced or unduly influenced to participate in this study? Did they have the right to refuse to participate or withdraw without penalty? Were vulnerable subjects used?
8. How were appropriate steps taken to safeguard the privacy of subjects? How have data been kept anonymous and/or confidential?

> **BOX 13.4 Examples of Legal and Ethical Content in Published Research Reports Found in the Appendices**
>
> - "The study was conducted under the standards and ethical criteria of the Helsinki declaration, and was submitted to the approval of the ethics & research Committee of the Bahia de Cadiz-La Janda Health District" (De la Fuente Coria et al., 2020) (Appendix B).
> - "Approval for this study was obtained through an affiliated university Institutional Review Board and the organization's Office of Research" (Flanders et al., 2020) (Appendix C).

When considering the special needs of vulnerable subjects, you should be sensitive to whether the special needs of groups, unable to act on their own behalf, have been addressed. For instance, has the right of self-determination been addressed by the informed consent protocol identified in the research report? How have the researchers addressed the need to align the language of the informed consent with the linguistic competency of the potential subjects?

When qualitative studies are reported, verbatim quotes from informants often are incorporated into the findings section of the article. In such cases, you will evaluate how effectively the author protected the informant's identity, either by using a fictitious name or by withholding information such as age, gender, occupation, or other potentially identifying data (see Chapters 5 to 7 for ethical issues related to qualitative research).

It should be apparent from the preceding sections that although the need for guidelines for the use of human subjects in research is evident and the principles themselves are clear, there are many instances when you must use your best judgment both as a patient advocate and as a research consumer when evaluating the ethical nature of a research project. When conflicts arise, you must feel free to raise suitable questions with appropriate resources and personnel. In an institution, these may include contacting the researcher first and then, if there is no resolution, the director of nursing research and the chairperson of the IRB. In cases where ethical considerations in a research article are in question, clarification from a colleague, agency, or IRB is indicated. You should pursue your concerns until satisfied that the patient's rights and your rights as a professional nurse are protected.

KEY POINTS

- Ethical and legal considerations in research first received attention after World War II during the Nuremberg Trials, from which developed the Nuremberg Code. This became the standard for research guidelines protecting the human rights of research subjects.
- The Belmont Report discusses three basic ethical principles (respect for persons, beneficence, and justice) that underlie the conduct of research involving human subjects.
- Protection of human rights includes (1) the right to self-determination, (2) the right to privacy and dignity, (3) the right to anonymity and confidentiality, (4) the right to fair treatment, and (5) the right to protection from discomfort and harm.
- Procedures for protecting human rights include gaining informed consent, which illustrates the ethical principle of respect, and obtaining IRB approval, which illustrates the ethical principles of respect, beneficence, and justice.

- Special consideration should be given to studies involving vulnerable populations, such as children, older adults, non–English-speaking individuals, prisoners, and those who are mentally or physically disabled.
- Nurses must be knowledgeable about the legal and ethical components of research so they can evaluate whether a researcher has ensured protection of patient rights.

CLINICAL JUDGMENT CHALLENGES

- A state government official interested in determining the number of infants infected with the human immunodeficiency virus (HIV) has approached your hospital to participate in a statewide-funded study. The protocol will include testing of all newborns for HIV, but the mothers will not be told that the test is being done, nor will they be told the results. Using the basic ethical principles found in Box 13.2, defend or refute the practice. How will the findings of the proposed study be affected if the protocol is carried out?
- As a research consumer, what kind of information related to the legal and ethical aspects of a research study would you expect to see written about in a published research study? How does that differ from the data the researcher would have to prepare for an IRB submission?
- A randomized controlled trial (RCT) testing the effectiveness of a new Lyme disease vaccine is being conducted as a multisite RCT. There are two vaccine intervention groups, each of which is receiving a different vaccine, and one control group that is receiving a placebo. Using the information in Table 13.2, identify the conditions under which the RCT would be halted as a result of potential legal and ethical issues for subjects.
- **IPE** Your interprofessional quality improvement team is asked to do a presentation about risk/benefit ratio and how it influences clinical decision making and resource allocation in your clinical organization. Think about the key elements to address.

REFERENCES

Amdur, R., & Bankert, E. A. (2011). *Institutional review board: Member handbook* (3rd ed.). Boston, MA: Jones & Bartlett.

American Nurses Association. (2015). *Code for nurses with interpretive statements*. Kansas City, MO: Author.

Brainard, J., & Miller, D. W. (2000). U.S. regulators suspend medical studies at two universities. *Chronicle of Higher Education*, A30.

Department of Health & Human Services. (2018a). Definitions. Common Rule. Federal Regulations, Title 45, Sections 160.103. Retrieved from https://www.govinfo.gov/content/CFR-2013-title45-vol1pdf/CFR-2013-title45-vol1-sec160-103.pdf.

Department of Health & Human Services. (2018b). Protection of Human subjects. Code of Federal Regulations, Title 45, Part 46. Retrieved from http://www.hhs.gov/ohrp/regulations and policy regulations/45-crf-46/index.html.

Code of Federal Regulations, (2009). Part 46, Vol. 1. http://www.accessdata.fda.gov/scripts/cdrh/cfdocs/cfcfr/cfresearch.cfm.

French, H. W. (1997, October 9). AIDS research in Africa: Juggling risks and hopes. *New York Times*, A1–A12.

Hershey, N., & Miller, R. D. (1976). *Human experimentation and the law*. Germantown, MD: Aspen.

Hilts, P. J. (1995, March 9). Agency faults a UCLA study for suffering of mental patients. *New York Times*, A1–A11.

Levine, R. J. (1986). *Ethics and regulation of clinical research* (2nd ed.). Baltimore, MD and Munich, Germany: Urban & Schwartzenberg.

National Commission for the Protection of Human Subjects of Biomedical and Behavioral Research. (1978). *Belmont report: ethical principles and guidelines for research involving human subjects, DHEW pub no 05.* Washington, DC: US Government Printing Office, 78–0012.

US Department of Health and Human Services (DHHS). (2009). 45 CFR 46. *Code of Federal Regulations: protection of human subjects.* Washington, DC: Author.

US Food and Drug Administration (FDA). (2020a). A guide to informed consent, Code of Federal Regulations, Title 21, Part 50. http://www.fda.gov/oc/ohrt/irbs/informedconsent.html.

US Food and Drug Administration (FDA). (2020b). Institutional Review Boards, Code of Federal Regulations, Title 21, Part 56. http://www.fda.gov/oc/ohrt/irbs/appendixc.html.

Wheeler, D. L. (1997). Three medical organizations embroiled in controversy over use of placebos in AIDS studies abroad. *Chronicle of Higher Education,* A15–A16.

Go to Evolve at **http://evolve.elsevier.com/LoBiondo/** for review questions, appraisal exercises, and additional research articles for practice in reviewing and appraisal.

14

Appraising Data Collection Methods

Susan Sullivan-Bolyai, Carol Bova

Go to Evolve at **http://evolve.elsevier.com/LoBiondo/** for review questions.

LEARNING OUTCOMES

After reading this chapter, you should be able to do the following:

- Define the types of data collection methods used in research.
- List the advantages and disadvantages of each data collection method.
- Compare how specific data collection methods contribute to the strength of evidence in a study.
- Identify potential sources of bias related to data collection.
- Discuss the importance of intervention fidelity in data collection.
- Critically evaluate the data collection methods used in published research studies.

KEY TERMS

anecdotes	fidelity	objective	reactivity
closed-ended questions	field notes	observation	respondent burden
concealment	intervention	open-ended questions	scale
consistency	interview guide	operational definition	scientific observation
content analysis	interviews	participant observation	self-report
debriefing	Likert-type scale	physiological data	systematic
demographic data	measurement	questionnaires	systematic error
existing data	measurement error	random error	

Nurses are always collecting information (or data) from patients. We collect data on blood pressure, age, weight, and laboratory values as part of our daily work. Data collected for practice purposes and for research have several key differences. Data collection procedures in research must be **objective**; free from researchers' personal biases, attitudes, and beliefs; and systematic. **Systematic** means that everyone who is involved in the data collection process collects the data from each subject in a uniform, consistent, or standard way. This is called **fidelity**. When reading a study, the data collection methods should be identifiable, transparent, and repeatable. Thus, when reading the research literature to inform your evidence-based practice, there are several issues to consider regarding data collection methods.

It is important that researchers carefully define the *concepts* or *variables* they measure. The process of translating a concept into a measurable variable requires development of an **operational definition**. An operational definition is how the researcher measures each variable. **Example:** ➤ Di Stasio and colleagues (2020) (see Appendix D) conceptually defined *caregiver burden* as an extreme perspective of being vulnerable that is associated with ongoing, relentless caregiving (in this case, with loved ones with Parkinson disease) and results in a negative effect on their own life. They operationally defined this caregiver burden and vulnerability as measured by the Stress Vulnerability Scale, a measurement scale that assesses adults' self-reported perspectives on feeling burdened and vulnerable in the past month.

The purpose of this chapter is to familiarize you with the ways that researchers collect data from subjects. The chapter provides you with the tools for evaluating data collection procedures commonly used in research, their strengths and weaknesses, how consistent data collection operations (fidelity) can increase study rigor and decrease bias that affects study internal and external validity (see Chapter 8), and how useful each technique is for providing evidence for nursing practice. This information will help you critique the research literature and decide whether the findings provide evidence that is applicable to your practice setting.

MEASURING VARIABLES OF INTEREST

Largely the success of a study depends on the fidelity (consistency and quality) of the data collection methods or measurement used. Determining what **measurement** to use in a study may be the most difficult and time-consuming step in study design. Thus the process of evaluating and selecting the instruments to measure variables of interest is of critical importance to the potential success of the study.

As you read research articles and the data collection techniques used, look for **consistency** with the study's aim, hypotheses, setting, and population. Data collection may be viewed as a two-step process. First, the researcher chooses the study's data collection method(s). An algorithm that influences a researcher's choice of data collection methods is diagrammed in the Critical Thinking Decision Path. The second step is deciding if the measurement scales are reliable and valid. Reliability and validity of instruments are discussed in Chapter 15 (for quantitative research) and in Chapter 6 (for qualitative research).

DATA COLLECTION METHODS

When reading a study, be aware that investigators decide early in the process whether they need to collect their own data or whether data already exist in the form of records or databases. This decision is based on a thorough literature review and the availability of existing data. If the researcher determines that no data exist, new data can be collected through **observation** (systematically viewing an activity in progress), self-report (interviewing or questionnaires), or collecting **physiological data** using standardized instruments or testing procedures (e.g., laboratory tests, x-rays). **Existing data** can be collected by extracting data from medical records or local, state, and national databases. Each of these methods has a specific purpose as well as pros and cons inherent in its use. It is important to remember that all data collection methods rely on the ability of the researcher to standardize these procedures to increase data accuracy and reduce measurement error.

CRITICAL THINKING DECISION PATH
Consumer of Research Literature Review

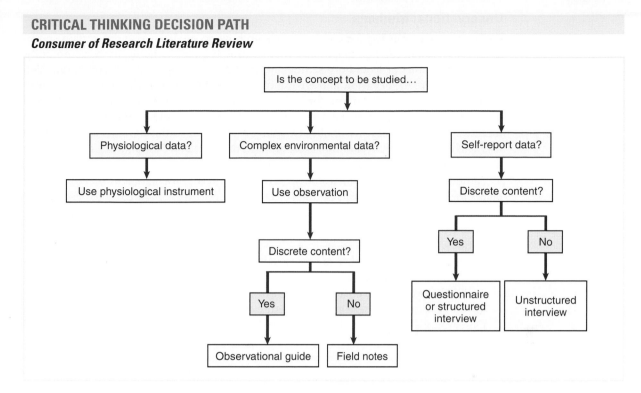

Measurement error is the difference between what really exists and what is measured in a study. Every study has some amount of measurement error. Measurement error can be random or systematic (see Chapter 15). Random error occurs when scores vary in a random way. Random error occurs when data collectors do not use standard procedures to collect data consistently among all subjects in a study. Systematic error occurs when scores are incorrect but in the same direction. An example of systematic error occurs when all subjects were weighed using a weight scale that is under by 3 pounds for all subjects in the study. Researchers attempt to design data collection methods that will be consistently applied across all subjects and time points to reduce measurement error.

HELPFUL HINT

Remember that the researcher may not always present complete information about the way the data were collected, especially when established instruments were used. To learn about the instrument that was used in greater detail, you may need to consult the original article describing the instrument.

To help decipher the quality of the data collection section in a research article, we will discuss the three main methods used for collecting data: observation, self-report, and physiological measurement.

EVIDENCE-BASED PRACTICE TIP

It is difficult to place confidence in a study's findings if the data collection methods are not consistent.

Observational Methods

Observation is a method for collecting data on how people behave under certain conditions. Observation can take place in a natural setting (e.g., in the home, in the community, on a nursing unit) or laboratory setting and includes collecting data on communication (verbal, nonverbal), behavior, and environmental conditions such as the home environment. Observation is also useful for collecting data that may have cultural or contextual influences associated with social determinants of health. **Example:** ➤ If a researcher wants to understand the emergence of obesity among immigrants in the United States, it may be useful to observe food preparation, exercise patterns, types of food resources, and shopping practices in the communities of the specific groups.

Although observing the environment is a normal part of living, **scientific observation** places a great deal of emphasis on the objective and systematic nature of the observation. The researcher is not merely looking at what is happening, but rather is watching with a trained eye for specific events. To be scientific, observations must fulfill the following four conditions:

1. Observations undertaken are consistent with the study's aims/objectives.
2. There is a standardized and systematic plan for observation and data recording.
3. All observations are checked and controlled.
4. The observations are related to scientific concepts and theories.

Observational methods may be structured or unstructured. Unstructured observation methods are not characterized by a total absence of structure but usually involve collecting descriptive information about the topic of interest. In participant observation, the observer keeps **field notes** (a short summary of observations) to record the activities as well as the observer's interpretations of these activities. Field notes usually are not restricted to any particular type of action or behavior; rather, they represent a narrative set of unstructured written notes intended to paint a picture of a social situation in a more general sense. Another type of unstructured observation is the use of anecdotes. **Anecdotes** are summaries of a particular observation that usually focus on the behaviors of interest and frequently add to the richness of research reports by illustrating a particular point (see Chapters 5 and 6 for more on qualitative data collection strategies). Structured observations involve specifying in advance what behaviors or events are to be observed. Typically standardized forms are used for recordkeeping and include categorization systems, checklists, or rating scales. Structured observation relies heavily on the formal training and standardization of the observers (see Chapter 15 for an explanation of interrater reliability).

Observational methods can also be distinguished by the role of the observer. The observer's role is determined by the amount of interaction between the observer and those being observed. These methods are illustrated in Fig. 14.1. **Concealment** refers to whether the subjects know they are being observed. Concealment has ethical implications for the study. Whether concealment is permitted in a study will be decided by an institutional review board (see Chapter 13). The decision will be based on the potential risk to the subjects, the scientific rationale for the concealment, as well as the plan to debrief the participants about the concealment once the study is completed. In data collection, **intervention** deals with whether the observer provokes actions from those who are being observed. Box 14.1 describes the basic types of observational roles implemented by the observer(s). These are distinguishable by the amount of concealment or intervention implemented by the observer.

Observing subjects without their knowledge may violate assumptions of informed consent, therefore researchers face ethical problems with this approach. However,

	Concealment	
	Yes	No
Intervention Yes	Researcher hidden An intervention	Researcher open An intervention
No	Researcher hidden No intervention	Researcher open No intervention

FIG 14.1 Types of observational roles in research.

sometimes there is no other way to collect such data, and the data collected are unlikely to have negative consequences for the subject. In these cases, the disadvantages of the study are outweighed by the advantages. Further, the problem is often handled by informing subjects after the observation, allowing them the opportunity to refuse to have their data included in the study, and discussing any questions they may have. This process is called debriefing.

When the observer is neither concealed nor intervening, the ethical question is not a problem. Here the observer makes no attempt to change the subjects' behavior and informs them that they are to be observed. Because the observer is present, this type of observation allows a greater depth of material to be studied than if the observer is separated from the subject by an artificial barrier, such as a one-way mirror. Participant observation is a commonly used observational technique in which the researcher functions as a part of a social group to study the group in question. The problem with this type of observation is reactivity (also referred to as the Hawthorne effect) or distortion created when the subjects change behavior because they know they are being observed (see Chapter 8).

BOX 14.1   Basic Types of Observational Roles

1. *Concealment without intervention.* The researcher watches subjects without their knowledge and does not provoke the subject into action. Often such concealed observations use hidden television cameras, audio recording devices, or one-way mirrors. This method is often used in observational studies of children and their parents. You may be familiar with rooms with one-way mirrors in which a researcher can observe the behavior of the occupants of the room without being observed by them. Such studies allow for the observation of children's natural behavior and are often used in developmental research.

2. *Concealment with intervention.* Concealed observation with intervention involves staging a situation and observing the behaviors that are evoked in the subjects as a result of the intervention. Because the subjects are unaware of their participation in a research study, this type of observation has fallen into disfavor and rarely is used in nursing research.

3. *No concealment without intervention.* The researcher obtains informed consent from the subject to be observed and then simply observes his or her behavior.

4. *No concealment with intervention.* No concealment with intervention is used when the researcher is observing the effects of an intervention introduced for scientific purposes. Because the subjects know they are participating in a research study, there are few problems with ethical concerns; however, *reactivity* is a problem in this type of study.

Scientific observation has several advantages, the main one being that observation may be the only way for the researcher to consistently study the variable of interest. **Example:** ➤ What people say they do often may not be what they really do. Therefore, if the study is designed to obtain substantive findings about human behavior, observation may be the only way to ensure the validity of the findings. In addition, no other data collection method can match the depth and variety of information that can be collected when using these techniques. Such techniques also are quite flexible in that they may be used in both experimental and nonexperimental designs. As with all data collection methods, observation also has its disadvantages. Data obtained by observational techniques are vulnerable to observer bias. Emotions, prejudices, and values can influence the way behaviors and events are observed and recorded. In general, the more the observer needs to make inferences and judgments about what is being observed, the more likely it is that distortions will occur. Thus in judging the adequacy of observation methods, it is important to consider how observation forms were constructed and how observers were trained and evaluated.

Ethical issues can also occur if subjects are not fully aware that they are being observed. For the most part, it is best to inform subjects of the study's purpose and the fact that they are being observed. However, in certain circumstances, informing the subjects will change behaviors (Hawthorne effect; see Chapter 8). **Example:** ➤ If a nurse researcher wants to study hand-washing frequency in a nursing unit, telling the nurses that they are being observed for their rate and quality of hand washing would likely increase the hand-washing rate and 20-second rule, thereby making the study results less valid. Therefore researchers must carefully balance full disclosure of all research procedures with the ability to obtain valid data through observational methods.

Self-Report Methods

Self-report methods require subjects to respond directly to either interviews or questionnaires about their experiences, behaviors, feelings, or attitudes. Self-report methods are commonly used in nursing research and are most useful for collecting data on variables that cannot be directly observed or measured by physiological instruments. Some variables commonly measured by self-report in nursing research studies include quality of life, satisfaction with nursing care, social support, pain, resilience, and functional status.

The following are some considerations when evaluating self-report methods:

- *Social desirability.* There is no way to know for sure if a subject is telling the truth. People are known to respond to questions in a way that makes a favorable impression.

Example: ➤ If a nurse researcher asks patients to describe the positive and negative aspects of nursing care received, the patient may want to please the researcher and respond with all positive responses, thus introducing bias into the data collection process. There is no way to tell whether the respondent is telling the truth or responding in a socially desirable way, so the accuracy of self-report measures is always open for scrutiny.

- *Respondent burden* is another concern for researchers who use self-report (Bromley et al., 2015). Respondent burden occurs when the length of the questionnaire or interview is too long or the questions are too difficult to answer in a reasonable amount of time considering respondents' age, health condition, or mental status. It also occurs when there are multiple data collection points, as in longitudinal studies when the same questionnaires must be completed multiple times. Respondent burden can result in incomplete or erroneous answers or missing data, jeopardizing the validity of the study findings.

Interviews and Questionnaires

Interviews are a method of data collection in which a data collector asks subjects to respond to a set of open-ended or closed-ended questions as described in Box 14.2. Interviews are used in both quantitative and qualitative research, but they are best used when the researcher may need to clarify the task for the respondent or obtain more personal information and/or nuances about the study focus from the respondent.

Open-ended questions allow more varied information to be collected and require a qualitative or content analysis method to analyze responses (see Chapter 6). Qualitative content analysis is a method of analyzing narrative or word responses to questions and either counting similar responses or grouping the responses into themes or categories (also used in qualitative research). Interviews may take place face to face, over the phone, or online via a an Internet-based format.

Questionnaires are paper-and-pencil instruments designed to gather data from individuals about knowledge, attitudes, beliefs, and feelings. Questionnaires, like interviews, may be open-ended or closed-ended, as presented in Box 14.2. Questionnaires are most useful when there is a finite set of questions. Individual items in a questionnaire must be clearly written so the intent of the question and the nature of the response options are clear. Questionnaires may be composed of individual items that measure different variables or

---

BOX 14.2 Uses for Open-Ended and Closed-Ended Questions

- **Open-ended questions** are used when the researcher wants the subjects to respond in their own words or when the researcher does not know all of the possible alternative responses. Interviews that use open-ended questions often use a list of questions and probes called an **interview guide**. Responses to the interview guide are often audio-recorded to capture the subject's responses. An example of an open-ended question is used for the interview in Appendix E.
- **Closed-ended questions** are structured, fixed-response items with a fixed number of responses. Closed-ended questions are best used when the question has a finite number of responses and the respondent is to choose the one closest to the correct response. Fixed-response items have the advantage of simplifying the respondent's task but result in omission of important information about the subject. Interviews that use closed-ended questions typically record a subject's responses directly on the questionnaire. An example of a closed-ended item is found in Box 14.3.

concepts (e.g., age, race, ethnicity, and years of education) or scales. Survey researchers rely almost entirely on questionnaires for data collection.

Questionnaires can be referred to as *instruments, measures, scales,* or *tools.* When multiple items are used to measure a single concept, such as quality of life or anxiety, and the scores on those items are combined mathematically to obtain an overall score, the questionnaire or measurement instrument is called a scale. The important issue is that each of the items must measure the same concept or variable. An intelligence test is an example of a scale that combines individual item responses to determine an overall quantification of intelligence.

Scales can have subscales or total scale scores. For instance, in the study by Flanders and colleagues (2020) (see Appendix C), the Professional Quality of Life scale (ProQOL) has subscales measuring compassion satisfaction and compassion fatigue. The latter subscale has two parts that measure secondary trauma stress and burnout. In this study, nurses self-reported how often they experienced these coping outcomes by responding on a 5-point scale with a 1 indicating never, 2 rarely, 3 sometimes, 4 often, and 5 very often. This type of response option is called a Likert-type scale.

EVIDENCE-BASED PRACTICE TIP

Scales used in research should have evidence of adequate reliability and validity so you feel confident that the findings reflect what the researcher intended to measure (see Chapter 15).

Box 14.3 shows three items from a survey of nursing job satisfaction. The first item is closed-ended and uses a Likert scale response format. The second item is also closed-ended, and it forces respondents to choose from a finite number of possible answers. The third item is open-ended, and respondents use their own words to answer the question, allowing an unlimited number of possible answers. Often researchers use a combination of Likert-type, closed-ended, and open-ended questions when collecting data in nursing research.

In most studies, demographic data are collected in addition to measurement data from surveys and other types of self-report instruments. Demographic data includes information that describes important characteristics about the subjects in a study (e.g., age, gender, race,

---

BOX 14.3   Examples of Open-Ended and Closed-Ended Questions

Open-Ended Questions

Please list the three most important reasons why you chose to stay in your current job:

1. _____
2. _____
3. _____

Closed-Ended Questions (Likert Scale)

How satisfied are you with your current position?

1	2	3	4	5
Very satisfied	Moderately satisfied	Undecided	Moderately dissatisfied	Very dissatisfied

Closed-Ended Questions

On average, how many patients do you care for in 1 day?

1. 1–3
2. 4–6
3. 7–9
4. 10–12
5. 13–15
6. 16–18
7. 19–20
8. More than 20

ethnicity, education, marital status). It is important to collect demographic data to describe and compare different study samples so you can evaluate how similar the sample is to your patient population. For instance, DiStasio and colleagues (2020, Appendix D) reported that the majority of their sample of caregivers of loved ones with Parkinson disease were female and older than 60 years of age. If working with patients with this diagnosis, you would be able to compare your family caregiver population needs with this sample to help inform your practice.

When reviewing articles with numerous questionnaires, remember (especially if the study deals with vulnerable populations) to assess if the author(s) addressed potential respondent burden such as the following:

- Language fluency
- Reading level (sixth grade, when possible)
- Questionnaire font size (14-point font)
- Need to read and assist some subjects
- Time it took to complete the questionnaire (30 minutes)
- Multiple data collection points

This information is very important for judging the respondent burden associated with study participation. It is important to examine the benefits and caveats associated with using interviews and questionnaires as self-report methods. Interviews offer some advantages over questionnaires. The response rate is almost always higher with interviews, and there are fewer missing data, which helps reduce bias.

HELPFUL HINT

Remember, sometimes researchers make trade-offs when determining the measures to be used. **Example:** ➤ A researcher may want to learn about an individual's attitudes regarding job satisfaction; however, practicalities may preclude using an interview, so a questionnaire may be used instead.

Another advantage of the interview is that vulnerable populations such as children, the blind, and those with low literacy may not be able to fill out a questionnaire. With an interview, the data collector knows who is giving the answers. When questionnaires are mailed, for example, anyone in the household could be the person who supplies the answers. Interviews also allow for some safeguards, such as clarifying misunderstood questions, and observing and recording the level of the respondent's understanding of the questions. In addition, the researcher has flexibility over the order of the questions.

With questionnaires, the respondent can answer questions in any order. Sometimes changing the order of the questions can change the response. Finally, interviews allow for richer and more complex data to be collected. This is particularly so when open-ended responses are sought. Even when closed-ended response items are used, interviewers can probe to understand why a respondent answered in a particular way. This is a particularly important strategy to consider when conducting research with a culturally diverse or recent immigrant population for whom English is a second language.

Questionnaires also have certain advantages. They are much less expensive to administer than interviews that require hiring and thoroughly training interviewers. Thus, if a researcher has a fixed amount of time and money, a larger and more diverse sample can be obtained with questionnaires. Questionnaires may allow for more confidentiality and anonymity with sensitive issues that participants may be reluctant to discuss in an interview. Finally, the fact that no interviewer is present assures the researcher and the reader that there will be no interviewer bias. *Interviewer bias* occurs when the interviewer unwittingly leads the respondent to answer in a certain way. This problem can be especially pronounced in studies that use open-ended questions. The tone used to ask the question and/or nonverbal interviewer responses such as a subtle nod of the head or facial expression could lead a respondent to change an answer to correspond with what the researcher wants to hear.

Finally, the use of Internet-based self-report data collection (both interviewing and questionnaire delivery) has gained momentum. The use of an online format is economical and can capture subjects from different geographical areas without the expense of travel or mailings. Open-ended questions are already typed and do not require transcription; closed-ended questions can often be imported directly into statistical analysis software and therefore reduce data entry mistakes. The main concerns with Internet-based data collection procedures involve the difficulty of ensuring informed consent (e.g., Is checking a box indicating agreement to participate the same thing as signing an informed consent form?) and the protection of subject anonymity, which is difficult to guarantee with any Internet-based venue. In addition, the requirement that subjects have computer access limits the use of this method in certain age groups and populations. However, the advantages of increased efficiency and accuracy make Internet-based data collection a growing trend among nurse researchers.

Physiological Measurement

Physiological data collection involves the use of specialized equipment to determine the physical and biological status of subjects. Such measures can be *physical,* such as weight or temperature; *chemical,* such as blood glucose level; *microbiological,* as with cultures; or *anatomical,* as in radiological examinations. What separates these data collection procedures from others used in research is that they require special equipment to make the observation.

Physiological or biological measurement is particularly suited to the study of many types of nursing problems. **Example:** ➤ Examining different methods for taking a patient's temperature or blood pressure or monitoring blood glucose levels may yield important information for determining the effectiveness of certain nursing monitoring procedures or interventions. However, it is important that the method be applied consistently to all subjects in the study. De la Fuente Coria and colleagues (2020, Appendix B) collected fasting blood glucose from each patient in their study at the same time each day and used the same laboratory to run the bloodwork to ensure consistency across the physiological measure. **Example:** ➤ Nurses are quite familiar with taking blood pressure measurements. However, for research studies that involve blood pressure measurement, the process must be standardized. The subject must be positioned (sitting or lying down) the same way for a specified period, the same blood pressure instrument must be used, and often multiple blood pressure measurements are taken under the same conditions to obtain an average value.

The advantages of using physiological data collection methods include the objectivity, precision, and sensitivity associated with these measures. Unless there is a technical malfunction, two readings of the same instrument taken at the same time by two different nurses are likely to yield the same result. Because such instruments are intended to measure the variable being studied, they offer the advantage of being precise and sensitive enough to pick up subtle variations in the variable of interest. It is also unlikely that a subject in a study can deliberately distort physiological information.

Physiological measurements are not without inherent disadvantages and include the following:

- Some instruments may be quite expensive to obtain and use.
- Physiological instruments often require specialized training to be used accurately.
- The variable of interest may be altered as a result of using the instrument. **Example:** ➤ An individual's blood pressure may increase just because a health care professional enters the room (called *white coat syndrome*).
- Although thought as being nonintrusive, the presence of some types of devices may change the measurement. **Example:** ➤ The presence of a heart rate monitoring device may make some patients anxious and increase their heart rate.
- All types of measuring devices are affected in some way by the environment. A simple thermometer can be affected by the subject drinking something hot or smoking a cigarette immediately before the temperature is taken. Thus it is important to consider whether the researcher controlled such environmental variables in the study.

Existing Data

The data collection methods discussed thus far concern the ways that researchers gather new data to study phenomena of interest. Sometimes existing data can be examined in a new way to study a problem. The use of records (e.g., medical records, care plans, hospital records, death certificates) and databases (e.g., US Census, National Cancer Database, Minimum Data Set for Nursing Home Resident Assessment and Care Screening) are frequently used to answer research questions about clinical problems. Typically, this type of research design is referred to as secondary analysis, and analysis of very large computerized data sets is sometimes referred to as *big data* (Brennan & Bakken, 2015).

The use of available data has advantages. First, data are already collected, thus eliminating subject burden and recruitment problems. Second, most databases contain large populations; therefore sample size is rarely a problem, and random sampling is possible. Larger samples allow the researcher to use more sophisticated analytic procedures, and random sampling enhances generalizability of findings. Some records and databases collect standardized data in a uniform way and allow the researcher to examine trends over time. Finally, the use of available records has the potential to save significant time and money.

On the other hand, institutions may be reluctant to allow researchers to have access to their records. If the records are kept so that an individual cannot be identified (known as *de-identified data*), this is usually not a problem. However, the Health Insurance Portability and Accountability Act (HIPAA), a federal law, protects the rights of individuals who may be identified in records (see Chapter 13). Recent escalation in the computerization of health records has led to discussion about the desirability of access to such records for research. Currently, it is not clear how much computerized health data will be readily available for research purposes.

Another problem that affects the quality of available data is that the researcher has access only to those records that have survived. If the records available are not representative of all of the possible records, the researcher may have to make an intelligent guess as to their accuracy. **Example:** ➤ A researcher may be interested in studying the social determinants of health, specifically, socioeconomic factors associated with the suicide rate. Frequently, these data are underreported because of the stigma attached to suicide, so the records would be biased.

> **EVIDENCE-BASED PRACTICE TIP**
>
> Critical appraisal of any data collection method includes evaluating the appropriateness, objectivity, and consistency of the method employed.

CONSTRUCTION OF NEW INSTRUMENTS

Sometimes researchers cannot locate an instrument with acceptable reliability and validity to measure the variable of interest (see Chapter 15). In this situation, a new instrument or scale must be developed.

Instrument development is complex and time-consuming. It consists of the following steps:

- Define the concept to be measured.
- Clarify the target population.
- Develop the items.
- Assess the items for content validity.
- Develop instructions for respondents and users.
- Pretest and pilot test the items.
- Estimate reliability and validity.

Defining the concept to be measured requires that the researcher develop expertise in the concept, which includes an extensive review of the literature and of all existing measurements that deal with related concepts. The researcher will use all of this information to synthesize the available knowledge so that the construct can be defined.

Once defined, the individual items measuring the concept can be developed. The researcher will develop many more items than are needed to address each aspect of the concept. The items are evaluated by a panel of experts in the field to determine whether the items measure what they are intended to measure (content validity) (see Chapter 15). Items will be eliminated if they are not specific to the concept. In this phase, the researcher must ensure consistency among the items as well as consistency in testing and scoring procedures.

Finally, the researcher pilot tests the new instrument to determine the quality of the instrument as a whole (reliability and validity) and the ability of each item to discriminate among individual respondents (variance in item response). Pilot testing can also yield important evidence about the reading level (too low or too high), length of the instrument (too short or too long), directions (clear or not clear), response rate (the percent of potential subjects who return a completed scale), and appropriateness of culture or context. The researcher also may administer a related instrument to see if the new instrument is sufficiently different from the older one (construct validity). Instrument development and testing is an important part of nursing science because our ability to evaluate evidence related to practice depends on measuring nursing phenomena in a clear, consistent, and reliable way (see Chapter 8).

▶▶ APPRAISAL FOR EVIDENCE-BASED PRACTICE
DATA COLLECTION METHODS

Assessing the adequacy of data collection methods is an important part of evaluating the results of studies that provide evidence for clinical practice. The data collection procedures provide a snapshot of the rigor with which the study was conducted. From an evidence-based practice perspective, you can judge if the data collection procedures would fit within your clinical environment and with your patient population. The manner in which the data were collected affects the study's internal and external validity. A well-developed "Methods" section in a study decreases bias in the findings. A key element for evidence-based practice is if the procedures were consistently completed. Also consider the following:

- If observation was used, was an observation guide developed, and were the observers trained and supervised until there was a high level of interrater reliability? How was the training confirmed periodically throughout the study to maintain fidelity and decrease bias?
- Was a data collection procedure manual developed and used during the study?
- If the study tested an intervention, was there interventionist and data collector training and supervision?
- If a physiological instrument was used, was the instrument properly calibrated throughout the study and the data collected in the same manner from each subject?
- If there were missing data, how were the data accounted for?

Some of these details may be difficult to discern in a research article because of space limitations imposed by the journal. Typically, the interview guide, questionnaires, or scales are not available for review. However, research articles should indicate the following:

- Type(s) of data collection method used (self-report, observation, physiological, or existing data)
- Evidence of training and supervision for the data collectors and interventionists
- Consistency with which data collection procedures were applied across subjects
- Any threats to internal validity or bias related to issues of instrumentation or testing
- Any sources of bias related to external validity issues, such as the Hawthorne effect
- Scale reliability and validity discussed
- Interrater reliability across data collectors and time points (if observation was used)

When you review the data collection "Methods" section of a study, it is important to think about the data strength and quality of the evidence. You should have confidence in the following:

- An appropriate data collection method was used
- Data collectors were appropriately trained and supervised
- Data were collected consistently by all data collectors
- Respondent burden, reactivity, and social desirability was avoided

You can critically appraise a study in terms of data collection bias being minimized, thereby strengthening potential applicability of the evidence provided by the findings. Because a research article does not always provide all of the details, it is not uncommon to contact the researcher to obtain added information that may assist you in using results in practice. Some helpful questions to ask are listed in the Critical Appraisal Criteria box.

CRITICAL APPRAISAL CRITERIA

Data Collection Methods

1. Are all of the data collection instruments clearly identified and described?
2. Are operational definitions provided and clear?
3. Is the rationale for their selection given?
4. Is the method used appropriate to the problem being studied?
5. Were the methods used appropriate to the clinical situation?
6. Was a standardized manual used to guide data collection?
7. Were all data collectors adequately trained and supervised?
8. Are the data collection procedures the same for all subjects?

Observational Methods

1. Who did the observing?
2. Were the observers trained to minimize bias?
3. Was there an observation guide?
4. Were the observers required to make inferences about what they saw?
5. Is there any reason to believe that the presence of the observers affected the subject's behavior?
6. Were the observations performed using the principles of informed consent?
7. Was interrater agreement between observers established?

Self-Report: Interviews

1. Is the interview schedule described adequately enough to know whether it covers the topic?
2. Is there clear indication that the subjects understood the task and the questions?
3. Who were the interviewers, and how were they trained?
4. Is there evidence of interviewer bias?

Self-Report: Questionnaires

1. Is the questionnaire described well enough to know whether it covers the topic?
2. Is there evidence that subjects were able to answer the questions?
3. Are the majority of the items appropriately closed-ended or open-ended?

Physiological Measurement

1. Is the instrument used appropriate to the research question or hypothesis?
2. Is a rationale given for why a particular instrument was selected?
3. Is there a provision for evaluating the accuracy of the instrument?

Existing Data: Records and Databases

1. Are the existing data used appropriately, considering the research question and hypothesis being studied?
2. Are the data examined in such a way as to provide new information?
3. Is there any indication of selection bias in the available records?

KEY POINTS

- Data collection methods are described as being both objective and systematic. The data collection methods of a study provide the operational definitions of the relevant variables.
- Types of data collection methods include observational, self-report, physiological, and existing data. Each method has advantages and disadvantages.
- Physiological measurement involves the use of technical instruments to collect data about patients' physical, chemical, microbiological, or anatomical status. They are suited

to studying patient clinical outcomes and how to improve the effectiveness of nursing care. Physiological measurements are objective, precise, and sensitive. Expertise, training, and consistent application of these tests or procedures are needed to reduce the measurement error associated with this data collection method.

- Observational methods are used in nursing research when the variables of interest deal with events or behaviors. Scientific observation requires preplanning, systematic recording, controlling the observations, and providing a relationship to scientific theory. This method is best suited to research problems that are difficult to view as a part of a whole. The advantages of observational methods are that they provide flexibility to measure many types of situations, and they allow for depth and breadth of information to be collected, often in natural settings like the community. Disadvantages include that data may be distorted as a result of the observer's presence, and observations may be biased by the person who is doing the observing.

- Interviews are commonly used data collection methods in nursing research. Either open-ended or closed-ended questions may be used when asking the subject questions. The form of the question should be clear to the respondent, free from suggestion, and grammatically correct.

- Questionnaires, or paper-and-pencil tests, are useful when there are a finite number of questions to be asked. Questions must be clear and specific. Questionnaires are less costly in terms of time and money to administer to large groups of subjects, particularly if the subjects are geographically widespread. Questionnaires also can be completely anonymous and prevent interviewer bias.

- Existing data in the form of records or large databases are an important source for research data. The use of available data may save the researcher considerable time and money when conducting a study. This method reduces problems with subject recruitment, access, and ethical concerns. However, records and available data are subject to problems of authenticity and accuracy.

CLINICAL JUDGMENT CHALLENGES

- When a researcher opts to use observation as the data collection method, what steps must be taken to minimize bias?

- In a randomized controlled trial investigating the differential effect of an educational video intervention in comparison with a phone counseling intervention, data were collected at four different hospitals by four different data collectors. What steps should the researcher take to ensure fidelity?

- What are the strengths and weaknesses of collecting data using existing sources such as records, charts, and databases?

- **IPE** Your interprofessional journal club just finished reading the research article by De la Fuente Coria and colleagues in Appendix B. As part of your critical appraisal of this study, your team needed to identify the strengths and weaknesses of the data collection section. Discuss the sources of bias in the data collection procedures and evidence of fidelity.

- How would the use of a training manual decrease the possibility of introducing bias into the data collection process, thereby increasing intervention fidelity?

REFERENCES

Brennan, P. F., & Bakken, S. (2015). Nursing needs big data and big data needs nursing. *Journal of Nursing Scholarship, 47*, 477–484. https://doi.org/10.1111/jnu.12159. Epub 2015 Aug 19.

Bromley, E., Mikesell, L., Jones, F., & Khodyakov, D. (2015). From subject to participant: Ethics and the evolving role of community in health research. *American Journal of Public Health, 105*(5), 900–908. https://doi.org/10.2105/AJPH.2014.302403.

Di Stasio, E., DiSimone, E., Galeti, A., & Donati, D. (2020). Stress-related vulnerability and usefulness of healthcare education in Parkinson's disease: The perception of a group of family caregivers, a cross sectional study. *Applied Nursing Research, 51*. https://doi.org/10.1016/j.apnr.2019.151186.

Flanders, Hampton, Missi, Ipsan, & Gruebbel (2020). Effectiveness of a staff resilience program in a pediatric intensive care unit. *Journal of Pediatric Nursing, 50*, 1–4. https://doi.org/10.1016/j.pedn.2019.10.007. 2020Epub 2019 Oct 25.

De la Fuente Coria, Cruz-Cobo, & Santi-Cano (2020). Effectiveness of a primary care nurse delivered educational intervention for patients with type 2 diabetes mellitus in promoting metabolic control and compliance with long-term therapeutic targets: Randomised controlled trial. *International Journal of Nursing Studies, 101*, 103417.

Go to Evolve at **http://evolve.elsevier.com/LoBiondo/** for review questions, appraisal exercises, and additional research articles for practice in reviewing and appraisal.

15

Appraising Reliability & Validity

Geri LoBiondo-Wood, Judith Haber

Go to Evolve at **http://evolve.elsevier.com/LoBiondo/** for review questions.

LEARNING OUTCOMES

After reading this chapter, you should be able to do the following:

- Discuss how measurement error can affect study outcomes.
- Discuss the purposes of reliability and validity.
- Define *reliability*.
- Discuss the concepts of stability, equivalence, and homogeneity as they relate to reliability.
- Compare and contrast the estimates of reliability.
- Define *validity*.
- Compare and contrast content, criterion-related, and construct validity.

- Identify the criteria for critiquing the reliability and validity of measurement instruments.
- Use the critical appraisal criteria to evaluate the reliability and validity of measurement instruments.
- Discuss how reliability and validity contribute to the strength and quality of evidence provided by the findings of a study.

KEY TERMS

chance (random) errors
concurrent validity
construct
construct validity
content validity
content validity index
contrasted-groups
   (known-groups)
   approach
convergent validity

criterion-related
   validity
Cronbach's alpha
divergent/discriminant
   validity
equivalence
error variance
face validity
factor analysis
homogeneity

hypothesis-testing
   approach
internal consistency
interrater reliability
item to total
   correlations
kappa
Kuder-Richardson
   (KR-20) coefficient
Likert scale

observed test score
predictive validity
reliability
reliability coefficient
split-half reliability
stability
systematic (constant)
   error
test-retest reliability
validity

The measurement of phenomena is a major focus of researchers. Unless measurement instruments validly (accurately) and reliably (consistently) reflect the concepts of the theory being tested, conclusions drawn from a study will be invalid or biased. Issues of reliability and validity are of central concern to researchers and to appraisers of research. From either perspective, instruments that are used in a study must be evaluated. Researchers often face the challenge of developing new instruments and, as part of that process, establishing the reliability and validity of those instruments.

When reading studies, you must assess the reliability and validity of the instruments to determine the soundness of these selections in relation to testing the concepts (concepts are often called **constructs** in instrument development studies) or variables under study. The appropriateness of instruments and the extent to which reliability and validity are demonstrated have a profound influence on the strength of the findings and the extent to which the findings are biased (see Chapter 8). Invalid measures produce invalid estimates of the relationships between variables, thus introducing bias, which affects the study's internal and external validity. As such, evaluating reliability and validity is an extremely important critical appraisal skill for assessing the strength and quality of evidence provided by the design, findings, and applicability of findings to practice. This chapter examines the types of reliability and validity and demonstrates the applicability of these concepts to the evaluation of instruments in research and evidence-based practice.

RELIABILITY, VALIDITY, AND MEASUREMENT ERROR

Reliability is the ability of an instrument to measure the attributes of a variable or construct *consistently*. **Validity** is the extent to which an instrument measures the attributes of a concept *accurately*. To understand reliability and validity, you must understand potential errors related to instruments. Researchers may be concerned about whether the scores that were obtained from a sample of subjects were consistent, true measures of the behaviors and thus an accurate reflection of the differences among individuals. The extent of variability in test scores that is attributable to error rather than a true measure of the behaviors is the **error variance**. Error in measurement can occur in multiple ways.

An **observed test score** derived from a set of items actually consists of the true score plus error (Fig. 15.1). The error may be either chance or random error, or it may be systematic or constant error. Validity is concerned with systematic error, whereas reliability is concerned with random error. **Chance** or **random errors** are errors that are difficult to control (e.g., a respondent's anxiety level at the time of testing). Random errors are unsystematic in nature; they are a result of a transient state in the subject, the context of the study, or the

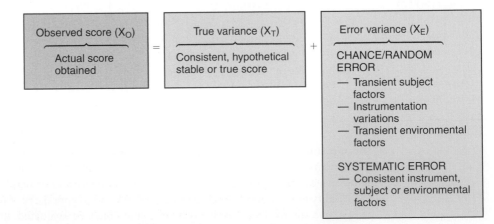

FIG 15.1 Components of observed scores.

administration of an instrument. **Example:** ➤ Perceptions or behaviors that occur at a specific point in time (e.g., anxiety) are known as *state* or *transient characteristics* and are often beyond the awareness and control of the examiner. Another example of random error is in a study that measures blood pressure. Random error resulting in different blood pressure readings could occur by misplacement of the cuff, not waiting for a specific time period before taking the blood pressure, or placing the arm randomly in relationship to the heart while measuring blood pressure.

Systematic or constant error is measurement error that is attributable to relatively stable characteristics of the study sample that may bias their behavior and/or cause incorrect instrument calibration. Such error has a systematic biasing influence on the subjects' responses and thereby influences the validity of the instruments. For instance, level of education, socioeconomic status, social desirability, response set, or other characteristics may influence the validity of the instrument by altering measurement of the "true" responses in a systematic way. **Example:** ➤ A subject is completing a survey examining attitudes about caring for older adult patients. If the subject wants to please the investigator, items may constantly be answered in a socially desirable way rather than reflecting how the individual actually feels, thus making the estimate of validity inaccurate. Systematic error also occurs also when a physiological instrument is improperly calibrated. Consider a scale that consistently gives a person's weight at 2 pounds less than the actual body weight. The scale could be quite reliable (i.e., capable of reproducing the precise measurement), but the result is consistently invalid.

The concept of error is important when appraising instruments in a study. The information regarding the instruments' reliability and validity is found in the "Instrument" or "Measures" section of a study, which can be separately titled or appear as a subsection of the "Methods" section of a research report, unless the study is a psychometric or instrument development study (see Chapter 10).

> ### HELPFUL HINT
>
> Research articles vary considerably in the amount of detail included about reliability and validity. When the focus of a study is instrument development, psychometric evaluation—including reliability and validity data—is carefully documented and appears throughout the article rather than briefly in the "Instruments" or "Measures" section, as in a research article.

VALIDITY

Validity is the extent to which an instrument measures the attributes of a concept accurately. When an instrument is valid, it reflects the concept it is supposed to measure. A valid instrument that is supposed to measure anxiety does so; it does not measure another concept, such as stress. A measure can be reliable but not valid. Let's say that a researcher wanted to measure anxiety in patients by measuring their body temperatures. The researcher could obtain highly accurate, consistent, and precise temperature recordings, but such a measure may not be a valid indicator of anxiety. Thus the high reliability of an instrument is not necessarily congruent with evidence of validity. A valid instrument, however, is reliable. An instrument cannot validly measure a variable if it is erratic, inconsistent, or inaccurate. There are three types of validity that vary according to the type of information provided and the purpose of the instrument (i.e., *content, criterion-related,* and *construct validity*).

As you appraise research articles, you will want to evaluate whether sufficient evidence of validity is present and whether the type of validity is appropriate to the study's design and the instruments used in the study.

As you read the instruments or measures sections of studies, you will notice that validity data are reported much less frequently than reliability data. DeVon and colleagues (2007) note that adequate validity is frequently claimed, but rarely is the method specified. This lack of reporting, largely caused by publication space constraints, shows the importance of critiquing the quality of the instruments and the conclusions (see Chapters 14 and 17).

EVIDENCE-BASED PRACTICE TIP

Selecting instruments that have strong evidence of validity increases your confidence in the study findings—that the researchers actually measured what they intended to measure.

Content Validity

Content validity represents the universe of content or the domain of a given variable/construct. The universe of content provides the basis for developing the items that will adequately represent the content. When an investigator is developing an instrument and issues of content validity arise, the concern is whether the measurement instrument and the items it contains are representative of the content domain that the researcher intends to measure. The researcher begins by defining the concept and identifying the attributes or dimensions of the concept. The items that reflect the concept and its domain are developed.

The formulated items are submitted to content experts who judge the items. **Example:** ➤ Researchers typically request that the experts indicate their agreement with the scope of the items and the extent to which the items reflect the concept under consideration. Box 15.1 provides an example of content validity.

Another method used to establish content validity is the content validity index (CVI). The CVI moves beyond the level of agreement of a panel of expert judges and calculates an index of interrater agreement or relevance. This calculation gives a researcher more confidence or evidence that the instrument truly reflects the concept or construct. When reading the instrument section of a research article, note that the authors will comment if a CVI

BOX 15.1 Published Examples of Content Validity and Content Validity Index

Content Validity

Garzon & Heredia (2019) developed the Treatment Adherence Questionnaire for Patients With Hypertension. The developers asked a panel of four experts based on academic preparation and on clinical experience over 5 years to evaluate each item as either essential, useful but not essential, or not necessary. Based on the data from the experts, all items were retained.

Content Validity Index

For the Chinese Illness Perception Questionnaire Revised Trauma (the Chinese IPQ-Revised-Trauma), the Item-level Content Validity Index (I-CVI) was calculated by a panel of five trauma content experts. An average of 88% for all subscale items was scored by the experts, indicating that the validity of the score was reguaranteed. A few words were fixed after expert checking. The ratings were on a four-point scale with a response format of 1 = *not relevant* to 4 = *highly relevant*. The I-CVI for each item was computed based on the percentage of experts giving a rating of 3 or 4, indicating item relevance (Lee et al., 2016).

was used to assess content validity. When reading a psychometric study that reports the development of an instrument, you will find great detail and a much longer section indicating how exactly the researchers calculated the CVI and the acceptable item cutoffs. In the scientific literature, there has been discussion of accepting a CVI of 0.78 to 1.0, depending on the number of experts (DeVon et al., 2007; Lynn, 1986). An example from a study that used CVI is presented in Box 15.1. A subtype of content validity is face validity, which is a rudimentary type of validity that basically verifies that the instrument gives the appearance of measuring the concept. It is an intuitive type of validity in which colleagues or subjects are asked to read the instrument and evaluate the content in terms of whether it appears to reflect the concept the researcher intends to measure.

EVIDENCE-BASED PRACTICE TIP

If face and/or content validity, the most basic types of validity, was (or were) the only type(s) of validity reported in a research article, you would not appraise the measurement instrument(s) as having strong psychometric properties, which would negatively influence your confidence about the study findings.

Criterion-Related Validity

Criterion-related validity indicates to what degree the subject's performance on the instrument and the subject's actual behavior are related. The criterion is usually the second measure, which assesses the same concept under study. Two forms of criterion-related validity are concurrent and predictive.

Concurrent validity refers to the degree of correlation of one test with the scores of another more established instrument of the same concept when both are administered at the same time. A high correlation coefficient indicates agreement between the two measures and evidence of concurrent validity.

Predictive validity refers to the degree of correlation between the measure of the concept and some future measure of the same concept. Because of the passage of time, the correlation coefficients are likely to be lower for predictive validity studies. Examples of concurrent and predictive validity as they appear in research articles are illustrated in Box 15.2.

Construct Validity

Construct validity is based on the extent to which a test measures a theoretical construct, attribute, or trait. It attempts to validate the theory underlying the measurement by testing of the hypothesized relationships. Testing confirms or fails to confirm the relationships that are predicted between and/or among concepts and, as such, provides more or less support for the construct validity of the instruments measuring those concepts. The establishment of construct validity is complex, often involving several studies and approaches. The hypothesis-testing, convergent and divergent, contrasted-groups, and factor analytical approaches are discussed in the following sections. Box 15.3 provides examples of different types of construct validity as it is reported in published research articles.

Hypothesis-Testing Approach

When the hypothesis-testing approach is used, the investigator uses the theory or concept underlying the measurement instruments to validate the instrument. The investigator does this by developing hypotheses regarding the behavior of individuals with varying scores on

BOX 15.2 Published Examples of Reported Criterion-Related Validity

Concurrent Validity

Concurrent validity of the Postpartum Childcare Stress Checklist (PCSC) was assessed by investigating correlations between the PCSC and multiple other theoretically related scales such as the 10-item Edinburgh Postnatal Depression Scale (EPDS) (Cox, Holden and Sagovsky, 1987) and the 20-item State-Trait Anxiety Inventory (STAI) (Spielberger, 1983) using Spearman's rho correlation coefficient. They expected that higher childcare stress at 4 weeks postpartum would be associated with higher depression and anxiety symptoms and lower partner-specific social support. The PCSC and its dimensions were significantly positively correlated with depressive (all $p < .001$) and anxiety (all $p < .001$) symptomatology and significantly negatively correlated with postpartum partner-specific social support (all $p < .001$). Partner-specific support correlated most strongly with the partner relationship dimension of the PCSC (Dennis et al., 2018).

Predictive Validity

The predictive validity of the Postpartum Childcare Stress Checklist (PCSC) was assessed by using Spearman's rho correlation coefficient to examine the correlation of the PCSC with theoretically related instruments at 8 weeks postpartum. The PCSC positively correlated with depressive and anxiety symptoms among those without depression and anxiety, respectively, at 1 and 4 weeks postpartum (all $p < .01$). The PCSC and its dimensions were also negatively correlated with both global and partner-specific social support at 8 weeks (all $p < .01$) (Dennis et al., 2018)

BOX 15.3 Published Examples of Reported Construct Validity

Contrasted Groups (Known Groups)

Oral anticoagulation therapy is effective for the management of thromboembolic disorders. An adequate level of knowledge of self-management is important for optimizing clinical outcomes. The Anticoagulation Knowledge Tool was developed to access patient knowledge. The psychometric properties of this instrument were established in English but not in other languages for non–English speakers. To assess the instrument, reliability and validity was assessed. To assess the validity of the instrument using contrasted groups methodology, three groups (health care providers, patients, and the general public) were administered the instrument. Based on the findings using this methodology across all three groups, the instrument was found to be valid (Magon et al., 2018).

Convergent Validity

Convergent construct validity of the electronic Frailty Index (eFI) and a standard frailty index (FI); the phenotype model of frailty; Clinical Frailty Scale (CFS); and Edmonton Frail Scale were assessed to estimate correlation coefficients and 95% confidence intervals (Brundle et al., 2019).

Divergent (Discriminant) Validity

The eFI was assessed for divergent (discriminant) validity. The researchers administered the instrument to different groups based on frailty scores. Statistically significant group differences were detected between normal and abnormal Karnofsky performance scale scores, quality-of-life scores, depression scores, and eFI scores (Brundle et al., 2019).

Factor Analysis

In a pilot study using the Irritability Scale-Initial Version (TISi) for assessing irritability of cancer patients on three dimensions (physical, affective, and behavioral), a confirmatory factor analysis was conducted on TISi at Time 1 using *Mplus 8.1*. The factor loadings generally supported the assignment of items to the three subscales of the TSIi if a cut-point of .4 is used to retain items. However, there is no stated consensus regarding an absolute cut-point value (Zhang and Ganocy, 2020).

Hypothesis Testing

In a study assessing the construct validity of the Multi-Source Interference Task (MSIT), a computerized neurophysiological test assessed cognitive function for use with heart failure (HF) patients at risk for impairment in directed attention, critical to performing HF self-care. The MSIT has not been used in HF studies. The construct validity was evaluated using a hypothesis testing approach. Hypotheses predicted that MSIT performance in HF is significantly worse than healthy adults, and performance on the MSIT is positively correlated with two other tests: Trail-Making and Stroop Tests, both assessing aspects of attention similar to the MSIT. *t*-tests and correlations were used to examine the differences between patients with HF ($n = 20$) and age and education-matched healthy adults and associations between the MSIT and other instruments. The findings reveal support for the hypotheses, thereby providing evidence of construct validity for the MSIT for use with patients with HF to examine directed attention (Jung et al., 2018).

the measurement instrument, collecting data to test the hypotheses, and making inferences on the basis of the findings concerning whether the rationale underlying the instrument's construction is adequate to explain the findings and thereby provide support for evidence of construct validity (see Box 15.2).

Convergent and Divergent Approaches

Strategies for assessing construct validity include convergent and divergent approaches. Convergent validity, sometimes called *concurrent validity*, refers to a search for other measures of the construct. Sometimes two or more instruments that theoretically measure the same construct are identified, and both are administered to the same subjects. A correlational analysis (i.e., test of relationship; see Chapter 16) is performed. If the measures are positively correlated, convergent validity is said to be supported.

Divergent validity, sometimes called discriminant validity, uses measurement approaches that differentiate one construct from others that may be similar. Sometimes researchers search for instruments that measure the opposite of the construct. If the divergent measure is negatively related to other measures, validity for the measure is strengthened.

HELPFUL HINT

When validity data about the measurement instruments used in a study are not included in a research article, you have no way of determining whether the intended concept is actually being captured by the instruments. In such a case, it is important to go back to the original primary source to check the instrument's validity before you use the results.

Contrasted-Groups Approach

When the contrasted-groups approach (sometimes called the known-groups approach) is used to test construct validity, the researcher identifies two groups of individuals who are suspected to score extremely high or low in the characteristic being measured by the instrument. The instrument is administered to both the high-scoring and the low-scoring group, and the differences in scores are examined. If the instrument is sensitive to individual differences in the trait being measured, the mean performance of these two groups should differ significantly, and evidence of construct validity would be supported. A *t* test or analysis of variance could be used to statistically test the difference between the two groups (see Box 15.2 and Chapter 16).

EVIDENCE-BASED PRACTICE TIP

When the instruments used in a study are presented, note whether the sample(s) used to develop the measurement instrument(s) is (are) similar to your patient population.

Factor Analytical Approach

A final approach to assessing construct validity is factor analysis. This is a procedure that gives the researcher information about the extent to which a set of items measures the same underlying concept (variable) of a construct. Factor analysis assesses the degree to which the individual items on a scale truly cluster around one or more concepts. Items designed to measure the same concept should load on the same factor; those designed to measure different concepts should load on different factors (Anastasi & Urbina, 1997;

Furr & Bacharach, 2008; Nunnally & Bernstein, 1993). This analysis, as illustrated in the example in Box 15.2, will also indicate whether the items in the instrument reflect a single construct or several constructs.

The Critical Thinking Decision Path will help you assess the appropriateness of the type of validity and reliability selected for use in a particular study.

CRITICAL THINKING DECISION PATH
Determining the Appropriate Type of Validity and Reliability Selected for a Study

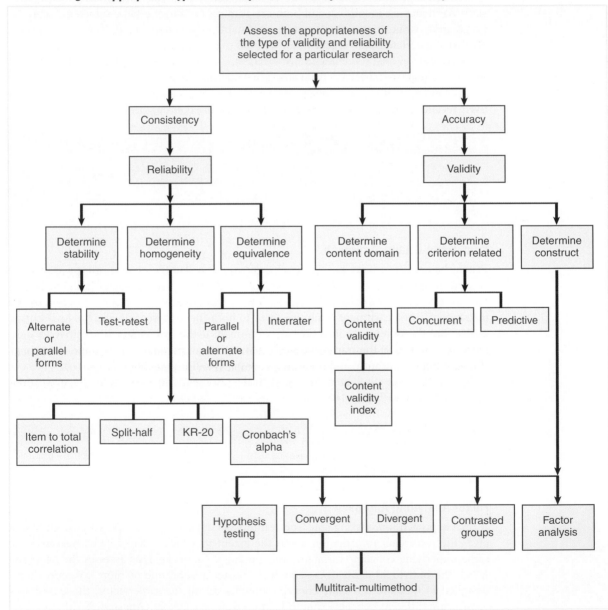

RELIABILITY

Reliable people are those whose behavior can be relied on to be consistent and predictable. Likewise, the **reliability** of an instrument is defined as the extent to which the instrument produces the same results if the behavior is repeatedly measured with the same scale. Reliability is concerned with consistency, accuracy, precision, stability, equivalence, and homogeneity. Concurrent with the questions of validity or after they are answered, you ask about the reliability of the instrument. Reliability refers to the proportion of consistency to inconsistency in measurement. In other words, if we use the same or comparable instruments on more than one occasion to measure a set of behaviors that ordinarily remain relatively constant, we would expect similar results if the instruments are reliable.

The main attributes of a reliable scale are stability, homogeneity, and equivalence. The **stability** of an instrument refers to the instrument's ability to produce the same results with repeated testing. The **homogeneity** of an instrument means that all of the items in an instrument measure the same concept, variable, or characteristic. An instrument is said to exhibit equivalence if it produces the same results when equivalent or parallel instruments or procedures are used. Each of these attributes and an understanding of how to interpret reliability are essential.

Reliability Coefficient Interpretation

Reliability is concerned with the degree of consistency between scores that are obtained at two or more independent times of testing and is expressed as a correlation coefficient. The reliability coefficient ranges from 0 to 1. The **reliability coefficient** expresses the relationship between the error variance, the true (score) variance, and the observed score. A zero correlation indicates that there is no relationship. When the error variance in a measurement instrument is low, the reliability coefficient will be closer to 1. The closer to 1 the coefficient is, the more reliable the instrument. **Example:** ➤ A reliability coefficient of an instrument is reported to be 0.89. This tells you that the error variance is small and the instrument has little measurement error. On the other hand, if the reliability coefficient of a measure is reported to be 0.49, the error variance is high and the instrument has a problem with measurement error. For a research instrument to be considered reliable, a reliability coefficient of 0.70 or above is necessary. If it is a clinical instrument, a reliability coefficient of 0.90 or higher is considered to be an acceptable level of reliability.

The tests of reliability used to calculate a reliability coefficient depend on the nature of the instrument. The tests are test-retest, item to total correlation, split-half, Kuder-Richardson (KR-20), Cronbach's alpha, and interrater reliability. These tests as they relate to stability, equivalence, and homogeneity are listed in Box 15.4, and examples of the types of reliability are shown in Box 15.5. There is no best means to assess reliability. The reliability method that the researcher uses should be consistent with the study's aim and the instrument's format.

BOX 15.4 **Measures Used to Test Reliability**		
Stability	**Homogeneity**	**Equivalence**
Test-retest reliability	Item to total correlation	Parallel or alternate form
Parallel or alternate form	Split-half reliability	Interrater reliability
	Kuder-Richardson coefficient	
	Cronbach's alpha	

BOX 15.5   Published Examples of Reported Reliability

Internal Consistency

A study by Kim and colleagues (2020a) examined whether baseline negative emotional states (depression and anxiety) would predict craving for cigarettes and other nicotine withdrawal symptoms in early abstinence and whether they would predict failure in quitting smoking among women living with human immunodeficiency virus (HIV). Anxiety was assessed at baseline using the Generalized Anxiety Disorder 7-Item Scale, an instrument with established reliability and validity (Spitzer, Kroenke, Williams and Lowe, 2006). Cronbach's alpha was 0.92 in the current study.

Test-Retest Reliability

A study by Zhang and Ganocy (2020) pilot-tested a new measure, the Irritability Scale-Initial Version (TISi), for assessing irritability of cancer patients on three dimensions: physical, affective, and behavioral. Spearman correlation analyses of test-retest reliability provided statistically significant ($p < .001$) correlations for IISI1 ($r = .69$) and its subscales (physical, $r = .61$; mood, $r = .76$; behavioral, $r = .67$). ICCs were high overall, .86, physical.81; mood.80; and behavioral .77. All ICC p values were $< .001$.

Kuder-Richardson (KR-20)

A study by Pai and colleagues (2019) was developed to validate the Psychosocial Assessment Tool-Hematopoietic Cell Transplant (PAT-HCT). The PAT-HCT was developed to screen family psychosocial risk when a member is experiencing the stressors of a Hematopoietic Stem Cell Transplant. One method employed in this study to validate the instrument was the use of Kuder-Richardson (KR-20). Based on the KR-20, internal consistency for the total scale and was strong (KR-20 = .88).

Interrater Reliability and Kappa

A study by Denny and Such (2018) explored the relationships between postoperative pain and subsyndromal delirium in older adults, which typically occurs between 24 and 72 hours after surgery. The Memorial Delirium Assessment Scale (MDAS), a clinician-rated scale, was used to assess delirium severity with acceptable interrater reliability (IRR = .92) (Breitbart et al., 1997). All research team members responsible for delirium assessments completed an educational module. The principal investigator and the research assistants evaluated interrater reliability using dual scoring of the participants and research assistants until scores were in agreement for two consecutive assessments before completing the MDAS independently.

Item to Total

Simpson and colleagues (2019) tested the internal consistency and test-retest reliability of the Atopic Dermatitis Control Tool (ADCT), a brief self-administered instrument used to assess how well symptoms of atopic dermatitis symptoms are controlled over the past week. Item to total correlations were estimated at baseline and at 1, 2, 3, and 6 months using the Pearson correlation coefficient. The Pearson correlation coefficient was PCC > 0.5, thus supporting the reliability of the scale.

Stability

An instrument is stable or exhibits stability when the same results are obtained on repeated administration of the instrument. Measurement over time is important when an instrument is used in a longitudinal study and therefore used on several occasions. Stability is also a consideration when a researcher is conducting an intervention study that is designed to effect a change in an outcome variable. In this case, the instrument is administered and then again later, after the experimental intervention has been completed. The tests that are used to estimate stability are test-retest and parallel or alternate form.

Test-Retest Reliability

Test-retest reliability is the administration of the same instrument to the same subjects under similar conditions on two or more occasions. Scores from repeated testing are compared. This comparison is expressed by a correlation coefficient, usually a Pearson *r* (see Chapter 16). The interval between repeated administrations varies and depends on the variable being measured. **Example:** ➤ If the variable that the test measures is related to the developmental stages in children, the interval between tests should be short. The amount of time over which the variable was measured should also be identified in the study.

> **HELPFUL HINT**
>
> When a longitudinal design with multiple data collection points is being conducted, look for evidence of test-retest reliability.

Internal Consistency/Homogeneity

Another attribute of an instrument related to reliability is the internal consistency or homogeneity. In this case, the items within the scale reflect or measure the same concept. This means that the items within the scale correlate or are complementary to each other. This also means that a scale is unidimensional. A unidimensional scale is one that measures one concept, such as self-efficacy. Box 15.5 provides several examples of how internal consistency is reported. Internal consistency can be assessed using one of four methods: item to total correlations, split-half reliability, Kuder-Richardson (KR-20) coefficient, or Cronbach's alpha.

> **EVIDENCE-BASED PRACTICE TIP**
>
> When the characteristics of a study sample differ significantly from the sample in the original study, check to see if the researcher has reestablished the reliability of the instrument with the current sample.

Item to Total Correlations

Item to total correlations measure the relationship between each of the items and the total scale. When item to total correlations are calculated, a correlation for each item on the scale is generated (Table 15.1). Items that do not achieve a high correlation may be deleted from the instrument. Usually in a research study, all of the item to total correlations are not reported unless the study is a report of a methodological study. The lowest and highest correlations are typically reported.

Cronbach's Alpha

The fourth and most commonly used test of internal consistency is Cronbach's alpha, which is used when a measurement instrument uses a Likert scale. Many scales used to measure psychosocial variables and attitudes have a Likert scale response format. A Likert scale format asks the subject to respond to a question on a scale of varying degrees of intensity between two extremes. The two extremes are anchored by responses ranging from "strongly agree" to "strongly disagree" or "most like me" to "least like me." The points between the two extremes may range from 1 to 4, 1 to 5, or 1 to 7. Subjects are asked to identify the response closest to how they feel. Cronbach's alpha simultaneously compares each item in the scale with the others. A total score is used in the data analysis, as illustrated in Box 15.6. Alphas above 0.70 are sufficient evidence for supporting the internal consistency of the instrument. Fig. 15.2 provides examples of items from an instrument that use a Likert scale format.

BOX 15.6   Examples of Cronbach Alpha

Kim, Y., Loewe & Hong (2021) used the Korean version of the Alcohol Use Disorders Identification Test (Park & Kim, 2010) to measure attitudes, subjective norms, perceived behavioral control (PBC) and intentions toward controlled drinking behavior to examine and compare predictors of controlled drinking behaviors. The scale demonstrated internal consistency of .96 for Korean American workers and .94 for Korean male workers.

Kuo et al. (2021) used a three item financial stress scale adapted from the Boston Longitudinal Study and found that the scale yielded a .82 Cronbach's alpha in the sample (Kuo et al., 2021).

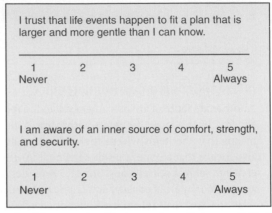

FIG 15.2 Examples of a Likert scale. (Redrawn from Roberts, K. T., & Aspy, C. B. (1993). Development of the serenity scale. *Journal of Nursing Measurement, 1*(2), 145–164.)

Split-Half Reliability

Split-half reliability involves dividing a scale into two halves and making a comparison. The halves may be odd-numbered and even-numbered items or may be a simple division of the first from the second half, or items may be randomly selected into halves that will be analyzed opposite one another. The split-half method provides a measure of consistency. The two halves of the test or the contents in both halves are assumed to be comparable, and a reliability coefficient is calculated. If the scores for the two halves are approximately equal, the test may be considered reliable. See Box 15.5 for an example.

Kuder-Richardson (KR-20) Coefficient

The Kuder-Richardson (KR-20) coefficient is the estimate of homogeneity used for instruments that have a dichotomous response format. A dichotomous response format is one in which the question asks for a "yes/no" or "true/false" response. The technique yields a correlation that is based on the consistency of responses to all items of a single form of a test that is administered one time. The minimum acceptable KR-20 score is $r = 0.70$ (see Box 15.5).

IPE HIGHLIGHT

Your team is critically appraising a study reporting on an innovative intervention for reducing the risk for hospital-acquired pressure ulcers. Data are collected using observation and multiple observers. You want to find evidence that the observers have been trained until there is a high level of interrater reliability so that you are confident that they were observing the subjects' skin according to standardized criteria and completing their checklist ratings in a consistent way across observers.

Equivalence

Equivalence either is the consistency or agreement among observers using the same measurement instrument or is the consistency or agreement between alternate forms of an instrument. An instrument is thought to demonstrate equivalence when two or more observers have a high percentage of agreement of an observed behavior or when alternate forms of a test yield a high correlation. There are two methods to test equivalence: interrater reliability and alternate or parallel form.

Interrater Reliability

Some measurement instruments are not self-administered questionnaires but are direct measurements of observed behavior. Instruments, often checklists, that depend on direct observation of a behavior that is to be systematically recorded must be tested for interrater reliability. To accomplish interrater reliability, two or more individuals should make an observation, or one observer should examine the behavior on several occasions. The observers should be trained or oriented to the definition and operationalization of the behavior to be observed. The consistency or reliability of the observations among observers is extremely important. Interrater reliability tests the consistency of the observer rather than the reliability of the instrument. Interrater reliability is expressed as a percentage of agreement between scorers or as a correlation coefficient of the scores assigned to the observed behaviors.

Kappa (κ) expresses the level of agreement observed beyond the level that would be expected by chance alone. κ ranges from +1 (total agreement) to 0 (no agreement). A κ of 0.80 or higher indicates good interrater reliability. κ between 0.80 and 0.68 is considered acceptable/substantial agreement; less than 0.68 allows tentative conclusions to be drawn at times when lower levels are accepted (McDowell & Newell, 1996) (see Box 15.5).

> **EVIDENCE-BASED PRACTICE TIP**
>
> Interrater reliability is an important approach to minimizing bias.

Parallel or Alternate Form

Parallel or alternate form was described in the discussion of stability in this chapter. Use of parallel forms is a measure of stability and equivalence. The procedures for assessing equivalence using parallel forms are the same.

CLASSICAL TEST THEORY VERSUS ITEM RESPONSE THEORY

The methods of reliability and validity described in this chapter are considered classical test theory (CTT) methods. There are newer methods that you will find described in research articles under the category of item response theory (IRT). The two methods share basic characteristics, but some feel that IRT methods are superior for discriminating test items. Several terms and concepts linked with IRT are Rasch models and one (or two) parameter logistic models. The methodology of these methods is beyond the scope of this text, but several references are cited for future use (DeVellis, 2012; Furr & Bacharach, 2008).

HOW VALIDITY AND RELIABILITY ARE REPORTED

When reading a research article, a lengthy discussion of how the different types of reliability and validity were obtained will typically not be found. What is found in the "Methods" section is the instrument's title, a definition of the concept/construct that it measures, and a sentence or two about reliability and/or validity of data. Examples of what you will see include the following:

- Jang and colleagues (2019) reported reliability for the Parenting Stress Scale (PSS), an instrument assessing overall parenting stress in the parent-child system. The scale had satisfactory internal consistency reliability (Cronbach's alpha = .83) and test-retest reliability (ICC = .81) (Berry and Jones, 1981). Cronbach's alpha was reestablished for the current sample (alpha = .87).
- The Brief Resilience Scale (BRS) (Smith et al., 2008), a six-item self-report with a 5-point Likert response scale that assesses a person's self-reported resilience (defined as the ability to recover from stress), was used in a study by Rodriguez-Rey and colleagues (2019). It has shown adequate internal consistency reliability (alpha = .80 to .90) and test-retest reliability (r = .62 to .69). The Spanish BRS (Rodriguez-Rey, Alonso-Tapia, and Hernansiaz-Garrido, 2016) showed adequate internal consistency (alpha = .83) and test-retest reliability (ICC = .69). The internal consistency for this study sample was alpha = .80.
- Kim and colleagues (2020) investigated the underlying mechanisms of health literacy's role in diabetes management among a group of Korean Americans with type 2 diabetes mellitus. Based on the well-established REALM health literacy instrument, they aimed to develop the diabetes-specific Rapid Estimate of Adult Literacy in Medicine (DM REALM) test for their pilot study. They used item-response theory to identify and remove items with potential cultural bias and duplicative content to produce a shorter version of the scale. The Korean version has a high internal consistency reliability (Cronbach's alpha = .98) and yielded adequate evidence of convergent validity by significant positive correlations with the functional Health Literacy (HL) scale (r = .49; p < .001).

▷ APPRAISAL FOR EVIDENCE-BASED PRACTICE
RELIABILITY AND VALIDITY

Reliability and validity are crucial aspects in the critical appraisal of a measurement instrument. Criteria for critiquing reliability and validity are presented in the Critical Appraisal Criteria box. When reviewing a research article, you must appraise each instrument's reliability and validity. In a research article, the reliability and validity for each measure should be presented, or a reference should be provided where it is described in more detail. If this information is not presented at all, you must seriously question the merit and use of the instrument and the evidence provided by the study's results.

The amount of information provided for each instrument will vary depending on the study type and the instrument. In a psychometric study (an instrument development study), you will find detail regarding how the researchers established the reliability and validity of the instrument. When reading a research article in which the instruments are used to test a research question or hypothesis, you may find only brief reference to the type of reliability and validity of the instrument. If the instrument is a well-known, reliable, and valid instrument, it is not uncommon that only a passing comment may be made, which is appropriate.

Example: ➤ A study by Poghosyan and colleagues (2020) studied the relationship between organizational support and nurse practitioner outcomes, including job satisfaction, intent to leave, and quality outcomes. Their survey tool, used in past surveys of nurse practitioners (Poghosyan, Liu, Shang and D'Aunno, 2017), contained validated measures of organizational support, nurse practitioner outcomes, and work characteristics. Previous research has documented the high predictive validity of the clinician self-reported quality of care measures (McHugh and Stimpfel, 2012). As in the previously provided example, authors often will cite a reference that you can locate if you are interested in detailed data about the instrument's reliability or validity. If a study does not use reliable and valid questionnaires, you must consider the sources of bias that may exist as threats to internal or external validity. It is very difficult to place confidence in the evidence generated by a study's findings if the measures used did not have established validity and reliability. The following discussion highlights key areas related to reliability and validity that should be evident as you read a research article.

CRITICAL APPRAISAL CRITERIA

Reliability and Validity

1. Was an appropriate method used to test the reliability of the instrument?
2. Is the reliability of the instrument adequate?
3. Was an appropriate method(s) used to test the validity of the instrument?
4. Is the validity of the measurement instrument adequate?
5. If the sample from the developmental stage of the instrument was different from the current sample, were the reliability and validity recalculated to determine whether the instrument is appropriate for use in a different population?
6. What kinds of threats to internal and/or external validity are presented by weaknesses in reliability and/or validity?
7. Are strengths and weaknesses of the reliability and validity of the instruments appropriately addressed in the "Discussion," "Limitations," or "Recommendations" sections of the report?
8. How do the reliability and/or validity affect the strength and quality of the evidence provided by the study findings?

The investigator determines which type of reliability procedures must be used in the study, depending on the nature of the measurement instrument and how it will be used. **Example:** ➤ If the instrument is to be administered twice, you would expect to read that test-retest reliability was used to establish the stability of the instrument. If an alternate form has been developed for use in a repeated-measures design, evidence of alternate form reliability should be presented to determine the equivalence of the parallel forms. If the degree of internal consistency among the items is relevant, an appropriate test of internal consistency should be presented. In some instances, more than one type of reliability will be presented, but as you assess the "Instruments" section of a research report, you should determine whether all are appropriate. **Example:** ➤ The Kuder-Richardson formula implies that there is a single right or wrong answer, making it inappropriate to use with scales that provide a format of three or more possible responses. In the latter case, another formula is applied, such as Cronbach's coefficient alpha. Another important consideration is the acceptable level of reliability, which varies according to the type of test. Reliability coefficients of 0.70 or higher are desirable. The validity of an instrument is limited by its reliability; that is, less confidence can be placed in scores from tests with low reliability coefficients.

Satisfactory evidence of validity will probably be the most difficult item for you to ascertain. It is this aspect of measurement information that is most likely to fall short as page count limitations often account for this brevity. Detailed validity data usually are only reported in studies focused on instrument development; therefore validity data are mentioned only briefly or, sometimes, not at all. The most common type of reported validity is content validity. When reviewing a study, you want to find evidence of content validity.

Once again, you will find the detailed reporting of content validity and the CVI in psychometric studies. Box 15.2 provides a good example of how content validity is reported in a psychometric study. Such procedures provide you with assurance that the instrument is psychometrically sound and that the content of the items is consistent with the conceptual framework and construct definitions. In studies in which several instruments are used, the reporting of content validity is either absent or very brief.

Construct validity and criterion-related validity are more precise statistical tests of whether the instrument measures what it is supposed to measure. Ideally an instrument should provide evidence of content validity as well as criterion-related or construct validity, before one invests a high level of confidence in the instrument. You will see evidence that the reliability and validity of a measurement instrument are reestablished periodically, as you can see in the examples that appear in Boxes 15.2 to 15.5. You would expect to see the strengths and weaknesses of instrument reliability and validity presented in the "Discussion," "Limitations," and/or "Recommendations" sections of an article. In this context, the reliability and validity may be discussed in terms of bias—that is, threats to internal and/or external validity that affect the study findings. **Example:** ➤ A study by Kim and colleagues (2020) evaluated the psychometric properties of the DM REALM health literacy instrument for use in a population of Korean American adults with type 2 diabetes mellitus. The authors noted that their findings should be interpreted with caution regarding generalization as the sample was relatively small, and internal consistency for one subscale was low (.66). Nevertheless, they concluded that the study findings have significant scientific implications for improving health literacy in a population of first-generation Korean older adult immigrants with type 2 diabetes mellitus whose primary language is not English and among the most vulnerable for low health literacy. Low health literacy is often a source of health disparities, and it is a major barrier to effective management of chronic conditions like type 2 diabetes among people with chronic illnesses.

The findings of any study in which the reliability and validity are sparse does limit generalizability of the findings, but also adds to our knowledge regarding future research directions. Finally, recommendations for improving future studies in relation to instrument reliability and validity may be proposed.

As you can see, the area of reliability and validity is complex. You should not feel intimidated by the complexity of this topic; use the guidelines presented in this chapter to systematically assess the reliability and validity aspects of a research study. Collegial dialogue is also an approach for evaluating the merits and shortcomings of an existing and a newly developed instrument that is reported in the nursing literature. Such an exchange promotes the understanding of methodologies as well as reliability and validity strategies, stimulates the acquisition of a basic knowledge of psychometrics, and encourages the exploration of alternative methods of observation and use of reliable and valid instruments in clinical practice.

KEY POINTS

- Reliability and validity are crucial aspects of conducting and critiquing research.
- Validity is the extent to which an instrument measures the attributes of a concept accurately. Three types of validity are content validity, criterion-related validity, and construct validity.
- The choice of a method for establishing reliability or validity is important and is made by the researcher on the basis of the characteristics of the measurement instrument and its intended use.

- Reliability is the ability of an instrument to measure the attributes of a concept or construct consistently. The major tests of reliability are test-retest, parallel or alternate form, split-half, item to total correlation, Kuder-Richardson, Cronbach's alpha, and interrater reliability.
- The selection of a method for establishing reliability or validity depends on the characteristics of the instrument, the testing method that is used for collecting data from the sample, and the kinds of data that are obtained.
- Critical appraisal of instrument reliability and validity in a research report focuses on internal and external validity as sources of bias that contribute to the strength and quality of evidence provided by the findings.

CLINICAL JUDGMENT CHALLENGES

- Discuss the types of validity that must be established before you invest a high level of confidence in the measurement instruments used in a research study.
- What are the major tests of reliability? Why is it important to establish the appropriate type of reliability for a measurement instrument?
- A journal club just finished reading the research report by De la Fuente and colleagues (2020) in Appendix B. As part of their critical appraisal of this study, they needed to identify the strengths and weaknesses of the reliability and validity section of this research report. If you were a member of this journal club, how would you assess the reliability and validity of the instruments used in this study?
- How does the strength and quality of evidence related to reliability and validity influence the applicability of findings to clinical practice?
- **IPE** When your quality improvement team finds that a researcher does not report reliability or validity data, which threats to internal and/or external validity should your team consider? In your judgment, how would these threats affect your evaluation of the strength and quality of evidence provided by the study and your team's confidence in applying the findings to practice (Chapter 8)?

REFERENCES

Anastasi, A., & Urbina, S. (1997). *Psychological testing* (7th ed.). New York, NY: Macmillan.

Brundle, C., Heaven, A., Brown, L., Teale, E., Young, J., West, R., & Clegg, A. (2019). Convergent validity of the electronic Frailty Index, doi: 10.1093/ageing/afy162.

Dennis, C., Brown, H. K., & Brennenstuhl, S. (2018). Development, psychometric assessment, and predictive validity of the postpartum childcare stress checklist. *Nursing Research, 67*(6), 439–446.

Denny, D. L., & Such, T. L. (2018). Exploration of relationships between postoperative pain and subsyndromal delirium in older adults. *Nursing Research, 67*(6), 421–429.

DeVon, F. A., Block, M. E., Moyle-Wright, P., et al. (2007). A psychometric toolbox for testing validity and reliability. *Journal of Nursing Scholarship, 39*(2), 155–164.

DeVellis, R. F. (2012). *Scale development: Theory and applications.* Los Angeles, CA: Sage Publications.

Furr, M. R., & Bacharach, V. R. (2008). *Psychometrics: An introduction.* Los Angeles, CA: Sage Publications.

Garzon, N. E., & Heredia, L. P. D. (2019). Validity and reliability of the treatment adherence questionnaire for patients with hypertension. *Investigation & Education en Enfermeria, 37*(3).

Jang, M., Brandon, D., & Vorderstrasse, A. (2019). Relationships among parental psychological distress, parental feeding practices, child diet, and child body mass index. *Nursing Research, 68*(4), 296–306.

Jung, M., Jonides, J., Berman, M. G., Northouse, L., Koeling, T. M., & Pressler, S. J. (2018). Construct validity of the multi-source interference task to examine attention in heart failure. *Nursing Research, 67*(6), 465–472.

Kim, S. S., Cooley, M. E., Lee, S. A., & DeMarco, R. F. (2020). Prediction of smoking abstinence in women living with Human Immunodeficiency virus infection. *Nursing Research, 69*(3), 167–175.

Kim, M. Y., Kim, K. B., Ko, J., Murry, N., Xie, B., Radhakrishnan, K., & Han, H. (2020). Health literacy and outcomes of a community-based self-help intervention: A case of Korean Americans with type 2 diabetes. *Nursing Research, 69*(3), 210–218.

Kim, Y., Lowe, J., & Hong, O. (2021). Controlled drinking behavior among Korean American and Korean male workers. *Nursing Research, 70*(2), 114–122.

Kuo, W., Oakley, L. D., Brown, R. L., Hagen, E. W., Barnet, J. H., & Peppard, P. E. (2021). *Nursing Research, 7*, 123–131.

Lee, C. E., VonAh, D., Szuck, B., & Lau, Y. J. (2016). Determinants of physical activity maintenance in breast cancer survivors after a community-based intervention. *Oncology Nursing Forum, 43*(1), 93–102.

Lynn, M. R. (1986). Determination and quantification of content validity. *Nursing Research, 35*, 382–385.

Magon, A., Arrigoni, C., Roveda, T., Grimodi, P., Dellafiore, F., Moia, M., Obamiro, K. O., & Caruso, R. (2018). Anticoagulation Knowledge Tool (AKT): Further evidence of validity in the Italian Population. *PLoS One, 13*(11), e0204534.

McDowell, I., & Newell, C. (1996). *Measuring health: A guide to rating scales and questionnaires.* New York, NY: Oxford Press.

Nunnally, J. C., & Bernstein, I. H. (1993). *Psychometric theory* (3rd ed.). New York, NY: McGraw-Hill.

Pai, A., Swain, A.M., Chen, F.F., Hwang, W., Vega, G., Carlosn, O., Ortiz, F.A., Carter, K., Joffe, N., Kolb, E.A., Davies, S.M., Chewning, J. H., Deatrick, J., Kazak, A.E. (2019). Screening for family psychosocial risk in pediatric hematopoietic stem cell transplantation with the psychosocial assessment toll. *Biology of Blood and Marrow Transplantation,* 1374–1381, doi: 10.1016/j.bbmt.2019.03.012.

Poghosyan, L., Ghaffari, A., Liu, J., & McHugh, M. D. (2020). Organizational support for nurse practitioners and workforce outcomes. *Nursing Research, 69*(4), 280–288.

Rodriguez-Rey, R., Garcia-Liana, H., Ruiz-Alvarez, M. P., Gomez-Gomez, A., delPeso, G., & Seigas, R. (2019). Multicenter validation of the emotional state instrument for dialysis patients. *Nursing Research, 68*(1), 39–47.

Simpson, E., Eckert, L., Gadkari, A., Mallya, U. G., Yang, M., Nelson, L., Brown, M., Reaney, M., Mahajan, P., Guillemin, I., Boguniewicz, M., & Pariser, D. (2019). Validation of the Atopic Dermatitis Control Tool (ADCT©) using a longitudinal survey of biologic-treated patients with atopic dermatitis. *BMC Dermatology, 19*, 15.

Zhang, A. Y., & Ganocy, S. J. (2020). Measurement of irritability in cancer patients. *Nursing Research, 69*(2), 91–99.

Go to Evolve at **http://evolve.elsevier.com/LoBiondo/** for review questions, appraisal exercises, and additional research articles for practice in reviewing and appraisal.

16

Appraising Data Analysis: Descriptive & Inferential Statistics

Susan Sullivan-Bolyai, Carol Bova

Go to Evolve at **http://evolve.elsevier.com/LoBiondo/** for review questions.

LEARNING OUTCOMES

After reading this chapter, you should be able to do the following:

- Differentiate between descriptive and inferential statistics.
- State the purpose of descriptive statistics.
- Identify the levels of measurement in a study.
- Describe a frequency distribution.
- List measures of central tendency and their use.
- List measures of variability and their use.
- State the purpose of inferential statistics.
- Explain the concept of probability as it applies to the analysis of sample data.
- Distinguish between a type I and type II error and its effect on a study's outcome.

- Distinguish between parametric and nonparametric tests.
- List some commonly used statistical tests and their purposes.
- Critically appraise the statistics used in published research studies.
- Evaluate the strength and quality of the evidence provided by the findings of a research study, and determine applicability to practice.

KEY TERMS

analysis of covariance
analysis of variance
categorical variable
chi-square (x^2)
continuous variable
correlation
degrees of freedom
descriptive statistics
dichotomous variable
factor analysis
Fisher exact probability test
frequency distribution

inferential statistics
interval measurement
levels of measurement
level of significance (alpha level)
mean
measurement
measures of central tendency
measures of variability
median
modality
mode

multiple regression
multivariate statistics
nominal measurement
nonparametric statistics
normal curve
null hypothesis
ordinal measurement
parameter
parametric statistics
Pearson correlation coefficient (Pearson *r*; Pearson product

moment correlation coefficient)
percentile
probability
range
ratio measurement
sampling error
scientific hypothesis
standard deviation
statistic
t statistic
type I error
type II error

It is important to understand the principles underlying statistical methods used in quantitative research. This understanding allows you to critically analyze the results of research that may be useful in practice. Researchers link the statistical analyses they choose with the type of research question, design, and level of data collected.

As you read a research article, you will find a discussion of the statistical procedures used in both the "Methods" and "Results" sections. In the "Methods" section, you will find the planned statistical analyses. In the "Results" section, you will find the data generated from testing the hypotheses or research aims/questions. The data are analyzed using both descriptive and inferential statistics.

Procedures that allow researchers to describe and summarize data are known as descriptive statistics. Descriptive statistics include measures of central tendency, such as mean, median, and mode; measures of variability, such as range and standard deviation (SD); and some correlation techniques, such as scatter plots. For example, De la Fuente Coria and colleagues (2020; Appendix B) used descriptive statistics to inform the reader about the 236 subjects with type 2 diabetes who participated in their study. They reported the means and standard deviations by the total sample, those randomized into the intervention and control groups (Table 16.1). Males made up 54.2% of the total sample, with an average age of 65.1 years and body mass index (BMI) of 7.6.

Statistical procedures that allow researchers to estimate how reliably they can make *predictions* and *generalize* findings based on the data are known as inferential statistics. Inferential statistics are used to analyze the data collected, test hypotheses, and answer the research questions/aims in a research study. With inferential statistics, the researcher is trying to draw conclusions that extend beyond the study's data.

This chapter describes how researchers use descriptive and inferential statistics in studies. This will help you determine the appropriateness of the statistics used and to interpret the strength and quality of the reported findings as well as the clinical significance and applicability of the results for your evidence-based practice.

LEVELS OF MEASUREMENT

Measurement is the process of assigning numbers to variables or events according to rules. Every variable in a study that is assigned a specific number must be similar to every other variable assigned that number. The measurement level is determined by the nature of the object or event being measured. Understanding the levels of measurement is an important first step when you evaluate the statistical analyses used in a study. There are four levels of measurement: nominal, ordinal, interval, and ratio (see Table 16.1). The level of measurement of each variable determines the statistic that can be used to answer a research question or test a hypothesis. The higher the level of measurement, the greater the flexibility the researcher has in choosing statistical procedures. The Critical Thinking Decision Path illustrates the relationship between levels of measurement and the appropriate use of descriptive statistics.

Nominal measurement is used to classify variables or events into categories. The categories are mutually exclusive; the variable or event either has or does not have the characteristic. The numbers assigned to each category are only labels; such numbers do not indicate more or less of a characteristic. Nominal level measurement is used to categorize a sample on such information as gender, marital status, or religious affiliation. For example, Di Stasio and colleagues (2020; Appendix D) measured gender using a nominal level

TABLE 16.1 Level of Measurement Summary Table

Measurement	Description	Measures of Central Tendency	Measures of Variability
Nominal	Classification	Mode	Modal percentage, range, frequency distribution
Ordinal	Relative rankings	Mode, median	Range, percentile, frequency distribution
Interval	Rank ordering with equal intervals	Mode, median, mean	Range, percentile, standard deviation
Ratio	Rank ordering with equal intervals and absolute zero	Mode, median, mean	All

CRITICAL THINKING DECISION PATH

Descriptive Statistics

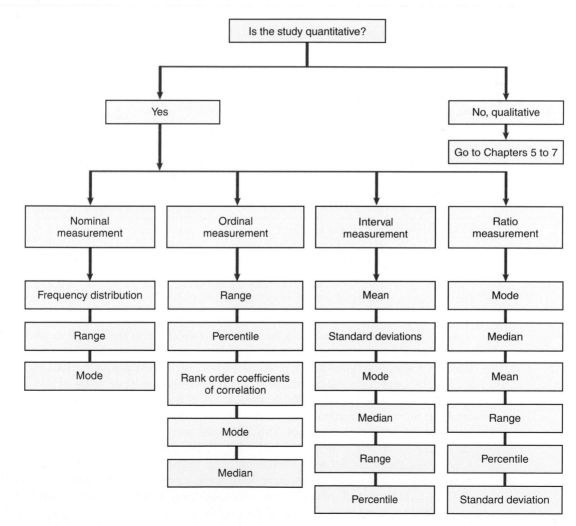

of measurement. Nominal-level measurement is the lowest level and allows for the least amount of statistical manipulation. When using nominal level variables, the frequency and percent are typically calculated. For example, Di Stasio and colleagues (2020) found that among their sample of caregivers, 71% were females and 29% were males (see Table 16.1).

A variable at the nominal level can also be categorized as either a dichotomous or a categorical variable. A **dichotomous** (nominal) **variable** is one that has *only two true values,* such as true/false or yes/no. For example, in the Di Stasio and colleagues (2020) example, the variable gender (male/female) is dichotomous because it has only two possible values. On the other hand, nominal variables that are **categorical** still have mutually exclusive categories but have *more than two true values,* such as current nursing degree (ADN, BSN, MSN) in the Flanders and colleagues (2020; Appendix C) study.

Ordinal measurement is used to show relative rankings of variables or events. The numbers assigned to each category can be compared, and a member of a higher category can be said to have more of an attribute than a person in a lower category. The intervals between numbers on the scale are not necessarily equal, and there is no absolute zero. For example, ordinal measurement is used to formulate class rankings, where one student can be ranked higher or lower than another. However, the difference in actual grade point average between students may differ widely. Another example is ranking individuals by their level of wellness or by their ability to carry out activities of daily living. Ordinal-level data are limited in the amount of mathematical manipulation possible. Frequencies, percentages, medians, percentiles, and rank order coefficients of correlation can be calculated for ordinal-level data.

Interval measurement shows rankings of events or variables on a scale with equal intervals between the numbers. The zero point remains arbitrary and not absolute. For example, interval measurements are used in measuring temperatures on the Fahrenheit scale. The distances between degrees are equal, but the zero point is arbitrary and does not represent the absence of temperature. Test scores also represent interval data. The differences between test scores represent equal intervals, but a zero does not represent the total absence of knowledge.

HELPFUL HINT

The term continuous variable is also used to represent a measure that contains a range of values along a continuum and may include ordinal, interval, and ratio level data (Plichta & Kelvin, 2013). An example is heart rate.

In many areas of science, including nursing, the classification of the level of measurement of scales that use Likert-type response options to measure concepts such as quality of life, depression, functional status, or social support is controversial, with some regarding these measurements as ordinal and others as interval. You must be aware of this controversy and look at each study individually in terms of how the data are analyzed. Interval level data allow more manipulation of data, including the addition and subtraction of numbers and the calculation of means. This additional manipulation is why many argue for classifying behavioral scale data as interval level. For example, Di Stasio and colleagues (2020) used the Stress-Related Vulnerability Scale (SVS) to measure vulnerability related to stressful situations, such as being the caregiver of a person with Parkinson disease. The SVS has nine items and uses a 4-point Likert scale with higher scores indicating greater vulnerability.

Ratio measurement shows rankings of events or variables on scales with equal intervals and absolute zeros. The number represents the actual amount of the property the object possesses. Ratio measurement is the highest level of measurement, but it is most often used in the physical sciences. Examples of ratio level data that are commonly used in nursing research are height, weight, pulse, and blood pressure. All mathematical procedures can be performed on data from ratio scales. Therefore the use of any statistical procedure is possible as long as it is appropriate to the design of the study.

HELPFUL HINT

Descriptive statistics assist in summarizing data. The descriptive statistics calculated must be appropriate to the purpose of the study and the level of measurement.

DESCRIPTIVE STATISTICS

Frequency Distribution

One way of organizing descriptive data is by using a frequency distribution. In a **frequency distribution**, the number of times each event occurs is counted. The data can also be grouped and the frequency of each group reported. Table 16.2 shows the results of an examination given to a class of 51 students. The results of the examination are reported in several ways. The columns on the left give the raw data tally and the frequency for each grade, and the columns on the right give the grouped data tally and grouped frequencies.

When data are grouped, it is necessary to define the size of the group or the interval width so no score will fall into two groups and each group will be mutually exclusive. The grouping of the data in Table 16.2 prevents overlap; each score falls into only one group. The grouping should allow for a precise presentation of the data without a serious loss of information.

Information about frequency distributions may be presented in the form of a table, such as Table 16.2, or in graphic form. Fig. 16.1 illustrates the most common graphic forms: the histogram and the frequency polygon. The two graphic methods are similar in that both plot scores, or percentages of occurrence, against frequency. The greater the number of points plotted, the smoother the resulting graph. The shape of the resulting graph allows for observations that further describe the data.

Measures of Central Tendency

Measures of central tendency are used to describe the pattern of responses among a sample. Measures of central tendency include the mean, median, and mode. They yield a single number that describes the middle of the group and summarize the members of a sample. Each measure of central tendency has a specific use and is most appropriate to specific kinds of measurement and types of distributions.

The **mean** is the arithmetical average of all of the scores (add all of the values in a distribution, and divide by the total number of values) and is used with interval or ratio data. The mean is the most widely used measure of central tendency. Most statistical tests of significance use the mean. The mean is affected by every score and can change greatly with extreme scores, especially in studies that have a limited sample size. The mean is generally considered the single best point for summarizing data when using interval or ratio level data. You can find the mean in research reports by looking for the symbol $\bar{x}$.

TABLE 16.2 **Frequency Distribution**

	INDIVIDUAL			GROUP		
Score	Tally	Frequency		Score	Tally	Frequency
90	|	1		>89	|	1
88	|	1		—	—	—
86	|	1		80–89	||||| ||||| |||||	15
84	||||| |	6		—	—	—
82	||	2		70–79	||||| ||||| ||||| ||||| |||	23
80	|||||	5		—	—	—
78	|||||	5		—	—	—
76	|	1		60–69	||||| |||||	10
74	||||| ||	7		—	—	—
72	||||| ||||	9		<59	||	2
70	|	1		—	—	—
68	|||	3		—	—	—
66	||	2		—	—	—
64	||||	4		—	—	—
62	|	1		—	—	—
60	—	0		—	—	—
58	|	1		—	—	—
56		0		—	—	—
54	|	1		—	—	—
52		0		—	—	—
50		0		—	—	—
Total		51		—	—	51

Mean, 73.1; standard deviation, 12.1; median, 74; mode, 72; range, 36 (54–90).

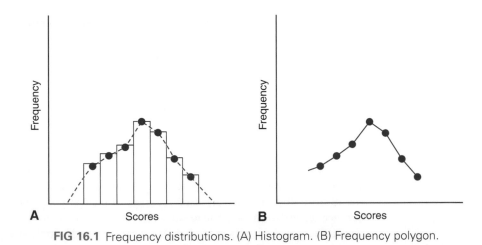

FIG 16.1 Frequency distributions. (A) Histogram. (B) Frequency polygon.

The **median** is the score where 50% of the scores are above it and 50% of the scores are below it. The median is not sensitive to extremes in high and low scores. It is best used when the data are skewed (see the "Normal Distribution" section later in this chapter) and the researcher is interested in the "typical" score. For example, if age is a variable and there is a wide range with extreme scores that may affect the mean, it would be appropriate to also report the median. The median is easy to find either by inspection or by calculation and can be used with ordinal, interval, and ratio level data.

The **mode** is the most frequent value in a distribution. The mode is determined by inspection of the frequency distribution (not by mathematical calculation). For example, in Table 16.2 the mode would be a score of 72 because nine students received this score, and it represents the score that was attained by the greatest number of students. It is important to note that a sample distribution can have more than one mode. The number of modes contained in a distribution is called the **modality** of the distribution. It is also possible to have no mode when all scores in a distribution are different. The mode is most often used with nominal data but can be used with all levels of measurement. The mode cannot be used for calculations, and it is unstable; that is, the mode can fluctuate widely from sample to sample from the same population.

> **HELPFUL HINT**
>
> Of the three measures of central tendency, the mean is affected by every score. The mean can only be calculated with interval and ratio data.

When you examine a study, the measures of central tendency provide you with important information about the distribution of scores in a sample. If the distribution is symmetrical and unimodal, the mean, median, and mode will coincide. If the distribution is skewed (asymmetrical), the mean will be pulled in the direction of the long tail of the distribution and will differ from the median. With a skewed distribution, all three statistics should be reported.

> **HELPFUL HINT**
>
> Measures of central tendency are descriptive statistics that describe the characteristics of a sample.

Normal Distribution

The concept of normal distribution is based on the observation that data from repeated measures of interval- or ratio-level data group themselves about a midpoint in a distribution in a manner that closely approximates the normal curve illustrated in Fig. 16.2. The **normal curve** is one that is symmetrical about the mean and is unimodal. The mean, median, and mode are equal. An additional characteristic of the normal curve is that a fixed percentage of the scores fall within a given distance of the mean. As shown in Fig. 16.2, about 68% of the scores or means will fall within 1 SD of the mean, 95% within 2 SD of the mean, and 99.7% within 3 SD of the mean. The presence or absence of a normal distribution is a fundamental issue when examining the appropriate use of inferential statistical procedures.

> **EVIDENCE-BASED PRACTICE TIP**
>
> Inspection of descriptive statistics for the sample will indicate whether the sample data are skewed.

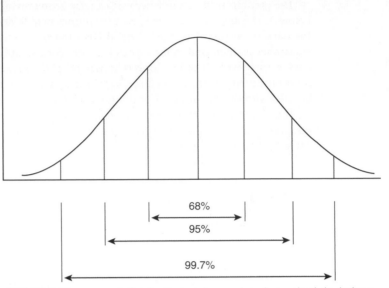

FIG 16.2 The normal distribution and associated standard deviations.

Interpreting Measures of Variability

Variability or dispersion is concerned with the spread of data. **Measures of variability** answer questions such as: "Is the sample homogeneous (similar) or heterogeneous (different)?" If a researcher measures oral temperatures in two samples, one sample drawn from a healthy population and one sample from a hospitalized population, it is possible that the two samples will have the same mean. However, it is likely that there will be a wider range of temperatures in the hospitalized sample than in the healthy sample. Measures of variability are used to describe these differences in the dispersion of data. As with measures of central tendency, the various measures of variability are appropriate to specific kinds of measurement and types of distributions.

> **HELPFUL HINT**
>
> The descriptive statistics related to variability will enable you to evaluate the homogeneity or heterogeneity of a sample.

The **range** is the simplest but most unstable measure of variability. Range is the difference between the highest and lowest scores. A change in either of these two scores would change the range. The range should always be reported with other measures of variability. The range in Table 16.2 is 36, but this could easily change with an increase or decrease in the high score of 90 or the low score of 54.

A **percentile** represents the percentage of cases a given score exceeds. The median is the 50th percentile, and in Table 16.2 it is a score of 74. A score in the 90th percentile is exceeded by only 10% of the scores. The zero percentile and the 100th percentile are usually dropped.

The **standard deviation** (SD) is the most frequently used measure of variability, and it is based on the concept of the normal curve (see Fig. 16.2). It is a measure of average deviation of the scores from the mean and as such should always be reported with the mean. The SD considers all scores and can be used to interpret individual scores. Table 16.1, in the De la Fuente Coria and colleagues (2020) study, uses a +/− symbol to indicate the SD for the major study variables by treatment group. For example, the SD for age in the total sample was +/− 9.5 years. The SD is used in the calculation of many inferential statistics.

> **HELPFUL HINT**
>
> Many measures of variability exist. The SD is the most useful because it helps you visualize how the scores disperse around the mean.

INFERENTIAL STATISTICS

Inferential statistics allow researchers to test hypotheses about a population using data obtained from probability samples. Statistical inference is generally used for two purposes: to estimate the probability that the statistics in the sample accurately reflect the population parameter, and to test hypotheses about a population.

A **parameter** is a characteristic of a *population,* whereas a **statistic** is a characteristic of a *sample.* We use statistics to estimate population parameters. Suppose we randomly sample 100 people with influenza and use an interval level scale to study the time to recovery in days. If the mean days to recovery for these subjects is 16, the mean represents the sample statistic. If we were able to study every subject with influenza, we could calculate an average time to recovery, and that score would be the parameter for the population. As you know, a researcher rarely is able to study an entire population, so inferential statistics provide evidence that allows the researcher to make statements about the larger population from studying the sample.

The example given alludes to two important qualifications of how a study must be conducted so that inferential statistics may be used. First, it was stated that the sample was selected using probability methods (see Chapter 12). Because you are already familiar with the advantages of probability sampling, it should be clear that if we wish to make statements about a population from a sample, the sample must be representative. All procedures for inferential statistics are based on the assumption that the sample was drawn with a known probability. Second, the scale used must be at either an interval or a ratio level of measurement. This is because the mathematical operations involved in calculating inferential statistics require this higher level of measurement. It should be noted that in studies that use nonprobability methods of sampling, inferential statistics are also used. To compensate for the use of nonprobability sampling methods, researchers use techniques such as sample size estimation using power analysis. The following two Critical Thinking Decision Paths examine inferential statistics and provide matrices that researchers use for statistical decision making.

CRITICAL THINKING DECISION PATH

Inferential Statistics—Difference Questions

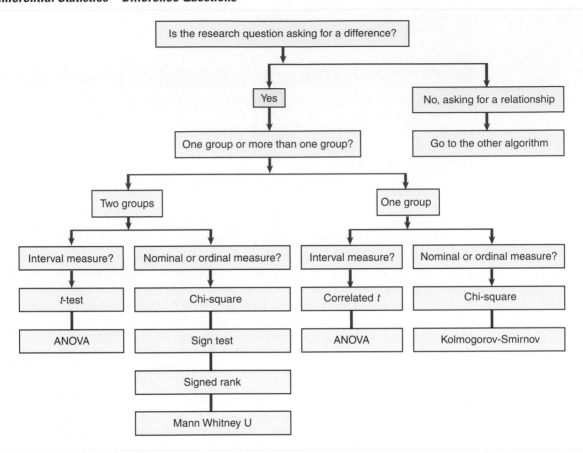

Hypothesis Testing

Inferential statistics are used for hypothesis testing. Statistical hypothesis testing allows researchers to make objective decisions about the data from their study. The use of statistical hypothesis testing answers questions such as "How much of this effect is the result of chance?", "How strongly are these two variables associated with each other?", and "What is the effect of the intervention?"

> **IPE HIGHLIGHT**
>
> Members of your interprofessional team may have diverse data analysis preparation. Capitalizing on everybody's background, try to figure out whether the statistical tests chosen for the studies your team is critically appraising are appropriate for the design, type of data collection, and level of measurement.

The procedures used when making inferences are based on principles of negative inference. In other words, if a researcher studied the effect of a new educational program for

CRITICAL THINKING DECISION PATH

Inferential Statistics—Relationship Questions

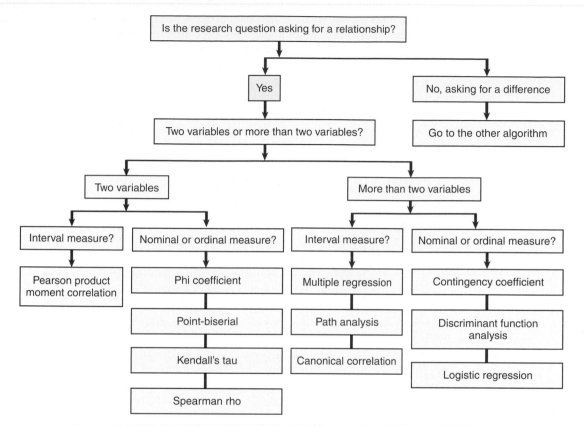

patients with chronic lung disease, the researcher would actually have two hypotheses: the scientific hypothesis and the null hypothesis. The research or **scientific hypothesis** is that which the researcher believes will be the outcome of the study. In our example, the scientific hypothesis would be that the educational intervention would have a marked effect on the outcome in the experimental group beyond that in the control group. The **null hypothesis**, which is the hypothesis that actually can be tested by statistical methods, would state that there is no difference between the groups. Inferential statistics use the null hypothesis to test the validity of a scientific hypothesis. The null hypothesis states that there is no relationship between the variables and that any observed relationship or difference is merely a function of chance.

> **HELPFUL HINT**
>
> Most samples used in clinical research are samples of convenience, but often researchers use inferential statistics. Although such use violates one of the assumptions of such tests, the tests are robust enough to not seriously affect the results unless the data are skewed in unknown ways.

Probability

Probability theory underlies all of the procedures discussed in this chapter. The probability of an event is its long-run relative frequency (0% to 100%) in repeated trials under similar conditions. In other words, what are the chances of obtaining the same result from a study that can be carried out many times under identical conditions? It is the notion of repeated trials that allows researchers to use probability to test hypotheses.

Statistical probability is based on the concept of sampling error. Remember that the use of inferential statistics is based on random sampling. However, even when samples are randomly selected, there is always the possibility of some error in sampling. Therefore the characteristics of any given sample may be different from those of the entire population. The tendency for statistics to fluctuate from one sample to another is known as *sampling error*.

EVIDENCE-BASED PRACTICE TIP

The strength and quality of evidence are enhanced by repeated trials that have consistent findings, thereby increasing generalizability of the findings and applicability to clinical practice.

Type I and Type II Errors

Statistical inference is always based on incomplete information about a population, and it is possible for errors to occur. There are two types of errors in statistical inference—type I and type II errors. A type I error occurs when a researcher rejects a null hypothesis when it is actually true (i.e., accepts the premise that there is a difference when actually there is no difference between groups). A type II error occurs when a researcher accepts a null hypothesis that is actually false (i.e., accepts the premise that there is no difference between the groups when a difference actually exists). The relationship of the two types of errors is shown in Fig. 16.3.

When critiquing a study to see if there is a possibility of a type I error having occurred (rejecting the null hypothesis when it is actually true), one should consider the reliability and validity of the instruments used. For example, if the instruments did not accurately measure the intervention variables, one could conclude that the intervention made a difference when in reality it did not. It is critical to consider the reliability and validity of all measurement instruments reported (see Chapter 15).

In a practice discipline, type I errors usually are considered more serious because if a researcher declares that differences exist when none are present, the potential exists for patient care to be affected adversely. Type II errors (accepting the null hypothesis when it is

Conclusion of test of significance	REALITY	
	Null hypothesis is true	Null hypothesis is not true
Not statistically significant	Correct conclusion	Type II error
Statistically significant	Type I error	Correct conclusion

FIG 16.3 Outcome of statistical decision making.

false) often occur when the sample is too small, thereby limiting the opportunity to measure *the treatment effect,* the true difference between two groups. A larger sample size improves the ability to *detect the treatment effect*—that is, the difference between two groups. If no significant difference is found between two groups with a large sample, it provides stronger evidence (than with a small sample) not to reject the null hypothesis.

Level of Significance

The researcher does not know when an error in statistical decision making has occurred. It is possible to know only that the null hypothesis is indeed true or false if data from the total population are available. However, the researcher can control the risk for making type I errors by setting the level of significance before the study begins (a priori).

The **level of significance (alpha level)** is the probability of making a type I error, the probability of rejecting a true null hypothesis. The minimum level of significance acceptable for most research is .05. If the researcher sets alpha, or the level of significance, at .05, the researcher is willing to accept the fact that if the study were done 100 times, the decision to reject the null hypothesis would be wrong 5 times out of those 100 trials. As is sometimes the case, if the researcher wants to have a smaller risk for rejecting a true null hypothesis, the level of significance may be set at .01. In this case, the researcher is willing to be wrong only once in 100 trials.

The decision as to how strictly the alpha level should be set depends on how important it is to avoid errors. For example, if the results of a study are to be used to determine whether a great deal of money should be spent in an area of patient care, the researcher may decide that the accuracy of the results is so important that an alpha level of .01 is needed. In most studies, however, alpha is set at .05.

Perhaps you are thinking that researchers should always use the lowest alpha level possible to keep the risk for both types of errors at a minimum. Unfortunately, decreasing the risk for making a type I error increases the risk for making a type II error. Therefore the researcher always must accept more of a risk for one type of error when setting the alpha level.

The level of statistical significance is often indicated by a p value. The p value represents the probability that the results of a statistical test were obtained by chance alone. The p value is most often set at $p < .05$ (the result is considered statistically significant). It is important to note that the alpha level is set *before* the study begins, and the p value is known only *after* completing the statistical analysis. De la Fuente Coria and colleagues (2020) found that length of time with diabetes in years and BMI at baseline were significantly different between the intervention and control groups ($p = .000$ and $p = .022$, respectively).

HELPFUL HINT

Decreasing the alpha level acceptable for a study increases the chance that a type II error will occur. When a researcher is doing many statistical tests, the probability of some of the tests being significant increases as the number of tests increases. Therefore, when a number of tests are being conducted, the researcher may decrease the alpha level to .01.

Clinical and Statistical Significance

It is important for you to realize that there is a difference between statistical significance and clinical significance. When a researcher tests a hypothesis and finds that it is statistically significant, it means that the finding is unlikely to have happened by chance. For example, if a study was designed to test an intervention to help a large sample of patients lose weight, and the researchers found that a change in weight of 1.02 pounds was statistically significant, one may find this questionable because few would say that a change in weight of just over 1 pound would represent a clinically significant difference. Therefore as a consumer of research, it is important to evaluate the clinical significance and the statistical significance of findings.

Some people believe that if findings are not statistically significant, they have no practical value. However, knowing that something does not work is important information to share with the scientific community. Unsupported hypotheses provide as much information about the intervention as supported hypotheses. Nonsignificant results (sometimes called *negative findings*) force the researcher to return to the literature and consider alternative explanations for why the intervention did not work as planned.

EVIDENCE-BASED PRACTICE TIP

You will study the results to determine whether the new treatment is effective, the size of the effect, and whether the effect is clinically important.

Parametric and Nonparametric Statistics

Tests of significance may be parametric or nonparametric. **Parametric statistics** have the following attributes:
1. Involve the estimation of at least one population parameter
2. Require measurement on at least an interval scale
3. Involve certain assumptions about the variables being studied

One important assumption is that the variable is normally distributed in the overall population.

In contrast with parametric tests, **nonparametric statistics** are not based on the estimation of population parameters, so they involve less restrictive assumptions about the underlying distribution. Nonparametric tests usually are applied when the variables have been measured on a nominal or ordinal scale, or when the distribution of scores is severely skewed.

HELPFUL HINT

Just because a researcher has used nonparametric statistics does not mean that the study is not useful. The use of nonparametric statistics is appropriate when measurements are not made at the interval level or the variable under study is not normally distributed.

There has been some debate about the relative merits of the two types of statistics. The moderate position taken by most researchers and statisticians is that nonparametric statistics are best used when data are not at the interval level of measurement, when the sample is small, and data do not approximate a normal distribution. However, most researchers prefer to use parametric statistics whenever possible (as long as data meet the assumptions) because they are more powerful and more flexible than nonparametric statistics.

Tables 16.3 and 16.4 list the commonly used inferential statistics. The test used depends on the level of the measurement of the variables in question and the type of hypothesis being studied. These statistics test two types of hypotheses: that there is a difference between

TABLE 16.3 Tests of Differences Between Means

Level of Measurement	One Group	TWO GROUPS			More Than Two Groups
		Related		Independent	
Nonparametric					
Nominal	Chi-square	Chi-square Fisher exact probability		Chi-square	Chi-square
Ordinal	Kolmogorov-Smirnov	Sign test Wilcoxon matched pairs Signed rank		Chi-square Median test Mann-Whitney *U* test	Chi-square
Parametric					
Interval or ratio	Correlated *t* ANOVA (repeated measures)	Correlated *t*		Independent *t* ANOVA	ANOVA ANCOVA MANOVA

ANOVA, Analysis of variance; *ANCOVA*, analysis of covariance; *MANOVA*, multiple analysis of variance.

TABLE 16.4 Tests of Association

Level of Measurement	Two Variables	More Than Two Variables
Nonparametric		
Nominal	Phi coefficient Point-biserial	Contingency coefficient
Ordinal	Kendall's tau Spearman rho	Discriminant function analysis
Parametric		
Interval or ratio	Pearson *r*	Multiple regression Path analysis Canonical correlation

groups (see Table 16.3) or that there is a relationship between two or more variables (see Table 16.4).

EVIDENCE-BASED PRACTICE TIP

Try to discern whether the test chosen for analyzing the data was chosen because it gave a significant *p* value. A statistical test should be chosen on the basis of its appropriateness for the type of data collected, not because it gives the answer that the researcher hoped to obtain.

Tests of Difference

The type of test used for any particular study depends primarily on whether the researcher is examining differences in one, two, or three or more groups and whether the data to be analyzed are nominal, ordinal, or interval (see Table 16.3). Suppose a researcher has conducted an experimental study (see Chapter 9). What the researcher hopes to determine is that the two randomly assigned groups are different after the introduction of the experimental treatment. If the measurements taken are at the interval level, the researcher would use the *t* test to analyze the data. If the *t* statistic was found to be high enough as to be unlikely to have occurred by chance, the researcher would reject the null hypothesis and conclude that the two groups were indeed more different than would have been expected on the basis of chance alone. In other words, the researcher would conclude that the experimental treatment had the desired effect.

EVIDENCE-BASED PRACTICE TIP

Tests of difference are most commonly used in experimental and quasi-experimental designs that provide Level II and Level III evidence.

The *t statistic* tests whether two group means are different. Thus this statistic is used when the researcher has two groups, and the question is whether the mean scores on some measure are more different than would be expected by chance. To use this test, the dependent variable (DV) must have been measured at the interval or ratio level, and the two groups must be independent. By *independent* we mean that nothing in one group helps determine who is in the other group. If the groups are related, as when samples are matched, and the researcher also wants to determine differences between the two groups, a paired or correlated *t* test would be used. The **degrees of freedom** (represents the freedom of a score's value to vary given what is known about the other scores and the sum of scores; often $df = N - 1$) are reported with the *t* statistic and the probability value (p). Degrees of freedom is usually abbreviated as *df*.

The *t* statistic illustrates one of the major purposes of research in nursing—to demonstrate that there are differences between groups. Groups may be naturally occurring collections, such as gender, or they may be experimentally created, such as treatment and control groups. Sometimes a researcher has more than two groups, or measurements are taken more than once, and then **analysis of variance** (ANOVA) is used. ANOVA is similar to the *t* test. Like the *t* statistic, ANOVA tests whether group means differ, but rather than testing each pair of means separately, ANOVA considers the variation between groups and within groups.

HELPFUL HINT

A research report may not always contain the test that was done. You can find this information by looking at the tables. For example, a table with *t* statistics will contain a column for *t* values, and an ANOVA table will contain *F* values.

Analysis of covariance (ANCOVA) is used to measure differences among group means, but it also uses a statistical technique to equate the groups under study on an important variable.

Nonparametric Statistics

When data are at the nominal level and the researcher wants to determine whether groups are different, the researcher uses the **chi-square** (x^2). Chi-square is a nonparametric statistic used to determine whether the frequency in each category is different from what would be expected by chance. As with the *t* test and ANOVA, if the calculated chi-square is high enough, the researcher would conclude that the frequencies found would not be expected on the basis of chance alone, and the null hypothesis would be rejected. Although this test is quite robust and can be used in many different situations, it cannot be used to compare frequencies when samples are small and expected frequencies are less than six in each cell. In these instances, the **Fisher exact probability test** is used.

When the data are ranks, or are at the ordinal level, researchers have several other nonparametric tests at their disposal. These include the *Kolmogorov-Smirnov test*, the *sign test*, the *Wilcoxon matched pairs test*, the *signed rank test for related groups*, the *median test*, and the *Mann-Whitney U test for independent groups*. Explanation of these tests is beyond the scope of this chapter; readers who desire further information should consult a general statistics book.

> ### HELPFUL HINT
>
> Chi-square is the test of difference commonly used for nominal-level demographic variables such as gender, marital status, religion, ethnicity, and others.

Tests of Relationships

Researchers often are interested in exploring the *relationship* between two or more variables. Such studies use statistics that determine the correlation, or the degree of association, between two or more variables. Tests of the relationships between variables are sometimes considered to be descriptive statistics when they are used to describe the magnitude and direction of a relationship of two variables in a sample and the researcher does not wish to make statements about the larger population. Such statistics also can be inferential when they are used to test hypotheses about the correlations that exist in the target population.

> ### EVIDENCE-BASED PRACTICE TIP
>
> You will often note that in the results or findings section of a research study, parametric measures (e.g., *t* tests, ANOVA) and nonparametric measures (e.g., chi-square, Fisher exact probability test) will be used to test differences among variables depending on their level of measurement. For example, chi-square may be used to test differences among nominal-level demographic variables, *t* tests will be used to test the hypotheses or research questions about differences between two groups, and ANOVA will be used to test differences among groups when there are multiple comparisons.

Null hypothesis tests of the relationships between variables assume that there is no relationship between the variables. Thus when a researcher rejects this type of null hypothesis, the conclusion is that the variables are in fact related. Suppose a researcher is interested in the relationship between the age of patients and the length of time it takes them to recover from surgery. As with other statistics discussed, the researcher would design a study to collect the appropriate data and then analyze the data using measures of association. In this example, age and length of time until recovery would be considered interval level measurements. The researcher would use a test called the Pearson correlation coefficient, Pearson *r*, or Pearson product moment correlation coefficient. Once the Pearson *r* is calculated, the researcher would consult the distribution for this test to determine whether the value obtained is likely to have occurred by chance. Again, the research reports both the value of the correlation and its probability of occurring by chance.

Correlation coefficients can range in value from −1.0 to +1.0 and also can be zero. A zero coefficient means that there is no relationship between the variables. *A perfect positive correlation* is indicated by a +1.0 coefficient, and a *perfect negative correlation* is indicated by a −1.0 coefficient. We can illustrate the meaning of these coefficients by using the example from the previous paragraph. If there were no relationship between the age of the patient and the time required for the patient to recover from surgery, the researcher would find a correlation of zero. However, if the correlation was +1.0, it would mean that the older the patient, the longer the recovery time. A negative coefficient would imply that the younger the patient, the longer the recovery time.

Of course, relationships are rarely perfect. The magnitude of the relationship is indicated by how close the correlation comes to the absolute value of 1. Thus a correlation of −.76 is just as strong as a correlation of +.76, but the direction of the relationship is opposite. In addition, a correlation of .76 is stronger than a correlation of .32. When a researcher tests hypotheses about the relationships between two variables, the test considers whether the magnitude of the correlation is large enough not to have occurred by chance. This is the meaning of the probability value or the *p* value reported with correlation coefficients. As with other statistical tests of significance, the larger the sample, the greater the likelihood of finding a significant correlation. Therefore researchers also report the *df* associated with the test performed.

Nominal and ordinal data also can be tested for relationships by nonparametric statistics. When two variables being tested have only two levels (e.g., male/female; yes/no), the *phi coefficient* can be used to test relationships. When the researcher is interested in the relationship between a nominal variable and an interval variable, the *point-biserial correlation* is used. *Spearman rho* is used to determine the degree of association between two sets of ranks, as is *Kendall's tau*. All of these correlation coefficients may range in value from −1.0 to +1.0.

EVIDENCE-BASED PRACTICE TIP

Tests of relationship are usually associated with nonexperimental designs that provide Level IV evidence. Establishing a strong statistically significant relationship between variables often lends support for replicating the study to increase the consistency of the findings and provide a foundation for developing an intervention study.

Advanced Statistics

Nurse researchers are often interested in health problems that are very complex and require that we analyze many different variables at once using advanced statistical procedures called **multivariate statistics**. Computer software has made the use of multivariate statistics quite accessible. When researchers are interested in understanding more about a problem than just the relationship between two variables, they often use a technique called **multiple regression**, which measures the relationship between one interval level dependent variable and several independent variables (IVs). Multiple regression is the expansion of correlation to include more than two variables, and it is used when the researcher wants to determine what variables contribute to the explanation of the DV and to what degree. For example, a researcher may be interested in determining what factors help women decide to breastfeed their infants. A number of variables, such as the mother's age, previous experience with breastfeeding, number of other children, and knowledge of the advantages of breastfeeding, may be measured and analyzed to see whether they separately and together predict the duration of breastfeeding. Such a study would require the use of multiple regression.

Another advanced technique often used in nursing research is **factor analysis**. There are two types of factor analysis: exploratory and confirmatory factor analysis. Exploratory factor analysis is used to reduce a set of data so that it may be easily described and used. It is also used in the early phases of instrument development and theory development. Factor analysis is used to determine whether a scale actually measured the concepts that it is intended to measure. Confirmatory factor analysis resembles structural equation modeling and is used in instrument development to examine construct validity and reliability and to compare factor structures across groups (Plichta & Kelvin, 2013).

Many studies use statistical modeling procedures to answer research questions. Causal modeling is used most often when researchers want to test hypotheses and theoretically derived relationships. *Path analysis, structured equation modeling (SEM), and linear structural relations analysis (LISREL)* are different types of modeling procedures used in nursing research.

Many other statistical techniques are available for nurse researchers. It is beyond the scope of this chapter to review all statistical analyses available. You should consider consulting statistical texts or websites as you sort through the evidence reported in studies that are important to your clinical practice.

⟫ APPRAISAL FOR EVIDENCE-BASED PRACTICE
DESCRIPTIVE AND INFERENTIAL STATISTICS

Nurses are challenged to understand the results of studies that use sophisticated statistical procedures. Understanding the principles that guide statistical analysis is the first step in this process. Statistics are used to describe the samples of studies and to test for hypothesized differences or associations in the sample. Knowing the characteristics of the sample of a study allows you to determine whether the results are potentially useful for your patients. For example, if a study sample was primarily White with a mean age of 42 years (SD 2.5), the findings may not be applicable if your patients are mostly older adults and African American. Cultural, demographic, or clinical factors of an older adult population of a different ethnic group may contribute to different results. Thus understanding the descriptive statistics of a study will assist you in determining the applicability of findings to your practice setting.

Statistics are also used to test hypotheses. Inferential statistics used to analyze data and the associated statistical significance level (p values) indicate the likelihood that the association or difference found in a study is caused by chance or a true difference among groups. The closer the p value is to zero, the less likely the association or difference of a study is a result of chance. Thus inferential statistics provide an objective way to determine whether the results of the study are likely to be a true representation of reality. However, it is still important for you to judge the clinical significance of the findings. Was there a big enough effect (difference between the experimental and control groups) to warrant changing current practice?

CRITICAL APPRAISAL CRITERIA

Descriptive and Inferential Statistics

1. Were appropriate descriptive statistics used?
2. Which level of measurement was used to measure each of the major variables?
3. Is the sample size large enough to prevent one extreme score from affecting the summary statistics used?
4. Which descriptive statistics are reported?
5. Were these descriptive statistics appropriate to the level of measurement for each variable?
6. Are there appropriate summary statistics for each major variable (e.g., demographic variables) and any other relevant data?
7. Does the hypothesis indicate that the researcher is interested in testing for differences between groups or in testing for relationships? What is the level of significance?
8. Does the level of measurement permit the use of parametric statistics?
9. Is the size of the sample large enough to permit the use of parametric statistics?
10. Has the researcher provided enough information to decide whether the appropriate statistics were used?
11. Are the statistics used appropriate to the hypothesis, the research question, the method, the sample, and the level of measurement?
12. Are the results for each of the research questions or hypotheses presented clearly and appropriately?
13. If tables and graphs are used, do they agree with the text and extend it, or do they merely repeat it?
14. Are the results understandable?
15. Is a distinction made between clinical significance and statistical significance? How is it made?

EVIDENCE-BASED PRACTICE TIP

A basic understanding of statistics will improve your ability to think about the effect of the IV on the DV and related patient outcomes for your patient population and practice setting.

There are a few steps to follow when critiquing the statistics used in studies (see the Critical Appraisal Criteria box). Before a decision can be made as to whether the statistics that were used make sense, it is important to return to the beginning of the research study and review the purpose of the study. Just as the hypotheses or research questions should flow from the purpose of a study, so should the hypotheses or research questions suggest the type of analysis that will follow. The hypotheses or the research questions should indicate the major variables that are expected to be tested and presented in the "Results" section. Both the summary descriptive statistics and the results of the inferential testing of each of the variables should be in the "Results" section with appropriate information.

After reviewing the hypotheses or research questions, you should proceed to the "Methods" section. Next, try to determine the level of measurement for each variable. From this information, it is possible to determine the measures of central tendency and variability that should be used to summarize the data. For example, you would not expect to see a mean used as a summary statistic for the nominal variable of gender. In all likelihood, gender would be reported as a frequency distribution. The means and SD should be provided for measurements performed at the interval level. The sample size is another aspect of the "Methods" section that is important to review when evaluating the researcher's use of descriptive statistics. The sample is usually described using descriptive summary statistics. Remember, the larger the sample, the less chance that one outlying score will affect the summary statistics. It is also important to note whether the researchers indicated that they did a power analysis to estimate the sample size needed to conduct the study.

If tables or graphs are used, they should agree with the information presented in the text. Evaluate whether the tables and graphs are clearly labeled. If the researcher presents grouped frequency data, the groups should be logical and mutually exclusive. The size of the interval in grouped data should not obscure the pattern of the data or create an artificial pattern. Each table and graph should be referred to in the text, but each should add to the text—not merely repeat it.

The following are some simple steps for reading a table:

1. Look at the title of the table and see if it matches the purpose of the table.
2. Review the column headings and assess whether the headings follow logically from the title.
3. Look at the abbreviations used. Are they clear and easy to understand? Are any non-standard abbreviations explained?
4. Evaluate whether the statistics contained in the table are appropriate to the level of measurement for each variable.

After evaluating the descriptive statistics, inferential statistics can then be evaluated. The best place to begin appraising the inferential statistical analysis of a research study is with the hypothesis or research question. If the hypothesis or research question indicates that a relationship will be found, you should expect to find tests of correlation. If the study is experimental or quasi-experimental, the hypothesis or research question would indicate that the author is looking for significant differences between the groups studied, and you would expect to find statistical tests of differences between means that test the effect of the intervention. Then as you read the "Methods" section of the paper, again consider which level of measurement the author has used to measure the important variables. If the level of measurement is interval or ratio, the statistics most likely will be parametric statistics. On the other hand, if the variables are measured at the nominal or ordinal level, the statistics used should be nonparametric. Also consider the size of the sample, and remember that samples must be large enough to permit the assumption of normality. If the sample is quite small (e.g., 5 to 10 subjects), the researcher may have violated the assumptions necessary for inferential statistics to be used. Thus the important question is whether the researcher has provided enough justification to use the statistics presented.

Finally, consider the results as they are presented. There should be enough data presented for each hypothesis or research question studied to determine whether the researcher actually examined each hypothesis or research question. The tables should accurately reflect the procedure performed and be in harmony with the text. For example, the text should not indicate that a test reached statistical significance while the tables indicate that the probability value of the test was above .05. If the researcher has used analyses that are not discussed in the text, you may want to refer to a statistics text or website to decide whether the analysis was appropriate to the hypothesis or research question and the level of measurement.

There are two other aspects of the data analysis section that you should appraise. The results of the study in the text of the article should be clear. In addition, the author should attempt to make a distinction between the clinical and statistical significance of the evidence related to the findings. Some results may be statistically significant, but their clinical importance may be doubtful in terms of applicability for a patient population or clinical setting. If this is so, the author should note it. Alternatively, you may find yourself reading a research study that is elegantly presented, but you come away with a "So what?" feeling. From an evidence-based practice perspective, a significant hypothesis or research question should contribute to improving patient care and clinical outcomes. The important question to ask is "What is the strength and quality of the evidence provided by the findings of this study and their applicability to practice?"

Note that the critical analysis of a research paper's statistical analysis is not done in a vacuum. It is possible to judge the adequacy of the analysis only in relationship to the other important aspects of the paper: the problem, the hypotheses, the research question, the design, the data collection methods, and the sample. Without consideration of these aspects of the research process, the statistics themselves have very little meaning.

KEY POINTS

- Descriptive statistics are a means of describing and organizing data gathered in research.
- The four levels of measurement are nominal, ordinal, interval, and ratio. Each has appropriate descriptive techniques associated with it.
- Measures of central tendency describe the average member of a sample. The mode is the most frequent score, the median is the middle score, and the mean is the arithmetical average of the scores. The mean is the most stable and useful of the measures of central tendency and, combined with the standard deviation, forms the basis for many of the inferential statistics.
- The frequency distribution presents data in tabular or graphic form and allows for the calculation or observations of characteristics of the distribution of the data, including skew symmetry, and modality.
- In nonsymmetrical distributions, the degree and direction of the off-center peak are described in terms of positive or negative skew.
- The range reflects differences between high and low scores.
- The SD is the most stable and useful measure of variability. It is derived from the concept of the normal curve. In the normal curve, sample scores and the means of large numbers of samples group themselves around the midpoint in the distribution, with a fixed percentage of the scores falling within given distances of the mean. This tendency of means to approximate the normal curve is called the *sampling distribution of the means.*
- Inferential statistics are a tool to test hypotheses about populations from sample data.
- Because the sampling distribution of the means follows a normal curve, researchers are able to estimate the probability that a certain sample will have the same properties as the total population of interest. Sampling distributions provide the basis for all inferential statistics.
- Inferential statistics allow researchers to estimate population parameters and to test hypotheses. The use of these statistics allows researchers to make objective decisions about the outcome of the study. Such decisions are based on the rejection or acceptance of the null hypothesis, which states that there is no relationship between the variables.
- If the null hypothesis is accepted, this result indicates that the findings are likely to have occurred by chance. If the null hypothesis is rejected, the researcher accepts the scientific hypothesis that a relationship exists between the variables that is unlikely to have been found by chance.
- Statistical hypothesis testing is subject to two types of errors: type I and type II.
- A type I error occurs when the researcher rejects a null hypothesis that is actually true.
- A type II error occurs when the researcher accepts a null hypothesis that is actually false.
- The researcher controls the risk for making a type I error by setting the alpha level, or level of significance; however, reducing the risk for a type I error by reducing the level of significance increases the risk for making a type II error.

- The results of statistical tests are reported to be significant or nonsignificant. Statistically significant results are those whose probability of occurring is less than .05 or .01, depending on the level of significance set by the researcher.
- Commonly used parametric and nonparametric statistical tests include those that test for differences between means, such as the *t* test and ANOVA, and those that test for differences in proportions, such as the chi-square test.
- Tests that examine data for the presence of relationships include the Pearson *r*, the sign test, the Wilcoxon matched pairs, the signed rank test, and multiple regression.
- The most important aspect of critiquing statistical analyses is the relationship of the statistics employed to the problem, design, and method used in the study. Clues to the appropriate statistical test to be used by the researcher should stem from the researcher's hypotheses. The reader also should determine whether all of the hypotheses have been presented in the paper.
- A basic understanding of statistics will improve your ability to think about the level of evidence provided by the study design and findings and their relevance to patient outcomes for your patient population and practice setting.

CLINICAL JUDGMENT CHALLENGES

- When reading a research study, what is the significance of applying findings if a nurse researcher made a type I error in statistical inference?
- What is the relationship between the level of measurement a researcher uses and the choice of statistics used? As you read a research study, identify the statistics, level of measurement, and the associated level of evidence provided by the design.
- When reviewing a study, you find that the sample size provided does not seem adequate. Before you make this final decision, think about how the design type (e.g., pilot study, intervention study), data collection methods, number of variables, and sensitivity of the data collection instruments can affect your decision.
- **IPE** When your team finishes critically appraising a research study, the team members responsible for the critique report that the findings are not statistically significant. Consider how these findings are or are not applicable to your practice.

REFERENCES

De la Fuente Coria, M. C., Cruz-Cobo, C., & Santi-Cano, M. J. (2020). Effectiveness of a primary care nurse delivered educational intervention for patients with type 2 diabetes mellitus in promoting metabolic control and compliance with long-term therapeutic targets: Randomized controlled trial. *International Journal of Nursing Studies, 101*, 1–8. https://doi.org/10.1016/j.ijnurstu.2019.103417.

Di Stasio, E., Di Simone, E., Galeti, A., et al. (2020). Stress-related vulnerability and usefulness of healthcare education in Parkinson's disease: The perception of a group of family caregivers, a cross-sectional study. *Applied Nursing Research, 51*, 1–5. https://doi.org/10.1016/j.apnr.2019.151186.

Flanders, S., Hampton, D., Missi, P., Ipsan, C., & Gruebbel, C. (2020). Effectiveness of a staff resilience program in a pediatric intensive care unit. *Journal of Pediatric Nursing, 50*, 1–4. https://doi.org/10.1016/j.pedn.2019.10.007.

Plichta, S. B., & Kelvin, E. (2013). *Munro's statistical methods for health care research* (6th ed). Philadelphia: Wolters Kluwer/Lippincott Williams & Wilkins.

Go to Evolve at **http://evolve.elsevier.com/LoBiondo/** for review questions, appraisal exercises, and additional research articles for practice in reviewing and appraisal.

17

Understanding Research Findings

Brennan Parmelee Streck, Geri LoBiondo-Wood

Go to Evolve at **http://evolve.elsevier.com/LoBiondo/** for review questions.

LEARNING OUTCOMES

After reading this chapter, you should be able to do the following:

- Discuss the difference between the "Results" and "Discussion" sections of a study.
- Determine whether the findings are objectively discussed.
- Describe how tables and figures are used in a research report.
- List the criteria of a meaningful table.
- Identify the purpose and components of the "Discussion" section of a study.

- Discuss the importance of including generalizability and limitations of a study in the report.
- Determine the purpose of including recommendations in the study report.
- Discuss how the strength, quality, and consistency of evidence provided by the findings are related to a study's results, limitations, generalizability, and applicability to practice.

KEY TERMS

confidence interval   generalizability   limitations   recommendations
findings

The ultimate goal of nursing research is to develop knowledge that advances evidence-based nursing practice and quality, cost-effective, and satisfying patient care. From a clinical perspective, highly important components of a study are: analysis, interpretation, discussion, and generalizability of the results. After analysis of the data, the researcher puts the final pieces of the jigsaw puzzle together to view the total research study with a critical eye. This process is analogous to evaluation, the last step in the nursing process. You may view these last steps as relatively easier for the investigator, but it is here that a most critical and creative process comes to the forefront. In the final sections of the report, after the statistical procedures have been applied, the researcher relates the findings to the research question or hypotheses, theoretical framework, literature review, methods, and analyses. The researcher reviews the findings for any potential bias and makes decisions about application of the findings to future research and/or practice.

The final sections of published studies are generally titled "Results" and "Discussion." Other topics include the following:

- Conclusions
- Limitations of the study
- Recommendations
- Implications for future research and nursing practice may be addressed separately or included in the "Results" or "Discussion" sections

The presentation format is a function of the author's and the journal's styles. The final sections will integrate all aspects of the research process and then discuss, interpret, and identify limitations, bias threats related to internal and external validity, and generalizability, thereby advancing evidence-based practice. The process that you and the investigator will use to assess the results of a study is depicted in the Critical Thinking Decision Path. The goal of this chapter is to introduce the purpose and content of the final sections of a research study, where data are presented, interpreted, discussed, and generalized.

FINDINGS

The **findings** of a study are the results, conclusions, interpretations, recommendations, and implications for future research and practice, which are addressed by separating the presentation into two major areas. These two areas are the results and the discussion of the results. The "Results" section focuses on the results or statistical findings of a study, and the "Discussion" section focuses on the remaining topics. For both sections, the rule applies—as it does to all other sections of a report—that the content must be presented clearly, concisely, and logically.

> **EVIDENCE-BASED PRACTICE TIP**
>
> Evidence-based practice is an active process that requires you to consider how, and if, research findings are applicable to your patient population and practice setting.

Results

The "Results" section is the data-bound section of the article; it is where the quantitative data or numbers generated by the descriptive and inferential statistical tests are presented. In reports of qualitative studies, the "Results" section includes non-numerical findings presented in narrative fashion; this is because the study was designed to capture non-numerical data (e.g., Hanna et al., 2020). Other headings that may be used for the results section are "Statistical Analyses," "Data Analysis," or "Analysis." The results of the data analysis set the stage for the "Interpretation" or "Discussion" and the "Limitations" sections that follow the results. The "Results" section should sequentially present and reflect analysis of each research question and/or hypothesis tested. The tests used to analyze the data should be identified. If the exact test that was used is not explicitly stated, the values obtained should be noted. The researcher does this by providing the numerical values of the statistics and stating the specific test value and probability level achieved (see Chapter 16). **Examples** ➤ of these statistical results can be found in Table 17.1. The numbers are important, but there is much more to the research process than the numbers. They are one piece of the whole. Chapter 16 conceptually presents the meanings of the numbers found in studies. Whether you only superficially understand statistics or have an in-depth knowledge of statistics, it should be apparent that the results are clearly stated, and the presence or lack of statistically significant results should be noted.

TABLE 17.1	**Examples of Reported Statistical Results**
Statistical Test	**Examples of Reported Results**
Mean	$m = 118.28$
Standard deviation	$SD = 62.5$, or given in parenthesis following the mean (± 62.5)
Pearson correlation	$r = .49$, $P < .01$
Analysis of variance	$F = 3.59$, $df = 2, 48$, $P < .05$
t test	$t = 2.65$, $P < .01$
Chi-square	$x^2 = 2.52$, $df = 1$, $P < .05$

CRITICAL THINKING DECISION PATH

Assessing Study Results

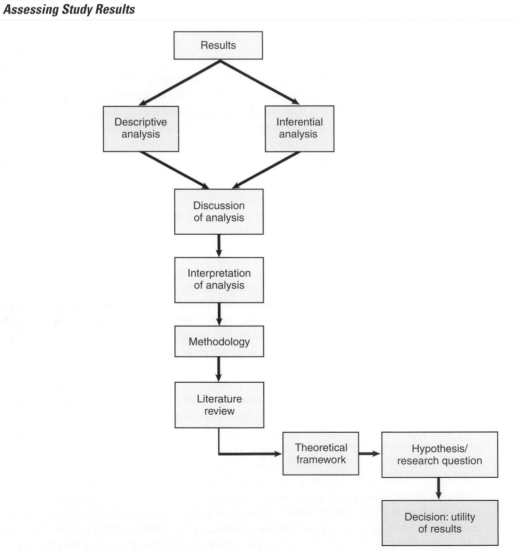

At times, the researchers will begin the "Results" or "Data Analysis" section by identifying the name of the statistical software program they used to analyze the data, although this is usually found in the "Methods" section. This is not a statistical test but a computer program specifically designed to analyze a variety of statistical tests. **Example:** ➤ De la Fuente Coria and colleagues (2020) state that, "For the statistical analysis, the IBM *SPSS* (version 24.0) program was used" (see Chapter 16). Information on the statistical tests used is presented after this information.

The researcher will present the data for all of the hypotheses tested or research questions (e.g., whether the hypotheses or research questions were accepted, rejected, supported, or partially supported). If the data supported the hypotheses or research questions, you may be tempted to assume that the hypotheses or research questions were *proven;* however, this is not true. It only means that the hypotheses or research questions were supported by the findings. The results suggest that the relationships or differences tested, derived from the theoretical framework, were statistically significant and probably logical for that study's sample. You may think that if a study's results are not supported statistically **or are only partially supported**, the study is irrelevant or possibly should not have been published, but this also is not true. If the data are not supported, you should not expect the researcher to bury the work in a file. It is as important for you and the researcher to review and understand studies where the hypotheses or research questions are not supported by the study findings. Information obtained from these studies is often as useful as data obtained from studies with supported hypotheses and research questions.

Studies that have findings that do not support one or more hypotheses or research questions can be used to suggest limitations (issues with the study's validity, bias, or study weaknesses) of particular aspects of a study's design and procedures. Findings from studies with data that do not support the hypotheses or research questions may suggest that current modes of practice or current theory may not be supported by research evidence and therefore must be reexamined, researched further, and not used at this time to support practice changes. Data help generate new knowledge and evidence and prevent knowledge stagnation. Generally, the results are interpreted in a separate section of the report. At times, you may find that the "Results" section contains the results and the researcher's interpretations, which are generally found in the "Discussion" section. Integrating the results with the discussion is the author's or journal editor's decision. Both sections may be integrated when a study contains several segments that may be viewed as fairly separate sub-problems of a major overall problem.

The investigator should also demonstrate objectivity in the presentation of the results. The investigators would be accused of lacking objectivity if they state the results in the following manner: "The results were not surprising as we found that the mean scores were significantly different in the comparison group, as we expected." Opinions or subjective statements about the data are therefore avoided in the "Results" section. Box 17.1 provides examples of objectively stated results. As you appraise a study, it is important to consider the following points when reading the "Results" section:

- Investigators responded objectively to the results in the presentation of the findings.
- Investigators interpreted the evidence provided by the results, with a careful reflection on all aspects of the study that preceded the results. Data presented are summarized. A

BOX 17.1 Examples of Results Section

- "With regard to the achievement of therapeutic objectives (Table 17.3), attaining the glycated hemoglobin target (<7%) was statistically higher after 24 months in the intervention group: 35.2% vs 24.7%, $p < 0.003$" (De la Fuente Coria et al., 2020).
- "RN turnover was reduced during the implementation year of the staff resilience program by 6%, although the decrease in turnover was not statistically significant ($p = .22$) (Flanders et al., 2020).

---

large amount of data are generated, but only the critical summary numbers for each test are presented. Examples of summarized demographic data are the means and standard deviations for age, education, and income. Including all data is too cumbersome. The results should be viewed as a summary.

- Reduction of data is provided in the text and through the use of tables and figures. Tables and figures facilitate the presentation of large amounts of data.
- Results for the descriptive and inferential statistics for each hypothesis or research question are presented. No data are omitted, even if they are not significant. Untoward events during the course of the study should be reported.

In their study, De la Fuente Corea and colleagues (2020; see Appendix B) developed tables to present the results visually. Table 17.2 provides a portion of the descriptive results about the subjects' demographics. Table 17.3 provides a portion of the compliance with study targets. Tables allow researchers to provide a more visually thorough explanation and discussion of the results. If tables and figures are used, they must be concise. Although the article's text is the major mode of communicating the results, the tables and figures serve a supplementary but independent role. The role of tables and figures is to report results with some detail what the investigator does not explore in the text. This does not mean that tables and figures should not be mentioned in the text. The amount of detail that an author uses in the text to describe the specific tabled data varies according to the needs of the author. A good table is one that meets the following criteria:

- Supplements and economizes the text
- Has precise titles and headings
- Does not repeat the text

TABLE 17.2 Baseline Data for Intervention and Control Groups

Variables	TG $n = 236$	IG $n = 97$	CG $n = 139$	P
Age (years)	65.1 ± 9.5	64.5 ± 9.6	65.5 ± 9.5	0.434
Males %(n)	54.2 (128)	54.6 (53)	54.0 (75)	1.000
Diabetes (years)	7.6 ± 4.1	8.8 ± 4.4	$6,7 \pm 3,6$	0.000[a]
BMI (kg/m^2)	30.8 ± 4.3	31.4 ± 4.5	29.3 ± 3.6	0.022
SBP (mm Hg)	135.91 ± 17.28	133.47 ± 16.79	138.22 ± 17.50	0.112
DBP (mm Hg)	77.19 ± 10.20	76.79 ± 9.10	77.57 ± 11.14	0.112

[a] Mann-Whitney U test.

BMI, Body mass index at beginning of study; *SBP,* systolic blood pressure at beginning of study; *DBP,* diastolic blood pressure at beginning of study; *TG,* total group; *IG,* intervention group; *CG,* control group.

From De la Fuente Coria, M., Cruz-Cobo, C., & Santi-Cano, M. (2020). Effectiveness of a primary care nurse delivered educational intervention for patients with type 2 diabetes mellitus in promoting metabolic control and compliance with long-term therapeutic targets: Randomised controlled trial. *International Journal of Nursing Studies, 101,* 103417.

TABLE 17.3	Compliance With Targets at 12 and 24 Months					
Variables %(n)	Total n = 236	IG n = 97	p within the IG[a]	CG n = 139	p within the CG[a]	p IG/CG
FBG baseline	41.6 (77)	38.2 (29)		44.0 (48)		0.452
12 months	48.3 (98)	53.4 (47)	0.031	44.3 (51)	1.000	0.206
24 months	51.5 (103)	25.5 (51)	0.008	26.0 (52)	0.424	0.203
Hb A_{1c} baseline	44.6 (75)	40.7 (33)		48.3 (42)		0.354
12 months	53.3 (104)	59.1 (55)	0.011	48.0 (49)	0.481	0.151
24 months	59.9 (109)	35.2 (64)	0.001	24.7 (45)	0.383	0.003

[a] McNemar.

IG, Intervention group; *CG,* control group; *BMI,* body mass index; *BP,* blood pressure; *FBG,* fasting blood glucose; *HbA$_{1c}$,* glycated hemoglobin.
From De la Fuente Coria, M., Cruz-Cobo, C., & Santi-Cano, M. (2020). Effectiveness of a primary care nurse delivered educational intervention for patients with type 2 diabetes mellitus in promoting metabolic control and compliance with long-term therapeutic targets: Randomised controlled trial. *International Journal of Nursing Studies, 101,* 103417.

Tables may be found in the study's appendices or embedded in the text. Each of these tables helps to economize and supplement the text clearly, with precise data that help you visualize the variables quickly and assess the results.

EVIDENCE-BASED PRACTICE TIP

As you reflect on the results of a study, think about how the results fit with previous research on the topic and the strength and quality of available evidence on which to base clinical practice decisions.

Discussion

In this section, the investigator interprets and discusses the study's results. The investigator makes the data come alive and gives meaning to and provides interpretations for the numbers in quantitative studies or the concepts in qualitative studies. This "Discussion" section contains a discussion of the findings, the study's limitations, and recommendations for practice, education, and future research. At times these topics are separated as stand-alone sections of the research report, or they may be integrated under the title of "Discussion." You may ask where the investigator extracted the meaning that is applied in this section. If the researcher does the job properly, you will find a return to the beginning of the study. The researcher returns to the earlier points in the study where the purpose, objective, and research question and/or a hypothesis was identified, and independent and dependent variables were linked on the basis of a theoretical framework and literature review (see Chapters 3 and 4). It is in this section that the researcher discusses:

- Significant and nonsignificant findings
- Strengths of the study design, methods (e.g., sampling strategy, instruments, intervention fidelity), and data analysis
- Limitations or weaknesses (threats to internal or external validity) of a study in light of the design, sample, instruments, data collection procedures, and fidelity
- How the theoretical framework was supported or not supported
- How the data may suggest additional or previously unrealized findings
- Strength and quality of the evidence provided by the study and its findings interpreted in relation to its applicability to practice, education, and future research

Even if the data are supported, this is not the final word. Statistical significance is not the endpoint of a researcher's thinking; statistically significant p values may not be necessarily indicative of research breakthroughs. It is important to think beyond statistical significance to clinical significance. This means that statistical significance for study findings do not always indicate that the results of a study are clinically significant. A key step in the evaluation process is the ability to critically analyze beyond the test of significance by assessing a research study's applicability to practice. Chapters 19 to 21 review the methods used to analyze the usefulness and applicability of research findings. Focal points of the nursing and health care literature is discussion of clinical significance, evidence-based practice, and quality improvement (Titler, 2012). As indicated throughout this text, many important pieces in the research puzzle must fit together for a study to be evaluated as a well-done study that has scientific rigor. The evidence generated by a study's findings are appraised to validate current practice or support the need for a change in practice (see Chapter 20). Results of unsupported hypotheses or research questions do not require the investigator to go on a fault-finding tour of each piece of the study—this can become an overdone process. All research studies have weaknesses and strengths. The final discussion is an attempt to identify the strengths and weaknesses as well as the potential bias in the study.

HELPFUL HINT

A well-written "Results" section is systematic, logical, concise, and drawn from all of the analyzed data. The writing in the "Results" section should allow the data to reflect the testing of the research questions and hypotheses. The length of this section depends on the scope and breadth of the analysis.

Researchers and appraisers should accept statistical significance with prudence. Statistically significant findings are not the sole means of establishing a study's merit. Remember that accepting statistical significance means accepting that the sample mean and its characteristics are the same as the population mean and characteristics (see Chapter 12). Another method to assess the merit of a study and determine whether the findings from one study can be generalized is to calculate a **confidence interval**. A confidence interval quantifies the uncertainty of a statistic or the probable value range within which a population parameter is expected to lie (see Chapter 19). The confidence interval provides the level of confidence (%) that a range of values contains the true population mean. The process used to calculate a confidence interval is beyond the scope of this text, but references are provided for further explanation (Altman, 2005; Altman et al., 2005; Kline, 2004). Other aspects, such as the sample, instruments, data collection methods, and fidelity, must also be considered.

Whether the results are or are not statistically supported, in this section the researcher returns to the conceptual/theoretical framework and analyzes each step of the research process to accomplish a discussion of the following issues:

- What are the possible or actual problems in the study?
- Whether hypotheses or research questions are supported or not supported, the researcher is obliged to review the study's processes.
- Was the theoretical thinking consistent with the hypotheses/research questions? (See Chapters 3 and 4.)
- Was the correct design chosen? (See Chapters 9 and 10.)

- Was the sample size adequate in terms of sampling methods (see Chapter 12)? Were inclusion and exclusion criteria clearly delineated?
- Did any bias arise during the course of the study (i.e., threats to internal and external validity)? (See Chapter 8.)
- Was data collection consistent, and did it demonstrate fidelity? (See Chapter 14.)
- Were the instruments sensitive to what was being tested, and were they reliable and valid? (See Chapters 14 and 15.)
- Were the analysis choices appropriate? (See Chapter 16.)

The purpose of this section is not to show humility or one's technical competence but rather to enable you to judge the validity of the interpretations drawn from the data and the general worth of the study. In this section, the researcher ties together all loose ends of the study and returns to the beginning to assess if the findings support, extend, or counter the theoretical framework of the study. It is from this point that you can begin to think about clinical relevance, the need for replication, or the germination of an idea for further research. The researcher also includes generalizability and recommendations for future research as well as a summary or a conclusion.

Generalizations (**generalizability**) are inferences that the data are representative of similar phenomena in a population beyond the study's sample. Rarely, if ever, can the findings of one study be the basis of a recommendation for action to implement a practice change. For example, a study by Haber and colleagues (2020) aimed to determine whether Nurse Family Partnership (NFP) nurse home visitors serving one geographical area who received oral health education increased their oral health knowledge and practice behaviors contributing to positive oral health outcomes for a racially/ethnically diverse Medicaid population sample of high-risk first-time pregnant women and their infants through 2 years of age. Although they report a significant change in oral health knowledge and health practice changes for nurse home visitors ($n = 10$) and mothers ($n = 27$), the researchers identified that the small sample size, lack of a client comparison group, and only one geographical area preclude the ability to generalize beyond this sample. Beware of research studies that may overgeneralize. Generalizations that draw conclusions and make inferences for a specific group in a particular situation and at a particular time are appropriate. Another **example** ➤ of such a limitation is drawn from the study conducted by De la Fuente Coria and colleagues (2020; Appendix B). The researchers appropriately noted the following:

> *Finally, the sample came from a single health centre. Therefore, the results cannot be generalized for the entire population.*

This type of statement is important for consumers of research. It helps guide our thinking in terms of a study's clinical relevance and also suggests areas for research. One study does not provide all of the answers, nor should it. In fact, the risk versus the benefit of the potential change in practice must be considered in terms of the strength and quality of the evidence (see Chapter 19). The greater the risk involved in making a change in practice, the stronger the evidence must be to justify implementing a practice change. The final steps of evaluation are critical links to the refinement of practice and the generation of future research. Evaluation of research, like evaluation of the nursing process, is not the last link in the chain but a connection between the strength of the evidence that may serve to improve patient care, inform clinical decision making, and support an evidence-based practice.

BOX 17.2 Examples of Research Recommendations and Practice Implications

Research Recommendations

- "More interviews with nonadherent people would be beneficial to gain a better understanding of nonadherence perspectives. Although the prevalence of MI is higher among men and it was convenient to recruit them, more women should be involved in this research" (Hanna et al., 2020).
- "Future research needs to be focused around using standardized tools to measure CF, compassion satisfaction, and resilience as well as specific interventions for pediatric intensive care nurses. Longitudinal studies would be helpful to determine the sustainability of the results over time" (Flanders et al., 2020).

Practice Implications

- "Education in diabetes can optimise glycemic control in patients, and ongoing diabetes education intervention can achieve favorable long-term results. Thus innovative strategies such as educational reinforcements and family involvement could increase glycemic control" (De la Fuente Coria et al., 2020).
- "Health care organizations should focus on providing resilience building interventions in high stress environments like the PICU, to promote compassion satisfaction and decrease CF [compassion fatigue] among nurses what work in the environments" (Flanders et al., 2020).

IPE HIGHLIGHT

Your team should remember the saying that a good study is one that raises more questions than it answers. So your team should not view a researcher's review of a study's limitations and recommendations for future research as evidence of the researcher's lack of research skills. Rather, it reflects the next steps in building a strong body of evidence.

The final element that the investigator integrates into the "Discussion" section is the recommendations. The **recommendations** are the investigator's suggestions for the study's application to practice, theory, and further research. This requires the investigator to reflect on the following questions:

- What contribution does this study make to clinical practice and future research?
- What are the strengths, quality, and consistency of the evidence provided by the findings?
- Does the evidence provided in the findings validate current practice or support the need for change in practice?

Box 17.2 provides **examples** ➤ of recommendations for future research and implications for nursing practice. This evaluation places the study into the realm of what is known and what must be known before being used. Nursing knowledge and evidence-based practice have grown tremendously over the last century through the efforts of many nurse researchers and scholars.

⟫ APPRAISAL FOR EVIDENCE-BASED PRACTICE
RESEARCH FINDINGS

The "Results" and the "Discussion" sections are the researcher's opportunity to examine the logic of the hypothesis (or hypotheses) or research question(s) posed, the theoretical framework, the methods, and the analysis (see the Critical Appraisal Criteria box). This final section requires as much logic, conciseness, and specificity as employed in the preceding steps of the research process. You should be able to identify statements of the type of analysis that was used and whether the data statistically supported the hypothesis or research question. These statements should be straightforward and should not reflect bias (see Tables 17.2 and 17.3). Auxiliary data or serendipitous findings also may be presented. If such auxiliary findings are presented, they should be as dispassionately presented as the hypothesis and research question data.

CRITICAL APPRAISAL CRITERIA
Research Findings

1. Are the results of each of the hypotheses or research questions presented?
2. Is the information regarding the results concisely and sequentially presented?
3. Are the tests that were used to analyze the data presented?
4. Are the results presented objectively?
5. If tables or figures are used, do they meet the following standards?
   a. They supplement and economize the text.
   b. They have precise titles and headings.
   c. They are not repetitious of the text.
6. Are the results interpreted in light of the hypotheses, research questions, theoretical framework, and all other steps that preceded the results?
7. If the hypotheses or research questions are supported, does the investigator provide a discussion of how the theoretical framework was supported?
8. How does the investigator attempt to identify the study's weaknesses (i.e., threats to internal and external validity) and strengths as well as suggest possible solutions for the research area?
9. Does the researcher discuss the study's clinical relevance?
10. Are any generalizations made and, if so, are they within the scope of the findings or beyond the findings?
11. Are any recommendations for future research stated or implied?
12. What is the study's strength of evidence?

The statistical test(s) used should also be noted. The numerical value of the obtained data should also be presented (see Tables 17.1 to 17.3). The presentation of the tests, the numerical values found, and the statements of support or nonsupport should be clear, concise, and systematically reported. For illustrative purposes that facilitate readability, the researcher should present extensive findings in tables. If the findings were not supported, you should—as the researcher did—attempt to identify, without finding fault, possible methodological problems (e.g., sample too small to detect a treatment effect).

From a consumer perspective, the "Discussion" section is very important for determining the potential application to practice. The "Discussion" section should interpret the study's data for future research and implications for practice, including its strength, quality, gaps, limitations, and conclusions of the study. Statements reflecting the underlying theory are necessary, whether or not the hypotheses or research questions were supported. Included in this discussion are the implications for practice. This discussion should reflect each step of the research process and potential threats to internal validity or bias and external validity or generalizability.

This discussion can help you begin to rethink clinical practice, provoke discussion in clinical settings (see Chapters 19 and 20), and find similar studies that may support or refute the phenomena being studied to more fully understand the problem. It is important to relate the current study's findings to previous work on the same topic, so that knowledge can build.

One study alone does not lead to a practice change. Evidence-based practice and quality improvement require you to critically read and understand each study—that is, the quality of the study, the strength of the evidence generated by the findings and its consistency with other studies in the area, and the number of studies that were conducted in the area. This assessment along with the active use of clinical judgment and patient preference leads to evidence-based practice.

KEY POINTS

- The analysis of the findings is the final step of a study. It is in this section that the results will be presented in a straightforward manner.
- All results should be reported whether or not they support the hypothesis. Tables and figures may be used to illustrate and condense data for presentation.
- Once the results are reported, the researcher interprets the results. In this presentation, usually titled "Discussion," readers should be able to identify the key topics being discussed. The key topics, which include an interpretation of the results, are the limitations, generalizations, implications, and recommendations for future research.
- The researcher draws together the theoretical framework and makes interpretations based on the findings and theory in the section on the interpretation of the results. Both statistically supported and unsupported results should be interpreted. If the results are not supported, the researcher should discuss the results, reflecting on the theory and the possible problems with the methods, procedures, design, and analysis.
- The researcher should present the study's limitations or weaknesses. This presentation is important because it affects the study's generalizability. The generalizations or inferences about similar findings in other samples also are presented in light of the findings.
- Be alert for sweeping claims or overgeneralizations. An overextension of the data can alert the consumer to possible researcher bias.
- The recommendations provide the consumer with suggestions regarding the study's application to practice, theory, and future research. These recommendations provide a final perspective on the utility of the investigation.
- The strength, quality, and consistency of the evidence provided by the findings are related to the study's limitations, generalizability, and applicability to practice.

CLINICAL JUDGMENT CHALLENGES

- Do you agree or disagree with the statement that "a good study is one that raises more questions than it answers"? Support your perspective with examples.
- As the number of resources such as the Cochrane Library, meta-analysis, systematic reviews, and evidence-based reports in journals grow, why is it necessary to be able to critically read and appraise the studies within the reports yourself? Justify your answer.
- **IPE** Engage your interprofessional team in a debate to defend or refute the following statement. "All results should be reported and interpreted whether or not they support the research question or hypothesis." If all findings are not reported, how would this affect the applicability of findings to your patient population and practice setting?
- How does a clear understanding of a study's discussion of the findings and implications for practice help you rethink your practice?

REFERENCES

Altman, D. G. (2005). Why we need confidence intervals. *World Journal of Surgery, 29*, 554–556.

Altman, D. G., Machin, D., Bryant, T., & Gardener, S. (2005). *Statistics with confidence: Confidence intervals and statistical guidelines* (2nd ed.). London: BMJ Books.

De la Fuente Coria, M., Cruz-Cobo, C., & Santi-Cano, M. (2020). Effectiveness of a primary care nurse delivered educational intervention for patients with type 2 diabetes mellitus in promoting metabolic control and compliance with long-term therapeutic targets: Randomised controlled trial. *International Journal of Nursing Studies, 101*, 103417. https://doi.org/10.1016/j.ijnurstu.2019.103417.

Flanders, S., Hampton, D., Missi, P., Ipsan, C., & Gruebbel, C. (2020). Effectiveness of a staff resilience program in a pediatric intensive care unit. *Journal of Pediatric Nursing, 50*, 1–4. https://doi.org/10.1016/j.pedn.2019.10.007.

Haber, J., Hartnett, E., Hille, A., & Cipollina, J. (2020). Promoting oral health for mothers and children: A nurse home visitor education program. *Pediatric Nursing, 46*(2), 70–76.

Hanna, A., Yael, E. M., Hadassa, L., Iris, E., Nikolsky, E., Lior, G., Carmit, S., & Liora. (2020). It's up to me with a little support": Adherence after myocardial infarction A qualitative study. *International Journal of Nursing Studies, 101*, 103416 1-10 vol. 101.

Kline, R. B. (2004). *Beyond significance testing: Reforming data analysis methods in behavioral research*. Washington, DC: American Psychological Association.

Titler, M. G. (2012). Nursing science and evidence-based practice. *Western Journal of Nursing Research, 33*(3), 291–295.

Go to Evolve at **http://evolve.elsevier.com/LoBiondo/** for review questions, appraisal exercises, and additional research articles for practice in reviewing and appraisal.

18

Appraising Quantitative Research

Carolynn Spera Bruno

Go to Evolve at **http://evolve.elsevier.com/LoBiondo/** for review questions.

LEARNING OUTCOMES

After reading this chapter, you should be able to do the following:

- Identify the purpose of the critical appraisal process.
- Describe the criteria for each step of the critical appraisal process.
- Describe the strengths and weaknesses of a research report.

- Assess the strength, quality, and consistency of evidence provided by a quantitative research report.
- Discuss applicability of the findings of a research report for evidence-based nursing practice.
- Conduct a critique of a research report.

The critical appraisal and interpretation of the findings of a research article is an acquired skill that is important for nurses to master as they learn to determine the usefulness of the published literature. As we strive to make recommendations to change or support nursing practice, it is important for you to be able to assess the strengths and weaknesses of a research article.

Critical appraisal is an evaluation of the quality, strength, and weaknesses of a study; it is not a "criticism" of the work, per se. It provides a structure for reviewing and evaluating the sections of a research study. This chapter presents critiques of two quantitative studies, a randomized controlled trial (RCT) and a cohort study, according to the critical appraisal criteria shown in Table 18.1. These studies provide Level II and Level IV evidence.

As reinforced throughout each chapter of this book, it is important not only to conduct and read research but to actively use research findings to inform evidence-based practice. As nurse researchers increase the depth (quality) and breadth (quantity) of studies, the data to support evidence-informed decision making regarding applicability of clinical interventions that contribute to quality outcomes are more readily available. This chapter presents critiques of two studies, each of which tests research questions reflecting different quantitative designs. Criteria used to help you judge the relative merit of a research study are found in previous chapters. An abbreviated set of critical appraisal questions presented in Table 18.1 summarize detailed criteria found at the end of each chapter and are used as a critical appraisal guide for the two sample research critiques in this chapter. These critiques are included to illustrate the critical appraisal process for quantitative studies and

TABLE 18.1 Summary of Major Content Sections of a Research Report and Related Critical Appraisal Guidelines

Section	Critical Appraisal Questions to Guide Evaluation
Background and Significance (see Chapters 2 and 3)	Does the background and significance section make it clear why the proposed study was conducted?
Research Question and Hypothesis (see Chapter 2)	1. What research question(s) or hypothesis (or hypotheses) are stated, and are they appropriate to express a relationship (or difference) between an independent and a dependent variable? 2. Has the research question(s) or hypothesis (or hypotheses) been placed in the context of an appropriate theoretical framework? 3. Has the research question(s) or hypothesis (or hypotheses) been substantiated by adequate experiential and scientific background material? 4. Has the purpose, aim(s), or goal(s) of the study been substantiated? 5. Is each research question or hypothesis specific to one relationship so that each can be either supported or not supported? 6. Given the level of evidence suggested by the research question, hypothesis, and design, what is the potential applicability to practice?
Review of the Literature (see Chapters 3 and 4)	1. Does the search strategy include an appropriate and adequate number of databases and other resources to identify key published and unpublished research and theoretical resources? 2. Is there an appropriate theoretical/conceptual framework that guides development of the research study? 3. Are both primary source theoretical and research literature used? 4. What gaps or inconsistencies in knowledge or research does the literature uncover so it builds on earlier studies? 5. Does the review include a summary/critique of the studies that includes the strengths and weakness or limitations of the study? 6. Is the literature review presented in an organized format that flows logically? 7. Is there a synthesis summary that presents the overall strengths and weaknesses and arrives at a logical conclusion that generates hypotheses or research questions?
Methods	
Internal and External Validity (see Chapter 8)	1. What are the controls for the threats to internal validity? Are they appropriate? 2. What are the controls for the threats to external validity? Are they appropriate? 3. What are the sources of bias, and are they dealt with appropriately? 4. How do the threats to internal and external validity affect the strength and quality of evidence? 5. Was the fidelity of the intervention maintained, and if so, how?
Research Design (see Chapters 9 and 10)	1. Which type of design is used in the study? 2. Is the rationale for the design appropriate? 3. Does the design used seem to flow from the proposed research question(s) or hypothesis (or hypotheses), theoretical framework, and literature review? 4. Which types of controls are provided by the design that increase or decrease bias?
Sampling (see Chapter 12)	1. Which type of sampling strategy is used? Is it appropriate for the design? 2. How was the sample selected? Was the strategy used appropriate for the design? 3. Does the sample reflect the population as identified in the research question or hypothesis? 4. Is the sample size appropriate? How is it substantiated? Was a power analysis necessary? 5. To which population may the findings be generalized?
Legal-Ethical Issues (see Chapter 13)	1. How have the rights of subjects been protected? 2. What indications are given that institutional review board approval has been obtained? 3. What evidence is given that informed consent of the subjects has been obtained?

Continued

TABLE 18.1 Summary of Major Content Sections of a Research Report and Related Critical Appraisal Guidelines—cont'd

Section	Critical Appraisal Questions to Guide Evaluation

Data Collection Methods and Procedures (see Chapter 14)	1. Physiological measurement:
	  a. Is a rationale given for why a particular instrument or method was selected? If so, what is it?
	  b. What provision is made for maintaining accuracy of the instrument and its use, if any?
	2. Observation:
	  a. Who did the observing?
	  b. How were the observers trained and supervised to minimize bias?
	  c. Was there an observation guide?
	  d. Was interrater reliability calculated?
	  e. Is there any reason to believe that the presence of observers affected the behavior of the subjects?
	3. Interviews:
	  a. Who were the interviewers? How were they trained and supervised to minimize bias?
	  b. Is there any evidence of interview bias, and if so, what is it? How does it affect the strength and quality of the evidence?
	4. Instruments:
	  a. What is the type and/or format of the instruments (e.g., Likert scale)?
	  b. Are the operational definitions provided by the instruments consistent with the conceptual definition(s)?
	  c. Is the format appropriate for use with this population?
	  d. Which type of bias is possible with self-report instruments?
	5. Available data and records:
	  a. Are the records or data sets used appropriate for the research question(s) or hypothesis (or hypotheses)?
	  b. What sources of bias are possible with use of records or existing data sets?
	6. Overall, how was intervention fidelity maintained?

Reliability and Validity (see Chapter 15)	1. Was an appropriate method used to test the reliability of the instrument(s)? 2. Was the reliability and validity of the instrument(s) adequate? 3. Was the appropriate method(s) used to test the validity of the instrument(s)? 4. Have the strengths and weaknesses related to reliability and validity of the instruments been presented? 5. What kinds of threats to internal and external validity are presented as weaknesses in reliability and/or validity? 6. How do the reliability and/or validity affect the strength and quality of evidence provided by the study findings?

Data Analysis (see Chapter 16)	1. Were the descriptive or inferential statistics appropriate to the level of measurement for each variable?
	2. Are the inferential statistics appropriate for the type of design, research question(s), or hypothesis (or hypotheses)?
	3. If tables or figures are used, do they meet the following standards?
	  a. They supplement and economize the text.
	  b. They have precise titles and headings.
	  c. They do not repeat the text.
	4. Did testing of the research question(s) or hypothesis (or hypotheses) clearly support or not support each research question or hypothesis?

TABLE 18.1   Summary of Major Content Sections of a Research Report and Related Critical Appraisal Guidelines—cont'd

Section	Critical Appraisal Questions to Guide Evaluation
Conclusions, Implications, and Recommendations (see Chapter 17)	1. Are the results of each research question or hypothesis presented objectively? 2. Is the information regarding the results concisely and sequentially presented? 3. If the data are supportive of the hypothesis or research question, does the investigator provide a discussion of how the theoretical framework was supported? 4. How does the investigator attempt to identify the study's weaknesses and limitations (e.g., threats to internal and external validity) and strengths and suggest possible research solutions in future studies? 5. Does the researcher discuss the study's relevance to clinical practice? 6. Are any generalizations made, and if so, are they made within the scope of the findings? 7. Are any recommendations for future research stated or implied?
Applicability to Nursing Practice (see Chapter 17)	1. What are the risks/benefits involved for patients if the findings are applied in practice? 2. What are the costs/benefits of applying the findings of the study? 3. Do the strengths of the study outweigh the weaknesses? 4. What are the strength, quality, and consistency of evidence provided by the study findings? 5. Are the study findings applicable in terms of feasibility? 6. Are the study findings generalizable? 7. Would it be possible to replicate this study in another clinical setting?

the potential applicability of research findings to clinical practice, thereby enhancing the evidence base for nursing practice.

For clarification, you are encouraged to return to earlier chapters for the detailed presentation of each step of the research process, key terms, and the critical appraisal criteria associated with each step of the research process. The criteria and examples in this chapter apply to quantitative studies using experimental and nonexperimental designs.

STYLISTIC CONSIDERATIONS

When you are reading research, it is important to consider the type of journal in which the article is published. Some journals publish articles regarding the conduct, methodology, or results of research studies (e.g., *Nursing Research*). Other journals (e.g., *Journal of Obstetric, Gynecologic, and Neonatal Nursing*) publish clinical, educational, and research articles. An author decides where to submit the manuscript based on the focus of the particular journal and its goodness of fit. Guidelines for publication, also known as "Information for Authors," are journal-specific and provide information regarding style, citations, and formatting. Typically research articles include the following:

- Abstract
- Introduction
- Background and significance
- Literature review (sometimes includes a theoretical framework)
- Methodology
- Results
- Discussion
- Conclusions

Critical appraisal is the process of identifying the methodological rigor of the research and the flaws or omissions that lead the reader to balance the precision of the research findings and evaluate the outcome(s) of the study based on its strengths and limitations. It is a process for objectively verifying that the study is sound and provides consistent, quality evidence that supports applicability to practice. Critical appraisal is the hallmark of promoting a sound evidence base for quality nursing practice.

CRITICAL APPRAISAL OF A QUANTITATIVE RESEARCH STUDY

THE RESEARCH STUDY

The study "Effectiveness of Music Therapy and Progressive Muscle Relaxation in Reducing Stress Before Exams and Improving Academic Performance in Nursing Students: A Randomized Trial," by Gallego-Gomez et al. (2020), published in *Nurse Education Today*, is presented in its entirety and followed by the critique. https://doi.org.proxy.library.nyu.edu/10.1016/j.nedt.2019.104217

Effectiveness of music therapy and progressive muscle relaxation in reducing stress before exams and improving academic performance in Nursing students: A randomized trial

Juana Inés Gallego-Gómez[a], Serafín Balanza[a], Jesús Leal-Llopis[a], Juan Antonio García-Méndez[a], José Oliva-Pérez[a], Javier Doménech-Tortosa[a], María Gómez-Gallego[a], Agustín Javier Simonelli-Muñoz[a]*[1], José Miguel Rivera-Caravaca[ab1]

Abstract

Background: Nursing students experiencing high stress levels before exams could suffer worse academic performance.

Objective: We evaluated an intervention combining Progressive Muscle Relaxation (PMR) and music therapy on the decrease of *before exams* stress and the improvement of academic results.

Design and methods: Randomized controlled trial including students from the Nursing Degree during the first semester of the 2017–2018 academic year. All participants were randomized to the control (CG) or the experimental group (EG). The CG took the exam as usual whereas in the EG, PMR and music therapy were performed before exams. Blood

[a]Faculty of Nursing, Catholic University of Murcia (UCAM), Murcia, Spain
[b]Department of Cardiology, Hospital Clínico Universitario Virgen de la Arrixaca, Instituto Murciano de Investigación Biosanitaria (IMIB-Arrixaca), CIBERCV, Murcia, Spain
*Corresponding author at: Faculty of Nursing, Catholic University of Murcia (UCAM), Campus de Guadalupe s/n, 30107 Murcia, Spain. *E-mail address:* agsimonelli@ucam.edu (A.J. Simonelli-Muñoz).
[1]Joint senior authors

samples were drawn to investigate variations in biochemical parameters. The academic performance was assessed by the score obtained in the "Clinical Nursing" exam.

Results: We included 112 students (75% females, mean age 24.3 ± 6.2 years, 56 students in every group). There were no differences in any parameter during the first measurement. Regarding the second measurement, we observed a reduction in heart rate for the EG and an increase in blood pressure, heart rate, and cortisol for the CG. Indeed, these parameters were significantly higher compared to the EG. The EG had a mean score of 5.07 ± 1.59 in the Clinical Nursing exam, which was significantly higher compared to the CG (4.42 ± 1.58, $p = 0.033$). The proportion of fails in the CG was also higher (62.5% vs. 42.9%, $p = 0.037$).

Conclusion: In this study including students from the Nursing degree, the combination of PMR and music therapy was effective for the control and decrease of stress before exams, and also demonstrated improvements in academic results.

Keywords

Progressive muscle relaxation	Exams
Music therapy	Academic performance
Stress	Nursing student

BACKGROUND

Academic stress, defined as a physiological, emotional, cognitive and behavioral reaction to stimuli, can affect the ability of the students to face the university environment (Dendle et al., 2018; Pozos-Radillo et al., 2018). Indeed, current studies have described high levels of stress in health sciences students such as Nursing, Medicine and Odontology (Crego et al., 2016; Silverstein and Kritz-Silverstein, 2010). Exams and clinical practices, as well as high academic workloads, negative interactions with the personnel and the faculty, financial problems and changes in their surroundings, social activities, feeding and rest habits, are stress factors that are more commonly found in this population (Quinn and Peters, 2017; Shudifat and Al-Husban, 2015; Silva-Sánchez, 2015). In this sense, recent studies have shown a significant relationship between the high levels of academic stress and psycho-physiological manifestations such as problems in concentration, mental blocks, chronic fatigue, somnolence and depression (Pozos-Radillo et al., 2016). Thus, Nursing students experiencing high levels of stress before exams could be incapable for demonstrating their knowledge (Prato and Yucha, 2013), and therefore, their academic performance could be impaired (Dendle et al., 2018).

Some authors consider that Nursing educators could use empirically-proven interventions to reduce stress and improve the abilities of coping (Labrague et al., 2017). In the last years, several studies have investigated the effectiveness of some interventions such as psychoeducational interventions (Labrague et al., 2017; McCarthy et al., 2018), music therapy (Ince and Çevik, 2014; Lee et al., 2016; Shih et al., 2016) and Progressive Muscle Relaxation (PMR) (Hashim and Zainol, 2015; Pal et al., 2014; Prato and Yucha, 2013), to cope with student anxiety or stress before academic exams, tests or evaluations. However, it is still unclear if any of these interventions have a real impact on the stress level of Nursing students.

Given that exams are a natural stressor with the ability to affect health, which can have negative repercussions on memory and test results (Maduka et al., 2015), the aim of this study was to evaluate the effectiveness of a prevention program that combines PMR and music therapy interventions on the decrease of stress during the exam period and the improvement of academic results.

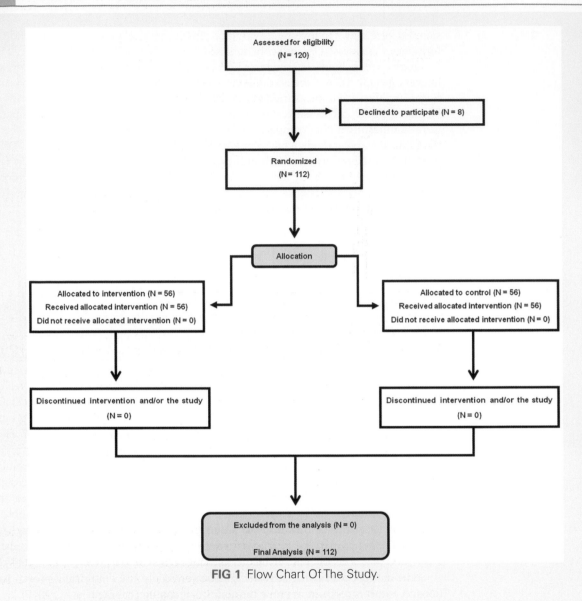

FIG 1 Flow Chart Of The Study.

DESIGN AND METHODS

This is a randomized controlled trial performed in students from the second year of the Nursing Degree that were going to take the Clinical Nursing exam during the first semester of the 2017–2018 academic year (i.e., from October 2017 to February 2018). All the participant students were part of the Nursing Degree from the Catholic University of Murcia.

All the students were considered as there were no specific inclusion or exclusion criteria. However, from the 120 screened students, 8 were excluded, as they did not want to participate in the study. The final sample size was 112 participants (Fig. 1).

Ethical issues

Before starting the study, the students were informed about the purpose of the study and signed an informed consent. This study followed the CONSORT guidelines and was approved by the Ethical Committee from the Catholic University of Murcia. The study was also performed with the ethical standards found in the 1964 Declaration of Helsinki and its later amendments.

Randomization

At inclusion, the participants were randomly assigned to the control group (CG) or the experimental group (EG) by using a simple randomized sampling. A total of 56 students were assigned to the CG, and another 56 to the EG group, with both groups age and sex-matched. The CG took the exam as usual, whereas in the EG, PMR and music therapy interventions were performed before the exam.

Visits, measurements, and experimental intervention

For each participant, two visits were scheduled. The first visit was performed in October 2017, during a non-exam period. The participants attended to this first visit fasted. A blood sample was drawn at 9 a.m., and clinical, sociodemographic and vital signs (heart rate, oxygen saturation, and blood pressure) parameters were recorded. The same procedure was performed in the CG and EG.

The second visit was carried out in February 2018, the same day as the exam. The CG was asked to attend at 9 a.m. (i.e. 1 h before the beginning of the exam) in fasting, and a new blood sample was drawn. The EG attended at 8 a.m. (2 h before the exam), in fasting. For 1 h, the experimental intervention was performed, and then a blood sample was also drawn. Before the exam, participants from both groups had enough time to have breakfast.

The experimental intervention consisted of a session of PMR and music therapy before taking the exam. This intervention was carried out in three classrooms with dimmed illumination, set up with chairs and mattresses for the better performing of the technique. The aim of the technique was to ease the tension and to achieve the relaxation of the main successive muscle groups. During the entire procedure, as well as during the exam, the EG listened to relaxing music. The music was listened using a CD player, without headphones, with an appropriate volume established at 50–60 dB. The intervention was performed by two nurses and a psychologist who had extensive experience with relaxation techniques and music therapy. Once the intervention was finished, a blood sample was drawn. Afterward, the students had breakfast and started the exam.

Analysis of the academic performance

An important part of the experimental intervention was to evaluate if this resulted in an improvement of academic performance. The academic performance was assessed by the score obtained by each student in the exam of the subject "Clinical Nursing." The score was classified as pass (≥ 5) or fail (< 5), with values ranging from 0 to 10.

Statistical analysis

For the randomization process, we used a random number generator using the software C4SDP-MAS v. 2.1 (Freeware: Study Design Pack, Glaxo Wellcome Biometry, S. A.). Participants were randomized into two groups with an allocation ratio of 1:1.

Categorical variables were expressed as frequencies and percentages. Continuous variables were presented as median and interquartile range (IQR), or mean $\pm$ standard deviation (SD) if distribution was normal according to the Kolmogorov-Smirnov test.

TABLE 1	Sociodemographic data		
	Experimental group N = 56	Control group N = 56	p-Value
Sex, n (%)			
Male	14 (25)	14 (25)	1.000
Female	42 (75)	42 (75)	1.000
Age (years), mean (SD)	24.24 (5.61)	24.53 (6.89)	0.802

SD = standard deviation.
p < 0.001]), heart rate (72.65 ± 12.11 bpm vs. 84.20 ± 16.80 bpm, p < 0.001) and cortisol levels (142.87 ± 65.81 ng/mL vs. 196.70 ± 79.85 ng/mL, p < 0.001).

The Pearson Chi-squared test was used to compare proportions. Differences between continuous and categorical variables were assessed using Student's *t*-test or Mann-Whitney *U* test, as appropriate, and correlations between continuous variables were assessed by the Pearson's correlation coefficient.

A p value < 0.05 was accepted as statistically significant. Statistical analyses were performed using SPSS v. 22.0 (SPSS, Inc., Chicago, IL, USA) for Windows.

RESULTS

We included 112 students, of which most were females (84, 75%), with a mean age of 24.3 ± 6.2 years. Patients were randomized in a 1:1 manner so that the CG was composed of 56 students and the EG was also composed of 56 students. Both groups included 42 (75%) females and the mean age was 24.53 ± 6.89 years and 24.24 ± 5.61 years (p = 0.802) for the CG and EG, respectively. Thus, both groups were balanced according to sex and age (Table 1).

We investigated variations in clinical and biochemical parameters in both groups of students as is summarized in Table 2. Of note, there were no differences in any of the parameters between the experimental and the control group during the first measurement. Thus, both groups were homogeneous also from this point of view.

Regarding the second measurement, we observed a significant reduction in the heart rate for the experimental group (79.26 ± 14.77 bpm to 72.65 ± 12.11 bpm, p = 0.001). Compared to the first measurement, the other parameters remained stable in this group. However, in the control group, blood pressure, heart rate, and cortisol levels were significantly increased in the second measurement compared with the first, whereas glucose levels were significantly reduced.

Importantly, we observed differences in several parameters between both groups when we analyzed the second measurement. These were significantly lower for blood pressure (both, systolic [115.15 ± 13.59 mmHg vs. 123.22 ± 16.55 mmHg, p = 0.007] and diastolic [68.02 ± 10.22 mmHg vs. 76.67 ± 11.85 mmHg, p < 0.001]), heart rate (72.65 ± 12.11 bpm vs. 84.20 ± 16.80 bpm, p < 0.001) and cortisol levels (142.87 ± 65.81 ng/mL vs. 196.70 ± 79.85 ng/mL, p < 0.001).

We also investigated the percentage of students that increased or reduced the values of the parameters from the first to the second measurement. Hence, most students of the experimental group suffered a reduction of the heart rate in the second measurement without significantly different increase or reduction in any of the other parameters. On contrary, a higher proportion of students from the control group increased the systolic and diastolic blood pressures, heart rate, and cortisol levels in the second measurement. As expected, glucose decreased in most students from both groups (Table 3).

TABLE 2 Values of the variables measured before and after the intervention: between both groups and intra-group variability			
	Experimental group	Control group	p-Value (inter-group)
Systolic blood pressure (mmHg), mean (SD)			
1st measurement	113.84 ± 14.77	112.59 ± 16.15	0.530
2nd measurement	115.15 ± 13.59	123.22 ± 16.55	0.007
p-Value (intra-group)	0.289	< 0.001	
Diastolic blood pressure (mmHg), mean (SD) 1st measurement	70.19 ± 9.79	66.09 ± 13.27	0.591
2nd measurement	68.02 ± 10.22	76.67 ± 11.85	< 0.001
p-Value (intra-group)	0.235	< 0.001	0.060
Heart rate (beats per minute), mean (SD) 1st measurement	79.26 ± 14.77	77.45 ± 16.15	
2nd measurement	72.65 ± 12.11	84.20 ± 16.80	< 0.001
p-Value (intra-group) Oxygen saturation (%), mean (SD)	0.001	< 0.001	
1st measurement	98.04 ± 1.80	98.05 ± 2.50	0.442
2nd measurement	98.12 ± 1.62	98.33 ± 1.15	0.442
p-Value (intra-group)	0.822	0.496	0.787
Cortisol (ng/mL), mean (SD) 1st measurement	148.60 ± 66.46	152.22 ± 77.03	
2nd measurement	142.87 ± 65.81	196.70 ± 79.85	< 0.001
p-Value (intra-group)	0.508	< 0.001	
Glucose (mg/dL), mean (SD) 1st measurement	83.34 ± 17.85	80.30 ± 8.13	0.241
2nd measurement	78.23 ± 21.93	76.90 ± 5.97	0.670
p-Value (intra-group)	0.056	0.002	

SD = standard deviation.

Finally, the academic performance was evaluated after having the scores of the exam. The experimental group had a mean score of 5.07 ± 1.59 points, which was significantly higher compared with the mean score of the control group (4.42 ± 1.58 points, p = 0.033). By categorizing the exam score as pass or fail, the proportion of fails in the control group was higher than in the experimental group (35 [62.5%] vs. 24 [42.9%], p = 0.037).

DISCUSSION

In the present study, the combined intervention of PMR and music therapy has demonstrated to avoid the increase in blood pressure, heart rate, and cortisol levels, which are strongly associated with higher stress. This intervention also improved the academic results in university students from the Nursing degree.

TABLE 3   **Experimental group: direction of the changes before (first measure) and after (second measure) the intervention**

		EXPERIMENTAL GROUP		CONTROL GROUP	
		N (%)	p-Value	N (%)	p-Value
Systolic blood pressure	Reduction from the first measure	21 (37.49)	0.369	12 (21.42)	< 0.001
	Increase from the first measure	31 (54.35)		44 (78.57)	
	Same as the first measure	4 (7.14)		0 (0.0%)	
Diastolic blood pressure	Reduction from the first measure	28 (49.99)	0.242	13 (23.21)	< 0.001
	Increase from the first measure	24 (42.85)		41 (73.21)	
	Same as the first measure	4 (7.14)		2 (3.57)	
Heart rate	Reduction from the first measure	37 (66.07)	0.003	14 (25.0)	< 0.001
	Increase from the first measure	17 (30.35)		42 (74.99)	
	Same as the first measure	2 (3.57)		0 (0.0)	
Oxygen saturation	Reduction from the first measure	19 (33.92)	0.883	20 (35.71)	0.984
	Increase from the first measure	23 (41.07)		20 (35.71)	
	Same as the first measure	14 (24.99)		16 (28.57)	
Cortisol	Reduction from the first measure	29 (51.78)	0.642	11 (19.64)	< 0.001
	Increase from the first measure	27 (48.21)		44 (78.56)	
	Same as the first measure	0 (0.0)		1 (1.78)	
Glucose	Reduction from the first measure	41 (73.21)	0.001	40 (71.42)	0.002
	Increase from the first measure	15 (26.78)		16 (28.57)	
	Same as the first measure	0 (0.0)		0 (0.0)	

Stress is a "physiological and/or psychological reaction to an event that is perceived as threatening or burdensome" (Riggio, 2015). The levels of stress in Nursing students vary from moderate to high, and several studies have pointed to exams as the main source of academic stress (Shukla et al., 2013; Yamashita et al., 2012), together with the relationship with professors (Bagcivan et al., 2015), heavy workloads (Suresh et al., 2013), and the academic sphere per se.

For these reasons, it is important to help Nursing students with appropriate and specific interventions that result in positive outcomes. With this regard, numerous studies have analyzed the effectiveness of diverse techniques for coping with the stress before exams. To date, most of them that studied the sources of stress and coping strategies used by Nursing students were cross-sectional and used self-administered tools that were very different in their quantity of elements, contents and even structure (Bagcivan et al., 2015; Graham et al., 2016; Khajehei et al., 2011), which may hinder the comparison and validation of the results. In addition, the results we present here include the serum cortisol and glucose levels. This is important, since adrenaline, blood glucose, the lipid profile and particularly cortisol have been previously related with stress in students before the exam period (Maduka et al., 2015). These objective parameters avoid the possible bias of subjective answers in self-administered questionnaire or scales to assess the level of stress.

To the best of our knowledge, this is the first study combining PMR and music therapy as a method for the control of academic stress. There are studies that have analyzed the efficacy of music therapy or relaxation therapy separately (Lee et al., 2016; Pal et al., 2014; Shih et al., 2016), and others analyzed the effects of this combined therapy, but in different contexts and populations. Thus, Zhou et al. showed the effects of two combined therapies on depression, anxiety, and the duration of the hospital stay on women with breast cancer after a radical mastectomy (Zhou et al., 2015). The results in this context were also positive. There are also studies on the effects of music on the brain, and more specifically on aspects such as cognition, emotional processing, anxiety, and stress. Menon and Levitin, and later Salimpoor et al. (Menon and Levitin, 2005; Salimpoor et al., 2011), studied young subjects showing that listening to music had an influence on the physiological responses controlled by the autonomous nervous system. All of these results allow us to consolidate the hypothesis that music therapy is an excellent, easy-to-use, useful, and accessible tool without negative secondary effects, applicable to various contexts and effective in the treatment of various psychiatric disorders in teenagers and youths, so it is deemed a safe and economical alternative treatment (Burrai et al., 2014; Melo et al., 2018; Mohammadi et al., 2014; Yinger and Gooding, 2015). A systematic review and meta-analysis has also corroborated the efficacy of music interventions on the treatment of hypertension (Kuhlmann et al., 2016), which also has been confirmed in our study, given that the control group had a significant increase in their blood pressure, whereas it remained stabilized in the experimental group.

On the other hand, the efficacy of PMR therapy for the decrease of the student's exam stress has been proven as well (Pal et al., 2014; Prato and Yucha, 2013).

Taking the above information into account, we have proved that the combination of two interventions included in the Nursing taxonomy (Butcher et al., 2017), PMR and music therapy, was effective for the control and decrease of stress before exams. While several parameters increased in the control group from the first to the second measurement, with our intervention, we were able to maintain constant all of these in the 56 students from experimental group. Thus, the level of stress was lower in this group and importantly, the academic results were better. This is in agreement with some authors who stated that academic stress negatively affects the student's performance (Crego et al., 2016; Labrague et al., 2017; Maduka et al., 2015). These results seem to evidence the need to establish strategies to prevent the occurrence of stress among the Nursing students before an exam or when facing other stressful situations from the discipline itself, such as oral exams, clinical practices, and the performing of invasive techniques.

LIMITATIONS

There are some limitations to acknowledge. First, this research included only students in their second year of Degree. We recognize that to include students of different years would enhance the generalizability of the study, and this is an issue that we will take in mind in the future. Second, this study was conducted only in Nursing students, and therefore our results must be prospectively validated in University students from a larger variety of academic sectors and involving other Universities.

CONCLUSION

In this study including university students from the Nursing degree, the combination of PMR and music therapy was effective for the control and decrease of stress before exams. This intervention also demonstrated to improve academic results in this population of students.

Funding source

None declared.

Ethical approval

Ethical Committee from the Catholic University of Murcia (UCAM).

Declaration of competing interest

The authors declare that they have not conflicts of interest.

REFERENCES

Bagcivan, G., Cinar, F. I., Tosun, N., & Korkmaz, R. (2015). Determination of nursing students' expectations for faculty members and the perceived stressors during their education. *Contemp. Nurse, 50*(1), 58–71. https://doi.org/10.1080/10376178.2015.1010259.

Burrai, F., Micheluzzi, V., Zito, M. P., Pietro, G., & Sisti, D. (2014). Effects of live saxophone music on physiological parameters, pain, mood and itching levels in patients undergoing haemodialysis. *J. Ren. Care, 40*(4), 249–256. https://doi.org/10.1111/jorc.12078.

Butcher, H. K., Bulechek, G. M., Dochterman, J. M., & Wagner, C. M. (2017). *Nursing Interventions Classification (NIC)*. Madrid: Elsevier, seventh edition.

Crego, A., Carrillo-Diaz, M., Armfield, J. M., & Romero, M. (2016). Stress and academic performance in dental students: the role of coping strategies and examination-related self-efficacy. *J. Dent. Educ., 80*(2), 165–172.

Dendle, C., Baulch, J., Pellicano, R., Hay, M., Lichtwark, I., Ayoub, S., & … Horne, K. (2018). Medical student psychological distress and academic performance. *Med. Teach.*, 1–7. https://doi.org/10.1080/0142159x.2018.1427222.

Graham, M. M., Lindo, J., Bryan, V. D., & Weaver, S. (2016). Factors associated with stress among second year student nurses during clinical training in Jamaica. *J. Prof. Nurs., 32*(5), 383–391. https://doi.org/10.1016/j.profnurs.2016.01.004.

Hashim, H. A., & Zainol, N. A. (2015). Changes in emotional distress, short term memory, and sustained attention following 6 and 12 sessions of progressive muscle relaxation training in 10–11 years old primary school children. *Psychol. Health Med., 20*(5), 623–628. https://doi.org/10.1080/13548506.2014.1002851.

Ince, S., & Çevik, K. (2014). The effect of listening to music about the anxiety of the nursing students during their first blood extraction experience. *Indian J. Physiol. Pharmacol., 58*(3), 298–301.

Khajehei, M., Ziyadlou, S., Hadzic, M., & Kashefi, F. (2011). The genesis and consequences of stress among midwifery students. *Br. J. Midwifery, 19*(6), 379–385.

Kuhlmann, A. Y., Etnel, J. R., Roos-Hesselink, J. W., Jeekel, J., Bogers, A. J., & Takkenberg, J. J. (2016). Systematic review and meta-analysis of music interventions in hypertension treatment: a quest for answers. *BMC Cardiovasc. Disord., 16*, 69. https://doi.org/10.1186/s12872-016-0244-0.

Labrague, L. J., McEnroe-Petitte, D. M., Gloe, D., Thomas, L., Papathanasiou, I. V., & Tsaras, K. (2017). A literature review on stress and coping strategies in nursing students. *J. Ment. Health, 26*(5), 471–480. https://doi.org/10.1080/09638237.2016.1244721.

Lee, K. S., Jeong, H. C., Yim, J. E., & Jeon, M. Y. (2016). Effects of music therapy on the cardiovascular and autonomic nervous system in stress-induced university students: a randomized controlled trial. *J. Altern. Complement. Med., 22*(1), 59–65. https://doi.org/10.1089/acm.2015.0079.

Maduka, I. C., Neboh, E. E., & Ufelle, S. A. (2015). The relationship between serum cortisol, adrenaline, blood glucose and lipid profile of undergraduate students under examination stress. *Afr. Health Sci., 15*(1), 131–136. https://doi.org/10.4314/ahs. v15i1.18.

McCarthy, B., Trace, A., O'Donovan, M., O'Regan, P., Brady-Nevin, C., O'Shea, M., & … Murphy, M. (2018). Coping with stressful events: a pre-post-test of a psycho-educational intervention for undergraduate nursing and midwifery students. *Nurse Educ. Today, 61*, 273–280. https://doi.org/10.1016/j.nedt.2017.11.034.

Melo, G. A. A., Rodrigues, A. B., Firmeza, M. A., Grangeiro, A. S. M., Oliveira, P. P., & Caetano, J. A. (2018). Musical intervention on anxiety and vital parameters of chronic renal patients: a randomized clinical trial. *Rev. Lat. Am. Enfermagem., 26*, e2978. https://doi.org/10.1590/1518-8345.2123.2978.

Menon, V., & Levitin, D. J. (2005). The rewards of music listening: response and physiological connectivity of the mesolimbic system. *Neuroimage, 28*(1), 175–184. https://doi.org/10.1016/j. neuroimage.2005.05.053.

Mohammadi, A., Ajorpaz, N. M., Torabi, M., Mirsane, A., & Moradi, F. (2014). Effects of music listening on preoperative state anxiety and physiological parameters in patients undergoing general surgery: a randomized quasi-experimental trial. *Cent. Eur. J. Nurs. Midw., 5*(4), 156–160.

Pal, G. K., Ganesh, V., Karthik, S., Nanda, N., & Pal, P. (2014). The effects of short-term relaxation therapy on indices of heart rate variability and blood pressure in young adults. *Am. J. Health Promot., 29*(1), 23–28. https://doi.org/10.4278/ajhp.130131-QUAN-52.

Pozos-Radillo, E., Preciado-Serrano, L., Plascencia-Campos, A., Valdez-Lopez, R., & Morales-Fernandez, A. (2016). Psychophysiological manifestations associated with stress in students of a public university in Mexico. *J. Child. Adolesc. Psychiatr. Nurs., 29*(2), 79–84. https://doi.org/10.1111/jcap.12142.

Pozos-Radillo, E., Preciado-Serrano, L., Plascencia-Campos, A., Morales-Fernandez, A., & Valdez-Lopez, R. (2018). Predictive study of academic stress with the irritable bowel syndrome in medicine students at a public university in Mexico. *Libyan J. Med., 13*(1), Article 1479599. https://doi.org/10.1080/19932820.2018.1479599.

Prato, C. A., & Yucha, C. B. (2013). Biofeedback-assisted relaxation training to decrease test anxiety in nursing students. *Nurs. Educ. Perspect., 34*(2), 76–81.

Quinn, B. L., & Peters, A. (2017). Strategies to reduce nursing student test anxiety: a literature review. *J. Nurs. Educ., 56*(3), 145–151. https://doi.org/10.3928/01484834-20170222-05.

Riggio, R. E. (2015). *Introduction to Industrial and Organizational Psychology* (6th ed). New York: Routledge.

Salimpoor, V. N., Benovoy, M., Larcher, K., Dagher, A., & Zatorre, R. J. (2011). Anatomically distinct dopamine release during anticipation and experience of peak emotion to music. *Nat. Neurosci., 14*(2), 257–262. https://doi.org/10.1038/nn.2726.

Shih, Y. N., Chien, W. H., & Chiang, H. S. (2016). Elucidating the relationship between work attention performance and emotions arising from listening to music. *Work, 55*(2), 489–494. https://doi.org/10.3233/wor-162408.

Shudifat, R. M., & Al-Husban, R. Y. (2015). Perceived sources of stress among first-year nursing students in Jordan. *J. Psychosoc. Nurs. Ment. Health Serv., 53*(6), 37–43. https://doi.org/10.3928/02793695-20150522-01.

Shukla, A., Kalra, G., & Pakhare, A. (2013). Understanding stress and coping mechanisms in Indian student nurses. *Sri Lanka Journal of Psychiatry, 4*(2), 29–33.

Silva-Sánchez, D. (2015). Stress in nursing students: a systematic review. *Science and Care, 12*(1), 119–133.

Silverstein, S. T., & Kritz-Silverstein, D. (2010). A longitudinal study of stress in first-year dentistry students. *J. Dent. Educ., 74*(8), 836–848.

Suresh, P., Matthews, A., & Coyne, I. (2013). Stress and stressors in the clinical environment: a comparative study of fourth-year student nurses and newly qualified general nurses in Ireland. *J. Clin. Nurs., 22*(5–6), 770–779. https://doi.org/10.1111/j.1365-2702. 2012.04145.x.

Yamashita, K., Saito, M., & Takao, T. (2012). Stress and coping styles in Japanese nursing students. *Int. J. Nurs. Pract., 18*(5), 489–496. https://doi.org/10.1111/j.1440-172X. 2012.02056.x.

Yinger, O. S., & Gooding, L. F. (2015). A systematic review of music-based interventions for procedural support. *J. Music. Ther., 52*(1), 1–77. https://doi.org/10.1093/jmt/thv004.

Zhou, K., Li, X., Li, J., Liu, M., Dang, S., Wang, D., & Xin, X. (2015). A clinical randomized controlled trial of music therapy and progressive muscle relaxation training in female breast cancer patients after radical mastectomy: results on depression, anxiety and length of hospital stay. *Eur. J. Oncol. Nurs., 19*(1), 54–59. https://doi.org/10.1016/j. ejon.2014.07.010.

THE CRITICAL APPRAISAL

Critical appraisal of this study aims to determine the rigor of the evidence presented and its applicability to nursing practice.

Review of the Literature

The authors provide a succinct summary of the literature related to studies that report interventions that reduce students' stress and enhance coping before taking exams in order to improve students' academic performance. The authors appropriately cite evidence from the literature to support high levels of academic stress for students in health professions programs. They accurately describe literature that reveals a gap about the actual impact of these interventions aimed at reducing stress during the exam period.

Research Questions

The literature review builds the case to support the purpose of this study: to evaluate a prevention program, an intervention of Progressive Muscle Relaxation (PMR) with music therapy, to investigate whether or not this combined intervention reduced high stress levels before exams and improves academic performance. The independent variable is the method of student preparation administered before taking an exam (which included PMR and music therapy for the experimental group and standard practice for the control group); the dependent variables are clinical and biochemical parameters that included heart rate, blood pressure, and cortisol and glucose levels. The population under study is clearly defined, and the results would be significant to better serve students' stress levels and academic performance in taking exams.

The research question is embedded in the aim of the study: to evaluate the effectiveness of a prevention program that combines PMR and music therapy interventions on the decrease of stress during the exam period and the improvement of academic results.

Research Design

In this RCT, providing Level II evidence, the researchers clearly included the three required elements of an RCT: manipulation of the independent variable, randomization, and control. Random assignment of subjects to an experimental group (EG) and a control group (CG) matched students in both groups by age and gender. A random number-generating software program was appropriately used.

Sample

A total sample size of 112 participants (females $n = 84$, 75% with a mean age of 24.3 +/– 6.2 years) from the second year of a nursing degree program from the Catholic University of Murcia were included in the study. Of note, there were no specific inclusion or exclusion criteria, nor was power analysis used to determine the sample size needed to detect a treatment effect. The researchers used a convenience sample to recruit students in the second year of their nursing curriculum but compensated for this by using random assignment. The authors appropriately report that there were no significant differences at baseline between these two student groups, CG and EG, as clearly presented in Table 18.1 based on sex and age.

Methods

Using randomization, participants were allocated on a 1:1 basis to a CG ($n = 56$), exam with no intervention, and EG ($n = 56$), exam using PMR and music therapy before test taking. Two nurses and a psychologist administered the experimental PMR and music, who had extensive experience with relaxation techniques and music therapy.

Both groups, control and experimental, had two scheduled visits to draw fasting blood work and to measure vital signs including heart rate, blood pressure, and oxygen saturation. Data were collected using a consistent protocol to maintain fidelity. The first data point measured all participants during a non-exam period. The second data point measured the blood work and vital signs on the day of an exam; the CG was drawn 1 hour before onset of the exam. In the EG, the intervention combining muscle relaxation and music therapy was administered for 1 hour, and the blood work was drawn after the intervention. Both groups ate breakfast before the exam. Academic performance of an exam on "Clinical Nursing" was measured by using each student's test score, which was classified as a failure < 5 or pass ≥ 5 (value range: 0 to 10).

Threats to Internal Validity

Threats to internal validity include selection of participants using a convenience sample; however, random assignment of participants to an intervention or CG helped control for selection bias. There is no mention to blinding of participants or researchers, which may represent a potential threat to internal validity. Another threat to internal validity specific to lack of power analysis is possible given the small sample size of the control and EGs; the small sample size increases the likelihood of a type II error, which can reduce the power of the study to detect the treatment effect. Maturation can also effect internal validity given the spacing of data collection points 4 months apart, occurring on October

2017 and February 2018, which may produce confounding effects. All participants were included in the study and data analysis, eliminating any attrition bias, another threat to internal validity.

Threats to External Validity

Researchers identified the following limitations and threat to external validity: subjects were second year students from only one university and the sample size was small, these issues limit the generalizability of the findings. Reactive effects of testing based on individual response may interfere with an individual participant's sensitivity to the experimental variable. Additionally, the sequencing of the concurrent curriculum was not explained; there may be some interaction effects if multiple exams were scheduled within the same data collection period. The Hawthorne effect may have altered participants' responses given they knew they were part of a program. In addition, the instructors likely surveyed students and collected these data.

Legal-Ethical Considerations

The study appropriately followed CONSORT guidelines and was reviewed and approved by the internal review board, the university's ethics committee. Informed consent was obtained from all participants before the study's initiation.

Instruments

Stress levels were examined using vital signs: blood pressure in mm Hg (systolic and diastolic), heart rate (beats per minute), oxygen saturation (%), cortisol (ng/mL), and glucose (mg/dL). These are appropriate instruments with established validity and reliability that provide valuable information regarding the students' level of stress and reduce the risk for instrumentation bias. The use of physiological data adds strength to measuring the impact of the intervention. It is important that physiological data were collected at baseline and at two subsequent data collection points. However, a weakness is that there were no baseline anxiety/stress measurements. These would be useful in comparing differences between participants in the experimental and CGs. Instead, intragroup variability was assessed. Although researchers acknowledge that quantitative indices to determine stress level avoid possible bias associated with self-report, it would have been important to measure students' perception of test anxiety before intervention to investigate whether or not it correlated with test performance. There are no baseline scores related to academic achievement aside from the Clinical Nursing exam that correlated with matching students, such that higher-performing students randomized into either EG continue to perform well despite the intervention. Another strength was the standardized relaxation protocol that was administered accompanied by relaxing music set at an appropriate and consistent volume of 50 to 60 dB.

Data Analysis

Statistical analysis was appropriately implemented to test for differences between the EG and CG. Categorical data were expressed in terms of frequencies and percentages, whereas continuous variables were identified using the Kolmogorov-Smirnov test. A Pearson's correlation coefficient was employed to examine correlations between these continuous variables. To assess differences between variables (continuous and categorical) a t test or Mann-Whitney U test were used. Statistical significance was deemed acceptable with a p value < 0.05.

Results

The findings for the EG reveal a significant decrease from baseline in heart rate, but not for other parameters. In contrast, the findings for the CG reveal that a significantly higher proportion of subjects from the CG had higher blood pressure, heart rate, and cortisol levels. Data for the second measurement reveals that a significant decrease in heart rate was observed among participants in the EG ($p < 0.001$) who received the combined PMR and music therapy intervention. In contrast, the CG demonstrated significant increases in blood pressure, heart rate, and cortisol levels. On the second measurement, both the EG and CG demonstrated significantly lower blood pressure (systolic, $p = 0.007$; and diastolic $p < 0.001$), heart rate ($p < 0.001$), and cortisol levels ($p < 0.001$); glucose decreased in both groups. The academic performance of the EG and CG provided support for the research question. The mean score of the EG was significantly higher compared with the CG ($p = 0.033$).

Conclusions, Implications, and Recommendations

Overall, nursing students receiving the intervention, a combination of PMR and music therapy, had lower measurements on physiological parameters associated with stress before taking an exam, and these students achieved higher academic scores on the Clinical Nursing exam than students in the CG.

This Level II RCT design included all of the required components (i.e., randomization, intervention, CGs, and manipulation of the independent variable) and rigor to be classified as a moderately well-designed RCT. RCTs allow investigators to determine causal relationships between the independent and dependent variables. In this case, strengths included a homogeneous sample with equivalence at baseline, random assignment, use of physiological measures, evidence of intervention fidelity, and consistency in data collection. Threats to external validity, as clearly described by the investigator, included concern for the study's generalizability given the small and homogeneous sample in which the research was limited to students in the second year of the curriculum and were nursing students in one program. Students coming from different academic programs or various types of universities may have different responses to the intervention.

This is a moderately well-designed and well-conducted RCT that provides Level II evidence. The strengths in the study design, data collection methods, and measures to address threats to internal and external validity make this Level II RCT a study providing evidence that adds to the evidence that students receiving PMR and music therapy before taking an exam experience a reduction in blood pressure, heart rate, and cortisol levels—all indices associated with level of stress. Additionally, students receiving the intervention scored higher on the academic exam than students in the CG. The interventions pose minimal risk and seem feasible to implement in larger studies of more heterogeneous populations.

CRITICAL APPRAISAL OF A QUANTITATIVE RESEARCH STUDY

THE RESEARCH STUDY

The study "Appropriate and Inappropriate Shocks in Hypertrophic Cardiomyopathy Patients with Subcutaneous Implantable Cardioverter-defibrillators: An International Multicenter Study" by Nazer et al. (2020), published in Heart Rhythm, is critiqued. The article is presented in its entirety to determine its usefulness and applicability for clinical practice and followed by the critique.

Appropriate and inappropriate shocks in hypertrophic cardiomyopathy patients with subcutaneous implantable cardioverter-defibrillators: An international multicenter study

Babak Nazer, MD[*], Zack Dale, MD[*], Gianmarco Carrassa, MD[†], Nosheen Reza, MD[‡], Tuna Ustunkaya, MD, PhD[‡], Nikolaos Papoutsidakis, MD, PhD[§], Andrew Gray, BS[*], Stacey J. Howell, MD[*], Miriam R. Elman, MS, MPH[*], Paolo Pieragnoli, MD[†], Giuseppe Ricciardi, MD[†], Daniel Jacoby, MD[§], David S. Frankel, MD, FHRS[‡], Anjali Owens, MD[‡], Iacopo Olivotto, MD[†], Stephen B. Heitner, MD[*]

ABSTRACT

Background: Subcutaneous implantable cardioverter-defibrillators (S-ICDs) are attractive for preventing sudden cardiac death in hypertrophic cardiomyopathy (HCM) as they mitigate risks of transvenous leads in young patients. However, S-ICDs may be associated with increased inappropriate shock (IAS) in HCM patients.

Objective: The purpose of this study was to assess the incidence and predictors of appropriate shock and IAS in a contemporary HCM S-ICD cohort.

Methods: We collected electrocardiographic and clinical data from HCM patients who underwent S-ICD implantation at four centers. Etiologies of all S-ICD shocks were adjudicated. We used Firth penalized logistic regression to derive adjusted odds ratios (aORs) for predictors of IAS.

Results: Eighty-eight HCM patients received S-ICDs (81 for primary and 7 for secondary prevention) with a mean follow-up of 2.7 years. Five patients (5.7%) had 9 IAS episodes (3.8 IAS per 100 patient-years) most often because of sinus tachycardia and/ or T-wave oversensing. Independent predictors of IAS were higher 12-lead electrocardiographic R-wave amplitude (aOR 2.55 per 1 mV; 95% confidence interval 1.15–6.38) and abnormal T-wave inversions (aOR 0.16; 95% confidence interval 0.02–0.97). There were 2 appropriate shocks in 7 secondary prevention patients and none in 81 primary prevention patients, despite 96% meeting Enhanced American College of Cardiology/American Heart Association criteria and the mean European HCM Risk-SCD score predicting 5.7% 5-year risk. No patients had sudden death or untreated sustained ventricular arrhythmias.

Conclusion: In this multicenter HCM S-ICD study, IAS were rare and appropriate shocks confined to secondary prevention patients. The R-wave amplitude increased IAS risk, whereas T-wave inversions were protective. HCM primary prevention implantable cardioverter-defibrillator guidelines overestimated the risk of appropriate shocks in our cohort.

[*]From the Knight Cardiovascular Institute, Oregon Health and Science University, Portland, Oregon
[†]Cardiomyopathy Unit, Careggi University, Florence, Italy
[‡]Cardiovascular Division, Perelman School of Medicine at the University of Pennsylvania, Philadelphia, Pennsylvania
[§]Cardiology Division, Yale University, New Haven, Connecticut.

Keywords
Hypertrophic cardiomyopathy
Inappropriate shocks
Risk stratification
Subcutaneous implantable cardioverter-defibrillator
Sudden cardiac death

Dr Olivotto was supported by the European Union's Horizon 2020 Research and Innovation Programme (grant no. 777204), the Italian Ministry of Health (RF-2013-02356787), and the Ente Cassa di Risparmio di Firenze (2016). Address reprint requests and correspondence: Dr Babak Nazer, Knight Cardiovascular Institute, Oregon Health and Science University, 3181 SW Sam Jackson Park Rd, Portland, OR 97239. E-mail address: nazer@ohsu.edu.
(Heart Rhythm 2020;17:1107–1114)

INTRODUCTION

Compared to other cardiovascular conditions, patients are diagnosed with hypertrophic cardiomyopathy (HCM) at a relatively young age (median 45.8 years; interquartile range 30.9–58.1 years) and may have an elevated risk of ventricular arrhythmias and sudden cardiac death (SCD).[1] The subcutaneous implantable cardioverter-defibrillator (EMBLEM S-ICD, EMBLEM MRI S-ICD, S-ICD, Boston Scientific, Natick, MA) is frequently considered for younger patients in whom an implantable cardioverter-defibrillator (ICD) but not pacing is indicated as a strategy to avoid risks of chronic indwelling transvenous leads.[2]

Despite these advantages, the S-ICD sensing algorithm, which makes use of three electrogram vectors analogous to the standard 12-lead electrocardiogram (ECG), may be prone to errors in arrhythmia detection leading to inappropriate shock (IAS)—most commonly via T-wave oversensing (TWOS). Indeed, in a contemporary review of S-ICD complications, an estimated 32% of all IAS were due to TWOS.[3] HCM patients frequently have pronounced QRS and T-wave abnormalities on their baseline ECGs, leading to a higher risk of TWOS and IAS. Preimplantation screening simulates the device's three sensing vectors and attempts to identify patients at risk of TWOS. This has resulted in 14%–38% of HCM patients being deemed inappropriate for S-ICD implantation.[4-7] Nevertheless, IAS has remained a significant issue for patients with HCM. The pooled EFFORTLESS (Evaluation oF FactORs ImpacTing CLinical Outcome and Cost EffectiveneSS of the S-ICD) and IDE (Investigational Device Exemption) cohort data for HCM patients demonstrated IAS incidence of 12.5% per year over a 22-month follow-up,[8] although more recent advances in sensing algorithms and device programming have led to reductions in the rates of IAS of up to 68%.[9]

In an evolving landscape of S-ICD utilization, the objectives of the present study were to determine the incidence of both appropriate and inappropriate device therapies in a multicenter cohort of HCM patients with an S-ICD and to determine predictors of IAS.

Methods
Study design and data collection

Consecutive patients with HCM implanted with an S-ICD between 2014 and 2019 at 4 centers (9–36 patients per center) were included in our cohort. Data on baseline patient characteristics, pre- and postimplant screening, and patient follow-up were retrospectively collected from electronic medical records. Pre-implant ECGs were analyzed systematically. QRS and QT intervals were electronically derived. R- and T-wave amplitudes were manually measured from isoelectric baseline to peak (or nadir if the T wave was predominantly negative). The maximum amplitude in all leads was recorded. T-wave inversions (TWIs; in leads other than V1 and AVR in which they are normal variants) were recorded. All data were anonymized and stored centrally. The study was conducted with approval of the institutional review boards at all sites.

Implant data and ICD programming

The decision to implant an S-ICD was based on clinical indication as determined by the treating clinician. Patients were screened with the three-lead surface ECG using the Boston Scientific screening tool and were required to pass at least one screening vector in at least the supine and standing positions. Additional screening in the prone position or with exercise testing was performed in 11 and 5 patients, respectively. The total number of combinations of body positions (including exercise) and sensing vectors screened was recorded as "number of vectors screened" for later analysis. The device was implanted using a standard two- or three-incision technique.[10,11] Defibrillation threshold testing was performed at the discretion of the implanting clinician. All devices were programmed with two therapy zones: a conditional shock zone variably set at 180–240 beats/min and a shock zone at 200–250 beats/min.

Stored electrograms of all shocks were reviewed independently by two investigators and adjudicated as appropriate or inappropriate. Etiology of IAS was determined by the investigators. Interobserver agreement was observed in each case. Episodes where multiple IAS were delivered sequentially as part of the same clinical encounter were counted as one IAS, provided that they occurred via the same mechanism.

Statistical analysis

Variables were selected a priori as potential risk factors for IAS on the basis of clinical experience and prior studies on IAS in S-ICD. Descriptive statistics were calculated for continuous variables using mean ± SD or median with interquartile range and categorical variables using frequency with percentage. To identify potential risk factors for IAS, we performed Firth penalized logistic regression. This modeling approach was used to reduce bias that may result from traditional logistic regression because of our small sample size and rare outcome.[12] Odds ratios (ORs) and 95% profile likelihood confidence intervals (CIs) were estimated from univariable and multivariable models. Complete case analyses were conducted using SAS 9.4 (SAS Institute, Inc., Cary, NC).

Results

Patient population and implant characteristics

The study cohort included 88 HCM patients (Table 1) who were followed for a mean of 2.7 ± 1.3 years after S-ICD implantation. The median age was 43.0 years (interquartile range 32.2–55.4 years; range 17.1–73.4 years), and 63 (71.5%) were male. Of these patients, 7 (7.9%) received S-ICD for secondary prevention and the remaining 81 (92%) for primary prevention. Ten patients received the first generation S-ICD (SQ-RX Model 1010 Boston Scientific; Natick, MA), 29 received EMBLEM S-ICD Model A209 (Boston Scientific; Natick, MA), and 49 received Model A219 (Boston Scientific; Natick, MA). Eighty-six leads were implanted in the left parasternal position and two in the right parasternal position. Upon implantation, all patients received dual-zone programming, with the conditional zone set

TABLE 1 Baseline characteristics

| | INAPPROPRIATE SHOCK | | |
Characteristic	Yes (n = 5)	No (n = 83)	P
Age (y)	36.1 (32.3–43.2)	43.9 (32.2–55.6)	.6873
Female sex	0 (0.0)	25 (30.1)	.3158
BMI (kg/m^2)	31.1 (23.2–32.4)	27.1 (23.9–30.1)	.5961
BSA (m^2)	2.2 (2.1–2.4)	2.0 (1.8–2.2)	.0954
Implant indication			
Primary	5 (100.0)	76 (91.6)	
Secondary	0 (0.0)	7 (8.4)	
HCM Risk-SCD score	6.6 (6.1–8.7)	4.5 (3.8–6.6)	.0293
Medications at baseline			
β-Blockers	3 (60.0)	59 (71.1)	.6298
Calcium channel blockers	2 (40.0)	14 (16.9)	.2227
β-Blocker or calcium channel blocker	5 (100.0)	65 (78.3)	.5787
Baseline QRS width (ms)	136.0 (94.0–144.0)	92.0 (86.0–102.0)	.0227
Baseline QTc interval (ms)	468.0 (447.0–507.0)	444.0 (424.0–463.0)	.0536
Baseline R-wave amplitude (all leads) (mV)	2.9 (2.2–3.1)	1.8 (1.3–2.4)	.0365
Baseline T-wave amplitude (all leads) (mV)	0.5 (0.4–0.6)	0.5 (0.3–0.6)	.4924
R/T-wave ratio (all leads)	18.6 (18.2–23.5)	25.0 (17.9–40.7)	.1896
Ejection fraction (%)	65.0 (57.0–65.0)	65.0 (60.0–70.0)	.3137
Presence of T-wave inversions	2 (40.0)	65 (78.3)	.0858
Maximal left ventricular wall thickness (mm)	22.6 (22.0–23.0)	18.0 (15.0–23.0)	.3722
Left ventricular mass (g)	282.0 (149.0–318.8)	187.0 (132.4–249.5)	.2505
LVOT pressure gradient (resting) (mm Hg)	6.0 (5.8–10.0)	7.0 (5.0–22.0)	.8215
LVOT pressure gradient (dynamic) (mm Hg)	57.5 (24.0–106.5)	14.0 (5.0–41.8)	.0915
Presence of LGE on CMR imaging	3 (60.0)	72 (86.7)	.1382
Presence of apical aneurysm	0 (0.0)	4 (4.8)	.9999
Vectors screened, number	9.0 (6.0–9.0)	6.0 (6.0–6.0)	.0903
Vectors passed screening, proportion	0.7 (0.4–1.0)	0.8 (0.7–1.0)	.3621
Conditional shock zone programming	210.0 (210.0–210.0)	210.0 (210.0–220.0)	.4066
Shock zone programming	220.0 (220.0–240.0)	240.0 (240.0–250.0)	.0987
SMARTPass programming used	3 (60.0)	57 (68.7)	.6003

Values are presented as median (interquartile range) or n (%).
BMI = body mass index; BSA = body surface area; CMR = cardiovascular magnetic resonance; HCM = hypertrophic cardiomyopathy; LGE = late gadolinium enhancement; LVOT = left ventricular outflow tract; QTc = corrected QT; SCD = sudden cardiac death.

at 207 ± 12 beats/min and the shock zone at 241 ± 11 beats/min. Defibrillation threshold testing was performed in all but six patients. SMARTPass was programmed on initially in 57 of 88 patients. Postimplant exercise QRS optimization occurred in seven patients.

IASs: Incidence, etiology, and clinical responses Five patients (5.7%) experienced a total of nine IAS over a mean follow-up of 2.7 ± 1.3 years (incidence 3.8 per 100 patient-years) (Figure 1 and Table 2). Seven of nine IAS (78%) occurred within a year of implantation (median time from implantation to first IAS 9.2 months). Five of nine IAS were due to TWOS, two of which occurred in the setting of rapidly conducted atrial fibrillation (AF) (Figure 2A) and three in the setting of sinus tachycardia (Figure 2B). Three IAS were due to sinus tachycardia during exercise without TWOS: one of these was in the conditional zone (inappropriately

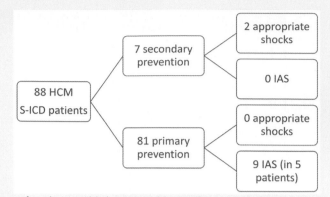

FIG 1 Flowchart of patients with hypertrophic cardiomyopathy and subcutaneous implantable cardioverter-defibrillator. Inappropriate shocks (IASs) occurred in five patients (5.7%) with an incidence of 3.8% per year.

discriminated) and two of these were in the shock zone (where morphology discrimination is not applied). One IAS was due to rapidly conducted AF with rates in the shock zone. Three IAS (all sinus tachycardia related) occurred in the setting of medication (b-blocker or calcium channel blocker) nonadherence, and all six sinus tachycardia–related IAS occurred during exercise (snowboarding and wakeboarding) or sexual intercourse. None of the patients who had received IAS had undergone preimplant exercise screening, but three had undergone screening in the prone position.

Clinical responses to IAS (Table 2) were increasing conditional zone rate (n53 IAS episodes), increasing shock zone rate (n52), changing sensing vector (n52), optimizing QRS morphology template during exercise (n53), medication changes (n55), and turning on SMARTPass filtering (in the one patient in whom it was not on previously). A detailed description of IAS events and responses can be found in Online Supplemental Table 1.

Predictors of IAS. In univariable analyses, potential risk factors associated with IAS were wider QRS complex (OR 1.08 per 1 ms; 95% CI 1.03–1.15), longer corrected QT interval (OR 1.03 per 1 ms; 95% CI 1.00–1.07), higher 12-lead ECG R-wave amplitude (maximal of all leads; OR 2.76 per 1 mV; 95% CI 1.14–7.11), and lower shock zone detection rate (OR

TABLE 2	Etiologies of inappropriate shocks and clinical response	
Etiology	**Number of patients (%)**	**Clinicians' response**
TWOS	5 (55%)	
During sinus tachycardia	3	Exercise QRS template (2), change sensing vector (2)
During AF	2	Turn on SMARTPass, AF rate control (2), change sensing vector
Sinus tachycardia without TWOS	3 (33%)	
In the shock zone	2	Increase shock zone rate
In the conditional zone (inappropriate discrimination)	1	Exercise QRS template, increase conditional zone rate
AF in the shock zone	1 (11%)	AF rate control

AF = atrial fibrillation; TWOS = T-wave oversensing.

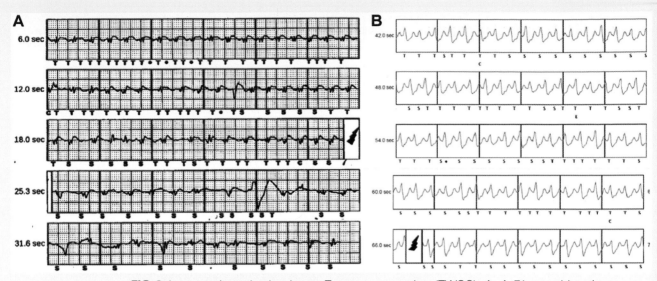

FIG 2 Inappropriate shocks due to T-wave oversensing (TWOS). A: A 74-year-old patient with TWOS during atrial fibrillation (AF) with device-detected rates in the shock zone (does not apply morphology discrimination). Clinician response was to change from the alternate to the secondary sensing vector and improve rate control for AF. B: A 32-year-old man with TWOS during sinus tachycardia while snowboarding, with device-detected rates in the conditional zone (not a morphology match by discrimination). Clinician response was to increase the conditional zone rate from 200 to 210 beats/min and perform exercise-based QRS template optimization of the device.

0.94 per beats/min; 95% CI 0.88–1.00) compared to those without IAS (Table 3). Multivariable analysis, however, identified only R-wave amplitude (adjusted OR 2.55 per 1 mV; 95% CI 1.15–6.38) and the presence of TWI (adjusted OR 0.16; 95% CI 0.02–0.97) as independent risk factors for IAS. The mean maximal R-wave amplitude in patients receiving IAS was 2.9 ± 1.0 mV (range 1.7–4.4 mV) compared with 1.960.8 mV (range 0.6–4.5 mV) in those who did not receive IAS (*P* = .016).

Appropriate shocks

Over an average of 2.7 ± 1.3 years of follow-up (237.6 patient-years), only 2 of 88 patients received appropriate shocks and both had undergone S-ICD implant for secondary prevention. None of the 81 primary prevention patients received an appropriate shock. The incidence of appropriate shocks was 0, 9.8, and 0.8 per 100 patient-years in the primary prevention cohort, secondary prevention cohort, and entire cohort, respectively.

Given the absence of appropriate shocks in primary prevention patients, we retrospectively applied HCM SCD risk stratification criteria to determine the preimplantation SCD risk and further investigate a potentially low threshold for primary prevention implantation (Figure 3). Of the 77 patients in whom the 2011 American College of Cardiology/American Heart Association HCM guidelines[13] could be applied, 62 patients (81%) met class IIa indication and 15 (19%) met class IIb or class III indication. The externally validated European HCM Risk-SCD score[14,15] predicted a 5.7% ± 3.4% 5-year risk of ventricular

Characteristic	UNIVARIABLE MODEL OR (95% CI)		MULTIVARIABLE MODEL OR (95% CI)	
TABLE 3	**Predictors of inappropriate shocks**			
Age (per 1 y)	1.00 (0.94–1.06)			
Female sex	0.21 (,0.01–1.95)			
BMI (per 1 kg/m²)	1.02 (0.89–1.11)			
BSA (per 1 m²)	5.37 (0.53–46.34)			
Presence of apical aneurysm	1.53 (0.01–17.64)			
β-Blocker at baseline	0.58 (0.11–3.65)			
Calcium channel blocker at baseline	3.42 (0.53–19.32)			
β-Blocker or calcium channel blocker at baseline	3.11 (0.33–414.88)			
HCM Risk-SCD score (per 1 unit)	1.17 (0.96–1.40)			
Baseline QRS width (per 1 ms)	1.08 (1.03–1.15)			
Baseline QTc interval (per 1 ms)	1.03 (1.00–1.07)			
Presence of T-wave inversions	0.20 (0.03–1.12)		0.16 (0.02–0.97)	
Maximal R-wave amplitude (all leads, per 1 mV)	2.76 (1.14–7.11)		2.55 (1.15–6.38)	
Maximal T-wave amplitude (all leads, per 1 mV)	3.31 (0.07–65.39)			
R/T-wave ratio (all leads, per 1 unit)	0.96 (0.87–1.02)			
Ejection fraction (per 1%)	0.94 (0.86–1.03)			
Maximal left ventricular wall thickness (per 1 mm)	1.05 (0.90–1.22)			
Left ventricular mass (per 1 g)	1.01 (0.99–1.03)			
LVOT pressure gradient (resting, per 1 mm Hg)	1.00 (0.90–1.02)			
LVOT pressure gradient (dynamic, per 1 mm Hg)	1.01 (0.99–1.02)			
Presence of LGE on CMR imaging	0.20 (0.03–1.34)			
Vectors screened (per 1 vector)	1.07 (0.83–1.28)			
Vectors passed screening (per 1 percent point)	0.06 (,0.01–3.82)			
Shock zone programming (per 1 beats/min)	0.94 (0.88–1.00)			
Conditional shock zone programming (per 1 beats/min)	0.97 (0.90–1.06)			
SMARTPass programming used	0.47 (0.09–3.03)			

AOR = adjusted odds ratio; BMI = body mass index; BSA = body surface area; CI = confidence interval; CMR = cardiovascular magnetic resonance; HCM = hypertrophic cardiomyopathy; LGE = late gadolinium enhancement; LVOT = left ventricular outflow tract; OR = odds ratio; QTc = corrected QT; SCD = sudden cardiac death.
Bolded text indicates that the variable met statistical significance.

arrhythmias. Using an "appropriateness" threshold of 4% risk, 55 patients (71%) were considered appropriate whereas 22 (29%) were not. Finally, applying the "Enhanced" American College of Cardiology/American Heart Association Strategy for prevention of SCD in high-risk patients with HCM proposed by Maron et al,[16] 73 (96%) satisfied an indication for ICD on the basis of these criteria whereas 3 (4%) did not. Sixty percent of patients satisfied

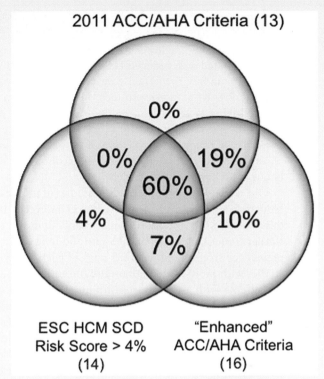

FIG 3 Preimplantation implantable cardioverter-defibrillator implantation risk stratification. Numbers reflect the proportion of the primary prevention cohort that satisfied each or multiple of the three risk stratification criteria. Two patients (3%) did not satisfy any of the criteria. ACC = American College of Cardiology; AHA = American Heart Association; ESC = European Society of Cardiology; HCM = hypertrophic cardiomyopathy; SCD = sudden cardiac death.

all three criteria, 85% satisfied at least two criteria, 97% satisfied at least one, and only two patients (3%) did not satisfy any criterion.

Other complications

Two patients ultimately underwent S-ICD extraction with implantation of a transvenous device: one due to sudden battery failure followed by failed defibrillation threshold testing after generator exchange and the second patient due to symptomatic 2:1 atrioventricular block that required pacing. There were no episodes of SCD or ventricular arrhythmias that were unsuccessfully treated by the S-ICD.

Discussion
IASs

In this multicenter study, 5.7% of 88 patients with HCM received IAS from the S-ICD over a mean follow-up of 2.7 years (w234 patient-years), with an IAS incidence of 3.8% per year. This is lower than described in earlier HCM S-ICD cohorts, which reported rates ranging from 6.2% to 12.5% over 17–22 months of follow-up.[6-8] A potential explanation is the use of SMARTPass filtering, which was used in 68% of our cohort, but was not yet available in prior studies.[6-8] The use of SMARTPass in our cohort was associated with an OR of 0.49 (95% CI 0.09–3.03) for IAS, but this did not achieve statistical significance. Another potential etiology for lower IAS rates in our study is dualzone programming, which has been associated with reduced IAS in the general S-ICD population as well as patients with HCM with an S-ICD.[8,17] Dual-zone programming was used in all our patients, but not uniformly (72%–84%) in prior studies.[7,8] Finally, contemporary ICD programming that trends toward higher tachycardia detection rates may have contributed to our lower IAS rates. In our study, our conditional and shock zones were set at 207 ± 12 and 241 ± 11 beats/min, respectively, compared with 200 ± 21 and 226 ± 18 beats/min in the EFFORTLESS S-ICD registry.[8] Indeed, a higher shock zone detection rate was associated with a reduction in IAS in our study's univariable models.

Our data correspond to trends in studies of the broader S-ICD population, which show a reduction of IAS from 11.7%–20.5% over 3–5 years of follow-up in earlier studies[18,19] down to 3.4% over a 2-year period[3] in more contemporary studies. Transvenous ICD studies show similar trends, as the era of high rate and long delay programming has decreased the IAS prevalence from the annualized rates of 6.4%–7.6% in older studies[20,21] down to 3.4% in studies with more contemporary programming.[22]

Patients with HCM present unique S-ICD IAS challenges in that they are younger, more likely to be physically active (thus more susceptible to sinus tachycardia), and have marked QRS and T-wave abnormalities. Indeed, in our study, six of nine IAS episodes were due to sinus tachycardia during exercise either resulting in TWOS or simply falling into S-ICD tachytherapy zones. Three of these were associated with medication nonadherence, which further predisposed patients to sinus tachycardia. This stresses the importance of dual-zone programming with higher rate cutoffs as well as regularly counseling on medication adherence as a means of avoiding IAS. In Figure 4 (and Online Supplemental Figure 1), we present an algorithmic approach to the management of IAS in patients with HCM.

Our study is the first to investigate predictors of IAS in patients with HCM and S-ICD. We identified the lower shock zone detection rate and prolonged QRS and QT intervals as univariable risk factors for IAS and higher R-wave amplitude as an independent multivariable risk factors for IAS (with TWIs being independently "protective" of IAS). Prior studies in the broader S-ICD population have corroborated that IAS is associated with prolonged QRS (particularly right bundle branch block) and corrected QT duration.[23] R-wave amplitude has not been previously shown to be an IAS risk factor. Our finding may seem paradoxical, as IAS are often due to TWOS in the setting of tall T waves relative to R-wave amplitude. However, there are two possible mechanisms. S-ICDs are designed, likely because of auto-decay sensing for the detection of VF, to sense a maximal QRS amplitude of 4.0 mV. Since the S-ICD rectifies the QRS signal (converting negative signal to positive), patients with particularly tall R waves may be sensitive to oversensing of Q or S complexes, which may simulate TWOS.[24] A second mechanism is that HCM patients with taller R waves likely have more aggressive forms/stages of the disease with greater hypertrophy and outflow tract obstruction and thus are more likely to have sinus tachycardia and AF, both of which were etiologies of IAS in our study. These two mechanisms may, in fact, be synergistic, as both higher R/T-wave ratios and advanced HCM have been associated with the failure of S-ICD preimplantation screening.[5] Our finding that TWIs were independently associated with *fewer* IAS is plausible, as it reduces the likelihood of double-counting T waves, but warrants further evaluation, as two of our five patients

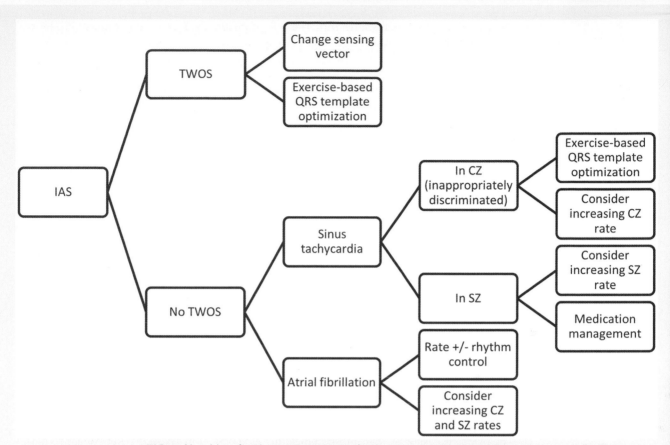

FIG 4 Algorithm for the management of subcutaneous implantable cardioveter-defibrillator inappropriate shocks (IASs) in hypertrophic cardiomyopathy (HCM) patients. This algorithm does not address non–T-wave oversensing (TWOS) forms of oversensing such as myopotentials, electromagnetic interference, or lead fracture, none of which occurred in our study. A more detailed algorithm is presented in Online Supplemental Figure 1. CZ = conditional shock zone; SZ = shock zone.

with IAS also had TWIs, and a prior study has associated TWIs with the failure of S-ICD preimplantation screening.[4]

While exercise testing has been associated with screen failure in up to 9% of patients with HCM,[5,25] no study has demonstrated a link between preimplant exercise screening and reduction in IAS. In our study, no patient who underwent prescreening with exercise testing had IAS, although the sample size is too limited to determine a direct relationship.

The role of routine postimplant exercise QRS template optimization is unclear; some studies have shown that routine exercise optimization does not reduce TWOS and IAS, although these studies did not primarily include HCM patients,[26] while others have shown prevention of recurrent TWOS by exercise QRS optimization in 87.5% of patients.[23] Five patients in our study underwent routine postimplant QRS template optimization and none of these patients experienced IAS because of TWOS or inappropriate discrimination (1 had an IAS for rapidly conducted AF in the shock zone). In addition, exercise QRS optimization was used in two patients *after* IAS. The role of postimplant exercise optimization merits further investigation.

Appropriate device therapy

The incidence of an appropriate S-ICD intervention was surprisingly low in our study, with the only two appropriate shocks in the whole cohort occurring in the seven patients implanted for secondary prevention. On the basis of the calculated European HCM Risk-SCD score (mean 5.7% 5-year risk), we anticipated seeing w3 appropriate shocks in our cohort of 81 patients implanted for primary prevention, although none occurred. To further investigate this low appropriate shock rate, we determined that the majority of S-ICDs in our study were "indicated," as 79 of 81 patients met at least one of the three established HCM primary prevention criteria.

Many prior studies that defined existing SCD risk factors in HCM ICD guidelines used appropriate ICD therapies as a surrogate end point for SCD.[14] Thus, SCD risks may be overestimated in older studies in which ICDs were traditionally programmed with shorter delays and lower rate thresholds. The typically higher heart rate cutoffs (mean shock zone 241 beats/min in our study) and longer charge times of S-ICDs may prevent seemingly "appropriate" therapies that would have previously been delivered for VT episodes that would have otherwise self-terminated. Our lower-than-expected appropriate shock rate, particularly in our patients implanted for primary prevention, warrants further investigation, as does the lack of agreement between the three established ICD criteria.

Study limitations

While we report on a relatively large cohort of patients with HCM with an S-ICD, the incidence of IAS in our study was low and limited our statistical power to detect independent IAS predictors. The duration of follow-up in our study, while longer than most other studies of IAS,[6–8] was shorter than most studies that assess SCD in HCM.[14,16] Retrospective data collection may limit completeness of data. The lack of a separate cohort of HCM patients with transvenous ICDs limits comparison between device types for both IAS and appropriate therapies. Lastly, we collected data from four high-volume geographically diverse HCM centers, and this may not be representative of community S-ICD utilization and experience.

Conclusion

In a multicenter international HCM S-ICD cohort, 5.7% of patients received IAS (3.8 IAS episodes per 100 patient-years), which is lower than previously reported. The ECG R-wave amplitude was independently associated with an increased risk of IAS, whereas TWIs were protective. IAS were often due to sinus tachycardia with and without TWOS in the setting of exercise. Particularly for patients with tall R waves, we recommend preimplantation S-ICD screening with exercise and considering postimplantation exercise-based QRS template optimization. The incidence of appropriate shocks was lower than expected, as there were none in 81 patients implanted for primary prevention, 97% of whom met the established HCM ICD criteria, which may warrant reassessment.

Appendix

Supplementary data

Supplementary data associated with this article can be found in the online version at https://doi.org/10.1016/j.hrthm.2020.02.008.

REFERENCES

1. Ho, CY, Day, SM, Ashley, EA, et al. (2018). Genotype and lifetime burden of disease in hypertrophic cardiomyopathy insights from the sarcomeric human cardiomyopathy registry (SHaRe). *Circulation, 138,* 1387–1398.

2. Al-Khatib, SM, Stevenson, WG, Ackerman, MJ, et al. (2018). 2017 AHA/ACC/HRS guideline for management of patients with ventricular arrhythmias and the prevention of sudden cardiac death: executive summary. *Heart Rhythm, 15,* e190–e252.

3. Zeitler, EP, Friedman, DJ, Loring, Z, et al. (2020). Complications involving the subcutaneous implantable cardioverter-defibrillator: lessons learned from MAUDE. *Heart Rhythm, 17,* 447–454.

4. Maurizi, N, Olivotto, I, Olde Nordkamp, LRA, et al. (2016). Prevalence of subcutaneous implantable cardioverter-defibrillator candidacy based on template ECG screening in patients with hypertrophic cardiomyopathy. *Heart Rhythm, 13,* 457–463.

5. Srinivasan, NT, Patel, KH, Qamar, K, et al. (2017). Disease severity and exercise testing reduce subcutaneous implantable cardioverter-defibrillator left sternal ECG screening success in hypertrophic cardiomyopathy. *Circ Arrhythm Electrophy- siol, 10.*

6. Weinstock, J, Bader, YH, Maron, MS, Rowin, EJ, & Link, MS. (2016). Subcutaneous implant- able cardioverter defibrillator in patients with hypertrophic cardiomyopathy: an initial experience. *J Am Heart Assoc, 5,* 1–7.

7. Olde Nordkamp, LRA, Brouwer, TF, Barr, C, et al. (2015). Inappropriate shocks in the sub- cutaneous ICD: incidence, predictors and management. *Int J Cardiol, 195,* 126–133.

8. Lambiase, PD, Gold, MR, Hood, M, et al. (2016). Evaluation of subcutaneous ICD early performance in hypertrophic cardiomyopathy from the pooled EFFORTLESS and IDE cohorts. *Heart Rhythm, 13,* 1066–1074.

9. Theuns, DAMJ, Brouwer, TF, Jones, PW, et al. (2018). Prospective blinded evaluation of a novel sensing methodology designed to reduce inappropriate shocks by the subcutaneous implantable cardioverter-defibrillator. *Heart Rhythm, 15,* 1515–1522.

10. Knops, RE, Olde Nordkamp, LRA, De Groot, JR, & Wilde, AAM (2013). Two-incision tech- nique for implantation of the subcutaneous implantable cardioverter-defibrillator. *Heart Rhythm, 10,* 1240–1243.

11. Kleijn, S, & Van Der Veldt, A (2010). An entirely subcutaneous implantable cardioverter-defibrillator. *N Engl J Med, 363,* 1577.

12. Firth, D. (1995). Amendments and corrections: bias reduction of maximum likelihood estimates. *Biometrika, 82,* 667.

13. Gersh, BJ, Maron, BJ, Bonow, RO, et al. (2011). 2011 ACCF/AHA guideline for the diagnosis and treatment of hypertrophic cardiomyopathy: executive summary. *J Thorac Cardiovasc Surg, 142,* 1303–1338.

14. O'Mahony, C, Jichi, F, Pavlou, M, et al. (2014). A novel clinical risk prediction model for sudden cardiac death in hypertrophic cardiomyopathy (HCM Risk-SCD). *Eur Heart J, 35,* 2010–2020.

15. O'Mahony, C, Jichi, F, Ommen, SR, et al. (2018). International external validation study of the 2014 European Society of Cardiology Guidelines on Sudden Cardiac Death Prevention in Hypertrophic Cardiomyopathy (EVIDENCE-HCM). *Circulation, 137,* 1015–1023.

16. Maron, MS, Rowin, EJ, Wessler, BS, et al. (2019). Enhanced American College of Cardiology/ American Heart Association strategy for prevention of sudden cardiac death in high-risk patients with hypertrophic cardiomyopathy. *JAMA Cardiol, 02111,* 1–14.

17. Weiss, R, Knight, BP, Gold, MR, et al. (2013). Safety and efficacy of a totally subcutaneous implantable-cardioverter defibrillator. *Circulation, 128,* 944–953.

18. Brouwer, TF, Yilmaz, D, Lindeboom, R, et al. (2016). Long-term clinical outcomes of sub- cutaneous versus transvenous implantable defibrillator therapy. *J Am Coll Cardiol, 68,* 2047–2055.

19. Boersma, L, Barr, C, Knops, R, et al. (2017). Implant and midterm outcomes of the subcu- taneous implantable cardioverter-defibrillator registry: the EFFORTLESS study. *J Am Coll Cardiol, 70,* 830–841.

20. Auricchio, A, Schloss, EJ, Kurita, T, et al. (2015). Low inappropriate shock rates in patients with single- and dual/triple-chamber implantable cardioverter-defibrillators using a novel suite of detection algorithms: PainFree SST trial primary results. *Heart Rhythm, 12*, 926–936.

21. Moss, AJ, Zareba, W, Hall, WJ, et al. (2002). Prophylactic implantation of a defibrillator in patients with myocardial infarction and reduced ejection fraction. *N Engl J Med, 346*, 6.

22. Moss, AJ, Schuger, C, Beck, CA, et al. (2012). Reduction in inappropriate therapy and mortality through ICD programming. *N Engl J Med, 367*, 2275–2283.

23. Kooiman, KM, Knops, RE, Olde Nordkamp, L, Wilde, AAM, & De Groot, JR (2014). Inappropriate subcutaneous implantable cardioverter-defibrillator shocks due to T-wave oversensing can be prevented: implications for management. *Heart Rhythm, 11*, 426–434.

24. Batul, SA, Yang, F, Wats, K, Shrestha, S, & Greenberg, YJ. (2017). Inappropriate subcutane- ous implantable cardioverter-defibrillator therapy due to R-wave amplitude variation: another challenge in device management. *HeartRhythm Case Rep, 3*, 78–82.

25. Francia, P, Adduci, C, Palano, F, et al. (2015). Eligibility for the subcutaneous implantable cardioverter-defibrillator in patients with hypertrophic cardiomyopathy. *J Cardi- ovasc Electrophysiol, 26*, 893–899.

26. Afzal, MR, Evenson, C, Badin, A, et al. (2017). Role of exercise electrocardiogram to screen for T-wave oversensing after implantation of subcutaneous implantable cardioverter-defibrillator. *Heart Rhythm, 14*, 1436–1439.

Review of the Literature

The introduction of the article clearly explains that younger adults (median age 45.8 years) diagnosed with hypertrophic cardiomyopathy (HCM) remain at increased for of ventricular arrhythmias and therefore sudden cardiac death (SCD). The preferred device among this population, a subcutaneous implantable cardioverter defibrillator (S-ICD), offers advantages compared with an implantable cardioverter-defibrillator (ICD) or pacemaker. Transvenous leads commonly associated with ICDs or pacemakers generate higher-risk secondary to chronic indwelling transvenous leads. Although S-ICDs present advantages, the authors highlight that patients with HCM frequently develop prominent QRS- and T-wave abnormalities on ECG, leading to a higher incidence of T-wave oversensing. Aberration in the S-ICDs sensing algorithm without concomitant device reprogramming can cause incidence of inappropriate shock (IAS). As such, 14% to 38% of patients diagnosed with HCM are deemed inappropriate for S-ICD implantation. Improvements in sensing algorithms and reprogramming function have led to significant reduction, up to 68%, in the rate of IAS. The researchers present a clear description of the indications of S-ICD implantation in this patient population based on a current review of the published literature. Yet there is a gap in the literature about the use of S-ICDs among younger adults diagnosed with HCM. The current study will address gaps in the literature associated specifically with IAS use among younger adults diagnosed with HCM.

Research Questions

The researchers clearly establish that patients with HCM are appropriate candidates for S-ICDs to mitigate the risks associated with use of transvenous leads seen in younger adult patients. However, the IAS among patients with S-ICDs may be higher. The research questions are embedded in the objectives of this study and clearly stated as follows: "to determine the incidence of both appropriate and inappropriate device therapies in a multicenter cohort of HCM patients with an S-ICD and to determine predictors of IAS."

Research Design

In this retrospective cohort study, providing Level IV evidence, the researchers examined the incidence, predictors, and potential risk factors a priori, associated with IAS in S-ICD patients.

This is a nonexperimental study because randomization was not used, there is no manipulation of the independent variable(s), and there is no CG. The relationship between the independent and dependent variable(s) is explored, but no causality can be inferred. It is important to note that although this study provides a lower level of evidence than an RCT, as long as the design is sound and appropriate for the research questions, it may provide important preliminary data to support future intervention studies. Because there is a gap in the literature, the findings of this study may provide the best available evidence.

Sample

A sample of 88 patients diagnosed with HCM who received an S-ICD between 2014 and 2019 across four international centers were enrolled in this retrospective cohort study. Of these, 81 participants received an S-ICD for primary prevention, and 7 participants received an ICD for secondary prevention. The authors clearly described the recruitment and enrollment process; inclusion criteria were appropriate for the design. The adequacy of the sample size was not justified with use of power analysis.

Methods

Electrocardiographic evidence (preimplant and postimplant) and clinical data were collected from a sample ($n = 88$) of consecutive patients diagnosed with HCM who received S-ICD implantation across four international HCM medical centers. Appropriate baseline data, including screening from preimplant and postimplant data (i.e., ECGs, specifically QRS and QT intervals; manual measurement of R- and T-wave amplitudes; and T-wave inversions) were collected using retrospective, an electronic medical record audit. The clinical indication to implant an S-ICD, as determined by the treating provider, was included in the study. Patients were screened using a standardized three-lead ECG screening tool manufactured by Boston Scientific and positioning screening vectors. Defibrillation threshold testing on implanted S-ICDs was performed on implantation with two therapy zones set at conditional shock at 180 to 240 beats per minute and shock zone set at 200 to 250 beats per minute. A strength was that review of shocks were independently reviewed by two investigators to determine whether these were inappropriate or appropriate. Any multiple IAS delivered sequentially was determined as one encounter for inclusion in the data analysis. The researchers adjusted for etiologies of all sustained S-ICD shocks.

Threats to Internal Validity

Cohort studies are useful in estimating the risk for disease, incidence rate, and relative risk. To generate statistical power for the accurate detection of IAS predictors, an adequate sample size is necessary. Therefore the small sample poses a threat to internal validity, and there was no power analysis reported to validate the adequacy of the sample size to determine significance. However, the possibility of detection bias was moderated based on clearly established protocols with two independent investigators validating data, such as ECG waveform measurements and screening criteria. The extensive use of physiological measures and outcome variables is a strength of the study and minimizes measurement bias. Although the researchers indicate that the follow-up data point for IAS studies was longer than most, it was shorter than most studies that examine sudden cardiac death in

HCM, which contributes to increased risk for bias. Investigators also identify limitations of the comparator group, a cohort of HCM patients with transvenous ICD implantation, for examining differences in IAS and appropriate shock. Retrospective cohort studies pose common threats, such as presenting limitations to the completeness of these data. However apparent threats from selection bias, recall bias, history, mortality (or attrition), maturation, instrumentation, or testing do not appear to be relevant in this study.

Threats to External Validity

Selection Effects

The researchers offer that collecting data among four HCM international centers that offer geographical variability but a small sample may not offer representative data of regional S-ICD clinical practice.

Instrumentation

In this retrospective cohort study, electrographic evidence and clinical data were collected from electronic health records (EHRs) among four HCM centers. A strength of the study is that baseline characteristics, screening preimplant and postimplant (decision to implant; screening tool; and threshold testing), and follow-up data were captured appropriately from retrospective EHR review. Well-established preimplantation ICD risk stratification criteria with high reliability and validity including the 2011 ACC/AHA HCM guidelines, European HCM Risk-SCD score, and "Enhanced" ACC/AHA Strategy were employed.

Legal-Ethical Considerations

The research was approved by appropriate institutional review boards across the four multisite centers. The data are collected from EHRs, so there is no risk to patients.

Data Analysis

The aim of the data analysis was to report baseline characteristics among HCM patients receiving inappropriate shock. Table 18.1 succinctly displays these data presented as median (interquartile range) or n (%). To express incidence, etiology, and clinical response to IAS among patients with S-ICD, a clearly presented flowchart is displayed in Fig. 18.1. Potential predictors of risk factors correlating with IAS (wider QRS complex, longer QTc interval, R-wave amplitude, and lower shock zone detection) were appropriately analyzed using univariate analysis, whereas, multivariate analysis examined R-wave amplitude and T-wave inversion. These data are clearly expressed as OR in Table 3. Three tables and three figures were appropriately used to visually display these data. The researchers state that statistical modeling was chosen to reduce bias associated with a small sample size and infrequent outcome. Appropriate use of odds ratios and 95% likelihood confidence intervals were reported. Case analyses were performed using SAS 9.4 version.

Results

The HCM study cohort ($n = 88$) were followed for a mean of 2.7 +/− 1.3 years after S-ICD implantation. Of the cohort, five patients (5.7%) received 9 IAS at follow up; seven of these (78%) received IAS within 1 year postimplant. Explanations for five of the nine IAS included T-wave oversensing, and two of these occurred in the context of atrial fibrillation (AFIB) with rapid ventricular response (RVR); three occurred secondary to sensing sinus tachycardia while on a β-blocker or calcium channel blocker.

Results of appropriate shocks were based on an analysis of three cohorts: primary prevention, secondary prevention, and entire sample. Based on appropriate shocks on average follow-up (2.7 +/− 1.3 years), only two patients from the sample received appropriate shocks (these had S-ICD implantation for secondary prevention); no patients received an appropriate shock who had an implant for primary prevention. Further rigorous risk stratification criteria were applied using the 2011 American College of Cardiology/American Heart Association (ACC/AHA) HCM guidelines given the absence of appropriate shocks among a primary prevention HCM SCD cohort. Of these 77 patients included in the analysis, 81% met indications for class IIa and 19% met either class IIb or class III. To predict the risk for ventricular arrhythmias, scores were further validated using the European HCM Risk-SCD score and demonstrated 5.7% +/− 3.4% 5-year risk. Further validation of appropriateness of implant using an "Enhanced" ACC/AHA Strategy for HCM patients at high-risk for sudden cardiac death showed that ICD was indicated in 96% of the sample; 60% satisfied all three of the screening tool's criteria, 85% met two criteria, and 97% met at least one criteria.

Conclusions, Implications, and Recommendations

Conclusions and implications for practice are clearly stated and are consistent with the reported results. Recommendations for future research are implied, but not overstated, in the discussion. Of this HCM cohort with S-ICD, 5.7% of patients received IAS; R-wave amplitude was found to be an independent associate of increased IAS risk, and T-wave inversions were reported as protective. The incidence of appropriate shocks among 81 patients who received S-ICD for primary prevention were found to be lower than what was expected.

Implications for Nursing Practice

This multicenter international retrospective cohort study provides data on incidence and predictors associated with appropriate and IAS after S-ICD implantation among HCM patients. Noteworthy is that younger adult patients are prone to increased physical activity patterns and sinus tachycardia along with marked QRS and T-wave irregularities. Noncompliance of medications were found in three patients, which predisposed them to sinus tachycardia. Considerations for patient education, reprogramming, and the use of SMARTPass algorithms lends useful information when applying the findings from this study to HCM patients with S-ICD. There was minimal to no risk associated with this study. Dissemination of the data from this study provides future researchers and clinicians a basis for future research which includes a larger sample size and a comparison group.

CLINICAL JUDGMENT CHALLENGES

- Discuss how the stylistic considerations of a journal affect the researcher's ability to present the research findings of a quantitative report.
- Discuss how the limitations of a research study affect generalizability of the findings.
- Discuss how you differentiate the "critical appraisal" process from simply "criticizing" a research report.
- Analyze how threats to internal and external validity affect the strength and quality of evidence provided by the findings of a research study.
- How would a staff nurse who has just critically appraised the study by Nazer et al. (2020) determine whether the findings of this study were applicable to practice?

PART IV

Application of Research: Evidence-Based Practice

Research Vignette: Shannon Munro and **Dian P. Baker**

RESEARCH VIGNETTE

COAST TO COAST: PREVENTING HARM BY REDUCING HOSPITAL ACQUIRED PNEUMONIA

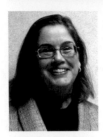

Shannon Munro, PhD, APRN, NP
Researcher
Diffusion of Excellence Initiative
Veterans Health Administration
Salem, Virginia

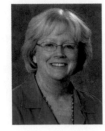

Dian P. Baker, PhD, APRN-BC
Professor, Nursing
California State University, Sacramento
Sacramento, California

It is estimated that only half of evidence-based practices ever reach widespread clinical application and directly affect public health (Bauer et al., 2015). To move research and best practice quickly to the bedside requires grit, determination, and interdisciplinary collaboration. From opposite coasts, this team of researchers joined forces to improve the health and quality of life of hospitalized patients and call attention to the preventable harm of non–ventilator-associated hospital-acquired pneumonia (NV-HAP).

NV-HAP is one of the most common hospital-acquired infections; however, most hospitals do not routinely conduct surveillance or implement NV-HAP prevention measures. Therefore the team is spreading the word about NV-HAP, an underappreciated, preventable patient safety issue that contributes to high health care costs, longer lengths of stay, and increased morbidity and mortality (Giuliano et al., 2018; Munro & Baker, 2018). Although some hospitalized patients are clearly at higher risk (e.g., medically fragile, immune compromised), all patients carry some risk of developing NV-HAP, including young, healthy patients (Baker & Quinn, 2018; Baker et al., 2019; Munro & Baker, 2018). Each NV-HAP case costs an estimated $40,000; thus, preventing 100 cases may save up to $400 million, 700 to 900 hospital days, and the lives of 20 to 30 patients (Quinn et al., 2014).

Because hospital-acquired pneumonia frequently originates from bacteria in the mouth that migrate to the lungs, the team chose to focus its efforts on improving oral hygiene. Poor oral care is a modifiable risk factor for NV-HAP and, frequently, a missed care opportunity in the hospital setting, with up to 82% of patients not receiving any oral care assistance during their stay (Kalisch et al., 2009; Kalisch & Xie, 2014).

Implementation science is never done in isolation, and this team has built on the work of many experts in the field with the support of partners in nursing, medicine, dentistry, speech and language pathology, health informatics, and other disciplines.

These two advanced practice nurses partnered to scale this program of research that translates research evidence to the bedside:

Dr. Dian Baker served as an investigator in five research studies, including a national 21-hospital study on the incidence of NV-HAP and the effect of prevention-related interventions like oral care. In addition, she studied Healthcare Cost and Utilization Project (HCUP) data for NV-HAP risks and outcomes and the relationship between sepsis and NV-HAP. Dr. Baker launched the international hospital-acquired pneumonia prevention implementation, evaluation, and research project. Her team has supported more than 50 nurses' efforts in leading NV-HAP prevention at their respective hospitals.

Dr. Shannon Munro successfully piloted, scaled, and spread local research on NV-HAP prevention as best practice in VA Medical Centers nationwide. The VA team significantly reduced the risk of developing NV-HAP by providing consistent oral hygiene during hospital admissions. As of August 2020, 75 VA hospitals and 256 units were implementing the practice, with additional spread planned for the future. The team is in the midst of a partnered evaluation of the implementation and dissemination process and health outcomes for veterans receiving care in the following types of units: medical-surgical and presurgical; intensive care; oncology, hospice, and palliative care; geriatrics and long-term care; spinal cord injury; blind rehabilitation; and inpatient mental health. Dr. Munro received support and funding from the Veterans Health Administration (VHA) Diffusion of Excellence Initiative; Quality Enhancement Research Initiative; Veterans Engineering Resource Center; Office of Strategic Integration; Center of Innovation for Veteran-Centered and Value-Driven Care; and the VHA Offices of Nursing, Dental, and Rural Health. Based on this research, national VA trends in NV-HAP rates decreased on acute care units between 2016 and 2020 based on electronic medical record coding data.

The work of this team is interconnected and can be summarized into these general areas:

1. Improving understanding of NV-HAP risk factors, including missed oral care (Munro & Baker, 2018; Munro et al., 2018)
2. Calculating the incidence of NV-HAP and related sequelae, such as sepsis (Giuliano & Baker, 2020; Giuliano et al., 2018; Munro & Baker, 2018)
3. Identifying barriers, challenges, and facilitators in launching a prevention initiative among multiple hospitals across private industry and the VHA (Baker et al., 2019; Munro & Baker, 2018; Munro et al., 2018)
4. Evaluating the oral care initiative to prevent NV-HAP, including the implementation process, tools and strategies, and health outcomes across a variety of health care settings (e.g., acute care, rehabilitation, long-term care units) (Baker et al., 2019; Munro & Baker, 2018; Munro et al., 2018)
5. Determining how nurse leaders affect patient safety and quality in large-scale quality improvement initiatives (Baker et al., 2019; Munro & Baker, 2018; Munro et al., 2018)
6. Developing a national research agenda, policy, and implementation strategy with VA leadership, the Centers for Disease Control and Prevention (CDC), The Joint Commission, the U.S. Food and Drug Administration (FDA), the American Dental Association (ADA), the Health Resources and Services Administration (HRSA), the Patient Safety

Movement Foundation, and private industry, along with experts in the fields of dentistry, geriatrics, implementation science, informatics, nursing, and medicine.

Nurses have the unique opportunity to address patient safety issues they see firsthand, work together to improve health outcomes, and spread promising evidence-based practice to the bedside nationwide. This team is excited to be partnering with national health care leaders to make oral care for hospitalized patients and long-term care residents the standard of care and to develop policies and strategies to continue scaling the initiative to reduce the risk of NV-HAP to improve the lives and health of generations to come.

REFERENCES

Baker, D., & Quinn, B. (2018). Hospital Acquired Pneumonia Prevention Initiative-2: Incidence of nonventilator hospital-acquired pneumonia in the United States. *American Journal of Infection Control, 46*(1), 2–7. https://doi.org/10.1016/j.ajic.2017.08.036.

Baker, D., Quinn, B., Ewan, V., & Giuliano, K. K. (2019). Sustaining quality improvement: Long-term reduction of nonventilator hospital-acquired pneumonia. *Journal of Nursing Care Quality, 34*(3), 223–229. https://doi.org/10.1097/NCQ.0000000000000359.

Bauer, M. S., Damschroder, L., Hagedorn, H., Smith, A. M., & Kilbourne, A. M. (2015). An introduction to implementation science for the non-specialist. *BMC Psychology, 3*(1), 32. https://doi.org/10.1186/s40359-015-0089-9.

Giuliano, K., & Baker, D. (2020). Sepsis in the context of nonventilator hospital-acquired pneumonia. *American Journal of Critical Care, 29*(1), 9–14.

Giuliano, K., Baker, D., & Quinn, B. (2018). The epidemiology of nonventilator hospital-acquired pneumonia in the United States. *American Journal of Infection Control, 46*(3), 322–327. https://doi.org/10.1016/j.ajic.2017.09.005.

Kalisch, B. J., Landstrom, G., & Williams, R. A. (2009). Missed nursing care: Errors of omission. *Nursing Outlook, 57*(1), 3–9. https://doi.org/10.1016/j.outlook.2008.05.007.

Kalisch, B. J., & Xie, B. (2014). Errors of omission: missed nursing care. *Western Journal of Nursing Research, 36*(7), 875–890. https://doi.org/10.1177/0193945914531859.

Munro, S., & Baker, D. (2018). Reducing missed oral care opportunities to prevent non-ventilator associated hospital acquired pneumonia at the Department of Veterans Affairs. *Applied Nursing Research, 44*, 48–53. https://doi.org/10.1016/j.apnr.2018.09.004.

Munro, S., Haile-Mariam, A., Greenwell, C., Demirci, S., Farooqi, O., & Vasudeva, S. (2018). Implementation and dissemination of a Department of Veterans Affairs oral care initiative to prevent hospital acquired pneumonia among non-ventilated patients. *Nursing Administration Quarterly, 42*(4), 363–372. https://doi.org/10.1097/NAQ.0000000000000308.

Quinn, B., Baker, D., Munro-Cohen, S., Stewart, J., Lima, C., & Parise, C. (2014). Basic nursing care to prevent non-ventilator hospital acquired pneumonia. *Journal of Nursing Scholarship, 46*(1), 11–19. https://doi.org/10.1111/jnu.12050.

19

Strategies and Tools for Developing an Evidence-Based Practice

Carl A. Kirton

Go to Evolve at **http://evolve.elsevier.com/LoBiondo/** for review questions.

LEARNING OUTCOMES

After reading this chapter, you should be able to do the following:

- Identify the key elements of a focused clinical question.
- Discuss the use of databases to search the literature.
- Review a research article for relevance and validity.
- Critically appraise study results and apply the findings to practice.
- Make clinical decisions based on evidence from the literature combined with clinical expertise and patient preferences.

KEY TERMS

confidence interval	negative likelihood ratio	odds ratio	relative risk
electronic index	negative predictive value	positive likelihood ratio	relative risk reduction
information literacy	null value	positive predictive value	sensitivity
likelihood ratio	number needed to treat	prefiltered evidence	specificity

In today's environment of knowledge explosion, new investigations that potentially affect maintaining a practice that is based on evidence can be challenging. However, the development of an evidence-based nursing practice is contingent on applying new and important evidence to clinical practice. A few simple strategies will help you move to a practice that is evidence oriented. This chapter will assist you in becoming a more efficient and effective reader of the literature. Through a few important tools and a crisp understanding of the important components of a study you will be able to use an evidence base to determine the merits of a study for your practice and for your patients.

Consider the case of a nurse who uses evidence from the literature to support her practice: Melody Tavares is a staff registered nurse who works in the pediatric clinic of a publicly funded city health system that serves a diverse population with few neighborhood supermarkets. The geographical area sometimes has been described as a "food desert," with a scarcity of food stores with fresh fruits and vegetables as well as other affordable healthy food choices.

As part of her nursing assessment, Melody obtains and records the body mass index (BMI) of all children. She routinely observes that most of her pediatric patients have a BMI in the 80th to 95th percentile for their age. Melody routinely provides education to parents of pediatric patients to avoid sweetened beverages as a weight-reduction strategy for children with a high BMI. Melody wants to be certain that consumption of SSBs in childhood is associated with obesity and decides to consult the literature to answer this question.

EVIDENCE-BASED STRATEGY #1: ASKING A FOCUSED CLINICAL QUESTION

Developing a focused clinical question will help Melody focus on the relevant issue and prepare her for subsequent steps in the evidence-based practice process (see Chapters 1 to 3). A focused clinical question using the PICO format (see Chapters 2 and 3) is developed by answering the following four questions:

1. What is the *population* I am interested in?
2. What is the *intervention* I am interested in?
3. What will this intervention be *compared* with? (Note: Depending on the study design, this step may or may not apply.)
4. How will I know if the intervention makes things better or worse (thus identifying an *outcome* that is measurable)?

As you recall from Chapters 2 and 3, the simple mnemonic PICO is used to develop a well-designed clinical question (Table 19.1). Using this format, Melody develops the following clinical question: *Does the consumption of sugar-sweetened beverages [intervention] in comparison to consumption of unsweetened beverages [comparison] during childhood [population] increase body weight [outcome]?*

Once a clinical question has been framed, it is useful to assign the question to a clinical category. These categories are predominately based on study designs that you read about in previous chapters. These categories help you search for the correct type of study to answer the clinical question. Being able to critically appraise research is an important skill in evidence-based practice. Because clinicians may feel they lack the skills to appraise published research, clinical category worksheets are available to guide your assessment of the extent to which the author implemented a well-designed study. It also helps you answer the important question of whether or not the study findings apply to your specific patient or group.

- **Therapy category:** When you want to answer a question about the effectiveness of a particular treatment or intervention, you will select studies that have the following characteristics:
  - An experimental or quasi-experimental study design (see Chapter 9)
  - Outcome known or of probable clinical importance observed over a clinically significant period

TABLE 19.1	**Using PICO to Formulate Clinical Questions**	
Patient population	What group do you want information on?	Children
Intervention (or exposure)	What event do you want to study the effect of?	Sugar-sweetened beverages
Comparison	Compared with what? Is it better or worse than no intervention at all or than another intervention?	No sugar-sweetened beverages
Outcomes	What is the effect of the intervention?	Body mass index

For studies in this category, you will use a therapy appraisal tool to evaluate the study. A therapy tool can be accessed at https://www.cebm.net/wp-content/uploads/2018/11/RCT.pdf.

- **Diagnosis category:** When you want to answer a question about the usefulness, accuracy, selection, or interpretation of a particular measurement instrument or laboratory test, you will select studies that have the following characteristics:
  - Cross-sectional/case control/retrospective study design (see Chapter 10) with individuals suspected to have the condition of interest
  - Administration to the patient of both the new instrument or diagnostic test and the accepted "gold standard" measure
  - Comparison of the results of the new instrument or test and the "gold standard"

For studies in this category, you will use a diagnostic test appraisal tool to evaluate the article. A diagnostic tool can be accessed at https://www.cebm.net/wp-content/uploads/2018/11/Diagnostic-Accuracy-Studies.pdf

- **Prognosis category:** When you want to answer a question about a patient's likely course for a particular disease state or identify factors that may alter the patient's prognosis, you will select studies that have the following characteristics:
  - Nonexperimental, usually a longitudinal/cohort/prospective study of a particular group for a specific outcome or disease (see Chapter 10)
  - Follow-up for a clinically relevant period (time is the exposure)
  - Determination of factors in those who do and do not develop a particular outcome

For studies in this category, you will use a prognosis appraisal tool (sometimes called a *cohort tool*) to evaluate the study. A prognosis tool can be accessed at https://www.cebm.net/wp-content/uploads/2018/11/Prognosis.pdf.

- **Harm category:** When you want to determine the cause(s) of a particular symptom, problem, or disorder, you will select studies that have the following characteristics:
  - Nonexperimental, usually longitudinal or retrospective (ex post facto/case control study designs over a clinically relevant period; see Chapter 10)
  - Assessment of whether or not the patient has been exposed to the independent variable

For studies in this category, you use a harm appraisal tool (sometimes called a case-control tool) to evaluate the study. A harm tool can be accessed at https://www.cebm.net/wp-content/uploads/2018/11/Diagnostic-Accuracy-Studies.pdf. This is the same tool as the one used for critical appraisal of diagnostic accuracy.

EVIDENCE-BASED STRATEGY #2: SEARCHING THE LITERATURE

All of the skills that Melody needs to consult the literature and answer a clinical question are conceptually defined as information literacy. Your librarian is the best person to help you develop the necessary skills to become information literate. Part of being information literate is having the skills necessary to electronically search the literature to obtain the best evidence for answering your clinical question.

The literature is organized into electronic indexes or *databases*. Chapter 3 discusses the differences among databases and how to use these databases to search the literature. *CINHAL* is a popular database for nursing and health-related literature. You can also learn how to effectively search this database through an Internet-based tutorial. A beginner-level CINHAL search tutorial can be accessed at https://www.youtube.com/watch?v=euBWwBYbFSM, and an advanced-level CINHAL search tutorial can be accessed at https://www.youtube.com /watch?v=OTvSwEZ1pP4.

Using the CINHAL database (https://www.ebscohost.com/nursing/products/cinahl -databases), Melody uses the search function and enters the term "sugar sweetened beverages AND children." This strategy provides her with 896 articles. Of course, there are too many articles for Melody to review, and she does a quick scan and realizes that many of the articles do not answer her clinical question. Many are not research studies, and some articles have nothing to do with sugar sweeteners consumed by children. She recalls that the CINHAL database has a filter option that helps her find citations that correspond to a specific clinical category. A careful perusal of the list of articles and a well-designed clinical question help Melody select the key articles.

EVIDENCE-BASED PRACTICE TIP

Prefiltered sources of evidence can be found in journals and electronic format. **Prefiltered evidence** is evidence in which an editorial team has already read and summarized articles on a topic and appraised its relevance to clinical care. Prefiltered sources include *Evidence-based Nursing,* available online at http://ebn.bmj.com/ and in print, and the Joanna Briggs Institute EBP Database, available online through University or institutional libraries.

EVIDENCE-BASED STRATEGY #3: SCREENING YOUR FINDINGS

Once you have searched and selected the potential articles, how do you know which articles are appropriate to answer your clinical question? This is accomplished by screening the articles for quality, relevance, and credibility by answering the following questions (Kloda et al., 2020; LoBiondo-Wood et al., 2019):

1. Is each study from a peer-reviewed journal? Studies published in peer-reviewed journals have been through an extensive review and editing process (see Chapter 3).
2. Are the setting and sample of each study similar to mine so that results, if valid, would apply to my practice or to my patient population (see Chapter 12)?
3. Are any of the studies sponsored by an organization that may influence the study design or results (see Chapter 13)?

Your responses to these questions can help you decide to what extent you want to appraise each article. **Example:** ➤ If the study population is markedly different from the one to which you will apply the results, you may want to consider selecting a more appropriate study. If an article is worth evaluating, you should use the category-specific tool identified in evidence-based strategy #1 to critically appraise the article.

Melody reviews the abstract of the articles retrieved from her CINHAL citation lists and selects the following article: "Consumption of sugar-sweetened beverages and obesity in SNAP-eligible children and adolescents" (Twarog et al., 2020). This study was published in 2020 in *Primary Care Diabetes,* a peer-reviewed journal. This is an observational study that has a longitudinal/cohort design and examines factors that lead to a specific outcome of interest (obesity). Melody reads the abstract and finds that the objective of the study was to examine the association between Supplemental Nutrition Assistance Program (SNAP) participation and self-reported sugar-sweetened beverage (SSB) consumption and the association between self-reported SSB consumption and overweight/obesity in low-income children. This was a population-based sample of US children, 2 to 17 years of age, who completed the Dietary Screener Questionnaire and had a physical examination as part of

National Health and Nutrition Examination Survey (NHANES) during the 2009 to 2010 period. Melody knows that because this is a population-based study, there is good generalizability (see Chapter 8). Further, many of her patients receive nutrition assistance under the SNAP program, which is an added benefit. Melody finds that there were no funding or conflict of interest issues noted; she decides that this study is worth evaluating and selects the prognosis category tool.

HELPFUL HINT

If you are selecting a therapy study, consider both studies with significant findings (treatment is better) and studies with nonsignificant findings (treatment is worse, or there is no difference). Studies reporting nonsignificant findings are more difficult to find but are equally important.

EVIDENCE-BASED STRATEGY #4: APPRAISE EACH ARTICLE'S FINDINGS

Applying study results to individual patients or to a specific patient population and communicating study findings to patients in a meaningful way are the hallmark of evidence-based practice. Common evidence-based practice conventions that researchers and research consumers use to appraise and report study results are identified by four different types of clinical categories: therapy, diagnosis (sensitivity and specificity), prognosis, and harm. The language common to meta-analysis was discussed in Chapter 11. An appraisal tool for a meta-analysis (systematic review) can be found at https://www.cebm.net/wp-content /uploads/2019/01/Systematic-Review.pdf. Familiarity with these evidence-based practice clinical categories will help Melody search for, screen, select, and appraise articles appropriate for answering clinical questions.

Therapy Category

In articles that belong to the therapy category (experimental, randomized controlled trials [RCTs], or intervention studies), investigators attempt to determine whether a difference exists between two or more interventions. The evidence-based language used in a therapy article depends on whether the numerical values of the study variables are *continuous* (a variable that measures a degree of change or a difference on a range, such as blood pressure) or *discrete*, also known as *dichotomous* (measuring whether or not an event did or did not occur, such as the number of children diagnosed with obesity) (Table 19.2).

TABLE 19.2 Difference Between Continuous and Discrete Variables

Researcher Objective	Variable	How the Outcome Is Described in the Research Article
Continuous Variables		
Researcher is interested in degree of change after exposure to an intervention	Pain score, levels of psychological distress, blood pressure, weight	Measures of central tendency (e.g., mean, median, or standard deviation)
Discrete Variables		
Researcher is interested in whether or not an "event" occurred or did not occur	Death, diarrhea, pressure ulcer, pregnancy: "Yes" or "No"	Measures of event probability (e.g., relative risk or odds ratio)

TABLE 19.3   Measures of Association for Trials That Report Discrete Outcomes

Measure of Association	Definition	Comment
Relative risk, also called risk ratio	Compares the probability of the outcome in each group.	The RR is calculated by dividing the EER by CER. If CER and EER are the same, the RR = 1 (this means there is no difference between the experimental and control group outcomes). If the risk of the event is reduced in EER compared with CER, RR < 1. *The further to the left of 1 the RR is, the greater the event, the less likely the event is to occur.* If the risk of an event is greater in EER compared with CER, RR > 1. *The further to the right of 1 the RR is, the greater the event is likely to occur.*
Relative risk reduction	Tells us the reduction in risk in relative terms. The RRR is an estimate of the percentage of baseline risk that is removed as a result of the therapy; it is calculated as the ARR between the treatment and control groups divided by the absolute risk among patients in the control group.	Percent reduction in risk that is removed after considering the percent of risk that would occur anyway (the control group's risk), calculated as EER − CER/CER
Odds ratio	Estimates the odds of an event occurring. The OR is usually the measure of choice in the analysis of nonexperimental design studies. It is the probability of a given event occurring to the probability of the event not occurring.	If the OR = 1.0, this means there is no difference in the probability of an event occurring between the experimental and control group outcomes. If the probability of the event is reduced between groups, the OR < 1.0 (i.e., the event is less likely in the treatment group than in the control group). If the odds of an event is increased between groups, the OR > 1.0 (i.e., the event is more likely to occur in the treatment group than in the control group).

Note: When the experimental treatment *increases* the probability of a *good outcome* (e.g., satisfactory hemoglobin A_{1c} levels), there is a **benefit increase** rather than a risk reduction. The calculations remain the same.
CER, Control group event rate; *EER,* experimental group event rate; *OR,* odds ratio; *RR,* relative risk; *RRR,* relative risk reduction.

Generally speaking, therapy studies measure outcomes using discrete variables and present results as measures of association as relative risk (RR), relative risk reduction, or odds ratio (OR), as illustrated in Table 19.3. Understanding these measures is challenging but particularly important because they are used by all health care providers to communicate with each other and to patients the risks and benefits or lack of benefits of a treatment (or treatments). They are particularly useful to nurses, as they inform decision making that validates current practice or provides evidence that supports the need for a clinical practice change.

Example: ➤ Liu et al. (2019) conducted a study to evaluate the effectiveness of a school-based comprehensive intervention for childhood obesity in China, including (1) whether the school-based intervention would be effective for reducing excess weight gain among children and (2) whether the intervention would be beneficial for improving healthy eating, improving physical activity, and reducing sedentary behaviors among children.

Investigators randomized the schools to either the intervention group or the control group using computer-generated randomization sequences. Among the many variables studied, student BMI (a continuous variable) and whether or not the students were overweight or obese (dichotomous variable) in the intervention and control groups were measured 6 and 12 months after randomization. For the continuous data, the author described mean differences in BMI between the intervention group and the control group and analyzed the difference as statistically significant or not significant using p values (see Chapters 9 and 16). For the measured BMI, there was no statistical difference between the intervention and control groups at 6 months (-0.06, p 0.64) and at 12 months (0.07, p 0.54). The categorical data revealed that students were much more likely to be overweight or obese at 6 months in the intervention group ($n = 306$) than in the control group ($n = 299$) (OR, 1.16; 95% CI, 0.70 to 1.92; p 0.58). Surprisingly, students who received the intervention were almost two times more likely to be obese at 6 months. Examining the p value, we easily see that these findings are not statistically significant (p 0.58). At 12 months, students were much more likely to be overweight or obese in the control group ($n = 314$) than in the intervention group ($n = 304$) (OR, 0.95; 95% CI, 0.57–1.58; p 0.85). The intervention group was less likely (OR is < 1) to be obese or overweight. Examining the p value, we easily see that these findings are not statistically significant (p 0.85).

Two other measures can help you determine whether the reported or calculated measures are clinically meaningful. They are the **number needed to treat** (NNT) and the **confidence interval** (CI). These measures allow you to make inferences about how realistically the results about the effectiveness of an intervention can be generalized to individual patients and to a population of patients with similar characteristics.

The NNT is a useful measure for determining intervention effectiveness and its application to individual patients. It is defined as the number of people who need to receive a treatment (or intervention) for one patient to receive benefit. The NNT may or may not be reported by the study researchers but is easily calculated. Using data from the study and an online calculator (https://clincalc.com/Stats/NNT.aspx), you can easily find the NNT. Interventions with a high NNT require considerable expense and human resources to provide any benefit or to prevent a single episode of the outcome, whereas a low NNT is desirable because it means that more individuals will benefit from the intervention. For the 2019 Liu study of a 12-month school-based intervention to reduce childhood overweight and obesity in school-age children, the online calculator provides an NNT of 250. The interpretation of the NNT is that we would have to provide 250 students with the study intervention for 1 student to benefit from the intervention. Viewed from this perspective, it hardly seems worth providing the intervention! This gives us a very different and clinically useful perspective of the intervention; obviously the lower the NNT, the better the intervention.

The second clinically useful measure is the CI. The CI is a range of values that is based on a random sample of the population. It often accompanies measures of central tendency and measures of association and provides a measure of precision or uncertainty about the sample findings. Typically investigators record the CI results as a 95% degree of certainty; at times you may also see the degree of certainty recorded as 99%. Journals often include CIs as one of the statistical methods used to interpret study findings. Even when CIs are not reported, they can be easily calculated from study data. The method for performing these calculations is widely available in statistical texts.

Returning to the Liu (2019) study, it was found that the OR for the categorial data of overweight/obesity revealed that students were much more likely to be overweight at

6 months, with an OR of 1.16 (95% CI, 0.70 to 1.92). At 12 months, the OR was 0.95 (95% CI, 0.57 to 1.58). The CI, the number in parentheses, helps us place the study results in context for all patients similar to those in the study (generalizability). It can be stated that in school-age Chinese children (the study population) we can be 95% certain that when they receive the study's specific intervention, the odds of being overweight or obese is between 0.70 and 1.92 at 6 months and between 0.57 and 1.58 at 12 months; this is the range of effectiveness of the intervention. Recall that the odds of something happening is the ratio between success and failure (or something happening or not happening). Thus, at a minimum, you can see that at both 6 and 12 months, students were "less likely" to be overweight or obese (OR is < 1), and they were also "more likely" to be overweight or obese (OR is > 1).

Another unique feature of the CI is that it can tell us whether or not the study results are statistically significant. When an experimental value is obtained that indicates there is no difference between the treatment and control groups (e.g., no difference in the rate of overweight/obesity in children who received the intervention and those who did not), we label that value *the value of no effect,* or the **null value**. The value of no effect varies according to the outcome measure.

When examining a CI, if the interval *does not* include the null value, the effect is said to be statistically significant. When the CI *does* contain the null value, the results are said to be nonsignificant because the null value represents the value of no difference—that is, there is no difference between the treatment and control groups. In studies of equivalence (e.g., a study to determine whether two treatments are similar), this is a desired finding, but in studies of superiority or inferiority (e.g., a study to determine whether one treatment is better than the other), this is not the case.

The null value varies depending on the outcome measure. For numerical values determined by proportions/ratio (e.g., RR, OR), the null value is 1. That is, if the CI does not include the value 1, the finding is statistically significant. If the CI does include the value 1, the finding is not statistically significant. For numerical values determined by a mean difference between the score in the intervention group and the control group (usually with continuous measures), the null value is zero. If we examine an actual result from Table 2 in Appendix B, we can see an excellent demonstration of this concept; the authors report the changes in several important clinical outcomes in the diabetic patient at 12 and 24 months. The outcomes are accompanied by *mean changes* and CIs (in parentheses, the lower and upper limits of the CI). Can you identify which outcomes are significant and which are not by examining the CIs? In this case, if the CI includes the null value of zero, the result is not statistically significant. If the CI does not include the null value of zero, the result is statistically significant, as illustrated in Fig. 19.1A–D.

Diagnosis Articles

In studies that answer clinical questions of diagnosis, investigators study the ability of screening or diagnostic tests, or components of the clinical examination to detect (or not detect) disease when the patient has (or does not have) the particular disease of interest. The accuracy of a test, or technique, is measured by its sensitivity and specificity (Table 19.4).

Sensitivity is the proportion of those with disease who test positive; that is, sensitivity is a measure of how well the test detects disease when it is really there—a highly sensitive test has few false negatives. **Specificity** is the proportion of those without disease who test negative. It measures how well the test rules out disease when it is really absent; a specific test has few false positives. Sensitivity and specificity have some deficiencies in clinical use, primarily because sensitivity and specificity are merely characteristics of the performance of the test.

Describing diagnostic tests in this way tells us how good the test is, but what is more useful is how well the test performs in a particular population with a particular disease prevalence. This is important because in a population in which a disease is quite prevalent, there are fewer incorrect test results (false positives) compared with populations with low disease prevalence, for which a positive test may truly be a false positive. Predictive values are a measure of accuracy that accounts for the prevalence of a disease. As illustrated in Table 19.4, a **positive predictive value** (PPV) expresses the proportion of those with positive test results who truly have disease, and a **negative predictive value** (NPV) expresses the proportion of those with negative test results who truly do not have disease. Let us observe how these characteristics of diagnostic tests are used in nursing practice.

Example: ➤ Mid–upper arm circumference (MUAC) is a valuable tool for screening nutritional state in children. Of all anthropometric measures, MUAC is the easiest to obtain and is simple, practical, and reliable. MUAC is a good alternative for BMI in determining overweight/obesity in children/adolescents but has not been well studied as an alternative.

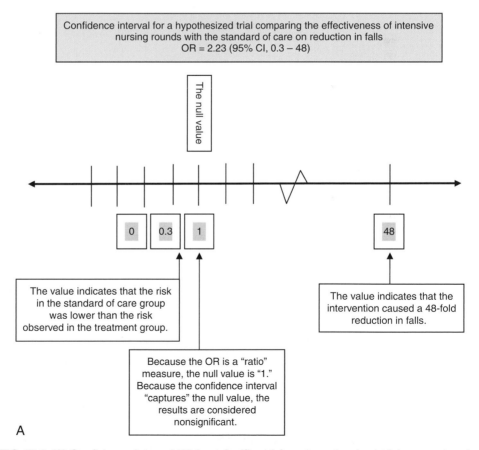

Confidence interval for a hypothesized trial comparing the effectiveness of intensive nursing rounds with the standard of care on reduction in falls
OR = 2.23 (95% CI, 0.3 – 48)

The null value

0   0.3   1   48

The value indicates that the risk in the standard of care group was lower than the risk observed in the treatment group.

The value indicates that the intervention caused a 48-fold reduction in falls.

Because the OR is a "ratio" measure, the null value is "1." Because the confidence interval "captures" the null value, the results are considered nonsignificant.

A

FIG 19.1 (A) Confidence interval (CI) (nonsignificant) for a hypothesized trial comparing the ratio of events in the experimental group and control group.

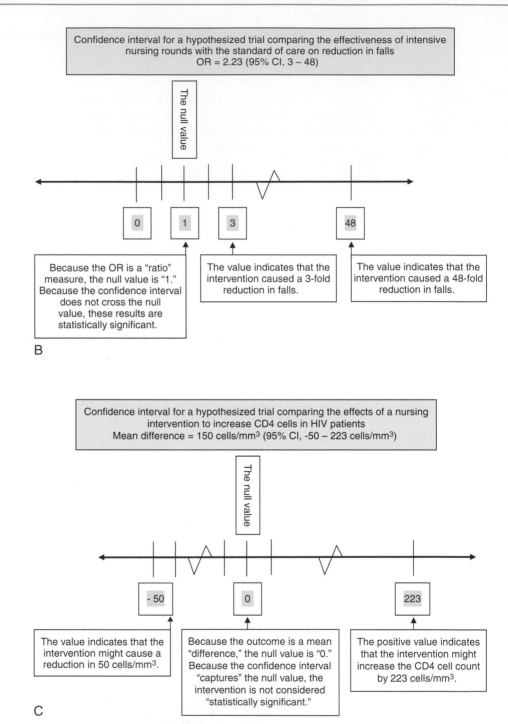

FIG 19.1, cont'd (B) CI (significant) for a hypothesized trial comparing the ratio of events in the experimental group and control group. (C) CI (nonsignificant) for a hypothesized control trial comparing the difference between two treatments.

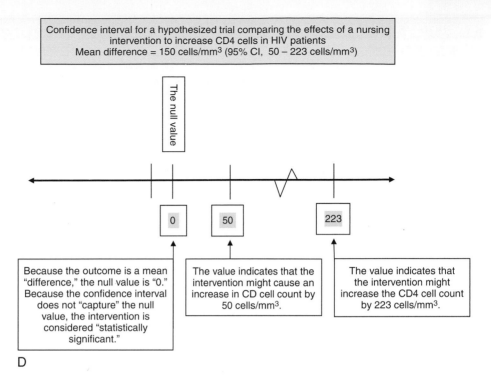

FIG 19.1, cont'd (D) CI (significant) for a hypothesized control trial comparing the difference between two treatments.

Talma et al. (2019) conducted a large national study that had as one of its aims to compare MUAC with BMI in a contemporary national sample to investigate the potential of MUAC in assessing overweight and obesity. A total of 6167 children were evaluated, BMI data was obtained, and the MUAC was measured by specifically trained health care professionals. The sensitivity and specificity data by age and gender is presented in Table 19.5.

Sensitivity ranged from 51.8% to 95.3%, and specificity ranged from 71.4% to 93.8%. Almost all sensitivities and specificities were high (>70%), except for sensitivity between 2 and 5 years of age. Therefore one-half of the children in this age group with overweight or obesity according to BMI were not detected by MUAC. This would suggest that MUAC can be used to detect obesity except in very young children.

Sensitivity and specificity apply to the diagnostic test and tell what portion of the individuals will have a positive or negative test. Clinicians and patients often want to know, when a test is negative or positive, what the probability is of actually having the disease. The PPV and NPV answer these questions. Table 19.4 shows how the PPV and NPV are calculated. In the study, the investigators did not supply the PPV or NPV, but it is easily calculated with the use of an online calculator (http://araw.mede.uic.edu/cgi-bin/testcalc.pl or http://www.pages.drexel.edu/~vk52/BSC.html).

Combining sensitivity, specificity, PPV, NPV, and prevalence to make clinical decisions based on the results of testing is cumbersome and complex. Fortunately, all of these measures can be described by one number, the **likelihood ratio** (LR). This value takes a pretest probability and, when the test is applied (either a positive test or a negative test), gives us a

TABLE 19.4 **Reporting the Outcome Results of Diagnostic Trials**

Measure of Accuracy	Definition	Comments
Sensitivity	A characteristic of a diagnostic test. It is the ability of the test to detect the proportion of people with the disease or disorder of interest. For a test to be useful in ruling out a disease, it must have a high sensitivity.	Formula for sensitivity: TP/(TP + FN), where TP and FN are number of true positive and false negative results, respectively.
Specificity	A characteristic of a diagnostic test. It is the ability of the test to detect the proportion of people without the disease or disorder of interest. For a test to be useful at confirming a disease, it must have a high specificity.	Formula for specificity: TN/(TN + FP), where TN and FP are number of true negative and false positive results, respectively.
PPV and NPV are closely related to sensitivity and specificity (how well the test performs) but differ in that sensitivity and specificity are fixed characteristics of a diagnostic test, whereas PPV and NPV consider how well the test performs in populations with a different prevalence of the disease it is testing.		
Positive predictive value	This is the proportion of people with a positive test who have the target disorder.	Formula for PPV: PPV = TP/(TP + FP)
Negative predictive value	This is the proportion of people with a negative test who do not have the target disorder.	Formula for NPV: NPV = TN/(TN + FN)
LR: A likelihood ratio is a measure that a given test result would be expected in a patient with the target disorder compared with the likelihood that the same result would be expected in a patient without the target disorder. It measures the power of a test to change the pretest into the posttest probability of a disease being present.		
Positive likelihood ratio	The LR of a positive test tells us how well a positive test result does by comparing its performance when the disease is present to that when it is absent. The best test to use for ruling in a disease is the one with the largest likelihood ratio of a positive test.	Formula for positive likelihood ratio: Sensitivity/(1 − Specificity)
Negative likelihood ratio	The LR of a negative test tells us how well a negative test result does by comparing its performance when the disease is absent to that when it is present. The better test to use to rule out disease is the one with the smaller likelihood ratio of a negative test.	Formula for negative likelihood ratio: (1 − Sensitivity)/Specificity

FN, False negative; *FP,* false positive; *LR,* likelihood ratio; *NPV,* negative predictive value; *PPV,* positive predictive value; *TN,* true negative; *TP,* true positive.

new probability. In other words, it tells us how much more we are certain the patient has the disease as a result of the test. As you can see from Table 19.4, the LR is calculated from the test's sensitivity and specificity, and with more training in determining disease prevalence (or pretest probability), you could actually state the numerical probability that a patient may have a disease based on the test's LR.

As illustrated in Table 19.6, a test with a large **positive likelihood ratio** (e.g., > 10), when applied, provides the clinician with a high degree of certainty that the patient has the suspected disorder. Conversely, a test with a very low positive likelihood ratio (e.g., < 2), when applied, provides little to no change in the degree of certainty that the patient has the suspected disorder.

When a test has an LR of 1 (the null value), the test will not contribute to decision making in any meaningful way and should not be used. A test with a large **negative likelihood ratio** provides the clinician with a high degree of certainty that the patient does not have the disease. The further away from 1 the negative LR is, the better the test will be for its use

TABLE 19.5   Sensitivity and Specificity of Mid–Upper Arm Circumference > 1.3 SDS in Predicting Overweight (Including Obesity) Classified by Body Mass Index International Obesity Task Force[26]

Age groups and gender	Sensitivity (%)	Specificity (%)
Male		
2–5 years	51.8	93.8
6–11 years	95.3	71.4
12–18 years	92.3	82.3
Female		
2–5 years	54.1	92.3
6–11 years	90.4	80.3
12–18 years	75.5	90.9

From Talma, H., van Dommelen, P., Schweizer, J. J., Bakker, B., Kist-van Holthe, J. E., Chinapaw, J. M. M., & Hirasing, R. A. (2019). Is mid-upper arm circumference in Dutch children useful in identifying obesity? *Archives of Disease in Childhood, 104*(2), 159–165.

TABLE 19.6   How Much Do Likelihood Ratio Changes Affect Probability of Disease?

Likelihood Ratio Positive	Likelihood Ratio Negative	Probability That Patient Has (LR) or Does Not Have (LR)
LR > 10	LR < 0.1	Large
LR 5–10	LR 0.1–0.2	Moderate
LR 2–5	LR 0.2–0.5	Small
LR < 2	LR > 0.5	Tiny
LR = 1.0	—	Test provides no useful information

LR, Likelihood ratio.

in ruling out disease (i.e., there will be few false negatives). More and more journal articles require authors to provide test LRs; they may also be available in secondary sources.

Prognosis Articles

In studies that answer clinical questions of prognosis, investigators conduct studies in which they want to determine the outcome of a particular disease or condition. Prognosis studies can often be identified by their longitudinal cohort design (see Chapter 10). At the conclusion of a longitudinal study, investigators statistically analyze data to determine which factors are strongly associated with the study outcomes, usually through a technique called *multivariate regression analysis* or simply *multiple regression* (see Chapter 16).

From this advanced statistical analysis, several factors are usually identified that predict the probability of developing the outcome or a particular disease. The probability is called an **odds ratio**. The OR (see Table 19.3) indicates how much more likely certain independent variables (factors) predict the probability of developing the dependent variable (outcome or disease).

Example: ➤ Returning to our case, Melody reviewed but did not select a prospective cohort longitudinal study of childhood obesity among low-income minority children. The authors conducted a 3-year prospective cohort analysis of parent-child pairs with children 3 to 5 years of age who were not obese (*n* = 605 pairs). The primary outcome was child obesity

TABLE 19.7	Measures of Association for Trials That Report Discrete Outcomes	
Measure of Association	**Definition**	**Comment**
Reporting Events in Terms of the Probability of It Occurring (Good or Bad)		
Odds ratio (OR)	We could estimate the odds of an event occurring. The OR is usually the measure of choice in the analysis of nonexperimental design studies. It is the probability of a given event occurring to the probability of the event not occurring.	If the OR = 1, this means there is no difference in the probability of an event occurring between the experimental and control group outcomes. If the probability of the event is reduced between groups, the OR is < 1 (i.e., the event is less likely in the treatment group than the control group). If the odds of an event is increased between groups, the OR > 1.0 (i.e., the event is more likely to occur in the treatment group than the control group).

at 36-month follow-up. Data collectors prospectively measured a child's weight and height five times over 3 years. These measurements were used to calculate a child's BMI, which was then classified as normal weight (BMI percentile >50th and <85th), overweight (BMI percentile >85th and <95th), or obese (BMI >95th). Participants were enrolled in a randomized controlled trial of a healthy lifestyle behavioral intervention. Multivariate logistic regression (the statistical method used to obtain an OR) was used to estimate the odds of obesity after 36 months. Predictors included age, sex, birth weight, gestational age, months of breastfeeding, ethnicity, baseline child BMI, energy intake, physical activity, food security, parent baseline BMI, and parental depression. These factors and their associated OR *(the dot)* and confidence intervals *(bars to the left and right of the dot)* are displayed in Fig. 19.2 (Heerman et al., 2019).

The interpretation of the ORs is described in Table 19.7. A higher OR indicates a greater probability of the development of the outcome. An OR less than 1 indicates that the probability of developing the outcome is reduced. Also recall from our discussion that whenever we are appraising CIs (to determine statistical significance), we must examine the CI for the presence of the null value. Because we are evaluating a "ratio," the null value is equal to 1. Thus any OR CI interval that contains a null value of 1 is not a significant finding. Looking at the horizontal line that represents the CIs in Fig. 19.2, can you tell which factors are and are not statistically significant? Any factors that do not contain the null value are statistically significant factors. Can you identify which factors are statistically significant? If you found that child age at enrollment (OR 2.11; 95% CI, 1.64 to 2.72), child baseline BMI (OR 3.37; 95% CI, 2.51 to 4.54), and parent (adult) baseline BMI (OR 1.36 for a 6-unit change; 95% CI, 1.09 to 1.70) all demonstrated statistically significant increased odds of childhood obesity at 36-month follow-up, you would have come to the same conclusion as the study authors.

HELPFUL HINT

Statistical significance does not always equal clinical significance.

Statistical significance is established by an analysis conducted by researchers. Although we always look to significant findings, the reader should be cautioned that nonsignificant findings may have some clinical significance. Clinical significance is established by experts in the field (including the same researchers) who decide if a statistically significant difference is clinically important or if a nonstatistically significant finding has some clinical significance.

Clinical significance is a subjective judgment and cannot be determined by a single study. This is why we need nurses and other clinical experts to read, evaluate, and interpret the evidence-based literature. Expert nurses may determine that materials, methods, or characteristics of the study population might have affected study results.

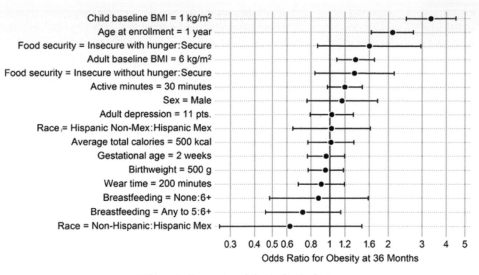

FIG 19.2 Example of Odds Ratio Data.

Using prognostic information with an evidence-based lens helps the nurse and patient focus on reducing factors that may lead to disease or disability. It also helps the nurse provide readily understood health literacy education and information with appropriate linguistic and reading level compatibility to patients and their families regarding the course of the condition.

IPE HIGHLIGHT

It is important that all members of your team understand the importance of being able to read tables included in research reports. The information you need to answer your clinical question should be contained in one or more of the tables.

Harm Articles

In studies that answer clinical questions of harm, investigators want to determine whether an individual has been harmed by being exposed to a particular event. Harm studies can be identified by their case-control design (see Chapter 10). In this type of study, investigators select the outcome they are interested in (e.g., pressure ulcers), and they examine if any one factor explains those who have and do not have the outcome of interest. The measure of association that best describes the analyzed data in case-control studies is the OR.

Example: ➤ Hu and colleagues (2019) used a case-control study design to investigate the association between television viewing and early childhood overweight/obese status. Table 19.8 presents data that shows results of this study. The interpretation of the data is relatively straightforward. You can see that most of the ORs are greater than 1. After controlling for family covariates and biological covariates (model 2), television viewing time was positively associated with children's overweight/obese status among the 4- to 5-year-old children (OR 1.81; 95% CI, 1.26 to 2.58). When further controlling for television viewing–related behaviors (model 3), the trends remained the same, but the OR decreased to 1.72 (95% CI, 1.16 to 2.54). Can you identify in which models and in which age group

TABLE 19.8 Odds Ratio and 95% CI for the Effects of TV Viewing on Childhood Overweight/Obesity Status Based on Age Group

TV viewing ≥ 1h per day	OVERWEIGHT/OBESE STATUS					
	1-TO 3-YEAR-OLD CHILDREN			4-TO 5-YEAR-OLD CHILDREN		
	OR	95% CI	p-value	OR	95% CI	p-value[a]
Model 1[b]	1.51	0.87–2.62	0.14	1.81	1.26–2.58	0.001
Model 2[c]	1.48	0.84–2.59	0.18	1.90	1.31–2.74	0.001
Model 3[d]	1.20	0.64–2.24	0.57	1.72	1.16–2.54	0.007

[a] CI and OR were obtained using conditional logistic regression model analysis.
[b] Adjusted for gender, maternal educational level, paternal educational level, family income.
[c] Model 1 + maternal weight status, paternal weight status, delivery mode.
[d] Model 2 + time spent by children in sporting activities, sleep duration of children, watching television while having meals, having snacks watching television, exposure to advertisements for junk food.
TV, Television, *OR* odds ratio, *CI* confidence interval.
From Hu, J., Ding, N., Yang, L., Ma, Y., Gao, M., & Wen, D. (2019). Association between television viewing and early childhood overweight and obesity: A pair-matched case-control study in China. *BMC Pediatrics, 19*(1), 184.

the results are not significant? Based on the previous discussion of CIs, you know that the CI can differentiate between findings that are significant and nonsignificant by examining whether or not the CI contains the null value; in the case of an OR, the null value is 1. The influence of television viewing on childhood overweight/obese status among 1- to 3-year-old children was not statistically significant in all models.

Harm data, with its measure of probabilities, help you identify factors that may or may not contribute to an adverse or beneficial outcome. This information will be useful for the nursing plan of care, program planning, or patient and family education.

Meta-Analysis

Meta-analysis statistically combines the results of multiple studies (usually RCTs) to answer a focused clinical question through an objective appraisal of carefully synthesized research evidence. The strength of a meta-analysis lies in its use of statistical analysis to summarize studies. As discussed in Chapter 11, a meta-analysis has the following characteristics:

- A clinical question is used to guide the process.
- All relevant studies, published and unpublished, on the question are gathered using preestablished inclusion and exclusion criteria to determine the studies to be used in the meta-analysis.
- At least two individuals independently assess the quality of each study based on preestablished criteria.
- Statistically combines the results of individual studies and presents a balanced and impartial quantitative and narrative evidence summary of the findings that represent a "state-of-the-science" conclusion about the strength, quality, and consistency of evidence supporting benefits and risks of a given health care practice (García-Perdomo, 2016).

A methodologically sound meta-analysis is more likely than an individual study to be successful in identifying the true effect of an intervention because it limits bias. An RR or, more commonly, the OR is the statistic of choice for use in a meta-analysis (see Tables 19.3 and 19.7). Meta-analysis can also report on continuous data; typically the mean difference in outcomes will be reported.

The typical manner of displaying data in a meta-analysis is by a pictorial representation known as a *blobbogram,* accompanied by a summary measure of effect size in RR, OR, or mean difference (see Chapter 11). Let us see how blobbograms (sometimes called *forest plots*) and ORs are used to summarize the studies in a systematic review by practicing with the data from a meta-analysis published in the *Journal of Pediatric Nursing* (Qiao et al., 2020). This meta-analysis was conducted to clarify the association between breastfeeding and the risk for preschoolers' obesity. Fig. 19.3 represents 14 studies that compared children who were breastfed versus children who were never breastfed. In the table, you can see a horizontal line that represents each trial in the analysis. The findings from each individual study are represented as a diamond and sometimes a square (the measured effect) on the horizontal line. Some analyses may also note each diamond or square as a bit different in size. This size reflects the weight the study has on the overall analysis. This is determined by the sample size and the quality of the study. The width of the horizontal line represents the 95% CI. The vertical line is the line of no effect (i.e., the null value), and we know that when the statistic is the OR, the null value is 1. In the next column, you will note the OR for each of the studies along with its CI. You will also note that horizontal line and diamond reflect the same information. The last column assigns a weight to each study based on the number of subject participants. The larger the sample size, the greater the weight assigned to the study for analysis purposes.

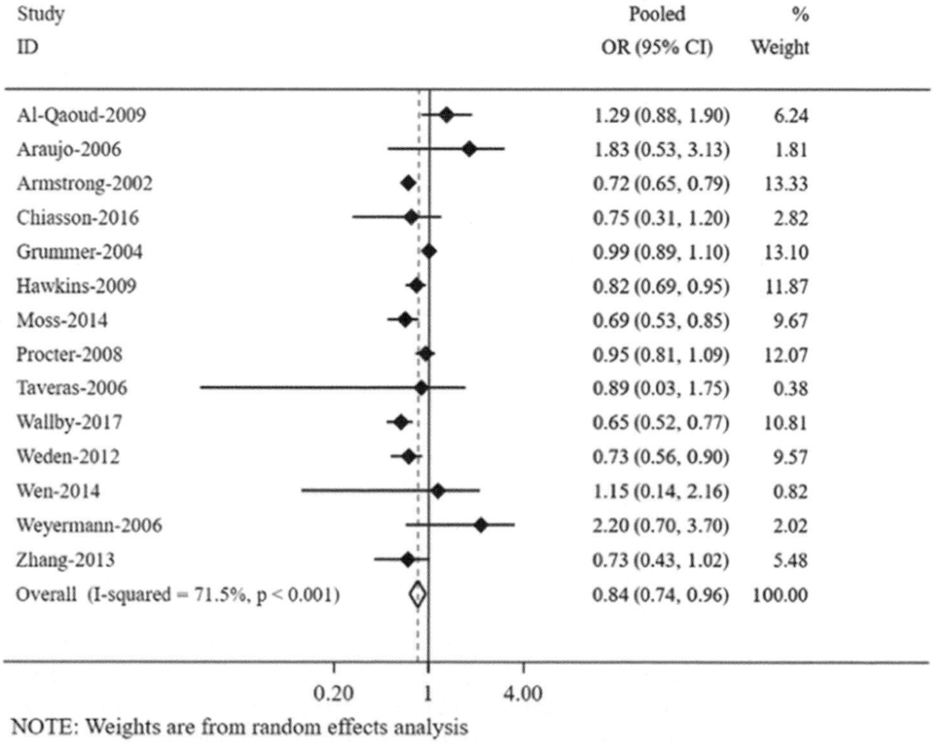

Study ID		Pooled OR (95% CI)	% Weight
Al-Qaoud-2009		1.29 (0.88, 1.90)	6.24
Araujo-2006		1.83 (0.53, 3.13)	1.81
Armstrong-2002		0.72 (0.65, 0.79)	13.33
Chiasson-2016		0.75 (0.31, 1.20)	2.82
Grummer-2004		0.99 (0.89, 1.10)	13.10
Hawkins-2009		0.82 (0.69, 0.95)	11.87
Moss-2014		0.69 (0.53, 0.85)	9.67
Procter-2008		0.95 (0.81, 1.09)	12.07
Taveras-2006		0.89 (0.03, 1.75)	0.38
Wallby-2017		0.65 (0.52, 0.77)	10.81
Weden-2012		0.73 (0.56, 0.90)	9.57
Wen-2014		1.15 (0.14, 2.16)	0.82
Weyermann-2006		2.20 (0.70, 3.70)	2.02
Zhang-2013		0.73 (0.43, 1.02)	5.48
Overall (I-squared = 71.5%, p < 0.001)		0.84 (0.74, 0.96)	100.00

0.20   1   4.00

NOTE: Weights are from random effects analysis

FIG 19.3 Example of a Forest plot.

When the CI of the result (horizontal line) touches or crosses the line of no effect (vertical line), we can say that the study findings did not reach statistical significance. If the CI does not cross the vertical line, we can say that the study results reached statistical significance. Can you tell which studies are significant and which ones are not? (Hint: There are only five significant studies. Be sure to check the CI column; sometimes pictures can be a bit misleading, especially when it is really close!

You will also notice other important information and additional statistical analyses that may accompany the blobbogram, such as a test to determine how well the results of each of the individual trials are mathematically compatible (heterogeneity, e.g., I-squared) and a test for overall effect. The reader is referred to a book of advanced research methods for discussion of these topics.

The empty diamond represents the summary ratio for all studies combined. In this case after statistically pooling the results of each of the trials, it shows that these studies, statistically combined, overall favor the treatment (children who were ever breastfed). You will note that the diamond almost appears as if it touches the line of no effect. Always validate your assessment by examining the confidence intervals that are often included in the table or text. The overall interpretation is that breastfeeding has some protective effect on childhood obesity. If this is a methodologically sound review, it can be used to support or change nursing practice or specific nursing interventions. A simple tool to help determine whether or not a systematic review is methodologically sound can be found at http://www.cebm.net/critical-appraisal/.

EVIDENCE-BASED STRATEGY #5: APPLYING THE FINDINGS

Evidence-based practice is about integrating individual clinical expertise and patient preferences with the best external evidence to guide clinical decision making (Sackett et al., 1996). With a few simple tools (see the links listed earlier in this chapter) and some practice, your day-to-day practice can be more evidence based. We know that using evidence in clinical decision making by nurses and all other health care professionals interested in matters associated with the care of individuals, communities, and health systems is increasingly important to achieving quality patient outcomes and cannot be ignored. Let us see how Melody uses evidence to validate her clinical question.

Melody critically appraises the article using the prognosis critical appraisal tool. Recall from Chapter 1 that the purpose of critical appraisal is to evaluate a research report's content for scientific merit and application to practice. Regardless of the tool used, most critical appraisal tools ask the examiner to answer several simple "yes," "no," or "not sure" questions. If most of the questions in your tool are answered with a "yes," it increases your confidence that the evidence has strong application to practice. "No" or "not sure" responses should prompt the appraiser to ask additional questions. It is important to consider whether or not the "no" or "not sure" responses represent a fatal flaw in the research or are something that is not significant or may be simply absent, for example, because of editorial page constraints.

Melody responds "yes" to all of the questions in the critical appraisal tool. The study results indicate that certain populations of children receiving SNAP benefits and consuming SSBs are more likely to be overweight or obese compared with their peers who receive SNAP benefits but do not consume SSBs. Melody decides that based on her initial observations, combined with support for her observation from high-quality evidence, she will continue to teach parents about the harms of SSBs. She decides that she will develop evidence-based health literacy handouts and also hold educational classes to help parents and children with identifying alternatives to SSBs.

SUMMARY

Clinical questions about nursing practice occur frequently; these questions come from nursing assessments, planning, and interventions; from patients; and from questions about the effectiveness of care. Nurses must think about how they can effectively review the literature for research evidence to answer a clinical question. It is important for nurses and all health care providers and the teams they are part of to be competent at using critical appraisal tools as a resource to evaluate clinical studies that can be used to inform clinical decision making about whether research findings are applicable to clinical practice. Nurses should understand and be able to interpret common measures of association, such as the OR and CIs, and apply this understanding to how data can be used to support current "best practices" or recommend evidenced-based changes in clinical care.

KEY POINTS

- Asking a focused clinical question using the PICO approach is an important evidence-based practice tool.
- Several types of evidence-based practice clinical categories used for evaluating research studies are therapy, diagnosis, prognosis, and harm. These categories focus on development of the clinical question, the literature search, and critical appraisal of research.
- An efficient and effective literature search, using information literacy skills, is critical in locating evidence to answer the clinical question.
- Sources of evidence (e.g., articles, evidence-based practice guidelines, evidence-based practice protocols) must be screened for relevance and credibility.
- Appraising the evidence generated by a study using an accepted critiquing tool is essential in determining the strength, quality, and consistency of evidence offered by a study.
- Studies that belong to the therapy category are designed to determine whether a difference exists between two or more treatments.

- Studies that belong to the diagnosis category are designed to investigate the ability of screening or diagnostic tests, tools, or components of the clinical examination to detect whether or not the patient has a particular disease using LRs.
- Studies in the prognosis category are designed to determine the outcomes of a particular disease or condition.
- Studies in the harm category are designed to determine whether an individual has been harmed by being exposed to a particular event.
- Meta-analysis is a research method that statistically combines the results of multiple studies (usually RCTs) and is designed to answer a focused clinical question through objective appraisal of synthesized evidence.

CLINICAL JUDGMENT CHALLENGES

- How would you use the PICO format to formulate a clinical question? Provide a clinical example.
- How can a nurse determine whether reported or calculated measures in a research study are clinically significant enough to inform evidence-based clinical decisions?
- How can a nurse in clinical practice determine whether the strength and quality of evidence provided by a diagnostic tool is sufficient to justify ordering it as a diagnostic test? Provide an example of a diagnostic test used to diagnose a specific illness.
- **IPE** How could your interprofessional quality improvement team use the PICO format to formulate a clinical question? Provide a clinical example from the quality improvement data from your unit.
- Choose a meta-analysis from a peer-reviewed journal, and describe how you as a nurse would use the findings of this meta-analysis in making a clinical decision about the applicability of a nursing intervention for your specific patient population and clinical setting.

REFERENCES

García-Perdomo, H. A. (2016). Evidence synthesis and meta-analysis: A practical approach. *International Journal of Urological Nursing, 10*(1), 30–36. https://doi.org/10.1111/ijun.12087.

Heerman, W. J., Sommer, E. C., Slaughter, J. C., Samuels, L. R., Martin, N. C., & Barkin, S. L. (2019). Predicting early emergence of childhood obesity in underserved preschoolers. *The Journal of Pediatrics, 213*, 115–120. https://doi.org/10.1016/j.jpeds.2019.06.031.

Hu, J., Ding, N., Yang, L., Ma, Y., Gao, M., & Wen, D. (2019). Association between television viewing and early childhood overweight and obesity: A pair-matched case-control study in China. *BMC Pediatrics, 19*(1), 184. https://doi.org/10.1186/s12887-019-1557-9.

Kloda, L. A., Boruff, J. T., & Soares Cavalcante, A. (2020). A comparison of patient, intervention, comparison, outcome (PICO) to a new, alternative clinical question framework for search skills, search results, and self-efficacy: A randomized controlled trial. *Journal of the Medical Library Association, 108*(2). https://doi.org/10.5195/jmla.2020.739.

Liu, Z., Li, Q., Maddison, R., Ni Mhurchu, C., Jiang, Y., Wei, D.-M., Cheng, L., Cheng, Y., Wang, D., & Wang, H.-J. (2019). A school-based comprehensive intervention for childhood obesity in China: A cluster randomized controlled trial. *Childhood Obesity, 15*(2), 105–115. https://doi.org/10.1089/chi.2018.0251.

LoBiondo-Wood, G., Haber, J., & Titler, M. (2019). *Evidence-based practice for nursing and healthcare quality improvement.* Elsevier.

Qiao, J., Dai, L.-J., Zhang, Q., & Ouyang, Y.-Q. (2020). A meta-analysis of the association between breastfeeding and early childhood obesity. *Journal of Pediatric Nursing, 53*, 57–66. https://doi .org/10.1016/j.pedn.2020.04.024.

Sackett, D. L., Rosenberg, W. M. C., Gray, J. A. M., et al. (1996). Evidence based medicine: What it is and what it isn't. *British Medical Journal, 312*, 71–72.

Talma, H., van Dommelen, P., Schweizer, J. J., Bakker, B., Kist-van Holthe, J. E., Chinapaw, J. M. M., & Hirasing, R. A (2019). Is mid-upper arm circumference in Dutch children useful in identifying obesity? *Archives of Disease in Childhood, 104*(2), 159–165. https://doi.org/10.1136 /archdischild-2017-313528.

Twarog, J. P., Peraj, E., Vaknin, O. S., Russo, A. T., Woo Baidal, J. A., & Sonneville, K. R. (2020). Consumption of sugar-sweetened beverages and obesity in SNAP-eligible children and adolescents. *Primary Care Diabetes, 14*(2), 181–185. https://doi.org/10.1016/j.pcd.2019.07.003.

Go to Evolve at **http://evolve.elsevier.com/LoBiondo/** for review questions, appraisal exercises, and additional research articles for practice in reviewing and appraisal.

20

Developing an Evidence-Based Practice

Marita Titler

Go to Evolve at **http://evolve.elsevier.com/LoBiondo/** for review questions.

LEARNING OUTCOMES

After reading this chapter, you should be able to do the following:

- Differentiate among conduct of research, evidence-based practice, and translation science.
- Describe the steps of evidence-based practice.
- Describe strategies for implementing evidence-based practice changes.
- Identify steps for evaluating an evidence-based change in practice.
- Use research findings and other forms of evidence to improve the quality of care.

KEY TERMS

conduct of research	evidence-based practice	implementation science	opinion leaders
dissemination	evidence-based	knowledge-focused	problem-focused triggers
evaluation	practice guidelines	triggers	translation science

A number of health care practices have an evidence base but are not yet part of the standard of care. Gaps between availability of evidence-based interventions and application in care delivery contribute to poor health outcomes such as obesity, health care–acquired infections, and fall injuries (Titler, 2018). Use of evidence-based practice (EBP) is an expected standard, as demonstrated by regulatory agencies such as The Joint Commission and the Centers for Medicare and Medicaid Services (CMS) (Titler et al., 2019). For example, non-payment for hospital-acquired events such as fall injuries and catheter-associated urinary tract infections (CAUTIs) are driven by a strong evidence base to prevent the occurrence of such events. Implementing EBP is a challenge, however, and requires the use of strategies that address the systems of care, individual practitioners, and senior leadership and will ultimately change health care cultures to be EBP environments (Brownson et al., 2018; Titler, 2018).

Translation of research into practice (TRIP) is a multifaceted, systemic process of promoting adoption of EBP in delivery of health care services that goes beyond dissemination of evidence-based guidelines (Titler, 2018). Dissemination activities take many forms, including publications, social media, conferences, consultations, and training programs, but promoting knowledge uptake and changing practitioner behavior requires active interchange with those in direct care (Titler, 2018, 2019; Titler et al., 2019). This chapter presents an overview of EBP and the process of applying evidence in practice to improve patient outcomes.

OVERVIEW OF EVIDENCE-BASED PRACTICE

The relationships among conduct, dissemination, and use of research are illustrated in Fig. 20.1. **Conduct of research** is the systematic investigation of a phenomenon to address research questions and test hypotheses that advance the state of the science (Titler, 2018). The conduct of research includes dissemination of findings from journals, social media, and scientific conferences (see Chapter 1).

Evidence-based practice is the conscientious and judicious use of current best evidence in conjunction with clinical expertise and patient values and circumstances to guide health care decisions (Straus et al., 2011; Titler, 2018). Best evidence includes findings from randomized controlled trials; evidence from other scientific approaches such as descriptive and qualitative research; and information from case reports and scientific principles. When adequate research evidence is available, practice is guided by research evidence in conjunction with clinical expertise and patient values (see Chapter 1). In some cases, however, a sufficient research base may not be available, and health care decision making is derived principally from evidence sources such as scientific principles, case reports, and quality improvement projects. As illustrated in Fig. 20.1, the application of research findings in practice may not only improve quality care but also create new and exciting questions to be addressed via the conduct of research.

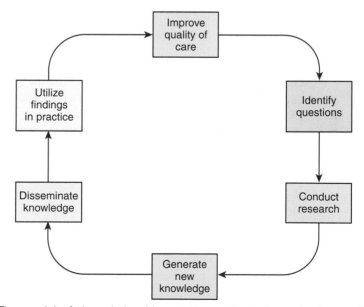

FIG 20.1 The model of the relationship among conduct, dissemination, and use of research. (From Weiler, K., Buckwalter, K., & Titler, M. [1994]. Debate: Is nursing research used in practice? In J. McCloskey, & H. Grace [Eds.], *Current issues in nursing* [4th ed.]. St Louis, MO: Mosby.)

In contrast, **translation science**, also more recently known as **implementation science**, focuses on testing implementation interventions to improve uptake and use of evidence to improve patient outcomes and population health and to explicate which implementation strategies work for whom, in which settings, and why (National Institutes of Health, 2020; Titler, 2018). An emerging body of knowledge in translation science provides an empirical base for guiding the selection of implementation strategies to promote adoption of EBP in real-world settings (Glegg et al., 2019; Titler, 2018). Thus *EBP* and *translation science,* though related, are not interchangeable terms; EBP is the actual application of evidence in practice (the "doing of" EBP), whereas translation science is the study of implementation strategies, factors, and contextual variables that effect knowledge uptake and use in practices and communities.

Models of Evidence-Based Practice

Multiple models of EBP and translation science are available (Birken et al., 2017; Titler, 2018). Although review of these models is beyond the scope of this chapter, implementing evidence in practice is best guided by a conceptual model.

The Iowa Model of Evidence-Based Practice

An overview of the Iowa Model of Evidence-Based Practice as an **example** ➤ of an EBP model is illustrated in Fig. 20.2. This model is widely used in academic and clinical settings (Titler et al., 2001; Iowa Model Collaborative, 2017). In this model, knowledge- and problem-focused "triggers" lead staff members to question current nursing practices and whether patient care can be improved through the use of research findings. If through the process of literature review and critique of studies it is found that there is an insufficient number of scientifically sound studies to use as a base for practice, consideration is given to conducting a study. Findings from such studies are then combined with findings from existing research to develop and implement these practices. If there is insufficient research to guide practice and conducting a study is not feasible, other types of evidence (e.g., case reports, scientific principles, theory) are used and/or combined with available research evidence to guide practice. Practice guidelines usually reflect research and nonresearch evidence and therefore are called **evidence-based practice guidelines** (Institute of Medicine [IOM], 2011; see Chapter 11).

Recommendations for practice are based on evidence synthesis. Sources of evidence-based recommendations may be a barrier to implementation if the recommendations are ambiguous or unclear. Potential users of EBP often complain that recommendations are vague, are nonspecific, and lack behaviorally specific terms (IOM, 2011). When your team is setting forth EBP recommendations, make sure they are clear, concise, actionable, and include sufficient information to carry out the recommendation; that is, detail precisely what the recommended action is and under what circumstances it is to be performed. Recommendations must be executable and worded so that adherence with the recommendation(s) can be evaluated. Consider the type of health care personnel the recommendations are targeting (e.g. physicians, nurses, community health workers, social workers). Include the underlying rationale (e.g., summary of relevant evidence, quality, quantity, and consistency of evidence), description of potential benefits and harms, and a rating of the strength of the evidence underpinning the recommendation (IOM, 2011).

The EBP recommendations derived from the evidence synthesis are then compared with current practice, and a decision is made about the necessity for a practice change. If a

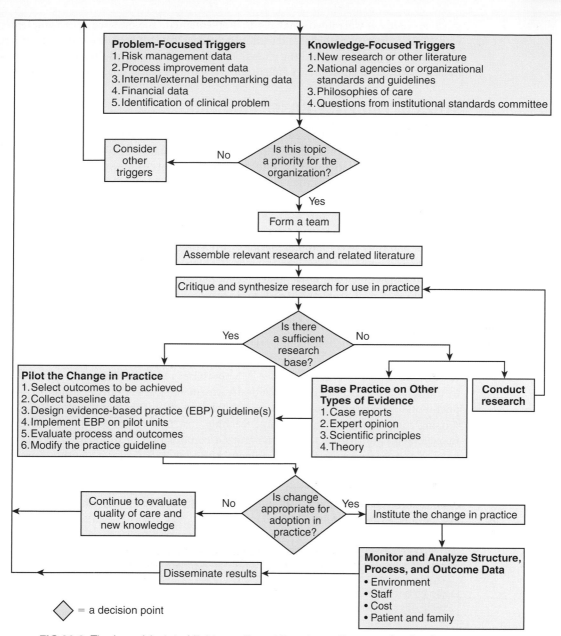

FIG 20.2 The Iowa Model of Evidence-Based Practice to Promote Quality Care. (From Titler, M. G., Kleiber, C., Steelman, V. J., et al. [2001]. The Iowa Model of Evidence-Based Practice to Promote Quality Care. *Critical Care Nursing Clinics of North America, 13*[4], 497–509.)

practice change is warranted, changes are implemented. The practice is first implemented with a small group of patients, and a pilot evaluation is conducted. The EBP is then refined based on evaluation data, and the change is implemented with additional patient populations for which it is appropriate. Patient/family, staff, and fiscal outcomes are monitored.

STEPS OF EVIDENCE-BASED PRACTICE

The Iowa Model of Evidence-Based Practice to Promote Quality Care (Titler et al., 2001; see Fig. 20.2), in conjunction with the Translating Research Into Practice (TRIP) Model (Fig. 20.3), derived from Rogers's Diffusion of Innovations framework (Rogers, 2003), provides steps for actualizing EBP. A team approach is most helpful in fostering adoption of a specific EBP.

Selection of a Topic

The first step is to select a topic. Ideas for EBP come from several sources categorized as problem- and knowledge-focused triggers. Problem-focused triggers are those identified by staff through quality improvement, risk surveillance, benchmarking data, financial data, or recurrent clinical problems. An example of a problem-focused trigger is increased incidence of central line occlusion in pediatric oncology patients.

Knowledge-focused triggers are ideas generated when staff read a research publication, listen to scientific papers at conferences, or encounter EBP guidelines published by federal agencies or specialty organizations. This includes those EBPs that the CMS expects to be implemented in practice, as the CMS now bases reimbursement of care on adherence to indicators of EBP. Examples include treatment of heart failure, community-acquired pneumonia, and prevention of nosocomial pressure ulcers. Each of these topics includes a nursing component, such as discharge teaching, instructions for patient self-care, or pain management. Sometimes topics arise from a combination of problem- and knowledge-focused triggers, such as family presence in the adult critical care setting. In selecting a topic, it is essential to consider how the topic fits with organization, department, and unit priorities to garner support from leaders within the organization and the necessary resources to successfully complete the project. Criteria to consider when selecting a topic are outlined in Box 20.1.

> **IPE   HIGHLIGHT**
>
> Regardless of which approach is used to select an EBP topic, it is critical that your team that will implement the potential practice change is involved in selecting the topic, developing the clinical question, and viewing it as contributing significantly to the quality of care for your patient population.

Forming a Team

A team is responsible for development, implementation, and evaluation of the EBP. A task force approach also may be used, in which a group is appointed to address a practice issue. The composition of the team is directed by the topic selected and should include interested stakeholders. **Example:** ➤ A team working on evidence-based pain management should be interdisciplinary and include pharmacists, nurses, physicians, and psychologists. In contrast, a team working on the EBP of bathing might include a nurse expert in skin care, assistive nursing personnel, and staff nurses. The engagement of patients, family members, and consumers as

---

BOX 20.1   Selection Criteria for an Evidence-Based Practice Project

1. Priority of the topic for nursing and for the organization
2. Magnitude of the problem (small, medium, large)
3. Applicability to several or few clinical areas
4. Likelihood of the change to improve quality of care, decrease length of stay, contain costs, or improve patient satisfaction
5. Potential issues associated with the topic and capability to diffuse them
6. Availability of baseline quality improvement or risk data that will be helpful during evaluation
7. Multidisciplinary nature of the topic and ability to create collaborative relationships to effect the needed changes
8. Interest and commitment of staff to the potential topic
9. Availability of a sound body of evidence, preferably research evidence

---

team members is important and is receiving more attention in EBP (Msowoya and Gephart, 2019; Shuman et al., 2016). Consider including a layperson as a team member who has experience with the topic. **Example:** ➤ A team focusing on prevention of **necrotizing enterocolitis** (NEC) in premature neonates may invite a parent to participate on the team because feeding breast milk (instead of formula) is one strategy to prevent NEC (Gephart et al., 2020).

In addition to forming a team, key stakeholders who can facilitate or put up barriers against successful implementation should be identified. A **stakeholder** is a key individual or group of individuals who will be directly or indirectly affected by the implementation of the EBP. Some of these stakeholders are likely to be members of the team. Others may not be team members but are key individuals within the organization or unit who can adversely or positively influence the adoption of the practice. Questions to consider in identification of key stakeholders include the following:

- How are decisions made in the areas where the EBP will be implemented?
- What types of system changes will be needed?
- Who is involved in decision making?
- Who is likely to lead and champion implementation of the EBP?
- Who can influence the decision to proceed with implementation of the practice?
- What type of cooperation is needed from stakeholders for the project to be successful?
- What kind of financial resources or other resources are needed?

Failure to involve or keep supportive stakeholders informed may place the success of the project at risk because they are unable to anticipate and/or defend the rationale for changing practice, particularly with resistors (e.g., nonsupportive stakeholders) who have a great deal of influence among their peer group. An important early task for the EBP team is to formulate the PICO question. This helps set boundaries around the project and assists in evidence retrieval. This approach is illustrated in Table 20.1 (see Chapters 1 to 3 and Chapter 19).

Evidence Retrieval

Once a topic is selected, relevant research and related literature must be retrieved (see Chapters 3 and 11). The Agency for Healthcare Research and Quality (AHRQ; http://www. AHRQ.gov) funds nine Evidenced-Based Practice Centers in the United States and sponsors development of Evidence-Based Reports that provide comprehensive, science-based information on a variety of health care topics. These reports are valuable sources of evidence to assist with clinical and policy decision making. Evidence sources can also be found in electronic databases such as the Cochrane Library (http://www.cochranelibrary.com) and the Centers

TABLE 20.1   Using PICO to Formulate the Evidence-Based Practice Question

	Patient/Population/ Problem	Intervention/ Treatment	Comparison Intervention	Outcome(s)
Tips for building the question	How would we describe a group of patients similar to ours?	Which main intervention are we considering?	What is the main alternative to compare with the intervention?	What can we hope to accomplish?
Example 1	Low rates of HPV vaccine (3-dose series) for preteen girls (11–12 years of age) for cervical cancer prevention. Pediatric practice.	Delivery of 3 series HPV vaccine to preteen girls. Provision of educational brochure for parents/ guardians. Clinician prompt to discuss HPV vaccine with parent and preteen. Telephone reminder for dose completion.	No HPV vaccine	Increased rates of HPV vaccine 3-dose series.
Example 2	Pain assessment of cognitively impaired elders	Pain assessment tool designed for assessing pain in cognitively impaired elders in long-term care setting.	Not assess pain Yes/no question	Regular pain assessment with treatment of pain

From University of Illinois at Chicago, P.I.C.O. Model for Clinical Questions, http://www.uic.edu/depts/lib/lhsp/resources/pico.shtml.

for Health Evidence (http://www.cche.net) (see Chapters 3 and 11). Once the literature is located, it is helpful to classify the articles as clinical (nonresearch), theory, research, systematic reviews, or EBP guidelines. Before reading and critiquing the research, it is useful to read background articles to have a broad view of the topic and related concepts and then critique the existing EBP guidelines. It is helpful to read and critique articles in the following order:

1. Clinical articles to understand the state of the practice
2. Theory articles to understand the theoretical perspectives and concepts that may be encountered in critiquing studies
3. EBP guidelines and evidence reports
4. Systematic reviews, meta-analyses, and synthesis reports to understand the state of the science
5. Primary research articles

Schemas for Grading the Evidence

There is no consensus regarding the best system to use to denote the type and quality of evidence or which grading schemas to use to denote the strength of a body of evidence (Balshem et al., 2011; IOM, 2011). See Table 20.2 for examples of grading and assessing quality of research studies. The GRADE website (http://www.gradeworkinggroup.org) provides important information that will help you understand the challenges and approaches for assessing the quality of evidence and strength of recommendations.

In grading the evidence, two important areas are essential to address: (1) the quality of the evidence (e.g., individual studies, systematic reviews, meta-analyses) and (2) the strength of the body of evidence. The domains and elements to include in grading the strength of the evidence are defined in Table 20.3. In Chapter 1, Fig. 1.1 provides an evidence hierarchy used for grading evidence that is an adaptation similar to the evidence hierarchies that appear in Table 20.2.

Critique and Synthesis of Research

Critique of evidence-based guidelines (see Chapter 11) and studies (see Chapters 8 to 10) should use the same methodology, and the critique process should be a shared responsibility. It is helpful, however, to have one individual provide leadership for the project and design strategies for completing critiques. A group approach to critiques is recommended because it distributes the workload, helps those responsible for implementing the changes understand the scientific base for the practice change, arms nurses with citations and research-based language to use in advocating for changes with peers and other disciplines, and provides novices an environment to learn how to critique

TABLE 20.2　**Examples of Evidence Rating Systems**	
Grade Working Group (http://www.gradeworkinggroup.org)	**US Preventative Services Task Force (USPSTF)** (http://www.uspreventiveservicestaskforce.org/)
Quality of the Evidence (Balshem et al., 2011; Guyatt et al., 2011, 2013) **High:** Very confident that the true effect lies close to that of the estimate of the effect. Scientific evidence provided by well-designed, well-conducted, controlled trials (randomized and non-randomized) with statistically significant results that consistently support the recommendation. **Moderate:** Moderately confident in the effect estimate: The true effect is likely to be close to the estimate of the effect, but there is a possibility that it is substantially different. **Low:** Confidence in the effect estimate is limited: The true effect may be substantially different from the estimate of the effect. **Very low:** Very little confidence in the effect estimate: The true effect is likely to be substantially different from the estimate of effect. **Note:** The type of evidence is first ranked as follows: Randomized trial = High Observational study = Low Any other evidence = Very low Quality may be downgraded as a result of design flaws/threats to internal validity (risk for bias), important inconsistency of results, uncertainty about the directness of the evidence, imprecise or sparse data, and high probability of publication bias, which can lower the evidence grade. Factors that may increase quality of evidence of observational studies: 1. Large magnitude of effect (direct evidence, relative risk [RR] = 2–5 or RR = 0.5–0.2 with no plausible confounders); very large with RR > 5 or RR < 0.2 and no serious problems with risk for bias or precision (sufficiently narrow confidence intervals); more likely to rate up if the effect is rapid and out of keeping with prior trajectory; usually supported by indirect evidence. 2. Dose-response gradient 3. All plausible residual confounders or biases would reduce a demonstrated effect, or suggest a spurious effect when results show no effect.	**Levels of Certainty Regarding Net Benefit (Quality of Evidence) (USPSTF, 2015)** **High:** Available evidence usually includes consistent results from a multitude of well-designed, well-conducted studies in representative primary care populations. These studies assess effects of the preventive service on health outcomes. This conclusion is therefore unlikely to be strongly affected by the results of future studies. **Moderate:** The available evidence is sufficient to determine the effects of the preventive service on health outcomes, but confidence in the estimate is constrained by factors such as: • Number, size, or quality of individual studies • Some heterogeneity of outcome findings or intervention models across the body of studies • Mild to moderate generalizability of findings to routine primary care practice As more information becomes available, the magnitude or direction of the observed effect could change, and this change may be large enough to alter the conclusion. **Low:** The available evidence is insufficient to assess effects on health outcomes. Evidence is insufficient because of one or more of the following: • Very limited number or size of studies • Inconsistency of direction or magnitude of findings across the body of evidence • Critical gaps in the chain of evidence • Findings not generalizable to routine primary care practice • Lack of information on prespecified health outcomes • Lack of coherence across linkages in the chain of evidence • More information may allow estimation of effects on health outcomes

Continued

TABLE 20.2 **Examples of Evidence Rating Systems—cont'd**

Grade Working Group (http://www.gradeworkinggroup.org)	US Preventative Services Task Force (USPSTF) (http://www.uspreventiveservicestaskforce.org/)
Strength of Recommendations (Andrews et al., 2013)	**Recommendation Grades (USPSTF, 2015)**
Strong: Confident that desirable effects of adherence to a recommendation outweigh undesirable effects.	A. The USPSTF recommends the service. There is high certainty that the net benefit is substantial.
Weak: Desirable effects of adherence to a recommendation probably outweigh undesirable effects, but developers are less confident.	B. The USPSTF recommends the service. There is high certainty that the net benefit is moderate or there is moderate certainty that the net benefit is moderate to substantial.
Note: Strength of recommendation is determined by the balance between desirable and undesirable consequences of alternative management strategies, quality of evidence, variability in values and preferences (trade-offs), and resource use.	C. The USPSTF recommends selectively offering or providing this service to individual patients based on professional judgment and patient preferences. There is at least moderate certainty that the net benefit is small.
	D. The USPSTF recommends against the service. There is moderate or high certainty that the service has no net benefit or that the harms outweigh the benefits.
	E. The USPSTF concludes that the current evidence is insufficient to assess the balance of benefits and harms of the service. Evidence is lacking, of poor quality, or conflicting, and the balance of benefits and harms cannot be determined.

TABLE 20.3 **Important Domains and Elements for Systems to Grade the Strength of Evidence**

Quality	The aggregate of quality ratings for individual studies, predicated on the extent to which bias was minimized
Quantity	Magnitude of effect, numbers of studies, and sample size or power
Consistency	For any given topic, the extent to which similar findings are reported using similar and different study designs
Relevance	Relevance of findings to characteristics of individual groups
Benefits and harms	The overall benefits and harms. Net benefits. Do the benefits outweigh the harms?

Modified from Institute of Medicine (IOM). (2011). *Clinical practice guidelines we can trust*. Washington, DC: The National Academies Press.

and apply research findings. Methods to make the critique process fun and interesting include the following:

- Using a journal club to discuss critiques done by each member of the group
- Pairing a novice and expert to do critiques
- Eliciting assistance from students who may be interested in the topic and want experience doing critiques
- Assigning the critique process to graduate students interested in the topic
- Making a class project to critique and synthesize the evidence for a given topic
- Using the critique criteria at the end of each chapter and the critique criteria summary tables in Chapters 6 and 18

> **HELPFUL HINT**
>
> Keep critique processes simple, and encourage participation by staff members who are providing direct patient care.

Once studies are critiqued, a decision is made regarding the use of each study in the synthesis of the evidence for application in practice. Factors that should be considered for inclusion of studies in the synthesis of findings are (1) overall scientific merit; (2) type of subjects enrolled (e.g., age, gender, pathology) and similarity to the patient population to which the findings will be applied; and (3) relevance of the study to the topic of question. **Example:** ➤ If the practice area is prevention of deep venous thrombosis in postoperative patients, a descriptive study using a heterogeneous population of medical patients is not appropriate for inclusion in the synthesis of findings.

To synthesize the findings from research critiques, it is helpful to use a summary table in which critical information from studies can be documented. Essential information to include in such a summary is as follows:

- Research questions/hypotheses
- Independent and dependent variables studied
- Description of the study sample and setting
- Type of research design
- Methods used to measure each variable and outcome
- Study findings

An **example** ➤ of a summary form is illustrated in Table 20.4.

> **HELPFUL HINT**
>
> Use of a summary form helps identify commonalities across studies with regard to study findings and the types of patients to which findings can be applied. It also helps in synthesizing the overall strengths and weakness of the studies as a group.

Setting Forth Evidence-Based Practice Recommendations

Based on the critique of practice guidelines and synthesis of research, recommendations for practice are set forth. The type and strength of evidence used to support the practice must be clearly delineated in your evidence table. Box 20.2 is another useful tool to assist with this activity.

Decision to Change Practice

After all evidence is critiqued and synthesized, the next step is to decide if the findings are appropriate for use in practice. Criteria to consider include the following:

- Relevance of evidence for practice
- Consistency in findings across studies and/or guidelines
- A significant number of studies and/or EBP guidelines with sample characteristics similar to those to which the findings will be used
- Consistency among evidence from research and other nonresearch evidence
- Feasibility for use in practice
- The risk/benefit ratio and cost (risk for harm versus potential benefit for the patient)

Synthesis of evidence may result in supporting current practice, making minor practice modifications, undertaking major practice changes, or developing a new area of practice.

TABLE 20.4   Example of a Summary Table for Research Critiques

Citation	Research Question	Study Design	Sample	Independent Variables and Measures	Dependent Variables and Measures	Results	General Strengths	General Weaknesses	Overall Quality of Study[a]	Summary Statements for Practice

[a] Use a consistent rating system (e.g., good, fair, poor).

BOX 20.2   Consistency of Evidence From Critiqued Research, Appraisals of Evidence-Based Practice Guidelines, Critiqued Systematic Reviews, and Nonresearch Literature

1. Are there replication of studies with consistent results?
2. Are the studies well designed?
3. Are recommendations consistent among systematic reviews, evidence-based practice guidelines, and critiqued research?
4. Are there identified risks to the patient by applying EBP recommendations?
5. Are there identified benefits to the patient?
6. Have cost analyses been conducted on the recommended action, intervention, or treatment?
7. Are there summary recommendations about assessments, actions, interventions/treatments from the research, systematic reviews, and evidence-based guidelines with an assigned evidence grade?

Development of Evidence-Based Practice

The next step is to document the evidence base of the practice using the agreed-on grading schema. When a critique and synthesis of evidence suggest a practice change, a written EBP standard (e.g., policy, standard of practice protocol, guideline) is warranted. This is necessary so individuals know (1) that the practices are based on evidence and (2) the type of evidence (e.g., randomized controlled trial, expert opinion) used in development of the practice.

It is imperative that once the EBP standard is written, key stakeholders have an opportunity to review it and provide feedback to the individual(s) responsible for developing it. Focus groups are a useful way to provide discussion about the EBP and to identify key areas that may be potentially troublesome during the implementation phase. Key questions that can be used in focus groups are listed in Box 20.3.

HELPFUL HINT

Use a consistent approach to developing EBP standards and referencing the research and related literature.

Implementing the Practice Change

If a practice change is warranted, the next step is implementation. This goes beyond writing a policy or procedure that is evidence based; it requires interaction among direct care providers to champion and foster evidence adoption, leadership support, and system changes.

The TRIP model is useful in selecting implementation strategies and illustrates that the rate and extent of adoption of evidence-based health care practices are influenced by four key areas: the nature of the innovation or EBP characteristics: Communication process; social system; EBP users; and rate and extent of adoption (see Fig. 20.3). Successful implementation requires implementation strategies to address each of these four areas (Titler, 2018).

Implementation Strategies to Address the Characteristics of the Evidence-Based Topic

Characteristics of an innovation or EBP that affect adoption include the relative advantage of the EBP (e.g., effectiveness, relevance to the task, social prestige); the compatibility with values, norms, work, and perceived needs of users; and complexity of the EBP

BOX 20.3   Key Questions for Focus Groups

1. What is needed by staff (e.g., nurses, physicians) to use this EBP in your setting?
2. In your opinion, how will this standard improve patient care in your unit/practice?
3. What modifications would you suggest in the EBP standard before using it in your practice?
4. Which content in the EBP standard is unclear? What needs revision?
5. What would you change about the format of the EBP standard?
6. Which part of this EBP change do you view as most challenging?
7. Do you have any other suggestions?

---

topic (Rogers, 2003; Titler, 2019). **Example:** ➤ EBP topics that are perceived by users as relatively simple (e.g., influenza vaccines for older adults) are more easily adopted in less time than those that are more complex (e.g., acute pain management for hospitalized older adults).

A key principle to use when planning implementation is that the attributes of the practice topic as perceived by users and stakeholders (e.g., ease of use, valued part of practice) are neither stable features nor sure determinants of their adoption. Rather, it is the interaction among the characteristics of the EBP topic, the intended users, and a particular context of practice that determines the rate and extent of adoption (Dogherty et al., 2012; Greenhalgh & Papoutsi, 2019). Implementation strategies that address characteristics of the EBP topic are quick reference guides (QRGs), electronic clinical decision support (CDS) tools, and key messaging at point-of-care delivery.

QRGs provide concise information targeted to clinicians implementing EBP (IOM, 2011; Titler et al., 2016; Titler, 2018). They concisely and accurately convey essential actions and information derived from EBP recommendations, and they are accessible at point-of-care delivery (Anderson & Titler, 2019). A variety of QRG formats are available such as laminated checklists and decision-making algorithms. The design and content of QRGs affect their use and subsequent implementation of EBP recommendations (Flodgren et al., 2016; Wilson et al., 2016). An example of a QRG is shown in Fig. 20.4.

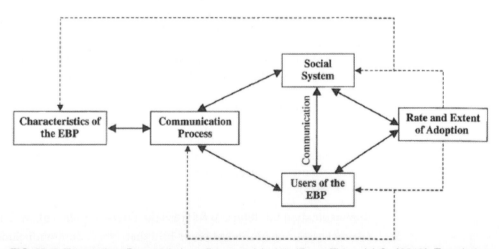

FIG 20.3 Translating Research into Practice Model. (From Titler, M.G. [2010]. Translation science and context. *Research Theory Nursing Practice, 24*[1].)

Risk factor
Compromised mobility, gait instability, or lower limb weakness

Indicators	Interventions	Hints and tips
• Unsteady/veering during transfers or walking • Reaching for walls or other supports while walking • Overbalancing, especially when reaching, bending, straightening, or turning • Unable to rise from chair without assistance	• Ambulate 3-4 times per day with assistance unless contraindicated • Refer patient to PT for assessment, gait, and strength training • Active or passive range of motion three times daily • Minimize use of immobilizing equipment (e.g., indwelling urinary catheters) • Assure proper assist equipment is readily available	• Seek advice from PT about safe exercises and activities the patient can perform on their own or with supervision • Ask patient's family and friends to assist with mobility interventions as appropriate • Without contraction muscle strength decreases by as much as 5% per day

FIG 20.4 Quick reference guide fall prevention: interventions to mitigate mobility risk factors. (From Titler, M. G., Conlon, P., Reynolds, M. A., et al. [2016]. The effect of translating research into practice intervention to promote use of evidence-based fall prevention interventions in hospitalized adults: a prospective pre-post implementation study in the U.S. *Applied Nursing Research, 31,* 52–59.)

Empirical support for evidence-based electronic clinical decision support interventions is mixed (IOM, 2011). Electronic reminders have small to modest effects on clinician behavior and appear to be more effective than alerts alone when included as a part of multifaceted implementation strategies (Arditi et al., 2012; Kahn et al., 2013). Attributes of computerized CDS tools effect adherence to EBP recommendations. Large to moderate improvements in EBP are demonstrated when CDS is automatic rather than on demand; the CDS is on-screen rather than on paper, and the CDS is patient-specific (rather than generic) (Van de Velde et al., 2018).

Conveying key messages about EBP recommendations at point-of-care delivery is another way to foster implementation. Distilling the recommendations to a few key points on visual displays can be very effective when designed appropriately. Examples include posters, infographics, and visual abstracts (Flodgren et al., 2016; Ibrahim et al., 2017).

Implementation Strategies to Address Communication

Communication is more than exchange of information; it is a transformational process of developing shared understanding through interactions and relationships (Manojlovich et al., 2015). Information and/or shared understanding moves through communication channels such as interactive communication routes (e.g. social media).

These communication channels serve as connectors among those implementing EBP recommendations (Rogers, 2003; Titler, 2019). Implementation strategies regarding communication are as follows:

- Social and mass media
- Education
- Opinion leadership
- Change champions
- Educational outreach/academic detailing

Mass media is communicating information in a directional message from one source to many individuals. Examples of mass media are television, radio, print materials, Internet sources, and digital technology (Brownson et al., 2018; Mosdøl et al., 2017). Professional societies and government organizations use mass media to impart informational messages to the public and stakeholder groups (Brownson et al., 2018). The effectiveness of mass media to align clinician practices with the evidence is equivocal and most likely increases awareness and persuasion early during implementation (Grimshaw et al., 2012).

The rapid growth of social media platforms such as Facebook and Twitter has led to increased use of *interactive* media in which communication channels are multidirectional in nature. Social media is a type of electronic communication using a variety of platforms (e.g., Facebook, Twitter) through which users create online communities for social networking to share information, ideas, and messages (Bardus et al., 2020; Kirton, 2019; Roland, 2018). Studies have demonstrated that use of social media increases users' knowledge about EBP (Frisch et al., 2014; Maloney et al., 2015; Tunnecliff et al., 2017). Use of social and mass media is important to consider when thinking about messaging such as the following:

- Knowing the audience
- Defining the customer
- Specifying the message and framing it
- Selecting the appropriate communication platforms

Education is necessary but not sufficient to change practice, and didactic continuing education alone does little to change practice behavior (Flodgren et al., 2013; Giguère et al., 2012). Compared with traditional learning, there is no evidence that e-learning (interactive online educational programs) makes a difference in health professionals' behaviors, knowledge, and skills. The general claims that e-learning is inherently more effective than traditional learning is misleading (Vaona et al., 2018). It is important that staff know the scientific basis for improvements in quality of care anticipated by the changes. Disseminating information to staff must be done creatively. A staff development program may not be the most effective method and may not reach the majority of the staff. Although it is unrealistic for all staff to have participated in the critical appraisal process or to have read all studies used, it is important that they know the myths and realities of the EBP. Staff education must also ensure competence in the skills necessary to carry out the new practice.

One method of communicating information to staff is through use of colorful posters that identify myths and realities or describe the essence of the change in practice (Anderson & Titler, 2019; Titler et al., 2016). Visibly identifying those who have learned the information and are using the EBP (e.g., via buttons, ribbons, pins) stimulates interest in others who may not have internalized the change. As a result, the "new" learner may begin asking questions about the practice and be more open to learning. Other educational strategies such as train-the-trainer programs, computer-assisted instruction, and competency testing are helpful in education of staff (Titler et al., 2016).

Studies and systematic reviews have demonstrated that opinion leaders are effective in changing behaviors of health care practitioners (Cranley et al., 2019; Dagenais et al., 2015; Flodgren et al., 2011; Nooraie et al., 2017), especially in combination with educational outreach or performance feedback. Opinion leaders are from the local peer group and are viewed as a respected source of influence, considered by associates as technically competent, and trusted to judge the fit between the EBP and the local situation (Dobbins et al., 2009; Flodgren et al., 2011). The key characteristic of an opinion leader is a trusted ability to evaluate new information in the context of group norms. To do this, an opinion leader must be considered by associates as technically competent and a full and dedicated member of the local group (Rogers, 2003).

Opinion leadership is multifaceted and complex, with role functions varying by circumstances, but few successful projects that have implemented EBP have managed without the input of identifiable opinion leaders. Social interactions such as "hallway chats," one-on-one discussions, and addressing questions are important yet often overlooked components of translation (Jordan et al., 2009). If the EBP that is being implemented is interdisciplinary, discipline-specific opinion leaders should be used to promote the practice change. Role expectations of an opinion leader are listed in Box 20.4.

Change champions are also helpful for implementing innovations (Dogherty et al., 2012). They are practitioners within the local group setting (e.g., clinic, patient care unit) who are expert clinicians, are passionate about the innovation, are committed to improving quality of care, and have a positive working relationship with other health professionals (Rogers, 2003). Important qualities of change champions are that they are in key linkage positions, understand the various interests of key stakeholders, and possess good interpersonal and negotiation skills (Bonawitz et al., 2020; Rogers, 2003). They circulate information, encourage peers to adopt the innovation, arrange demonstrations, and orient staff to the innovation (Titler et al., 2016). The change champion believes in an idea; will not take "no" for an answer; is undaunted by insults and rebuffs; and, above all, persists. They often broker change through their advocacy skills and personal network relationships (Bonawitz et al., 2020; Ploeg et al., 2010).

Multiple studies have demonstrated the effectiveness of educational outreach, also known as *academic detailing,* in improving clinicians' practice behaviors (Avorn, 2010; National Academy of Medicine [NAM], formally IOM, 2011; Wilson et al., 2016). Educational outreach involves interactive face-to-face education of practitioners in their setting by an individual (usually a clinician) with EBP expertise in a particular topic (e.g., cancer pain management). Academic detailers explain the research foundations of the EBP recommendations and respond convincingly to specific questions, concerns, or challenges that a practitioner might raise. An academic detailer can also deliver feedback on provider or team performance with respect to an EBP recommendation (e.g., frequency of pain

---

BOX 20.4 Role Expectations of an Opinion Leader

1. Be/become an expert in the evidence-based practice.
2. Provide organizational/unit leadership for adopting the evidence-based practice.
3. Implement various strategies to educate peers about the evidence-based practice.
4. Work with peers, other disciplines, and leadership staff to incorporate key information about the evidence-based practice into organizational/unit standards, policies, procedures, and documentation systems.
5. Promote initial and ongoing use of the evidence-based practice by peers.

assessment). The individual conducting the educational outreach must have attributes of shared learning, positive reinforcement for aligning practices with evidence, listening to challenges regarding implementation, and group problem solving. Clinicians' perceptions of educational outreach are quite positive and perceived as helpful in overcoming implementation barriers (Wilson et al., 2016).

Implementation Strategies to Address Users

Members of a social system (e.g., nurses, physicians, community health workers) influence how quickly and widely EBP is adopted (Rogers, 2003). When selecting implementation strategies, it is essential to first delineate the target audience(s) and key stakeholders that will use the EBP as well as the nature of the context where they work (e.g., primary care) and interact with the specified population (e.g. older adults with dementia). Implementation strategies that have demonstrated effectiveness in improving EBP of the users include the following (Hysong, 2009; Hysong et al., 2018; Ivers et al., 2012, 2014; Stacey et al., 2017; Titler & Anderson, 2019):

- Audit and feedback
- Performance gap assessment (PGA)
- Trying the EBP
- Engaging with recipients of the EBP
- Implementation team meetings to address barriers and acknowledge success

Performance gap assessment (PGA) provides information of current practices relative to recommended EBP at the beginning of a practice change. This implementation strategy is used to engage clinicians in discussions of practice issues and to select strategies for promoting alignment of practice with EBP recommendations. Specific practice indicators selected for PGA are derived from the EBP recommendations for the specified topic such as every-4-hour pain assessment for acute pain management. Studies have demonstrated improvements in performance when PGA is part of multifaceted implementation strategies (see Chapters 19 and 21) (Titler et al., 2016; Yano, 2008).

Audit and feedback (A/F) is ongoing auditing of performance indicators, aggregating data into reports, and discussing the findings with practitioners during the practice change (Ivers et al., 2012; Hysong et al., 2012; Wilson et al., 2016). This strategy helps staff know and see how their efforts to improve care and patient outcomes are progressing throughout the implementation process (Ivers et al., 2014). A/F reports are more effective when distributed regularly and discussed with clinicians rather than by passive dissemination to an individual or posting on a website (Hysong et al., 2012, 2018; Ivers et al., 2014).

Users of an innovation usually try it for a period before adopting it in their practice. When "trying an EBP" (i.e., piloting a change) is incorporated as part of the implementation process, users have an opportunity to use it, provide feedback to those in charge of implementation, and modify the practice if necessary. Piloting the practice as part of implementation has a positive influence on the extent of adoption of the new practice (Rogers, 2003).

An important part of implementing EBP is engaging with recipients of the EBP to address their values and preferences. EBP is applied *with* individuals, groups, and populations, not *to* them. Putting the patient, family, and community at the center of health care decisions is essential to address their values, characteristics, cultures, and other contextual factors that are important to them (Msowoya and Gephart, 2019). Use of patient decision-making aids is one approach to promote shared decision making, a process by which patients/consumers and health care workers partner to make informed health decisions that benefit the patient and are aligned with their knowledge and values (Msowoya and Gephart, 2019). Patient decision-making aids (also called *shared decision-making aids*) that promote health literacy are evidence-based documents or tools that support patients by making decisions explicit and providing information about options and their associated benefits and harms. Health literacy products that are decision-making aids should be targeted to the stakeholder end user(s) and be culturally relevant, reading-level appropriate, and linguistically aligned. They help clarify congruence between decisions and personal values (Msowoya and Gephart, 2019; Stacey et al., 2017). Use of patient decision-making aids provide the following guidance (Stacey et al., 2017):

- Increases patients' knowledge, the accuracy of their risk perceptions, and congruency between care choices and their values
- Decreases decisional conflict, indecisions about personal values, and the proportion of individuals who were passive in decision making
- Improves patient-clinician communication and satisfaction with their decision and the decision-making process

Examples of patient decision-making aids are available from the Ottawa Hospital Research Institute (https://decisionaid.ohri.ca/index.html).

Regular meetings with key stakeholders and those implementing the EBP recommendations help track the process of implementation, provide guidance for questions and challenges that arise, and facilitate sharing of implementation strategies that are working. Meetings are usually 45 to 60 minutes and can be via teleconference, face-to-face, or webinar. The meeting leader must facilitate regular attendance by the participants and ensure that each person has a "voice at the table." Meeting minutes and accountability for actions after the meeting are important to engage participants and move implementation forward (Titler & Anderson, 2019).

Implementation Strategies to Address the Social System

Clearly, the social system or context of care delivery matters when implementing EBPs (Rogers, 2003; Squires et al., 2015; Titler & Anderson, 2019; Yousefi-Nooraie et al., 2014). **Example:** ➤ Investigators demonstrated the effectiveness of a prompted voiding intervention for urinary incontinence in nursing homes, but sustaining the intervention in day-to-day practice was limited when the responsibility of carrying out the intervention was shifted to nursing home staff (rather than the investigative team) and required staffing levels in excess of a majority of nursing home settings (Engberg et al., 2004). This illustrates the importance of embedding interventions into ongoing care processes.

Context is gaining increased attention in EBP implementation. **Context** is the characteristics of the physical setting and the social dynamic practice factors in which implementation processes occur (May et al., 2016; Squires et al., 2015). The physical setting is composed of the key structural characteristics such as staffing, unit size, annual visit volume, and types of patients receiving care. The dynamic factors includes the roles, relationships, and dynamics among individuals and groups in the practice setting (Shuman et al., 2018). Contextual factors that affect implementation are described in Table 20.5.

Implementation strategies that target the social system or context include the following:
- Conducting an environmental scan,
- Meeting with key leadership stakeholders,
- Revising practice standards and documentation systems, and
- Providing recognition and rewards.

TABLE 20.5 **Contextual Factors That Affect Implementation**		
Context Factor	**Definition**	**Descriptions**
Organizational Capacity for EBP	Availability of resources, structures, and workforce to plan, deliver, and evaluate evidence-based interventions and programs (Brownson et al., 2018). Components of organizational capacity for EBP include (Tilter and Anderson, 2019): • Strong leadership • Clear strategic vision • Good managerial relations • Visionary staff in key positions • A climate conducive to experimentation and risk taking • Effective data-capture systems	Capacity-building involves intentional, coordinated, and mission-driven efforts to strengthen the activities, management, and governance of organizations to improve their performance (e.g., delivery of EBP) and impact (improved health care outcomes) (Brownson et al., 2018).
Leadership support (also called *implementation leadership*)	A strategic approach of organizational leaders characterized by a set of influencing behaviors that result in positive outcomes for implementation of EBP (Castiglione, 2020; Stetler et al., 2014)	• Leadership support is expressed verbally and through the provision of resources, materials, and time to enact EBP. Key behaviors include (Bianchi et al., 2018; Gifford et al., 2018; Stetler et al., 2014; Titler & Anderson, 2019): • Setting forth a mission, vision, and strategic plan for EBP • Using performance expectations for all employees that explicate the work of EBP • Using EBP language in verbal and written communication and in organizational documents • Role-modeling the use of evidence in clinical and administrative decision making • Establishing explicit expectations that midlevel managers foster microsystems that value and support clinical inquiry and EBP
Practice climate for use of EBP	Shared perceptions of staff regarding the practices, policies, procedures, and clinical behaviors rewarded, supported, and expected to facilitate effective implementation of EBP (Ehrhart et al., 2014; Shuman et al., 2018)	The extent to which a practice unit or setting prioritizes and values EBP in the following areas (Ehrhart et al., 2014): • Focus on EBP • Educational support for EBP • Recognition for EBP • Rewards for EBP • Selection of staff for EBP knowledge and skills • Selection of staff for openness
EBP competencies	Knowledge and skills of staff regarding all aspects of EBP. Competencies vary by role (e.g., nurse manager, staff nurse), job description, and educational level	Expected level of purposeful performance regarding use of evidence to improve care delivery. This requires the integration of knowledge, skills, and judgment about EBP (Shuman et al., 2018)

EBP, Evidence-based practice.

An environmental scan assesses internal strengths and challenges for a specific topic; in this case, EBP implementation. Environmental scans provide information about the structure and function of an organization and how work is done within this structure. Two purposes of an environmental scan are to understand the mission, vision, and values and to articulate how specific EBP contributes to the overall mission and goals of the organization. A third purpose is to become knowledgeable about the governance structure and senior leaders with whom you may need to interact for implementation. Specifically, you will want to understand the purpose of the various councils and committees that compose the governance structure and evaluate which ones you must work with for implementation. For example, many organizations have standards and quality improvement committees in their governance; it is likely that you will need to work with them as part of implementation. It is critical that you understand the governance of the organization, foster positive working relationships with those leading key governance committees, and listen to descriptions about how change occurs in the system. As part of your environmental scan, you may want to assess key context factors such as unit climate and leadership behaviors for EBP implementation. Several assessment tools are available (Titler & Anderson, 2019). These assessments provide insight for tailoring implementation strategies such as educational approaches and fostering leadership behaviors that promote EBP.

Meeting with key leaders from various disciplines is essential for implementation (Titler & Anderson, 2019). As part of your environmental scan, identify these key leaders and make a plan to meet with them. Initially, you will want to meet with the chief nurse executive (CNE) to describe the project and the overall goals related to quality and safety. Be prepared to discuss and illustrate with data the current practice, synthesis of the current evidence (see Chapter 11), practices that can be improved to align with the current evidence, and potential practice sites for implementation. The CNE is a valuable resource who can provide recommendations for involvement of key stakeholders, additional implementation team members, and individuals to serve as opinion leaders. The CNE also is a valuable resource for allocation of financial or other resources that are essential to effective implementation of the EBP. Establish the preferred methods for ongoing communication with the CNE such as e-mail updates, face-to-face meetings, and/or quarterly reports. In some cases, the EBP may be driven by the CNE to address a quality-of-care issue. In this case, the meeting would focus on understanding the CNE's perspective and focus of the project (Titler & Anderson, 2019). Midlevel managers through whom EBP will be implemented are key to success (Titler & Anderson, 2019). These individuals have different titles depending on the site of implementation (e.g., nurse managers, directors) but are characterized as a licensed clinician (e.g., RN) who is the direct supervisor of staff on the unit and has responsibility and accountability for unit-level operations. It is important that you garner the support of the nurse manager(s) where implementation is planned and that you keep them informed throughout the process.

As part of the work of implementing EBP, it is important that the social system (e.g., unit, service line, clinic) ensure that policies, procedures, standards, clinical pathways, and documentation systems support the use of the EBP (Titler & Anderson, 2019). Documentation forms or clinical information systems may need revision to support practice changes; documentation systems that fail to readily support the new practice thwart change. **Example:** ➤ If staff members are expected to reassess and document pain intensity within 30 minutes after administration of an analgesic agent, documentation forms must reflect this practice standard. It is the role of leadership to ensure that organizational documents and systems are flexible and supportive of EBP.

Recognition and rewards are important to acknowledge staff's investment in delivery of evidence-based care. Recognition can be achieved through organizational publications, personal thank-you notes from key leaders, presenting the work at system-level quality-improvement meetings, and nominating the team for excellence awards offered by the health system and professional nursing organizations. Rewards may include bonus payments, salary increases, and/or educational funds to be used at the discretion of the implementation team and/or practice unit (Titler & Anderson, 2019).

In summary, making an evidence-based change in practice is nonlinear and involves a series of iterative steps. Implementation strategies that promote the use of EBP include audit and feedback, use of clinical reminders and practice prompts, opinion leaders, change champions, interactive education, educational outreach, and addressing the context of care delivery (e.g., leadership, learning, questioning).

Evaluation

Evaluation is a structured approach to evaluate the impact of the EBP that is implemented. It is a key component of piloting the change in practice and when EBP is extended to additional practice areas (Titler & Medvec, 2019). The importance of the evaluation cannot be overemphasized; it provides information for performance gap assessment, audit, and feedback, and it provides information necessary to determine whether the EBP should be retained, modified, or eliminated.

An outcome achieved in a controlled environment (as when a researcher is implementing a study protocol for a homogeneous group of study patients) may not result in the same outcome when the practice is implemented in the clinical setting by several caregivers to a more heterogeneous patient population. Steps of the evaluation process are summarized in Box 20.5.

Evaluation includes both process and outcome measures (Titler & Medvec, 2019). The process component focuses on use of EBP being implemented. It is important to know if staff are using the practice and implementing the practice as noted in the EBP guidelines. Evaluation of the process also should note (1) barriers that staff encounter in carrying out the practice (e.g., lack of information, skills, or necessary equipment), (2) differences in opinions among health care providers, and (3) difficulty carrying out the steps of the

---

BOX 20.5 Steps of Evaluation for Evidence-Based Projects

1. Identify process and outcome variables of interest.
   Example: Process variable—Patients will have a fall risk assessment every 12 hours
   Outcome variables—Fall rates, Fall injury rate, Severity of fall injuries
2. Determine methods and frequency of data collection.
   Example: Process variable—Chart audit of all patients on [name unit] 1 day per month.
   Outcome variables—Calculated by month by the quality improvement and risk department
3. Determine baseline and follow-up sample sizes.
4. Design data collection forms.
   Example: Chart audit abstraction form for fall risk assessment (may be available electronically from electronic medical record).
   Outcome variable—Standardized risk or incident reports for adverse events such as falls
5. Establish content validity of data collection forms.
6. Train data collectors.
7. Assess interrater reliability of data collectors.
8. Collect data at specified intervals.
9. Provide staff regular feedback of measures (e.g., every 3 months) to illustrate progress in achieving the practice change.
10. Use data to assist staff in modification and/or integration of EBP change.
11. Provide final evaluation to staff and senior executives.
12. Write a final evaluation report.

TABLE 20.6 Examples of Evaluation Measures

	NURSES' SELF-RATING				
Example Process Questions	SD	D	NA/D	A	SA
I feel well prepared to use the Braden scale with older adult patients.	1	2	3	4	5
Malnutrition increases patient risk for pressure ulcer development.	1	2	3	4	5
Example Outcome Question	**Patient**				
On a scale of 0 (no pain) to 10 (worst possible pain), how much pain have you experienced over the past 24 hours?					

A, Agree; *D*, disagree; *NA/D*, neither agree nor disagree; *SA*, strongly agree; *SD*, strongly disagree.

practice as originally designed (e.g., shutting off tube feedings 1 hour before aspirating contents for checking placement of nasointestinal tubes). Process data can be collected from staff and/or patient self-reports, medical record audits, or observation of clinical practice. Examples of process and outcome questions are shown in Table 20.6.

Outcome data are an equally important part of evaluation. The purpose of outcome evaluation is to assess whether the patient, staff, and/or fiscal outcomes expected are achieved. Therefore it is important that baseline data be used for a preintervention/postintervention comparison (Titler & Medvec, 2019). Outcome variables should be those that are projected to change as a result of changing practice. **Example:** ➤ Research demonstrates that less restricted family visiting practices in critical care units result in improved satisfaction with care. Thus patient and family member satisfaction should be an outcome that is evaluated as part of changing visiting practices in adult critical care units. Outcomes should be assessed before the change in practice is implemented, after implementation, and every 3 to 6 months thereafter. Findings must be provided to clinicians to reinforce the impact of the change and to ensure that they are incorporated into quality-improvement programs. When collecting process and outcome data, it is important that data collection tools are user-friendly, short, concise, and easy to complete and that they have content validity. Focus on collecting the most essential data. Those responsible for collecting evaluative data must be trained on data collection methods and be assessed for interrater reliability (see Chapters 14 and 15).

One question that often arises is how much data are needed to evaluate a change. The preferred number of patients (*N*) is somewhat dependent on the size of the patient population affected by the practice change (Titler & Medvec, 2019). **Example:** ➤ If the practice change is for families of critically ill adult patients and the organization has 1000 adult critical care patients annually, 50 to 100 satisfaction responses preimplementation, and 25 to 50 responses postimplementation, 3 and 6 months should be adequate to look for trends in satisfaction and possible areas that must be addressed in continuing this practice (e.g., more bedside chairs in patient rooms). The rule of thumb is to keep the evaluation simple because data often are collected by busy clinicians who may lose interest if the data collection, analysis, and feedback are too long and tedious. It is also important to check with your institution's guidelines for collecting data related to practice changes because institutional approval may be needed.

The evaluation process includes planned feedback to staff who are making the change. The feedback includes verbal and/or written appreciation for the work and visual demonstration of progress in implementation and improvement in patient outcomes. The key to effective evaluation is to ensure that the EBP is warranted (e.g., will improve quality of care) and safe.

> **HELPFUL HINT**
>
> Include patient outcome measures (e.g., pressure ulcer prevalence) and cost (e.g., cost savings, cost avoidance) in evaluation practice projects.

FUTURE DIRECTIONS

Multiple health care systems, professional organizations, and regulatory agencies expect that patients receive evidence-based health care. Challenges to meet these expectations include building organizational capacity, education of clinicians and leaders to foster use of EBP, and engaging patients and families as part of the implementation team. An emerging body of knowledge in translation science provides an empirical foundation for implementation strategies to assure that we deliver high-quality, evidence-based care. Each of us must make the commitment to critically question current practices and improve care through implementation of the latest evidence.

KEY POINTS

- *EBP* and *translation science,* though related, are not interchangeable terms; EBP is the actual application of evidence in practice (the "doing of" EBP), whereas translation science is the study of implementation interventions, factors, and contextual variables that effect knowledge uptake and use in practices and communities.
- There are several models of EBP. A key feature of all models is the judicious review and synthesis of research and other types of evidence to develop an EBP standard.
- The steps of EBP using the Iowa Model of Evidence-Based Practice are as follows: (1) selecting a topic, (2) forming a team, (3) retrieving the evidence, (4) grading the evidence, (5) developing an EBP standard, (6) implementing the EBP, and (7) evaluating the effect on staff, patient, and fiscal outcomes.
- Adoption of EBP requires education of staff and the use of implementation strategies such as opinion leaders, change champions, educational outreach, performance gap assessment, and audit and feedback.
- It is important to evaluate the change. Evaluation provides data for performance gap assessment, audit, and feedback, and it provides information necessary to determine whether the practice should be retained.
- Evaluation includes both process and outcome measures.
- It is important for organizations to create a culture of EBP. Creating this culture requires an interactive process. Organizations must provide access to information, access to individuals who have skills necessary for EBP, and a written and verbal commitment to EBP in the organization's operations.

CLINICAL JUDGMENT CHALLENGES

- Discuss the differences among nursing research, EBP, and translation science. Support your discussion with examples.
- Why would it be important to use an EBP model, such as the Iowa Model of Evidence-Based Practice, to guide a practice project focused on justifying and implementing a change in clinical practice?

- **IPE** You are a staff nurse working on a cardiac step-down unit. You are asked to join an interprofessional quality-improvement team for the cardiac division. You find that many of your colleagues from other disciplines do not understand EBP. How would you help your colleagues understand the relevance of EBP to providing care that addresses the Triple Aim for this patient population?
- What barriers do you see to applying EBP in your clinical setting? Discuss strategies to use in overcoming these barriers.

REFERENCES

Anderson, C., & Titler, M. G. (2019). Launching implementation. In G. LoBiondo-Wood, J. Haber, & M. G. Titler (Eds.), *Evidence-based practice for healthcare and quality improvement* (pp. 197–205). Philadelphia, PA: Elsevier.

Andrews, J., Guyatt, G., Oxman, A. D., et al. (2013). GRADE guidelines: 14. Going from evidence to recommendations: The significance and presentation of recommendations. *Journal of Clinical Epidemiology, 66,* 719–725. https://doi.org/10.1016/j.jclinepi.2012.03.013. PMID: 23312392.

Arditi, C., Rege-Walther, M., Wyatt, J. C., et al. (2012). Computer-generated reminders delivered on paper to healthcare professionals: Effects on professional practice and health care outcomes. *Cochrane Database of Systematic Reviews, 12.* https://doi.org/10.1002/14651858.CD001175.pub3.

Avorn, J. (2010). Transforming trial results into practice change: The final translational hurdle: comment on "Impact of the ALLHAT/JNC7 Dissemination Project on thiazide-type diuretic use." *Archives of Internal Medicine, 170*(10), 858–860. https://doi.org/10.1001/archinternmed.2010.125.

Balshem, H., Helfand, M., Schunemann, H. J., et al. (2011). GRADE guidelines: 3. Rating the quality of evidence. *Journal of Clinical Epidemiology, 64*(4), 401–406. https://doi.org/10.1016/j.jclinepi.2010.07.015.

Bardus, M., Chahrour, M., Raslan, A. S., Meho, L. I., & Akl, E. A. (2020). The use of social media to increase the impact of health research: Systematic review. *Journal of Medical Internet Research, 22*(7).

Bianchi, M., Bagnasco, A., Bressan, V., et al. (2018). A review of the role of nurse leadership in promoting and sustaining evidence-based practice. *Journal of Nursing Management, 26,* 918–932.

Birken, S. A., Powell, B. J., Shea, C. M., Haines, E. R., Kirk, M. A., Leeman, J., Rohweder, C., Damschroder, L., & Presseau, J. (2017). Criteria for selecting implementation science theories and frameworks: Results from an international survey. *Implementation Science, 12*(124). https://doi.org/10.1186/s13012-017-0656-y.

Bonawitz, K., Wetmore, M., Heisler, M., et al. (2020). Champions in context: Which attributes matter for change efforts in healthcare? *Implementation Science, 15,* 62.

Brownson, R. C., Eyler, A., Harris, J. K., Moore, J., & Tabak, R. (2018). Getting the word out: New approaches for disseminating public health science. *Journal of Public Health Management and Practice, 24*(2), 102–111.

Brownson, R. C., Fielding, J. E., & Green, L. W. (2018). Building capacity for evidence-based public health: Reconciling the pulls of practice and the push of research. *Annual Review of Public Health, 39,* 27–53.

Castiglione, S. A. (2020). Implementation leadership: A concept analysis. *Journal of Nursing Management, 28,* 94–101.

Cranley, L. A., Keefe, J., Taylor, D., et al. (2019). Understanding professional advice networks in long-term care: An outside-inside view of best practice pathways for diffusion. *Implementation Science, 14,* 10.

Dagenais, C., Laurendeau, M.-C., & Briand-Lamarche, M. (2015). Knowledge brokering in public health: A critical analysis of the results of a qualitative evaluation. *Evaluation and Program Planning, 53*, 10–17. https://doi.org/10.1016/j.evalprogplan.2015.07.003.

Dobbins, M., Robeson, P., Ciliska, D., et al. (2009). A description of a knowledge broker role implemented as part of a randomized controlled trial evaluating three knowledge translation strategies. *Implementation Science, 4*, 23. https://doi.org/10.1186/1748-5908-4-23.

Dogherty, E. J., Harrison, M. B., Baker, C., & Graham, I. D. (2012). Following a natural experiment of guideline adaptation and early implementation: A mixed methods study of facilitation. *Implementation Science, 7*, 9. https://doi.org/10.1186/1748-5908-7-9.

Ehrhart, M. G., Aarons, G. A., & Farahnak, L. R. (2014). Assessing the organizational context for EBP implementation: The development and validity testing of the Implementation Climate Scale (ICS). *Implementation Science, 9*(1), 157.

Engberg, S., Kincade, J., & Thompson, D. (2004). Future directions for incontinence research with frail elders. *Nursing Research, 53*(Suppl 6), S22–S29. PMID: 15586144.

Flodgren, G., Conterno, L. O., Mayhew, A., et al. (2013). Interventions to improve professional adherence to guidelines for prevention of device-related infections. *Cochrane Database of Systematic Reviews*, 3. https://doi.org/10.1002/14651858.CD006559.pub2. PMID: 23543545.

Flodgren, G., Hall, A. M., Goulding, L., et al. (2016). Tools developed and disseminated by guideline producers to promote the uptake of their guidelines. *Cochrane Database of Systematic Reviews, 8* (Article No. CD010669).

Flodgren, G., Parmelli, E., Doumit, G., et al. (2011). Local opinion leaders: effects on professional practice and health care outcomes. *Cochrane Database of Systematic Reviews, 8*. https://doi.org/10.1002/14651858.CD000125.pub4. Article No. CD000125. PMID: 21833939, PMCID: PMC4172331.

Frisch, N., Atherton, P., Borycki, E., et al. (2014). Growing a professional network to over 3000 members in less than 4 years: Evaluation of InspireNet, British Columbia's Virtual Nursing Health Services Research Network. *Journal of Medical Internet Research, 16*(2), e49.

Gephart, S. M., Newnam, K., Wyles, C., Bethel, C., Porter, C., Quinn, M. C., Canvasser, J., Umberger, E., & Titler, M. (2020). Development of the NEC-Zero Toolkit: Supporting reliable implementation of necrotizing enterocolitis prevention and recognition. *Neonatal Network: NN, 39*(1), 6–15.

Gifford, W. A., Squires, J. E., Angus, D. E., et al. (2018). Managerial leadership for research use in nursing and allied health care professions: A systematic review. *Implementation Science, 13*, 127.

Giguère, A., Légaré, F., Grimshaw, J., et al. (2012). Printed educational materials: Effects on professional practice and healthcare outcomes. *Cochrane Database of Systematic Reviews, 10*. https://doi.org/10.1002/14651858.CD004398.pub3. Article No. CD004398. PMID: 23076904.

Glegg, S. M. N., Jenkins, E., & Kothan, A (2019). How the study of networks informs knowledge translation and implementation: A scoping review. *Implementation Science, 14*, 34.

Greenhalgh, T., & Papoutsi, C. (2019). Spreading and scaling up innovation and improvement. *BMJ, 365*, 12068.

Grimshaw, J. M., Eccles, M. P., Lavis, J. N., Hill, S. J., & Squires, J. E. (2012). Knowledge translation of research findings. *Implementation Science, 7*(50).

Guyatt, G. H., Oxman, A. D., Sultan, S., et al. (2013). GRADE guidelines: 11. Making an overall rating of confidence in effect estimates for a single outcome and for all outcomes. *Journal of Clinical Epidemiology, 66*(2), 151–157. https://doi.org/10.1016/j.jclinepi.2012.01.006.

Guyatt, G. H., Oxman, A. D., Sultan, S., et al. (2011). GRADE guidelines: 9. Rating up the quality of evidence. *Journal of Clinical Epidemiology, 64*(12), 1311–1316. https://doi.org/10.1016/j.jclinepi.2011.06.004.

Hysong, S. J. (2009). Meta-analysis: Audit and feedback features impact effectiveness on care quality. *Medical Care, 47*(3), 356–363.

Hysong, S. J., Smitham, K., SoRelle, R., Amspoker, A., Hughes, A. M., & Haider, P. (2018). Mental models of audit and feedback in primary care settings. *Implementation Science, 13*(73).

Hysong, S. J., Teal, C. R., Khan, M. J., & Haidet, P. (2012). Improving quality of care through improved audit and feedback. *Implementation Science, 7*, 45. https://doi.org/10.1186/1748-5908 -7-45. PMID: 22607640, PMCID: PMC3462705.

Ibrahim, A. M., Lillemoe, K. D., Klingensmith, M. E., & Dimick, J. B. (2017). Visual abstracts to disseminate research on social media: A prospective, case-control crossover study. *Annals of Surgery, 266*(6), 46–48.

Institute of Medicine (IOM). (2011). *Clinical practice guidelines we can trust.* Washington, DC: The National Academies Press. https://doi.org/10.17226/13058. PMID: 24983061.

Iowa Model Collaborative. (2017). Iowa model of evidence-based practice: Revisions and validation. *Worldviews on Evidence-Based Nursing, 14*(3), 175–182.

Ivers, N., Jamtvedt, G., Flottorp, S., et al. (2012). Audit and feedback: Effects on professional practice and healthcare outcomes. *Cochrane Database of Systematic Reviews, 6.* https://doi. org/10.1002/14651858.CD000259.pub3. Article No. CD000259. PMID: 22696318.

Ivers, N. M., Sales, A., Colquhoun, H., et al. (2014). No more "business as usual" with audit and feedback interventions: Towards an agenda for a reinvigorated intervention. *Implementation Science, 9*, 14. https://doi.org/10.1186/1748-5908-9-14.

Jordan, M. E., Lanham, H. J., Crabtree, B. F., et al. (2009). The role of conversation in health care interventions: Enabling sensemaking and learning. *Implementation Science, 4*, 15. https://doi. org/10.1186/1748-5908-4-15. PMID: 19284660, PMCID: PMC2663543.

Kahn, S. R., Morrison, D. R., Cohen, J. M., et al. (2013). Interventions for implementation of thromboprophylaxis in hospitalized medical and surgical patients at risk for venous thromboembolism. *Cochrane Database of Systematic Reviews, 7.* https://doi. org/10.1002/14651858.CD008201.pub2. PMID: 23861035.

Kirton, C. (2019). Dissemination. In G. LoBiondo-Wood, J. Haber, & M. G. Titler (Eds.), *Evidence-based practice for healthcare and quality improvement* (pp. 242–250). Philadelphia, PA: Elsevier.

Maloney, S., Tunnecliff, J., Morgan, P., et al. (2015). Translating evidence into practice via social media: A mixed-methods study. *Journal of Medical Internet Research, 17*(10), e242.

Manojlovich, M., Squires, J. E., Davies, B., & Graham, I. D. (2015). Hiding in plain sight: Communication theory in implementation science. *Implementation Science, 10*, 58.

May, C. R., Johnson, M., & Finch, T. (2016). Implementation, context and complexity. *Implementation Science., 11*(1), 141.

Mosdøl, A., Lidal, I. B., Straumann, G. H., & Vist, G. E. (2017). Targeted mass media interventions promoting healthy behaviours to reduce risk of non-communicable diseases in adult, ethnic minorities. *Cochrane Database of Systematic Reviews*, 2. (Article No. CD011683).

Msowoya, A. L., & Gephart, S. M. (2019). Patient-centered evidence-based practices. In G. LoBiondo-Wood, J. Haber, & M. G. Titler (Eds.), *Evidence-based practice for healthcare and quality improvement* (pp. 219–230). Philadelphia, PA: Elsevier.

National Institutes of Health (2020). Dissemination and implementation research in health. PAR-19-274. https://grants.nih.gov/grants/guide/pa-files/PAR-19-274,8/7/2020.

Nooraie, R. Y., Marin, A., Hanneman, R., Lohfeld, L., & Dobbins, M. (2017). Implementation of evidence-informed practice through central network actors: A case study of three public health units in Canada. *BMC Health Services Research, 17*, 208.

Ploeg, J., Skelly, J., Rowan, M., et al. (2010). The role of nursing best practice champions in diffusing practice guidelines: A mixed methods study. *Worldviews on Evidence-Based Nursing, 7*(4), 238–251.

Rogers, E. M. (2003). *Diffusion of innovations* (5th ed.). New York, NY: Free Press.

Roland, D. (2018). Social media, health policy, and knowledge translation. *Journal of the American College of Radiology, 15*(1PB), 149–152.

Shuman, C., Liu, X., Banaszak-Holl, J., Aebersold, M., Tschannen, D., & Titler, M. G. (2018). Associations among unit leadership and unit climates for implementation in acute care: A cross-sectional study. *Implementation Science, 13*, 62–72.

Shuman, C. J., Liu, J., Montie, M., et al. (2016). Patient perception and experiences with falls during hospitalization and after discharge. *Applied Nursing Research, 31*, 79–85. https://doi.org/10.1016/j.apnr.2016.01.009. PMID: 27397823.

Squires, J. E., Graham, I. D., Hutchinson, A. M., et al. (2015). Identifying the domains of context important to implementation science: A study protocol. *Implementation Science, 10*(1), 135. https://doi.org/10.1186/s13012-015-0325-y. PMID: 26416206, PMCID: PMC4584460.

Stacey, D., Légaré, F., Lewis, K., et al. (2017). Decision aids for people facing health treatment or screening decisions. *Cochrane Database of Systematic Reviews*, 4. (Article No. CD001431).

Stetler, C. B., Ritchie, J. A., Rycroft-Malone, J., & Charns, M (2014). Leadership for evidence-base practice: Strategic and functional behaviors for institutionalizing EBP. *Worldviews on Evidence-Based Nursing, 11*(4), 219–226.

Straus, E., Richardson, R. B., Glasziou, P., et al. (2011). *Evidence-based medicine: How to practice and teach* (4th ed.). New York, NY: Elsevier.

Titler, M. G. (2018). Translation research in practice: An introduction. *The Online Journal of Issues in Nursing, 23*(2). https://doi.org/10.3912/OJIN.Vol23No02Man01.

Titler, M. G. (2019). Planning for success. In G. LoBiondo-Wood, J. Haber, & M. G. Titler (Eds.), *Evidence-based practice for healthcare and quality improvement* (pp. 183–196). Philadelphia, PA: Elsevier.

Titler, M. G., & Anderson, C. (2019). Implementation strategies: The social system and users of the evidence-based practices. In G. LoBiondo-Wood, J. Haber, & M. G. Titler (Eds.), *Evidence-based practice for healthcare and quality improvement* (pp. 206–218). Philadelphia, PA: Elsevier.

Titler, M. G., Conlon, P., Reynolds, M. A., et al. (2016). The effect of translating research into practice intervention to promote use of evidence-based fall prevention interventions in hospitalized adults: A prospective pre-post implementation study in the U.S. *Applied Nursing Research, 31*, 52–59. https://doi.org/10.1016/j.apnr.2015.12.004.

Titler, M. G., Kleiber, C., Steelman, V. J., et al. (2001). The Iowa model of evidence-based practice to promote quality care. *Critical Care Nursing Clinics of North America, 13*(4), 497–509. PMID: 11778337.

Titler, M. G., LoBiondo-Wood, G., & Haber, J. (2019). Evidence-based practice overview. In G. LoBiondo-Wood, J. Haber, & M. G. Titler (Eds.), *Evidence-based practice for healthcare and quality improvement* (pp. 1–19). Philadelphia, PA: Elsevier.

Titler, M. G., & Medvec, B. R (2019). Evaluating the impact of implementing evidence-based practices. In G. LoBiondo-Wood, J. Haber, & M. G. Titler (Eds.), *Evidence-based practice for healthcare and quality improvement* (pp. 231–241). Philadelphia, PA: Elsevier.

Tunnecliff, J., Weiner, J., Gaida, J. E., et al. (2017). Translating evidence to practice in the health professions: A randomized trial of Twitter vs Facebook. *Journal of Medical Informatics Association, 24*(2), 403–408.

USPSTF. (2015). U.S. Preventative Services Task Force procedure manual. U.S. *Preventative Services Task Force*. December 2015. Retrieved August 2020 from https://www.uspreventiveservicestaskforce.org/uspstf/about-uspstf/methods-and-processes.

Van de Velde, S., Heselmans, A., Delvaux, N., et al. (2018). A systematic review of trials evaluating success factors of interventions with computerized clinical decision support. *Implementation Science, 13*(114).

Vaona, A., Banzi, R., Kwag, K. H., et al. (2018). E-learning for health professionals. *Cochrane Database of Systematic Reviews, 1*. (Article No. CD011736).

Wilson, D. S., Montie, M., Conlon, P., et al. (2016). Nurses' perceptions of implementing fall prevention interventions to mitigate patient-specific fall risk factors. *Western Journal of Nursing Research, 38*(8), 1012–1034. https://doi.org/10.1177/0193945916644995. PMID: 27106881.

Yano, E. M. (2008). The role of organizational research in implementing evidence-based practice: QUERI series. *Implementation Science, 3*, 29. https://doi.org/10.1186/1748-5908-3-29. PMID: 18510749, PMCID: PMC2481253.

Yousefi-Nooraie, R., Dobbins, M., & Marin, A. (2014). Social and organizational factors affecting implementation of evidence-informed practice in a public health department in Ontario: A network modeling approach. *Implementation Science, 9*, 29. https://doi.org/10.1186/1748-5908-9-29.

Go to Evolve at **http://evolve.elsevier.com/LoBiondo/** for review questions, appraisal exercises, and additional research articles for practice in reviewing and appraisal.

21

Quality Improvement

Maja Djukic, Mattia J. Gilmartin

Go to Evolve at **http://evolve.elsevier.com/LoBiondo/** for review questions.

LEARNING OUTCOMES

After reading this chapter, you should be able to do the following:

- Discuss the characteristics of quality health care defined by the Institute of Medicine.
- Compare the characteristics of the major quality improvement (QI) models used in health care.
- Identify two databases used to report health care organizations' performance to promote consumer choice and guide clinical QI activities.
- Describe the relationship between nursing-sensitive quality indicators and patient outcomes.
- Describe the steps in the improvement process, and determine appropriate QI tools to use in each phase of the improvement process.
- List four themes for improvement to apply to the unit where you work.
- Describe ways that nurses can lead QI projects in clinical settings.
- Use the SQUIRE Guidelines to critically appraise a journal article reporting the results of a QI project.

KEY TERMS

accreditation	flowchart	public reporting	social determinants of
benchmarking	Lean	quality health care	health
Clinical Microsystems	nursing-sensitive	quality improvement	SQUIRE Guidelines
common cause and	quality indicators	root cause analysis	value-based care
special cause variation	Plan-Do-Study-Act	run chart	
control chart	Improvement Cycle	Six Sigma	

TOTAL QUALITY MANAGEMENT/CONTINUOUS QUALITY IMPROVEMENT

The Institute of Medicine (IOM, 2001) defines **quality health care** as care that is safe, effective, patient-centered, timely, efficient, and equitable (Box 21.1). The quality of the health care system was brought to the forefront of national attention in several important reports (IOM, 1999, 2001), including Crossing the Quality Chasm, which concluded that "between the health care we have and the care we could have lies not just a gap, but a chasm"

> **BOX 21.1 Six Dimensions and Definitions of Health Care Quality**
>
> 1. Safe: Avoiding injuries to patients from the care that is intended to help them.
> 2. Effective: Providing services based on scientific knowledge to all who could benefit, and refraining from providing services to those not likely to benefit.
> 3. Patient-centered: Providing care that is respectful of and responsive to individual patient preferences, needs, and values, and ensuring that patient values guide all clinical decisions.
> 4. Timely: Reducing waits and sometimes harmful delays for both those who receive care and those who give care.
> 5. Efficient: Avoiding waste, including waste of equipment, supplies, ideas, and energy.
> 6. Equitable: Providing care that does not vary in quality because of personal characteristics such as gender, ethnicity, geographical location, and socioeconomic status.

(IOM, 2001, p. 1). The report notes that "the performance of the health care system varies considerably. It may be exemplary, but often is not, and millions of Americans fail to receive effective care" (IOM, 2001, p. 3).

Since the IOM (2001) report was published, the Agency for Healthcare Research and Quality (AHRQ) was mandated by Congress to provide a comprehensive overview of health care quality and disparities in care experienced by different racial and socioeconomic groups, including a total of 250 structure, process, and access measures. According to the latest AHRQ report, from 2000 to 2017, close to 70% of patient-centered care measures and over 50% of access to care, patient safety, effective treatment, and healthy living measures were improving. There were no changes in health care affordability measures. Further, the latest data showed persisting health care disparities. In 2017, Blacks, American Indian and Alaska Natives, and Native Hawaiians/Pacific Islanders received poorer care than Whites for 40% of quality measures (AHRQ, 2020). Hispanics received poorer care than Whites for 35% of quality measures, and Asians received poorer care than Whites for 28% of measures (AHRQ, 2020).

Despite these quality issues, the United States spends twice as much on health care per capita per year at $10,224 (Sawyer & Cox, 2018) compared with other developed nations, while ranking last in health care quality in comparison with 10 other countries (Schneider et al., 2017). It is this gap between high cost relative to quality that is making the US health care system a low-value system; we are paying a lot for not such great quality. To turn the low-value health care system to a high-value health care system, health care providers must improve quality while keeping costs constant or lower than they currently are.

The purpose of this chapter is to introduce you, the future health care provider, to the principles of **quality improvement** (QI) and provide examples of how to apply these principles in your practice so you can be better prepared to effectively contribute to needed health care improvements in a cost-conscious manner. QI uses data to monitor the outcomes of care processes and improvement methods to design and test changes to continuously improve the quality and safety of health care systems (Cronenwett, 2012).

NURSES' ROLE IN HEALTH CARE QUALITY IMPROVEMENT

Florence Nightingale championed QI by systematically documenting high rates of morbidity and mortality resulting from poor sanitary conditions among soldiers serving in the Crimean War of 1854 (McDonald, 2012). She used statistics to document changes in soldiers' health, including reductions in mortality resulting from a number of nursing interventions such as hand hygiene, instrument sterilization, changing of bed linens, ward sanitation, ventilation, and proper nutrition (McDonald, 2012). Today, nurses continue to be vital to health system improvement efforts (IOM, 2015). One main initiative developed to bolster nurses' education in health system improvements is *Quality and Safety Education for Nurses* (QSEN) (Cronenwett, 2012). The overall goal of this project is to help build nurses' competence in the areas of QI, patient-centered care, teamwork and collaboration, patient safety, informatics, and evidence-based practice (EBP). Other initiatives, such as the Care Innovation and Transformation Program (American Organization for Nursing Leadership, 2020), have been developed to increase nurses' engagement in QI. To effectively influence improvements in the work setting and ensure that all patients consistently receive excellent care, it is important to do the following:

- Align national, organizational, and unit-level goals for QI.
- Recognize external drivers of quality, such as accreditation, payment, and performance measurement.
- Develop skills to apply QI models and tools.

NATIONAL GOALS AND STRATEGIES FOR HEALTH CARE QUALITY IMPROVEMENT

The National Quality Strategy, first published in 2011 and established by the Affordable Care Act to pursue the triple health care improvement aim of better care, affordable care, and healthy people/healthy communities (AHRQ, 2017), set aims and priorities for QI (Box 21.2). Achieving these national quality targets requires major redesign of the health care system.

The redesign of the health care system is led by a change in the overall philosophy of care delivery from volume-based care to value-based care (*NEJM* Catalyst, 2017). In the currently predominant model of volume-based care, providers are paid by the government and private insurers based on the number of services provided and the number of patients treated. In this paradigm, there is little financial incentive for providers to keep people healthy by focusing on disease prevention and health care promotion (*NEJM* Catalyst, 2017). On the

---

BOX 21.2 National Quality Aims and Priorities

National Quality Aims

- Better Care: Improve the overall quality of care by making health care more patient-centered, reliable, accessible, and safe.

- Healthy People/Healthy Communities: Improve the health of the US population by supporting proven interventions to address behavioral, social, and environmental determinants of health in addition to delivering higher-quality care.

- Affordable Care: Reduce the cost of quality health care for individuals, families, employers, and government.

National Quality Priorities for Achieving the Aims

- Make care safer by reducing harm caused in the delivery of care.
- Ensure that all people and families are engaged as partners in their care.
- Promote effective communication and care coordination.
- Promote the most effective prevention and treatment practices for the leading causes of mortality, starting with cardiovascular disease.
- Work with communities to promote wide use of best practices to enable healthy living.
- Make quality care more affordable for individuals, families, employers, and governments by developing and spreading new health care delivery models.

other hand, a **value-based care** paradigm financially rewards providers for keeping their patient population healthy, therefore reducing overall costs of health care, while improving overall quality of health (*NEJM* Catalyst, 2017).

In the value-based care paradigm, health care providers are encouraged to achieve better value by expanding their QI focus on **social determinants of health** (SDOH). SDOH span five main categories: (1) economic stability (e.g., employment, food insecurity, housing instability); (2) education (e.g., enrollment in early childhood education, high school graduation, language, and literacy; (3) social and community context (e.g. discrimination, incarceration); (4) health and health care (e.g., access to primary care, health literacy); and (5) neighborhood and built environment (e.g., access to healthy foods, presence of crime and violence in a neighborhood, or absence of safe walking routes and playgrounds in a neighborhood) (Office of Disease Prevention and Health Promotion, 2020).

In essence, keeping healthy is difficult if a person is jobless, lacks access to healthy foods, lacks access stable housing, or is exposed to violence at home or in the neighborhood. Therefore as future health care providers, nurses must embrace the practice of integrating social and health services by screening their patient populations for social needs during every health care encounter and making referrals to appropriate social service agencies in the community. For example, Project Nurture integrated maternity care with substance use treatment and social service coordination to improve health outcomes for babies born to women with substance use disorders who were Medicaid beneficiaries (McConnell et al., 2020).

Addressing social determinants of health may feel overwhelming to a novice nurse. A simple first step you can take to contribute to health system redesign is to familiarize yourself with the national QI priorities, corresponding improvement goals, and national initiatives (Table 21.1) and use them to guide improvements in your work setting. As you gain clinical competence and feel more comfortable in your nursing role, you can begin to expand your QI reach to include SDOH.

> **HELPFUL HINT**
>
> To plan QI interventions focused on SDOH, you can review the *HealthyPeople 2030* list of interventions and resources for SDOH at https://www.healthypeople.gov/2020/topics-objectives/topic/social-determinants-health/interventions-resources.

QUALITY STRATEGY LEVERS

QI relies on aligning institutional priorities with several strategy levers that drive QI. The National Quality Strategy encourages multiple members of the health care community, including individuals, family members, payers, providers, and employers, to collaborate on using one or more of the nine strategy levers (AHRQ, 2017); we describe briefly how each lever is used for QI:

1. **Measurement and feedback**—Provide performance feedback to plans and providers to improve care. National health care performance standards are developed using a consensus process in which stakeholder groups, representing the interests of the public, health professionals, payers, employers, and government, identify priorities, measures, and reporting requirements to document and manage the quality of care (National Quality Forum [NQF], 2004). See Box 21.3 for examples of groups responsible for developing measurement standards.

TABLE 21.1 National Quality Strategy Priorities, Improvement Goals, and Related Initiatives

National Quality Strategy Priority	Long-Term Goals	Related National Initiatives
Patient safety	1. Reduce preventable hospital admissions and readmissions. 2. Reduce the incidence of adverse health care–associated conditions. 3. Reduce harm from inappropriate or unnecessary care.	Children's Hospitals' Solutions for Patient Safety Network (SPS Network) Michigan Health and Hospital Association Keystone Center
Patient- and family-centered care	1. Improve patient, family, and caregiver experience of care related to quality, safety, and access across settings. 2. In partnership with patients, families, and caregivers—and using a shared decision-making process—develop culturally sensitive and understandable care plans. 3. Enable patients and their families and caregivers to navigate, coordinate, and manage their care appropriately and effectively.	Better Health Partnership SisterLove, Inc. PatientsLikeMe VA Homelessness: Homeless Patient Aligned Care Teams Age-Friendly Health Systems Initiative
Effective communication and care coordination	1. Improve the quality of care transitions and communications across care settings. 2. Improve the quality of life for patients with chronic illness and disability by following a current care plan that anticipates and addresses pain and symptom management, psychosocial needs, and functional status. 3. Establish shared accountability and integration of communities and health care systems to improve quality of care and reduce health disparities.	GRACE Team Care VA Homelessness: Homeless Patient Aligned Care Teams
Prevention and treatment of leading causes of morbidity and mortality	1. Promote cardiovascular health through community interventions that result in improvement of social, economic, and environmental factors. 2. Promote cardiovascular health through interventions that result in adoption of the most healthy lifestyle behaviors across the life span. 3. Promote cardiovascular health through receipt of effective clinical preventive services across the life span in clinical and community settings.	Reversing the Trend: New York State Health Foundation's Diabetes Campaign Connecticut Association School-Based Health Centers
Health and well-being of communities	1. Promote healthy living and well-being through community interventions that result in improvement of social, economic, and environmental factors. 2. Promote healthy living and well-being through interventions that result in adoption of the most important healthy lifestyle behaviors across the life span. 3. Promote healthy living and well-being through receipt of effective clinical preventive services across the life span in clinical and community settings.	Better Health Greater Cleveland Healthy Kids, Healthy Communities Healthy Hawaii Initiative
Making quality care more affordable	1. Ensure affordable and accessible high-quality health care for people, families, employers, and governments. 2. Support and enable communities to ensure accessible, high-quality care while reducing waste and fraud.	HRSA's Flex Medicare Beneficiary Quality Improvement Program Blue Cross Blue Shield of Massachusetts (BCBSMA) Quality Contract

From the Agency for Healthcare Research and Quality. (2017). About the *National Quality Strategy*. Retrieved from https://www.ahrq.gov/workingforquality/about/index.html.

> ### BOX 21.3   Performance Measurement Standard Setting Groups
>
> **Introduction to Performance Measurement Standards**
>
> **National Quality Forum (NQF)** is a nonprofit organization that seeks to measure and improve the quality of health care in the United States by establishing national health care quality and safety goals and priorities. The NQF's evidence-based measure endorsement process is the gold standard for health care quality measurement. The NQF endorsement process is a transparent, consensus-based model that brings together stakeholders from the private and public sectors to foster quality improvement. Approximately 300 NQF-endorsed measures are used by federal public and private pay-for-performance programs and by private-sector and state health care quality programs.[a]
>
> **Agency for Healthcare Research and Quality, Quality Indicators (AHRQ).** The AHRQ Quality Indicators are standardized, evidence-based measures of the quality of hospital care that are readily available using hospital administrative data. There are 101 Quality Indicators organized into the four main categories of inpatient quality for adult and pediatric patients; preventative quality indicators for ambulatory care and avoidable complications. Approximately one-half of the AHRQ quality indicators are endorsed by the National Quality Forum and used to support hospital quality improvement, health system planning, and pay-for-performance initiatives.[b]

[a] National Quality Forum. (2015). *National Quality Forum, What We Do* (http://www.qualityforum.org/what_we_do.aspx).
[b] Agency for Healthcare Research and Quality. (2015). *About AHRQ Quality Indicators* (http://qualityindicators.ahrq.gov/FAQs_Support/FAQ_QI_Overview.aspx).

2. Public reporting—Compare treatment results, costs, and patient experience for the consumer. Several major public reporting systems are described in Box 21.4.
3. **Learning and technical assistance**—Foster learning environments that offer training, resources, tools, and guidance to help organizations achieve QI goals.
4. **Certification,** accreditation, **regulation**—Adopt or adhere to approaches to meet safety and quality standards. Several accrediting bodies are listed in Box 21.5.
5. **Consumer incentives and benefits designs**—Help consumers adopt healthy behaviors and make informed decisions.
6. **Payment**—Reward and incentivize providers to deliver high-quality, patient-centered care. Box 21.6 shows examples of payment incentives.
7. **Health information technology**—Improve communications, transparency, and efficiency for better coordinated health and health care.
8. **Innovation and diffusion**—Foster innovation in health care QI, and facilitate rapid adoption within and across organizations and communities.
9. **Workforce development**—Invest in people to prepare the next generation of health care professionals and support lifelong learning for providers.

Measuring Nursing Care Quality

Nurses deliver the majority of health care and therefore have a substantial influence on its overall quality (IOM, 2015). However, nursing's contribution to the overall quality of health care has been difficult to quantify, resulting in part from insufficient standardized measurement systems capable of capturing nursing care contribution to patient outcomes. The Robert Wood Johnson Foundation has funded the NQF to recommend nursing-sensitive consensus standards to be used to set standards for public accountability and QI. The work of the NQF (2004) resulted in the endorsement of 15 nursing-sensitive quality indicators (Table 21.2). Since the endorsement of "NQF 15," several data reporting mechanisms have been established for performance sharing internally among providers to identify areas

BOX 21.4 Public Reporting Systems

- Hospital Compare allows consumers to compare information on hospitals. The database includes performance measures on timely and efficient care, readmissions and deaths, complications, use of medical imaging, survey of patients' experiences, and payment and value of care. For more information, visit https://www.medicare.gov/hospitalcompare/.
- Nursing Home Compare allows consumers to compare information about nursing homes. It contains quality of care information on every Medicare and Medicaid-certified nursing home in the country. The database includes performance measures on health inspections, staffing, and clinical quality. For more information, visit https://www.medicare.gov/nursinghomecompare/search.html?
- Home Health Compare has information about the quality of care provided by Medicare-certified home health agencies that meet federal health and safety requirements throughout the nation. For more information, visit https://www.medicare.gov/homehealthcompare/search.html.
- Hospital Consumer Assessment of Healthcare Providers and Systems (HCAHPS). Developed by the Agency for Healthcare Research and Quality, the HCAHPS is a standardized survey and data collection method for measuring patients' perspectives on hospital care. The HCAHPS survey contains 32 questions about patient perspectives on care for eight key topics: communication with doctors; communication with nurses; responsiveness of hospital staff; pain management; communication about medicines; discharge information; cleanliness of the hospital environment; and quietness of the hospital environment, posthospital transitions, admissions through the emergency room, and mental and emotional health. HCAHPS performance is used to calculate incentive payments in the Hospital Value-Based Purchasing program for hospital discharges. For more information, visit https://www.medicare.gov/hospitalcompare/Data/Overview.html
- The Quality Payment Program is a CMS initiative that was implemented with passage of the Medicare Access and CHIP Reauthorization Act of 2015 (MACRA). With this program, the CMS is able to reward high-value, high-quality Medicare clinicians and reduce payments to those clinicians who are not able to meet performance standards. Clinicians can choose from two payment tracks: the Merit Based Incentive Payment System (MIPS) or Advanced Alternative Payment Models. For more information, visit https://qpp.cms.gov/about/qpp-overview.
- The Leapfrog Group is an initiative of organizations that buy health care who are working to improve the safety, quality, and affordability of health care for Americans. The Leapfrog Group conducts a survey for comparing hospitals' performance on the national standards of safety, quality, and efficiency that are most relevant to consumers and purchasers of care. For more information, visit https://www.leapfroggroup.org.

CMS, Center for Medicare and Medicaid Services.

in need of improvement, externally for purposes of accreditation and payment, and with health care consumers so they can choose providers based on the quality of services provided. Examples include the following:

The National Database of Nursing Quality Indicators is a proprietary database of the Press Ganey. The database collects and evaluates unit-specific nurse-sensitive data from hospitals in the United States. Participating facilities receive unit-level comparative data reports to use for QI purposes. For more information, visit https://www.pressganey.com/solutions/clinical-excellence/capture-nursing-specific-measures.

HELPFUL HINT

To find out how your hospital compares in nursing-sensitive quality indicators such as pressure ulcers, infections, and falls with another hospital in your area, go to https://www.medicare.gov/hospitalcompare/search.html? Identify high-performing organizations in your area from which you can learn.

BOX 21.5 Quality Improvement Accrediting Organizations

- **Joint Commission:** Responsible for ensuring a minimum standard of structures, processes, and outcomes for patient care. Accreditation by the Joint Commission is voluntary, but it is required to receive reimbursement for patient care services. For more information, see www.jointcommission.org/.
- **National Committee for Quality Assurance Accreditation for Health Plans (NCQA):** A private not-for-profit organization dedicated to improving health care quality. The NCQA is responsible for accrediting health insurance programs. Accredited health insurance programs are exempt from many or all elements associated with annual state audits. The NCQA developed and maintains the Healthcare Effectiveness Data and Information Set (HEDIS).
- **The Healthcare Effectiveness Data and Information Set (HEDIS):** A tool used by most health plans in the United States to measure performance on important dimensions of care and service. HEDIS allows for comparison of performance across health plans. For more information, visit http://www.ncqa.org/HEDISQualityMeasurement.aspx.
- **Commission on the Accreditation of Rehabilitation Facilities:** A nonprofit standard setting and accreditation group overseeing quality of care in the health and human services sector. Offers accreditation programs for Aging Service, Behavioral health, Child and Youth Services, Medical Rehabilitation, and Opioid Treatment Services. For more information, visit http://www.carf.org/Programs/.
- **American Nurses' Credentialing Center (ANCC) Organizational Recognition Program:** A nonprofit national certification organization that recognizes health care organizations that provide the very best in nursing care and uphold the tradition of professional nursing practice. Magnet, Pathways to Excellence, and Continuing Professional Development Accreditation. For more information about the ANCC's accreditation programs, visit https://www.nursingworld.org/organizational-programs/.

BOX 21.6 Financial Incentives to Promote Quality in the Health Care Sector

Capitation: A payment arrangement for health care services. Pays a provider (physician or nurse practitioner) or provider group a set amount for each enrolled person assigned to them, per period of time, whether or not that person seeks care. These providers generally are contracted with a type of health maintenance organization (HMO). Payment levels are based on average expected health care use of a particular patient, with greater payment for patients with significant medical history.[a]

Bundled Payments Initiative: Links payments for multiple services that patients receive during an episode of care. Payments seek to align incentives for hospitals, post–acute care providers, doctors, and other practitioners to improve the patient's care experience during a hospital stay in an acute care hospital through postdischarge recovery.[b]

Pay for Performance: An emerging movement in health insurance in which providers are rewarded for meeting preestablished targets for health care delivery services. This model rewards physicians, hospitals, medical groups, and other health care providers for meeting certain performance measures for quality and efficiency.[c]

Value-Based Health Care Purchasing: A project of participating health plans, including the CMS, where buyers hold providers of health care accountable for both cost and quality of care. Value-based purchasing brings together information on health care quality, patient outcomes, and health status, with data on the dollar outlays going toward health. The focus is on managing health care system use to reduce inappropriate care and to identify and reward the best-performing providers.[d]

Accountable Care Organization (ACO): A payment and care delivery model that seeks to tie provider reimbursements to quality metrics and reductions in the total cost of care for an assigned population of patients. A group of coordinated health care providers form an ACO, which then provides care to a group of patients. The ACO may use a range of payment models (e.g., capitation, fee-for-service). The ACO is accountable to the patients and the third-party payer for the quality, appropriateness, and efficiency of the health care provided.[e]

CMS, Center for Medicare and Medicaid Services.

[a] American Medical Association. (2012). Capitation (http://www.ama-assn.org/ama/pub/advocacy/state-advocacy-arc/state-advocacy-campaigns /private-payer-reform/state-based-payment-reform/evaluating-payment-options/capitation.page).

[b] Centers for Medicare and Medicaid Services. (2016). Bundled payments for care improvement initiative: General information (https://innovation.cms .gov/initiatives/Bundled-Payments/index.html).

[c] Integrated Healthcare Association. (2013). National pay for performance issue brief (http://www.iha.org/sites/default/files/resources/issue-brief-value -based-p4p-2013.pdf).

[d] Damberg, C. L., Sorbero, M. E., Lovejoy, S. L., et al. (2014). Measuring success in health care value-based purchasing programs: Summary and recommendations. Santa Monica, CA: RAND Corporation, RR-306/1-ASPE (http://www.rand.org/pubs/research_reports/RR306z1.html).

[e] American Hospital Association. (2014). Accountable care organizations: Findings from the survey of care systems and payment (http://www.aha.org /content/14/14aug-acocharts.pdf).

TABLE 21.2 **National Voluntary Standards for Nursing-Sensitive Care**

Framework Category	Measure	Description
Patient-centered outcome measures	Death among surgical inpatients with treatable serious complications (failure to rescue) Pressure ulcer prevalence[a] Falls prevalence[a] Falls with injury Restraint prevalence (vest and limb only) Urinary catheter–associated UTI for ICU patients Central line catheter–associated bloodstream infection rate for ICU and HRN patients[a] Ventilator-associated pneumonia for ICU and HRN patients[a]	Percent of major surgical inpatients who experience hospital-acquired complications (e.g., sepsis, pneumonia, gastrointestinal bleeding, shock/cardiac arrest, deep vein thrombosis/pulmonary embolism) that result in death Percent of inpatients who have hospital-acquired pressure ulcers (Stage 2 or greater) Number of inpatient falls per inpatient days Number of inpatient falls with injuries per inpatient days Percent of patients who have a vest or limb restraint Rate of UTI associated with use of urinary catheters for ICU patients Rate of bloodstream infections associated with use of central line catheters for ICU or HRN patients Rate of pneumonia associated with use of ventilators for ICU and HRN patients
Nursing-centered intervention measures	Smoking cessation counseling for AMI [a]Smoking cessation counseling for HFA Smoking cessation counseling for pneumonia	Percent of AMI inpatients with smoking history in the past year who received smoking cessation advice or counseling during hospitalization Percent of HF inpatients with smoking history within the past year who received smoking cessation advice or counseling during hospitalization Percent of pneumonia inpatients with smoking history within the past year who received smoking cessation advice or counseling during hospitalization
System-centered measures	Skill mix (RN, LVN/LPN, UAP, and contract) Nursing care hours per inpatient day (RN, LVN/LPN, and UAP) PES-NWI (composite and five subscales) Voluntary turnover	• Percent of RN care hours to total nursing care hours • Percent of LVN/LPN care hours to total nursing care hours • Percent of UAP care hours to total nursing care hours • Percent of contract hours (RN, LVN/LPN, and UAP) to total nursing care hours • Number of RN care hours per patient day • Number of nursing staff hours (RN, LVN, LPN, UAP) Composite score and mean presence scores for each of the following subscales derived from PES-NWI: • Nurse participation in hospital affairs • Nursing foundations for quality of care • Nurse manager ability, leadership, and support of nurses • Staffing and resource adequacy • Collegial nurse-physician relations Number of voluntary uncontrolled separations during the month for RNs and advanced practice nurses, LVN/LPNs, and nurse assistant/aides.

[a] NQF-endorsed national voluntary consensus standard for hospital care.
AMI, Acute myocardial infarction; *HF,* heart failure; *HRN,* high-risk nursery; *ICU,* intensive care unit; *LVP/LPN,* licensed vocational nurse/licensed practical nurse; *PES-NWI,* practice environment scale–nursing work index; *RN,* registered nurse; *UAP,* unlicensed assistive personnel; *UTI,* urinary tract infection.

Benchmarking

The measurement of quality indicators must be done methodically using standardized tools. Standardized measurement allows for benchmarking, which is "a systematic approach for gathering information about process or product performance and then analyzing why and how performance differs between business units" (Massoud et al., 2001, p. 74). Benchmarking is critical for QI because it helps identify when performance is below an agreed-on standard and signals the need for improvement. For example, when you record assessment of your patient's risk for falls using one of the standardized assessment tools such as the Hendrich II Fall Risk Model, Morse Fall Scale, and newly identified patient-reported risk factors such as fall at home 3 months before hospitalization, concern of falling, and lack of patient activation (Kiyoshi-Teo et al., 2019), it allows for comparison of your assessment to those of providers in other organizations who provide care to a similar patient population and who use the same tools to document assessments. Tracking changes in the overall fall risk score over time allows you to intervene if the score falls below a set standard, indicating high risk for falls. Equally, after you implement needed interventions focused on altered elimination, mental status, musculoskeletal weakness, or patient activation, you can track changes in the fall risk score to determine whether the interventions were effective in reducing the risk for falls. Therefore standardized measurement can tell you when changes in care are needed and whether implemented interventions have resulted in the actual improvement of patient outcomes.

When all clinical units document care in the same way, it is possible to document pressure ulcer care across units. These performance data are useful for benchmarking efforts where clinical teams learn from each other how to apply best practices from high-performing units to the care processes of lower-performing units. Benchmarking (Massoud et al., 2001, p. 75) can be used to do the following:

- Develop plans to address improvement needs.
- Borrow and adapt successful ideas from others.
- Understand what has already been tried.

COMMON QUALITY IMPROVEMENT PERSPECTIVES AND MODELS

QI as a management model is both a philosophy of organizational functioning and a set of statistical analysis tools and change techniques used to reduce variations in the quality of goods or services that an organization produces (Nelson et al., 2007). The QI model emphasizes customer satisfaction, teams and teamwork, and the continuous improvement of work processes. Other defining features of QI include the use of transformational leadership by leaders at all levels to set performance goals and expectations, use of data to make decisions, and standardization of work processes to reduce variation across providers and service encounters (Nelson et al., 2007). The key principles associated with QI are shown in Table 21.3.

Although QI has its roots in the manufacturing sector, many of the ideas, tools, and techniques used to measure and manage quality have been applied in health care organizations to improve clinical outcomes and reduce waste (McConnell et al., 2016). The major QI models used in health care include the following:

- Total Quality Management/Continuous Quality Improvement (TQM/CQI)
- Six Sigma

TABLE 21.3   Principles of Quality Improvement

Improvement Principle	Key Benefits
Principle 1—Customer focus/patient focus Health care organizations rely on patients and therefore should understand current and future patient needs, should meet patient requirements, and strive to exceed patient expectations.	• Increased customer value • Increased revenue and market share obtained through flexible and fast responses to market opportunities • Increased effectiveness in the organization's resources use to enhance patient satisfaction • Improved patient loyalty leading to repeat business
Principle 2—Leadership Leaders establish unity of purpose, and the organization's direction should create and maintain an internal environment in which people can become fully involved in organization's objectives achievement.	• People understand and are motivated toward the organization's goals and objectives • Activities are evaluated, aligned and implemented in a unified way • Miscommunication between organization levels are minimized
Principle 3—Engagement of people People at all levels are the essence of an organization and are essential to enhance organizational capability to create and deliver value.	• Motivated, committed, and involved people within the organization • Innovation and creativity further the organization's objectives • People are accountable for own performance • Enhanced involvement of people in improvement activities
Principle 4—Process approach Consistent results are achieved with more efficiently and effectively when activities are understood and managed as a system of interrelated processes.	• Lower costs and shorter cycle times through effective use of resources • Improved, consistent, and predictable results through a system of aligned processes • Focused and prioritized improvement opportunities
Principle 5—Improvement Successful organizations have an ongoing focus on improvement. Continual improvement is essential creating new opportunities.	• Performance advantage through improved organizational capabilities • Focus on root-cause analysis, followed by prevention and corrective action • Consideration of incremental and breakthrough improvements
Principle 6—Evidence-based decision making Effective decisions are based on the analysis and evaluation of data and information are more likely to produce desired results.	• Improved decision-making processes • Increased ability to demonstrate effectiveness of past decisions • Increased ability to review, challenge, and change opinions and decisions
Principle 7—Relationship management An organization and its suppliers are interdependent and a mutually beneficial relationship enhances ability of both to create value.	• Increased capability to create value for both parties by sharing resources and managing quality-related risks • A well-managed supply chain that provides a stable flow of goods and services • Optimization of costs and resources

From International Organization for Standardization. (2015). ISO 9001 quality management principles (https://www.iso.org/publication/PUB100080.html).

- Lean
- Clinical Microsystems

The key characteristics of each of these models are described in Table 21.4. Because QI uses a holistic approach, leaders often select one quality model that is used to guide the organization's overarching improvement agenda.

It is important to note that health care organizations have adopted principles and practices associated with the industrial QI approach relatively recently. Historically, the quality of health care was assessed retrospectively using the quality assurance (QA) model. The

TABLE 21.4	Overview of Quality Improvement Models Used in Health Care	
Model	**Main Characteristics**	**Related Resources**
TQM/CQI (Ogrinc et al., 2018)	• A holistic management approach used to improve organizational performance • Seeks to understand and manage variation in service delivery • Emphasizes customer satisfaction as an important performance measure • Relies on teamwork and collaboration among workers to deliver technically excellent and customer/patient-centered services • Quality management science uses tools and techniques from statistics, engineering, operations research, management, market research, and psychology • TQM/CQI tools and techniques are applied to specific performance problems in the form of improvement projects • The extent to which unit-level QI projects align with larger organizational quality goals is related to their success and sustainability	Institute for Healthcare Improvement: http://www.ihi.org/resources/Pages/default.aspx
Six Sigma (Henrique & Godinho, 2020)	• Developed at Motorola in the 1980s • Six Sigma takes its name from the statistical notation of sigma (σ) used to measure variation from the mean • Emphasizes meeting customer requirements and eliminating errors or rework with the goal of reducing process variation • Focuses on tightly controlling variations in production processes with the goal of reducing the number of defects to 3.4 units per 1 million units produced • Process control achieved by applying DMAIC improvement model • DMAIC includes: defining, measuring, analyzing, improving, and controlling • Practitioners achieve mastery levels using statistical tools to measure and manage process variation (e.g., yellow-belt, green-belt, black-belt)	AHRQ Innovations Exchange: www.innovations.ahrq.govhttps://innovations.ahrq.gov/qualitytools/lean-hospitals-six-sigma-and-lean-healthcare-forms
Lean (Henrique & Godinho, 2020)	• Sometimes referred to as the Toyota Quality Model • Focus: Eliminating waste from the production system by designing the most efficient and effective system • Production controlled through standardization and placing the right person and materials at each step of the process • Uses the PDSA improvement cycle • Statistical tools include value stream mapping and Kanban, or a visual cue, used to warn clinicians that there is a process problem • Performance measures vary from project to project and may inform the creation of new performance measures • Uses a master teacher ("Sensei") to spread the practices of Lean though the organizational culture	Institute for Healthcare Improvement: www.ihi.org/knowledge/Pages/IHIWhitePapers/GoingLeaninHealthCare.aspx
Clinical Microsystems (Nelson et al., 2007)	• Model of service excellence developed specifically for health care • Clinical microsystem is considered the building block of any health care system and is the smallest replicable unit in an organization • Members of a clinical microsystem are interdependent and work together toward a common aim	Clinical Microsystems: www.clinicalmicrosystem.org/

AHRQ, Agency for Healthcare Research and Quality; *CQI*, continuous quality improvement; *PDSA*, plan-do-study-act; *QI*, quality improvement; *TQM*, total quality management.

QA model uses chart audits to compare care against a predetermined standard. Corrective actions associated with QA focus on assigning individual blame and correcting deficiencies in operations. Another model commonly associated with health care QI is the Structure-Process-Outcome Framework (Donabedian, 1966). This framework is used to examine the resources that make up health care delivery services, clinicians' work practices, and the outcomes associated with the structure and processes. The evolution of the key perspectives used to understand and manage QI in health care organizations is summarized in Table 21.5.

QUALITY IMPROVEMENT STEPS AND TOOLS

Similar to the nursing process, which you use to guide your assessment, diagnoses, and treatment of patient problems, you can use the QI process steps (Massoud et al., 2001) for the following:

1. Assessing health system performance by collecting and monitoring data
2. Analyzing data to identify a problem in need of improvement
3. Developing a plan to treat the identified problem
4. Testing and implementing the improvement plan

Several tools facilitate each step of the QI process (Table 21.6). You can use these tools to assist with collecting and analyzing data and to identify and test improvement ideas. A case example, Nurse Response Time to Patient Call Light Requests (Box 21.7), is presented to introduce the steps of the improvement process and apply several basic QI tools used to measure and manage system performance. Using the QI process and tools enables nurses on the front lines to successfully lead interprofessional teams of providers in improving metrics that matter. For example, Ferrari and Taylor (2019) applied standardized QI process and tools in their organization to reduce central-line–associated bloodstream infections by 48% over 1 year.

Forming a Lead Quality Improvement Team

QI is inherently an interprofessional team process and requires contributions from various perspectives to assess the potential causes of system malfunction and improvement ideas (Nelson et al., 2007). A lead QI team should be composed of representatives from multiple professions involved in patient care, support staff, patients, and families. Although all professional staff, support staff, and patients should be involved throughout the improvement process, members of the lead team are responsible for planning, coordinating, implementing, and evaluating improvement efforts. To maintain a productive lead team, it is important to set a meeting schedule and use effective meeting tools such as the following (Nelson et al., 2007):

- Meeting agenda
- Meeting roles
- Ground rules
- Brainstorming
- Multivoting

Other tools that can help with project management to keep team and activities organized and focused include action plans and Gantt charts (Nelson et al., 2007). To download templates of meeting agendas, meeting role cards, action plans, and Gantt charts, go to the Clinical Microsystems website at https://clinicalmicrosystem.org/knowledge-center/worksheets/.

TABLE 21.5 Evolution of Quality Improvement Perspectives in Health Care

Model	Key Features	Quality Monitoring Mechanisms	Representative Research Questions
1920s–1980s QA Used to correct differences between what should be and what actually is (Chassin & Loeb, 2011)	• Uses external standards to guide quality • Quality assessed after the fact • Corrective action is punitive • The focus is on symptoms, individual failures, and compliance with standards	• Accreditation • Chart audit • Morbidity and mortality rounds	Did the implementation of Fall Champion Audits reduce fall rates on an inpatient acute care unit? (Loresto et al., 2020)
1960s–2010s Structure-Process-Outcome Framework examines system components that lead to health care quality (Donabedian, 1966)	• Stresses professional responsibility for evaluating care quality • Structure focuses on provider and organizational characteristics • Process focuses on how care is delivered • Outcome focuses on the end results of medical care	• Accreditation • Work redesign • Benchmarking • Professional education and credentialing	What are common and unique predictors of nurse-reported safety and quality of care? (Stimpfel et al., 2019)
1990s–2010s TQM/CQI Model used to continually improve services and organizational performance (Bigelow & Arndt, 1995)	• Systems approach to improve efficiency • Incorporates clinical, financial, administrative, and patient satisfaction perspectives • Focuses on meeting actual and unanticipated patient needs • Uses statistical analysis to reduce variation in service processes • Relies on team work and data-based decisions	• Accreditation • Benchmarking (HCAHPS) • Clinical practice guidelines • PDSA cycles • Process redesign • Lean • Six Sigma	How do P-D-S-A cycles of change that incorporate peer-reviewed evidence improve patient-centeredness, teamwork, communication, and safety in a 16-bed medical and surgical pediatric intensive care unit?(Modified from Tripathi et al., 2015).
2000s–2010s Patient Safety Systems approach to reduce harm to patients (Chassin & Loeb, 2011)	• Applies safety science methods to design health care delivery systems • Focuses on reducing or avoiding adverse events • Domains include patients; providers; care routines; system design	• Accreditation • Sentinel event reporting • National Patient Safety Goals • High-reliability organization model • Root cause analysis	What is the relationship between employee engagement and the dimensions of patient safety culture in critical care units? (Modified from Collier et al., 2016)
2010s to Present High Reliability Organizing (Day et al., 2018)	• A subset of safety focusing on organization performance in high-risk industries • Focus on identifying and catching errors before they cause harm • Integrates principles and practices of teams, psychological safety, mindfulness, Lean, and Six Sigma • Goal is zero harm or catastrophic events	• Safety culture • Lean and Six Sigma analyses • Employee empowerment to identify and respond to potential safety issues • Operational systems to focus on optimal care • Routines and communication patterns	What are the definitions and epidemiology of neonatal safety risk in the perioperative environment using the nonroutine events (NRE) framework and methodology? (Question adapted, France et al., 2020)

CQI, Continuous quality improvement; *HAPU,* hospital-acquired pressure ulcers; *HCAHPS,* Hospital consumer assessment of health care providers and systems; *PDSA,* plan-do-study-act; *QA,* quality assurance; *TQM,* total quality management.

TABLE 21.6	**Quality Improvement Tools and Activities**			
Basic Tools and Activities	**Step 1 Assess**	**Step 2 Analyze**	**Step 3 Plan and Implement**	**Step 4 Test and Evaluate**
Data collection	X	X	X	X
Flowcharts	X	X	X	X
Cause-and-effect analysis	—	X	—	—
Bar and pie charts	X	X	—	X
Run charts	X	X	—	X
Control charts	X	X	—	X
Histograms	X	X	—	X
Pareto charts	X	X	—	X
Benchmarking	X	—	—	X
Gantt charts	—	X	—	X

From Massoud R, Askov K, Reinke J, et al. (2001). A modern paradigm for improving healthcare quality. *QA Monograph Series 1*(1). Bethesda, MD: Published for the US Agency for International Development by the Quality Assurance Project.

After the lead team is assembled and team processes established, the team can begin assessment of the health system. To access resources on how to best facilitate interprofessional teamwork, visit The National Center for Interprofessional Practice and Education at https://nexusipe.org.

IPE HIGHLIGHT

To keep the interprofessional QI lead team engaged and on schedule, hold team meetings at least weekly, and display a timeline of QI activities, such as data collection, analysis, and results of Plan-Do-Study-Act (PDSA) cycles, with completion progress for each activity where all team members can see it.

Improvement Process Step 1: Assessment

In the assessment phase, the first step is to complete a structured assessment to understand more about performance patterns. The improvement team typically begins with a series of broad questions that are used to guide data collection. Common methods used to collect system performance data include check sheets and data sheets to understand performance patterns and surveys, focus groups, and interviews to gather information about patient and staff perceptions of system performance. Commonly collected data elements include information about the following (Nelson et al., 2007):

- Patients: What are the average age, gender, top diagnoses, and satisfaction scores?
- Professionals: What is the level of staff satisfaction? What is their skill set?
- Processes and patterns: What are the processes for admitting and discharging patients?
- Common performance metrics: What are the rates of pressure ulcers and falls with injury?

For useful data collection templates, visit https://clinicalmicrosystem.org/knowledge-center/worksheets/.

BOX 21.7 Applying the Quality Improvement Steps to a Clinical Performance Problem

A Case Study of a Call Bell Response Time Improvement Project

Case Study Background

After reviewing a year of HCAHPS patient satisfaction data, the QI team on the 6 East orthopedic unit noticed that the unit's scores were consistently below the hospital average on call bell response time. In addition to the somewhat mediocre patient satisfaction scores, the nurses were also frustrated with the way the unit staff responded to patient calls. Using the patient and staff satisfaction HCAHPS data as a starting point, the QI team selected call bell response time as an opportunity for improvement.

Improvement Step 1: Assessment

The goal of the 6 East QI project was to understand and manage system variation associated with patient satisfaction with call bell response times. The QI team began the improvement project by asking the following broad questions:
- What time of day is associated with a higher frequency of call bell use?
- What is the average time that it takes a staff member to answer a call bell?
- Are there variations in call bell response time based on the location of the patient's room in relation to the central nursing station?

The QI team designed a check sheet to collect data on the number of call bell requests each hour by patient room number. The charge nurse and unit clerk took turns recording call bell requests during a 24-hour period. The QI team downloaded data from the call bell system to gain information about the average response time and about unit staffing patterns and patient's admitting diagnoses.

Improvement Step 2: Analysis

To begin, the QI team tallied the call response time with a histogram using 5-minute intervals. In graphing the data, a clear pattern emerged. The patient wait times fell into three groups:
- One group waited an average of 8 minutes.
- The second group waited an average of 12 minutes.
- A third group waited an average of 20 minutes for a member of staff to respond to the call bell request.

Upon further analysis of the data, the QI team discovered that the patients with the longest waiting times were in rooms that are the furthest from the central nursing station. The QI team constructed a Pareto diagram to understand the nature and frequency of the patients' requests. This analysis revealed that the three most frequently occurring patient requests were:
- Pain medication
- Assistance with repositioning or toileting
- Assistance with opening and positioning food on the tray table during mealtime

Finally, the team constructed a fishbone diagram to identify the factors associated with the 20-minute response delays. Using these data, the QI team was able to identify the likely cause of the problem and its symptoms.

Improvement Step 3: Develop a Plan for Improvement

The QI team worked with the hospital librarian to identify relevant studies to develop their improvement project plan. The QI team reviewed several research studies about patient requests and response rates from both the patient and nurse perspectives. The team also reviewed studies about work redesign to involve the food service team more directly into the unit's workflow. Based on a critical appraisal of the evidence, the QI team decided to try two interventions for the improvement project:
1. Hourly nurse rounding to improve responsiveness for pain medication requests
2. Role redesign for the dietary staff to reduce patients' requests for meal assistance

The QI team agreed on the specific aim statements to guide the project:
1. In 30 days, we aim to reduce the number of call bell requests for pain medication from 15 per hour to 3 per 8-hour shift.
2. In 30 days, we aim to decrease average wait time for pain medication from 12 minutes to 5 minutes.

Improvement Step 4: Test and Implement the Improvement Plan

Case Study Continues: The QI team tested the two change ideas using PDSA cycles over 2 successive weeks. Hourly nurse rounding was tested using three nurses on the day and evening shift with patients admitted to three randomly assigned rooms for a 3-day period. During the hourly rounds, the nurses conducted pain assessments and administered medication and other pain management interventions. The nurses recorded their interventions on a data collection sheet in each patient's bedside chart. The unit clerk collected the call bell frequency and response

Continued

BOX 21.7 **Applying the Quality Improvement Steps to a Clinical Performance Problem**

A Case Study of a Call Bell Response Time Improvement Project—cont'd

time from the central system for the patients in the randomly assigned rooms during the PDSA testing period. During the testing period, the improvement team reviewed the data at the end of each shift to assess changes in performance.

During the next week, the improvement team piloted the change in the dietary aide's work responsibilities to include opening food trays at the bedside, positioning patients to eat, and filling water pitchers at the time meals were served. The change in dietary aide job responsibilities required training in infection control and body mechanics and creation of a new sign system to alert the dietary staff about the patients' dietary restrictions. This change idea was piloted using the same number of staff members, duration, patient rooms, and unit clerk documentation responsibilities as the PDSA cycle for the hourly nurse rounds. Staff feedback about the strengths and drawbacks of the hourly rounding and expanded food preparation responsibilities for the dietary aides, including suggestions for improving the practice changes, were collected.

Finally, to evaluate the effectiveness of the change ideas, the QI team used a run chart to track performance for the unit's call bell response time. The run chart was annotated to include the days that the team implemented the PDSA cycles to refine the process used for hourly nurse rounding and the change in the dietary aide's responsibilities to set up patients' meal trays. At the end of 1 month of experimentation, the QI team was able to reduce the number of call bell requests for pain medication from a high of 15 per hour at the beginning of the project to 3 per shift. Similarly, the average time that patients waited for their pain medication dropped from 12 minutes to 5 minutes. The team was able to achieve similar reductions in the call bell requests at mealtime by expanding the role of the dietary aide to include meal setup. Based on the performance data, the QI team recommended that hourly nurse rounding and meal setup by the dietary aides become the standard of practice on the unit.

To embed the new practices into the unit routines, the QI team supervised PDSA cycles until the entire unit reached the performance goal in the specific aim statement. The run chart data suggested that the call bell response process was mostly stable, with some variation attributed to new staff hired for the weekend day shift who were not fully oriented to the new routines for hourly nurse rounding and meal tray setup.

HELPFUL HINT

To reduce data collection burden related to QI projects, when starting the assessment phase of the QI process, first identify what performance data already exist in your organization. For example, find out if your organization is participating in the Press Ganey program, which collects quarterly data on pressure ulcers, infections, falls, staff satisfaction, and other quality indicators.

Improvement Step 2: Analysis

The next phase of the improvement process focuses on data analysis. Because QI uses a team problem-solving approach, data are displayed in graphic form so all team members can see how the system is performing and generate ideas for what to improve. Several tools exist to help display and analyze performance data.

Trending Variation in System Performance With Run and Control Charts

If quality health care means that the right care is delivered to the right people, in the right way, at the right time, for every individual, during each clinical encounter, it is important to learn when criteria are not met and why (IOM, 2001). One method is to track performance over time and understand sources of variation in system performance, which can guide improvement activities to design a better-functioning health system. Minimizing performance variation is one of the main QI goals. There are two main types of system variation (Nelson et al., 2007, p. 346):

- **Common cause variation** occurs at random and is considered a characteristic of the system. For example, you may never leave your house in time for prompt arrival to class. In this case, you must work on better managing multiple random causes of tardiness, such as getting up late or taking too long to shower, dress, and eat to improve your overall punctuality record.

- **Special cause variation** arises from a special situation that disrupts the causal system beyond what can be accounted for by random variation. An example may be that you usually leave your house on time for a prompt arrival to class, but special circumstances such as road construction or a broken elevator delay your arrival to class. Once these special causes of tardiness are resolved, you will arrive to class on time.

Variations in system performance over time are commonly displayed with run charts and control charts. A **run chart** is a graphical data display that shows trends in a measure of interest; trends reveal what is occurring over time (Nelson et al., 2007). The vertical axis of the run chart depicts the value of the measure of interest, and the horizontal axis depicts the value of each measure running over time. A run chart shows whether the outcome of interest is running in a targeted area of performance and how much variation there is from point to point and over time. For example, a patient newly diagnosed with diabetes can record blood glucose levels over 1 month using a run chart. By regularly charting blood glucose levels, the patient is able to reveal when blood glucose runs higher or lower than the target level of less than 100 mg/dL for a fasting plasma glucose (FPG) test. The run chart in Fig. 21.1 shows that FPG levels are consistently higher than the target, with a median FPG of 130 mg/dL; the trend of FPG readings in the first 19 days of the month is indicative of common cause variation. These random variations in FPG readings are likely caused by a confluence of several factors such as diet, exercise, and medication adherence. To correct the undesirable variation, the patient can assess which factors may be influencing the higher FPG values and then work with the primary health care provider to develop necessary interventions to better control blood glucose by better managing multiple causal factors. To determine whether interventions were successful, the patient and provider should continue to document blood glucose levels and then compare the median FPG values before and after interventions are implemented.

In addition, special cause variation in FPG is evident on days 19 to 28, where nine consecutive FPG readings are above the median line. It turns out that on these days, the patient had run out of glucose-lowering medication; this special circumstance caused increased

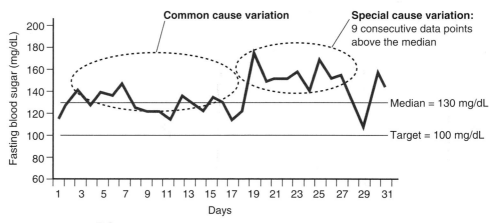

FIG 21.1 Run chart of daily fasting plasma glucose levels.

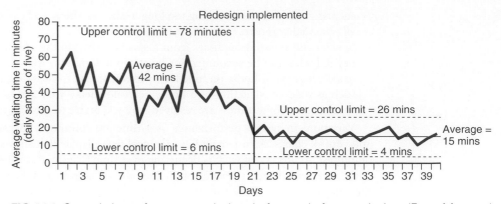

FIG 21.2 Control chart of average wait time before and after a redesign. (From Massoud R, Askov K, Reinke J, et al. [2001]. A modern paradigm for improving healthcare quality. *QA Monograph Series 1*[1]. Bethesda, MD: Published for the US Agency for International Development by the Quality Assurance Project.)

FPG. Although various rules exist for accurately determining the presence of special cause variation, generally special cause variation is present if the following are true (Nelson et al., 2007, p. 349):

- Eight data points in a row are above or below the median or mean.
- Six data points in a row are going up.
- Six data points in a row are going down.

Determining common and special causes of variation is important because treatment strategies for eliminating each type of variation will vary.

A **control chart** (Fig. 21.2) is also used to track system performance over time, but it is a more sophisticated data tool than a run chart (Nelson et al., 2007). A control chart includes information on the average performance level for the system depicted by a center line displaying the system's average performance (the mean value), and the upper and lower limits depicting one to three standard deviations from average performance level. The rules to detect special cause variation are the same for run charts and control charts, except that for control charts the upper and lower limits are additional tools used to detect special cause variation. Any point that falls outside the control limit is considered an outlier that merits further examination.

HELPFUL HINT

Use a run chart in step 2 of the QI process to analyze causes of variation in fasting plasma glucose (FPG) levels from the target level of 100 mg/dL and in step 4 of the QI process to evaluate if changes in diet, exercise, and medication adherence helped the patient achieve the targeted FPG.

Graphs

Graphs commonly used to understand system performance, displayed in Fig. 21.3, include pie **charts**, **bar charts**, and **histograms**. Selecting the appropriate chart depends on the type of data collected and the performance pattern the improvement team is trying to understand. A bar chart is used to display categorical-level data. A Pareto diagram is a special type of bar chart used to understand the frequency of factors that contribute to a common

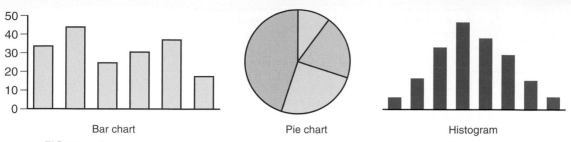

FIG 21.3 Examples of bar chart, pie chart, and histogram. (From Massoud R, Askov K, Reinke J, et al. [2001]. A modern paradigm for improving healthcare quality. *QA Monograph Series 1*[1]. Bethesda, MD: Published for the US Agency for International Development by the Quality Assurance Project.)

effect. It is used to display the Pareto Principle, sometimes referred to as the 80-20 Rule, or the Law of the Few (Massoud et al., 2001), which states that 80% of variation in a problem originates with 20% of cases. In a Pareto diagram, the bars are displayed in descending order of frequency. A histogram is another type of bar chart used for continuous-level data to show the distribution of the data around the mean, commonly called a *bell curve* (Massoud et al., 2001).

Cause-and-Effect Diagrams

More sophisticated visual data displays include **cause-and-effect diagrams** used to identify and treat the causes of performance problems. Two common tools in this category are a fishbone or Ishikawa diagram and a tree diagram (Massoud et al., 2001). The **fishbone diagram** facilitates brainstorming about potential causes of a problem by grouping potential causes into the categories of environment, people, materials, and process (Fig. 21.4). Fishbone diagrams can be used proactively to prevent quality defects, including errors, and retrospectively to identify factors that potentially contributed to quality defect or an error that has already occurred. An example of when a fishbone diagram is used retrospectively is during **root cause analyses** (RCAs) to identify system design failures that caused errors.

An RCA is a structured method used to understand sources of system variation that lead to errors or mistakes, including sentinel events, with the goal of learning from mistakes and mitigating hazards that arise as a characteristic of the system design (Hagley et al., 2019). An RCA is conducted by a team that includes representatives from nursing, medicine, management, QI, or risk management and the individual(s) involved in the incident (sometimes including the patient or family members in the discovery process), and it emphasizes system failures while avoiding individual blame (Hagley et al., 2019). An RCA seeks to answer three questions to learn from mistakes:

- What happened?
- Why did it happen?
- What can be done to prevent it from happening again?

Because the RCA is viewed as an opportunity for organizational learning and improvement, the most effective RCAs include a change in practice or work system design to lessen the chances of similar errors occurring in the future. Properly conducted RCA demands substantial time, expertise, and human resources, which are not always readily available. Alternative methods of incident reporting and analysis, in lieu of traditional RCA, should

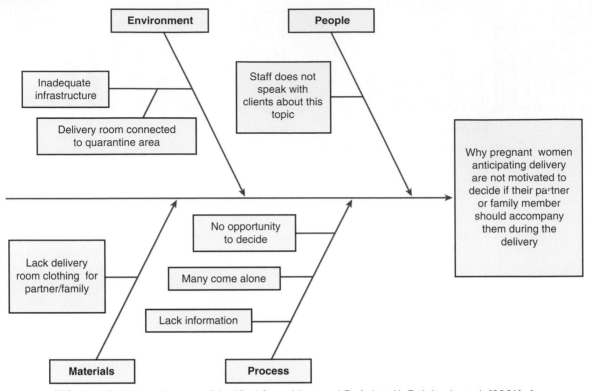

FIG 21.4 Fishbone diagram. (Modified from Massoud R, Askov K, Reinke J, et al. [2001]. A modern paradigm for improving healthcare quality. *QA Monograph Series 1*[1]. Bethesda, MD: Published for the US Agency for International Development by the Quality Assurance Project.)

be considered to better accommodate available time and human resources needs. Hagley et al. (2019) provide a review of alternative RCA approaches such as After-Action Review, Adverse Event Debriefing and Huddles, and Concise Incident Analysis.

A **tree diagram** is particularly useful for identifying the chain of causes, with the goal of identifying the root cause of a problem. For example, consider medication errors. The improvement team could use the **Five Whys** method to establish the chain of causes leading to the medication error:

- Question 1: Why did the patient receive the incorrect medicine?
  Answer 1: Because the prescription was wrong.
- Question 2: Why was the prescription wrong?
  Answer 2: Because the physician made the wrong decision.
- Question 3: Why did the physician make the wrong decision?
  Answer 3: Because he did not have complete information in the patient's chart.
- Question 4: Why wasn't the patient's chart complete?
  Answer 4: Because the physician's assistant had not entered the latest laboratory report.
- Question 5: Why hadn't the physician's assistant charted the latest laboratory report?
  Answer 5: Because the laboratory technician telephoned the results to the receptionist, who forgot to tell the assistant.

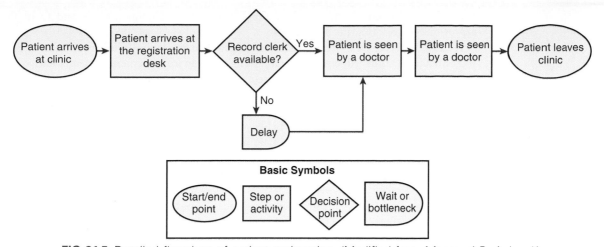

FIG 21.5 Detailed flowchart of patient registration. (Modified from Massoud R, Askov K, Reinke J, et al. [2001]. A modern paradigm for improving healthcare quality. *QA Monograph Series 1*[1]. Bethesda, MD: Published for the US Agency for International Development by the Quality Assurance Project.)

In this case using the Five Whys technique suggests that a potential solution for avoiding wrong prescriptions in the future may be to develop a system for tracking laboratory reports (Massoud et al., 2001).

Flowcharting

A flowchart depicts how a process works, detailing the sequence of steps from the beginning to the end of a process (Massoud et al., 2001). Several types of flowcharts exist, including the most simple (high level), a detailed version (detailed), and one that also indicates the people involved in the steps (deployment or matrix). Fig. 21.5 shows an example of a detailed flowchart. Massoud and colleagues (2001, p. 59) suggest using flowcharts to do the following:

- Understand processes
- Consider ways to simplify processes
- Recognize unnecessary steps in a process
- Determine areas for monitoring or data collection
- Identify who will be involved in or affected by the improvement process
- Formulate questions for further research

When flowcharting, it is important to identify a start point and an end point of a process, and then make a record of the actual, not the ideal, process. To obtain an accurate picture of the process, perform direct observation of the process steps and communicate with people who are directly part of the process to clarify all of the steps.

Improvement Step 3: Develop a Plan for Improvement

By identifying potential sources of variation, the improvement team can pinpoint the problem areas in need of improvement. The next phase is to treat the performance problem. This phase involves developing and testing a plan for improvement. A simple yet powerful model for developing and testing improvement is the **Model for Improvement** (Ogrinc et al., 2018). It begins with three questions to guide the change process and focus the improvement work (Ogrinc et al., 2018):

1. **Aim**. What are we trying to accomplish? Set a clear aim with specific measurable targets.
2. **Measures**. How will we know that the change is an improvement? Use qualitative and quantitative measures to support real improvement work to guide change progress toward the stated goal.
3. **Changes**. What changes can we make that will result in an improvement? Develop a statement about what the team believes they can change to cause improvement.

The **change ideas** reflect the team's hypotheses about what could improve system performance. There are several ways in which change ideas can be generated. The change ideas can be identified from the root causes of the performance problems that are identified during cause-and-effect and process analyses using a fishbone diagram, the Five Whys, and flowcharting tools in the analysis step of the improvement process. Another approach is to select common areas for change associated with the goals and philosophy of QI. Common **change topics**, also referred to as **themes for improvement**, include the following (Ogrinc et al., 2018):

- Eliminating waste
- Improving work flow
- Optimizing inventory
- Changing the work environment
- Managing time more effectively
- Managing variation
- Designing systems to avoid mistakes
- Focusing on products or services

Change ideas can also come from the evidence provided by your review of the available literature. This is where your EBP skills will be most helpful. You will need to critically appraise both research studies and QI studies of interventions that can be applied to remedy the identified problem. To help you decide whether a journal article is a research study or a QI study, see the critical decision tree in Fig. 21.6. Because QI studies capture the experiences of a particular organization or unit, the results of these studies are usually not generalizable. In an effort to promote knowledge transfer and learning from others' improvement experiences, the Standards for Quality Improvement Reporting Excellence, or the **SQUIRE Guidelines** (Ogrinc et al., 2015), were developed to promote the publication and interpretation of this type of applied research. The SQUIRE Guidelines are presented in Table 21.7; you should use them to evaluate QI studies.

Improvement Step 4: Test and Implement the Improvement Plan

The improvement changes that are identified in the planning phase are tested using the **Plan-Do-Study-Act** (PDSA) **Improvement Cycle**, which is the last step of the Improvement Model (Ogrinc et al., 2018; Massoud et al., 2001) depicted in Fig. 21.7. The focus of PDSA is experimentation using small and rapid tests of change. Actions involved in each phase of the PDSA cycle are detailed in Fig. 21.7. In this step, you evaluate the success of the intervention in bringing about improvement. It is important for the team to monitor the intended and unintended changes in system performance, the patient and staff perceptions of the change, and, ideally, the costs of the change. Also, in this phase of the improvement process, it is useful to track the stability and sustainability of the new work process by monitoring system performance over time. Results data should be presented in graphic data displays (explained earlier in the chapter) and compared with the baseline performance.

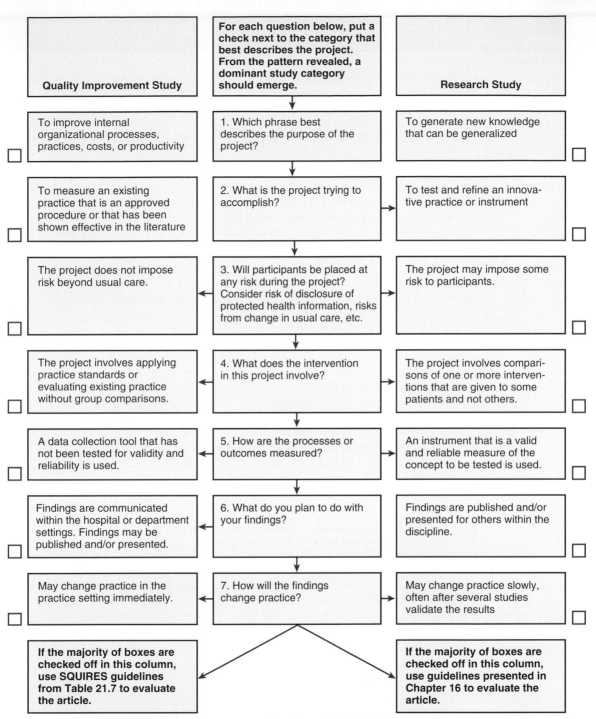

FIG 21.6 Differentiating QI from research projects. SQUIRE, Standards for Quality Improvement Reporting Excellence. (Modified with permission from King, D. L. [2008]. Research and quality improvement: Different processes, different evidence. *Medsurg Nursing, 17*[3], 167.)

TABLE 21.7 **Revised SQUIRE Guidelines Standards for Quality Improvement Reporting Excellence (Squires 2.0)**

Title and Abstract

Title	Indicate that the manuscript concerns an initiative to improve health care (broadly defined to include the quality, safety, effectiveness, patient-centeredness, timeliness, cost, efficiency, and equity of health care).
Abstract	a. Provide adequate information to aid in searching and indexing
	b. Summarize all key information from various sections of the text using the abstract format of the intended publication or a structured summary such as background, local problem, methods, interventions, results, and conclusions

Introduction—Why did you start?

Problem description	Nature and significance of the local problem.
Available knowledge	Summary of what is currently known about the problem, including relevant previous studies.
Rationale	Informal or formal frameworks, models, concepts, and/or theories used to explain the problem; any reasons or assumptions that were used to develop the intervention(s); and reasons why the intervention(s) was expected to work.
Specific aims	Purpose of the project and of this report.

Methods—What did you do?

Context	Contextual elements considered important at the outset of introducing the intervention(s).
Intervention(s)	a. Description of the intervention(s) in sufficient detail that others could reproduce it
	b. Specifics of the team involved in the work
Study of intervention(s)	a. Approach chosen for assessing the impact of the intervention(s)
	b. Approach used to establish whether the observed outcomes were a result of the intervention(s)
Measures	a. Measures chosen for studying processes and outcomes of the intervention(s), including rationale for choosing them, their operational definitions, and their validity and reliability
	b. Description of the approach to the ongoing assessment of contextual elements that contributed to the success, failure, efficiency, and cost
	c. Methods employed for assessing completeness and accuracy of data
Analysis	a. Qualitative and quantitative methods used to draw inferences from the data
	b. Methods for understanding variation within the data, including the effects of time as a variable
Ethical considerations	Ethical aspects of implementing and studying the intervention(s) and how they were addressed, including, but not limited to, formal ethics review and potential conflict(s) of interest.

Results—What did you find?

Results	a. Initial steps of the intervention(s) and their evolution over time (e.g., timeline diagram, flowchart, or table), including modifications made to the intervention during the project
	b. Details of the process measures and outcomes
	c. Contextual elements that interacted with the intervention(s)
	d. Observed associations between outcomes, interventions, and relevant contextual elements
	e. Unintended consequences such as unexpected benefits, problems, failures, or costs associated with the intervention(s)
	f. Details about missing data

Discussion—What does it mean?

Summary	a. Key findings, including relevance to the rationale and specific aims
	b. Particular strengths of the project
Interpretation	a. Nature of the association between the intervention(s) and the outcomes
	b. Comparison of results with findings from other publications
	c. Impact of the project on people and systems
	d. Reasons for any differences between observed and anticipated outcomes, including the influence of context
	e. Costs and strategic trade-offs, including opportunity costs

TABLE 21.7	**Revised SQUIRE Guidelines Standards for Quality Improvement Reporting Excellence (Squires 2.0)—cont'd**
Limitations	a. Limits to the generalizability of the work
	b. Factors that may have limited internal validity such as confounding, bias, or imprecision in the design, methods, measurement, or analysis
	c. Efforts made to minimize and adjust for limitations
Conclusions	a. Usefulness of the work
	b. Sustainability
	c. Potential for spread to other contexts
	d. Implications for practice and for further study in the field
	e. Suggested next steps
Other Information	
Funding	Sources of funding that supported this work and role, if any, of the funding organization in the design, implementation, interpretation, and reporting.

Note: Visit http://www.squire-statement.org/ for more information on publishing QI studies.
From Ogrinc G, Davies L, Goodman D, et al. (2015). SQUIRE 2.0 (Standards for Quality Improvement Reporting Excellence): revised publication guidelines from a detailed consensus process. *BMJ Quality and Safety, 0,* 1–7. doi:10.1136/bmjqs-2015-004411.

TAKING ON THE QUALITY IMPROVEMENT CHALLENGE AND LEADING THE WAY

Hospital leaders and other key stakeholders agree that enabling nurses to lead and participate in QI is vital for strengthening our health system's capacity to provide high-quality patient care (IOM, 2015). Nurses are on the front lines of delivering care, and they offer unique perspectives on the root causes of dysfunctional care and which interventions may work reliably and sustainably in everyday clinical practice to achieve best care. However, multiple barriers to nurses' participation in QI exist, including lack of organizational involvement in decision making and educational preparation for knowledgeable and meaningful QI involvement (Djukic et al., 2018). For nurses to contribute their knowledge and expertise to patient care delivery and the organization's quality enterprise, nursing leadership must engage in the following (Berwick, 2011, p. 326):

- Setting aims and building the will to improve
- Measurement and transparency
- Finding better systems
- Supporting PDSA activities, risk, and change
- Providing resources

Several common elements that make improvement work possible are captured in two bodies of knowledge (Berwick, 2011). One is **professional knowledge**, which includes knowledge of one's discipline, subject matter, and values of the discipline. The other is **knowledge of improvement,** which includes knowledge of complex systems functioning through dynamic interplay among various technical and human elements; knowledge of how to detect and manage variation in system performance; knowledge of managing group processes through effective conflict resolution and communication; and knowledge of how to gain further knowledge by continual experimentation in local settings through rapid tests of change. Linking these two knowledge systems promotes continuous improvement in health care. This chapter provides a starting point for you to develop basic knowledge and skills for the improvement work so you can better meet the challenges and expectations of a contemporary nursing practice.

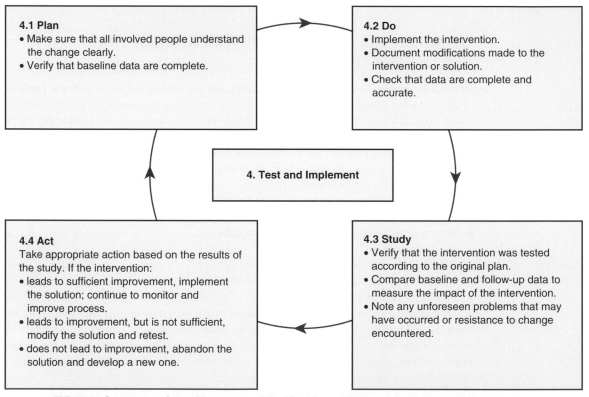

1. Assess	Activities • Define a specific goal for improvement. • Decide who needs to be on the problem-solving team. • Achieve group consensus on improvement goals.

2. Analyze	Activities • Analyze available and readily accessible data and information. • Identify indicators (measures of improvement). • Collect data prior to the intervention if necessary.

3. Develop	Activities • Generate possible interventions. • Rank interventions according to priority and feasibility. • If possible, test interventions sequentially (one at a time).

4.1 Plan
- Make sure that all involved people understand the change clearly.
- Verify that baseline data are complete.

4.2 Do
- Implement the intervention.
- Document modifications made to the intervention or solution.
- Check that data are complete and accurate.

4. Test and Implement

4.4 Act
Take appropriate action based on the results of the study. If the intervention:
- leads to sufficient improvement, implement the solution; continue to monitor and improve process.
- leads to improvement, but is not sufficient, modify the solution and retest.
- does not lead to improvement, abandon the solution and develop a new one.

4.3 Study
- Verify that the intervention was tested according to the original plan.
- Compare baseline and follow-up data to measure the impact of the intervention.
- Note any unforeseen problems that may have occurred or resistance to change encountered.

FIG 21.7 Summary of the QI process. (Modified from Massoud R, Askov K, Reinke J, et al. [2001]. A modern paradigm for improving healthcare quality. *QA Monograph Series 1*[1]. Bethesda, MD: Published for the US Agency for International Development by the Quality Assurance Project.)

KEY POINTS

- There is much room for improvement in the quality of health care in the United States.
- The quality of health care is evaluated in terms of its effectiveness, efficiency, access, safety, timeliness, and patient-centeredness.
- As the largest group of health professionals, nurses play a key role in leading QI efforts in clinical settings.
- Accreditation, payment, and performance measurement are external incentives used to improve the quality of care delivered by hospitals and health professionals. One example of this is The Joint Commission accreditation for health care delivery organizations.
- The National Quality Forum "15" (NQF 15) is a set of 15 nursing-sensitive measures to assess and improve the quality of nursing care delivered in the United States.
- Standardized measures such as patient fall rates are used to compare performance across nursing units and organizations.
- Health care payers use quality performance measures such as 30-day readmission rates as a basis for paying hospitals and providers.
- QI is both a philosophy of organizational functioning and a set of statistical analysis tools and change techniques used to reduce variation.
- The major approaches used to manage quality in health care are Total Quality Management/Continuous Quality Improvement, Lean, Six Sigma, and the Clinical Microsystems model.
- The defining characteristics of QI are focus on patients/customers; teams and teamwork to improve work processes; and use of data and statistical analysis tools to understand system variation.
- QI uses benchmarking to compare organizational performance and learn from high-performing organizations.
- QI tools, techniques, and principles are applied to clinical performance problems in the form of improvement projects, such as using a presurgical checklist to prevent wrong-side surgeries, a national patient safety goal.
- Unit-level improvement projects should align with organizational-level improvement priorities to promote the sustainability of the unit-level projects.
- There are four major steps in the QI process: assessment, analysis, improvement, and evaluation.
- Patient safety focuses on designing systems to remove factors known to cause errors or adverse events.
- Barriers exist that impede nurses' participation in QI, including insufficient staffing, lack of leadership support, and nurses' unfamiliarity with QI principles and practices.
- In the era of value-based care, nurses will be expected to expand their health care QI interventions to include not just improvement of clinical care and processes, but also improvement of SODH by screening their patients for social care needs and making appropriate community referrals.

CRITICAL THINKING CHALLENGES

- **IPE** Have your team discuss the similarities and differences among total QI, Lean, Six Sigma, and the Clinical Microsystems models. Choose one of the models for your team to use to guide your improvement project.

- Consider your unit's performance on the HCAHPS (Hospital Consumer Assessment of Healthcare Providers and Systems) Survey. What suggestions do you have for applying QI principles to improve your unit's score on these key performance indicators?
- Why is it important to document nurse-sensitive care outcomes using standardized performance measurement systems? How does performance measurement relate to QI activities?
- What barriers do you see for participating in unit-level QI initiatives? What suggestions do you have for overcoming these barriers?
- In which ways do QI studies differ from research studies? How would you use the results of a QI study to inform a change in practice on your unit?
- Reflect on SDOH in the economic, education, and built environment domains that you have observed in your patient population. What community referrals and resources are available for your patients to help them address their social care needs that can ultimately improve their health outcomes?

REFERENCES

Agency for Healthcare Research and Quality (AHRQ). (2020). *2018* National *healthcare quality and disparities report.* Retrieved from https://www.ahrq.gov/research/findings/nhqrdr/nhqdr18/index.html.

Agency for Healthcare Research and Quality (AHRQ). (2017). About the National Quality Strategy. Retrieved from https://www.ahrq.gov/workingforquality/about/index.html.

American Organization for Nursing Leadership. (2020). *Care innovation and transformation program.* Retrieved from https://www.aonl.org/education/cit.

Berwick, D. M. (2011). Preparing nurses for participation in and leadership of continual improvement. *Journal of Nursing Education, 50*(6), 322–327.

Bigelow, B., & Arndt, M. (1995). Total quality management: Field of dreams? *Health Care Management Review, 20*(4), 15–25.

Chassin, M. R., & Loeb, J. M. (2011). The ongoing quality improvement journey: Next stop, high reliability. *Health Affairs, 30*(4), 559–568. https://doi.org/10.1377/hlthaff.2011.0076.

Cronenwett, L. R. (2012). A national initiative: Quality and Safety Education for Nurses (QSEN). In G. Sherwood, & J. Barnsteiner (Eds.), *Quality and safety in nursing: A competency approach to improving outcomes* (pp. 49–64). Hoboken, NJ: Wiley-Blackwell.

Day, R. M., Demski, R. J., Pronovost, P. J., Sutcliffe, K. M., Kasda, E. M., Maragakis, L. L., … Winner, L. (2018). Operating management system for high reliability: Leadership, accountability, learning and innovation in healthcare. *Journal of Patient Safety and Risk Management, 23*(4), 155–166.

Djukic, M., Witkoski Stimpfel, A., Fletcher, J., & Kovner, C. (2018). Bachelor's degree nurse graduates report better quality and safety educational preparedness than associate degree graduates. *The Joint Commission Journal on Quality and Patient Safety, 45*(3), 180–186. https://doi.org/10.1016/j.jcjq.2018.08.008.

Donabedian, A. (1966). Evaluating the quality of medical care. *The Milbank Memorial Fund Quarterly, 44*(3), 166–206.

Ferrari, S., & Taylor, K. (2019). Effect of a systemwide approach to a reduction in central line–associated bloodstream infections. *Journal of Nursing Care Quality, 35*(1), 40–44. https://doi.org/10.1097/NCQ.0000000000000410.

France, D. J., Slagle, J., Schremp, E., Moroz, S., Hatch, L. D., Grubb, P., … Robinson, J. (2020). Defining the Epidemiology of Safety Risks in Neonatal Intensive Care Unit Patients Requiring Surgery. *Journal of Patient Safety.* https://doi.org/10.1097/PTS.0000000000000680. (Published on-line ahead of print).

Hagley, G., Mills, P., Watts, B. V., & Wu, A. W. (2019). Review of alternatives to root cause analysis: Developing a robust system for incidence report analysis. *BMJ Open Quality, 8*, e000646. https://doi.org/10.1136/bmjoq-2019-000646.

Henrique, D. B., & Godinho, M. (2020). A systematic literature review of empirical research in Lean and Six Sigma in healthcare. *Total Quality Management and Business Excellence, 31*(3-4), 429–449.

Institute of Medicine (IOM). (1999). *To err is human: Building a safer health system: executive summary*. Washington, DC: The National Academies Press. Retrieved from http://www.books.nap.edu/openbook.php?record_id=http://9728.

Institute of Medicine (IOM). (2001). *Crossing the quality chasm: A new health system for the 21st century: Executive summary*. Washington, DC: The National Academies Press. Retrieved from http://www.books.nap.edu/catalog/10027.html.

Institute of Medicine (IOM). (2015). *Assessing progress on the IOM report The Future of Nursing*. Washington, DC: The National Academies Press.

Kiyoshi-Teo, H., Northrup-Snyder, K., Cohen, D. J., Dieckmann, N., Stoyles, S., Winters-Stone, K., & Eckstrom, E. (2019). Older hospital inpatients' fall risk factors, perceptions, and daily activities to prevent falling. *Geriatric Nursing, 40*(3), 290–295.

Loresto, F. L., Grant, C., Solberg, J., & Eron, K. (2020). Assessing the Efect of Unit Champion-Initiatied Audits on Fall Rates: Improving Awareness. *Journal of Nursing Care Quality, 35*(3), 227–232. http://doi.org/10.1097/NCQ0000000000000449.

Massoud, R., Askov, K., Reinke, J., et al. (2001). A modern paradigm for improving healthcare quality. *QA Monograph Series 1*(1). Bethesda, MD: The Quality Assurance Project.

McConnell, J. K., Kaufman, M. R., Grunditz, J. I., Bellanca, H., Risser, A., & Rodriguez, M. I. (2020). Project Nurture integrates care and services to improve outcomes for opioid-dependent mothers and their children. *Health Affairs, 39*(4), 595–602. https://doi.org/10.1377/hlthaff.2019.01574.

McConnell, J. K., Lindrooth, R. C., Wholey, D. R., et al. (2016). Modern management practices and hospital admissions. *Health Economics, 25*, 470–485. https://doi.org/10.1002/hec.3171.

McDonald, L. (2012). *Florence Nightingale and Hospital Reform: Collected Works of Florence Nightingale* (Vol. 16). Wilfrid Laurier University Press.

National Quality Forum (NQF). (2004). *National voluntary consensus standard for nursing-sensitive care: an initial performance measure set*. Retrieved from http://www.qualityforum.org/Publications/2004/10/National_Voluntary_Consensus_Standards_for_Nursing-Sensitive_Care__An_Initial_Performance_Measure_Set.aspx.

NEJM Catalyst. (2017). What is value-based healthcare? Retrieved from https://www.catalyst.nejm.org/doi/full/10.1056/CAT.17.0558.

Nelson, E. C., Batalden, P. B., & Godfrey, M. M. (2007). *Quality by design: A clinical microsystems approach*. San Francisco, CA: Jossey-Bass.

Office of Disease Prevention and Health Promotion. (2020). Healthy People 2020: Social determinants of health. Retrieved from https://www.healthypeople.gov/2020/topics-objectives/topic/social-determinants-of-health.

Ogrinc, G., Davies, L., Goodman, D., et al. (2015). SQUIRE 2.0 (Standards for Quality Improvement Reporting Excellence): Revised publication guidelines from a detailed consensus process. *BMJ Quality and Safety, 0*, 1–7. https://doi.org/10.1136/bmjqs-2015-004411.

Ogrinc, G. S., Headrick, L. A., Barton, A. J., Dolansky, M. A., Madigosky, W. S., & Miltner, R. S. (2018). *Fundamentals of health care improvement: A guide to improving your patient's care* (3rd ed.). The Joint Commission and the Institute for Healthcare Improvement.

Sawyer, B., and Cox, C. (2018). How does health spending in the U.S. compare to other countries? Retrieved from https://www.healthsystemtracker.org/chart-collection/health-spending-u-s-compare-countries/#item-average-wealthy-countries-spend-half-much-per-person-health-u-s-spends.

Schneider, E. C., Sarnak, D. O., Squires, D., Shah, A., Doty, M. M. (2017). *Mirror, Mirror 2017: International Comparison Reflects Flaws and Opportunities for Better U.S. Health Care.* Retrieved from https://www.commonwealthfund.org/publications/fund-reports/2017/jul/mirror-mirror-2017-international-comparison-reflects-flaws-and.

Stimpfel, A. W., Djukic, M., Brewer, C. S., & Kovner, C. T. (2019). Common predictors of nurse-reported quality of care and patient safety. *Health Care Management Review, 44*(1), 57–66.

Tripathi, S., Arteaga, G., Rohlik, G., et al. (2015). Implementation of patient-centered bedside rounds in the pediatric intensive care unit. *Journal of Nursing Care Quality, 30*(2), 160–166.

US Department of Health and Human Services (USDHHS). (2020). *Hospital Compare.* Retrieved from https://www.medicare.gov/hospitalcompare/search.html.

Go to Evolve at **http://evolve.elsevier.com/LoBiondo/** for review questions, appraisal exercises, and additional research articles for practice in reviewing and appraisal.

International Journal of Nursing Studies 101 (2020) 103396

Contents lists available at ScienceDirect

International Journal of Nursing Studies

journal homepage: www.elsevier.com/ijns

Continuity of care interventions for preventing hospital readmission of older people with chronic diseases: A meta-analysis

Gabriella Facchinetti[a], Daniela D'Angelo[a,e,*], Michela Piredda[b], Tommasangelo Petitti[c], Maria Matarese[b], Alice Oliveti[d], Maria Grazia De Marinis[b]

[a] School of Nursing, Faculty of Medicine, Department of Biomedicine and Prevention, Tor Vergata University, Via Montpellier, 1 00133, Rome, Italy
[b] Research Unit Nursing Science, Campus Bio-Medico di Roma University, Via Alvaro del Portillo 21, 00128, Rome, Italy
[c] Research Unit Hygiene, Statistics and Public Health, Campus Bio-Medico di Roma University, Via Alvaro del Portillo 21, 00128, Rome, Italy
[d] Health management, Villa Betania Clinic, Via Pio IV 42, 00165, Rome, Italy
[e] National Center for Clinical Excellence, Quality and the Safety of Care (CNEC)', Istituto Superiore di Sanità, via Giano della Bella 34, Rome, Italy

ARTICLE INFO

Article history:
Received 1 February 2019
Received in revised form 1 August 2019
Accepted 6 August 2019

Keywords:
Aged
Continuity of patient care
Chronic disease
Meta-Analysis
Patient readmission

ABSTRACT

Background: Hospital readmission after discharge is a frequent, burdensome and costly event, particularly frequent in older people with multiple chronic conditions. Few literature reviews have analysed studies of continuity of care interventions to reduce readmissions of older inpatients discharged home over the short and long term.
Objective: To evaluate the effectiveness of continuity of care interventions in older people with chronic diseases in reducing short and long term hospital readmission after hospital discharge.
Design: Meta-analysis of randomized controlled trials.
Data sources: A comprehensive literature search on the databases PubMed, Medline, CINAHL and EMBASE was performed on 27 January 2019 with no language and time limits.
Review methods: RCTs on continuity of care interventions on older people discharged from hospital having hospital readmission as outcome, were included. Two reviewers independently screened the studies and assessed methodological quality using the Cochrane Risk of Bias tool. Selected outcome data were combined and pooled using a Mantel-Haenszel random-effects model.
Results: Thirty RCTs, representing 8920 patients were included. Results were stratified by time of readmissions. At 1 month from discharge, the continuity interventions were associated with lower readmission rates in 207/1595 patients in the experimental group (12.9%), versus 264/1645 patients in the control group (16%) (Relative Risk [RR], 0.84 [95% CI, 0.71-0.99]). From 1 to 3 months, readmission rates were lower in 325/1480 patients in the experimental group (21.9%), versus 455/1523 patients in the control group (29.8%) (RR 0.74 [95% CI, 0.65-0.84]). A subgroup analysis showed that this positive effect was stronger when the interventions addressed all of the continuity dimensions. After 3 months this impact became inconclusive with moderate/high statistical heterogeneity.
Conclusions: Continuity of care interventions prevent short term hospital readmission in older people with chronic diseases. However, there is inconclusive evidence about the effectiveness of continuity interventions aiming to reduce long term readmission, and it is suggested that stronger focus on it is needed.

What is already known about the topic?

- Older people with chronic conditions are associated with the highest rates of hospital readmission.
- The most-studied timeframe measuring hospital readmission is 30-day, probably due to the financial penalties introduced in Europe and US. Therefore, late hospital readmissions are understudied.
- A recent systematic review classifying interventions to reduce 30-day readmissions in older people could not identify effective any one intervention or bundle of interventions.

What this paper adds

- Continuity of care interventions prevent short term hospital readmission in older people with chronic diseases, and those

* Corresponding author.
  E-mail address: dangelo@iss.it (D. D'Angelo).
  @gabriel02689525 (G. Facchinetti)

http://dx.doi.org/10.1016/j.ijnurstu.2019.103396
0020-7489/© 2019 Elsevier Ltd. All rights reserved.

2 G. Facchinetti et al./International Journal of Nursing Studies 101 (2020) 103396

interventions that cover all continuity dimensions are more effective.

- It is paramount that healthcare systems should be designed to support long term care of chronicity, moving beyond the 30-day standard risk readmission rate.

1. Introduction

Chronic diseases are characterized by long duration and slow progression (World Health Organization, 2014) and are often related to multimorbidity status (Lalkhen and Mash, 2015; Pengpid and Peltzer, 2017). Older people living with a chronic disease have continuing complex care needs (Coleman, 2003) that require multiple care settings. Their life-pattern is characterized by frequent transitions in health (Naylor, 2012), high rates of hospital readmission (Berry et al., 2018) and involvement of patients, families and several healthcare providers in their care over a long period of time (Naylor, 2012). Chronic diseases can decrease quality of life and productivity and, if they are not effectively managed, result in acute and long-term complications requiring expensive hospitalizations and readmissions (Dye et al., 2018).

Effective management of chronicity includes continuity of care interventions with the goal of connecting and coordinating care between patients and providers across time and settings (Russell et al., 2011; van Servellen et al., 2006; Yang et al., 2017). Continuity of care occurs when healthcare events are experienced by patients as coherent, connected and consistent with their complex care needs (Haggerty et al., 2003). It is composed of three dimensions of continuity: *relational* (a patient-provider relationship over time), *informational* (the effective transfer and use of patients' past and current personal information) and *management* (consistent and timely coordination of care and services) (Haggerty et al., 2003). These elements are closely interrelated and should be all integrated by effective healthcare organizations (Guthrie et al., 2008). Moreover, two "core elements" distinguish continuity of care from other attributes of care: a focus on the patients' experience and the timeframe.

Most of the efforts spent on ensuring continuity of care aim at the reduction of hospital readmissions (Pacho et al., 2017), which are a common burden to healthcare systems (Gerhardt et al., 2013; Unruh et al., 2017), and undesirable events for patients (Kripalani et al., 2014). Older people perceived readmission to hospital as a challenge and a negative experience; they also felt that their existential, emotional and psychological wellbeing was not addressed by healthcare professionals (Blakey et al., 2017).

In literature, the most-studied timeframe measuring hospital readmission is 30-day, (Kristensen et al., 2015) probably due to the financial penalties introduced in Europe and US that forced hospitals to reduce early readmissions (Gupta and Fonarow, 2018) through pre and post-discharge continuity interventions. A number of publications exist on continuity of care interventions to reduce hospital readmission in adult patients but few reviews were conducted of studies on older people with chronic diseases. A systematic review aimed at classifying interventions to reduce 30-day readmissions in older people could not identify an intervention or bundle of interventions that reliably reduced readmissions (Hansen et al., 2011). Indeed, the effectiveness of continuity of care interventions in reducing hospital readmission in older people, in particular in the long-term, is still understudied. To date, the only metanalysis on the effectiveness of continuity of care intervention in the short and long term was conducted on adult patients with Chronic Obstructive Pulmonary Disease discharged home, with conflicting results (Yang et al., 2017). Therefore, the evidence on continuity of care interventions that effectively reduce both early and long term hospital readmission in older people with chronic diseases is sparse.

This systematic review of randomized controlled trials (RCTs) aims to evaluate the effectiveness of continuity of care interventions in older people with chronic diseases in reducing short and long term hospital readmission after hospital discharge.

2. Method

This review was reported in accordance with PRISMA statement guidance (Liberati et al., 2009). The protocol was previously registered on PROSPERO, registration number CRD42016050755. Preliminary searches of main databases could not find any existing or ongoing systematic reviews with this aim.

2.1. Eligibility criteria and search strategy

This review included only RCT with following inclusion criteria:

Types of participants: older patients ($\geq$ 65 years) diagnosed with one or more chronic diseases (World Health Organization, 2014), who were discharged home from hospital. Studies on cancer or psychiatric patients were excluded due to the particular illness trajectories characterizing those patients.

Types of intervention: continuity of care interventions provided by any healthcare professional during and after hospital discharge. Continuity of care interventions are defined as those focusing on the connection and coordination between patients and providers across time and settings and classified in informational, management, and relational continuity interventions (Reid et al., 2002). To be included, the interventions had to address at least one type of continuity (informational, management or relational) (Further details in Table 1).

Table 1
Characteristics of continuity of care dimensions.

Continuity of care dimensions (Reid et al., 2002)
Relational continuity
Relational continuity refers to an established relationship between patient and provider that extends across illnesses over time. An ongoing patient-provider relationship helps bridge discontinuous events and provides patients and caregivers with a sense of predictability and coherence. Relational continuity interventions usually refer to the strength of interpersonal relationships including the level of communication, comfort, trust and belief.
Informational continuity
Informational continuity is the transfer and use of information from previous events and conditions to plan appropriate interventions. The availability and use of data from prior events are a prerequisite for coordination of care, and accumulated knowledge is important for bridging separate care events and ensuring that services are responsive to patients' needs. Informational continuity interventions are related to the availability of documentation and to the comprehensiveness of information transfer between providers and settings.
Management continuity
Management continuity is achieved when interventions are delivered in a complementary and timely manner. When care is long term, the ability to provide consistent, predictable care is pivotal and care needs to be flexible enough to respond to changing patient health status and needs. Outreach and on-going monitoring are important to adapt the care strategy to the changing needs of the patients with a focus on individualized care plans and to increase patients'/caregivers' self-care.

G. Facchinetti et al./International Journal of Nursing Studies 101 (2020) 103396 3

Specifically, if the care was provided longitudinally with an ongoing therapeutic relationship with one or more providers who connect care over time, the interventions were considered as relational continuity. For example, the presence of a transitional care nurse who follows patients from hospital into their homes and guarantees the liaison with healthcare providers and the primary care hub.

If the information about patient's health was available and transferred from one provider to another throughout the follow-up period, the interventions were considered as informational continuity. For example, the use of interventions to record information such as electronic record charts, referral forms, and written discharge plans. As well as strategies to empower patients in their care through informational booklets or medication reconciliation.

When the care was provided with tailored and shared interventions to ensure consistency during treatment, the interventions were considered as management continuity. For example, the presence of a case manager who plays a vital role in patients/caregivers training and coaching with the aim to enhance their self-confidence in monitoring and managing the symptoms.

Since continuity of care is a result of the interconnection of all three dimensions, the more the interventions address different dimensions of continuity, the greater is the likelihood of the patients' experiencing continuity of care (Reid et al., 2002).

Types of outcome: all-cause hospital readmissions measured as the number of patients readmitted in both experimental and control groups during the follow up of 1 month, 1< months ≤3; 3< month ≤6, and 6< month ≤12 from discharge.

To enhance homogeneity, only studies in which the duration of intervention was as long as the readmission timeframe considered were included. For example, the studies included in the results of "readmission at 1 month" evaluated readmission at 1 month and interventions carried out in the course of 1 month; the studies included in the results of "readmission 1< months ≤3" evaluated readmission from 1 up to 3 months and interventions carried out in the course of up to three months, and so on.

A comprehensive literature search on the databases PubMed, Medline, CINAHL and EMBASE was performed on 27 January 2019 with no language and time limits. Medical subject headings and free-terms were searched for the following keywords: chronic disease, aged, continuity of patient care, hospital readmission (Appendix 1). Search strategies were checked by three reviewers (GF, DD, MP).

2.2. Study selection and data collection

Study screening was conducted independently by two reviewers (GF, DD). First, titles and abstracts and then full-texts selected from the first round were reviewed based on the inclusion criteria. To maximize search sensitivity a snowball method was used and the reference lists of the full-texts included were screened. Conflicts regarding study inclusion were resolved by mutual agreement between reviewers. The data from the full-texts selected were extracted independently by two authors (DA, AO) and checked by a third author (GF). Extracted data included first author, publication year, country, sample size, patient disease, interventions, follow-up time, type of continuity dimension, and principal healthcare provider involved in the intervention.

2.3. Quality assessment

Two reviewers independently evaluated the methodological quality and reliability of the findings through the risk of bias tool (Higgins et al., 2011). Study quality was assessed with the following criteria: selection, performance, detection, attrition, reporting and other biases. Each criterion was evaluated assigning zero for low risk, one point for unclear, and two points for high risk of bias. The potential total score ranged 0–14, in which a low score indicated higher quality level, and a high score indicated lower quality (Massimi et al., 2017). Based on this score, the studies were classified in three levels: low (> 3), moderate (2–3) and high (0–1) quality. Only moderate and high quality studies were included in review, to limit heterogeneity and improve the reliability of the study.

2.4. Definition of outcome

The primary outcome was the effectiveness of continuity of care interventions in reducing hospital readmissions of older patients with chronic diseases in the time sections of 1 month; 1< months ≤3; 3< months ≤6, and 6< months ≤12 months from discharge.

2.5. Data synthesis and analysis

Double data entry was performed by two reviewers (GF, DD). The number of patients readmitted in each group were reported and combined for the analysis. A meta-analysis was conducted using Review Manager software version 5.3 to pool data at different outcomes. For each study, we computed the relative risk (RR) of readmission at different outcomes. Pooled risk ratios and 95% of confidence intervals (CI) were computed by means of a Mantel-Haenszel random-effects modeltest (Mantel and Haenszel, 1959). Statistical heterogeneity was assessed using the standard chi-square (Cochran, 1954) and I-square with a value of greater than 50% indicating substantial heterogeneity (Higgins et al., 2003). Egger's test was used to detect funnel plot asymmetry (Higgins, 2011) and to assess potential publication bias. Subgroup analyses were planned on the time of follow-up (short and long term). Subgroup analyses were conducted to explore whether readmission risk at different time sections varied according to the number of continuity dimensions (three versus any) addressed by the interventions.

A post-hoc sensitivity analysis was conducted excluding those studies in which the randomization process was not clearly reported, multi-component continuity interventions were not employed, and the readmission rate was considered as a secondary outcome.

3. Results

The selection process is illustrated in Fig. 1. The search strategy yielded 854 articles. After duplicate removal and titles, abstracts and full-texts review, 36 studies were evaluated for methodological quality, 30 of which resulted eligible for the review and metanalysis.

3.1. Study and patient characteristics

A total of 8920 older patients discharged from hospital to home were included. All the studies were published in English in peer-reviewed journals from 1993 to 2018, and were mostly conducted in the USA (n = 10), China (n = 5), and Australia (n = 3). Patients were affected by chronic heart failure in 16 studies (53%), chronic obstructive pulmonary disease in 3 studies (10%), chronic obstructive pulmonary disease plus chronic heart failure in 2 studies (7%) and chronic lung disease in 1 study (3%). The remaining 8 studies (27%) coded patients' diseases under the broader classification of multi chronic disease (Table 2).

3.2. Intervention characteristics

The number of interventions carried out per each study ranged from 1 to 6. Eighteen different types of interventions were identified among which home visits (N = 17), telephone follow-up

4   *G. Facchinetti et al./International Journal of Nursing Studies 101 (2020) 103396*

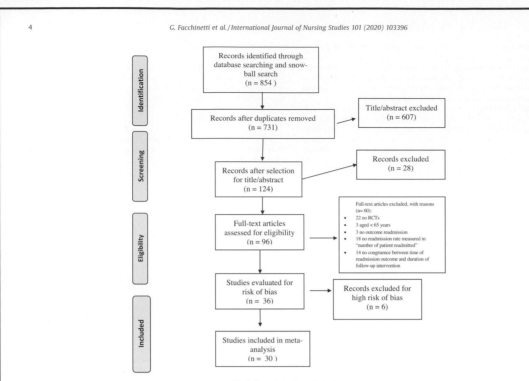

Fig. 1. Flow chart of search strategy.

(N = 16), self-management (N = 15), and transitional care models (N = 7) were prevalent (Table 2).

Most interventions were carried out by nurses with advanced competences (specialist nurse, case manager, health visitor, transition nurse, cardiac nurse, community nurse) in collaboration with other providers (n = 23 studies; 77%).

Eleven (37%) studies considered all three continuity dimensions. In particular, interventions of informational, management, and relational continuity were reported in 19 (63%), 29 (97%), and 18 (60%) studies, respectively.

3.3. Quality assessment

Of the 36 studies meeting our inclusion criteria, 6 had low quality and were excluded from the meta-analysis. Methodological quality was high in 10 (33%) and moderate in 20 (67%) studies. The double-blind procedure was not sufficiently detailed in 14 studies (47%) or absent in 6 studies (20%), where it might have been infeasible due to the nature of the intervention.

3.4. Readmission rates

The studies included presented readmission rates as primary (26, 87%), or secondary (4, 13%) outcomes. Fig. 2 shows our results in terms of all-cause readmissions, over a follow-up period from 1 to 12 months from discharge. The results were stratified by time sections (1 month; 1< months $\leq$3; 3< month $\leq$6, and 6< month $\leq$12). In addition, a subgroup analyses were performed to analyse the risk of hospital readmission stratified by number of continuity of care dimensions (Table 3).

3.5. Short term readmission

In this group eleven different and concurrent types of interventions were identified. Of these the most frequent were: telephone follow-up (82%), home visit (82%), self-management (72%), and patient education (27%).

3.5.1. Readmissions at 1 month

Data for readmission rates within 1 month were reported in 10 studies. The control and experimental groups included 3240 patients diagnosed with multi chronic diseases (n = 7; 70%), chronic obstructive pulmonary disease (n = 1; 10%), chronic heart failure (n = 1; 10%), and chronic obstructive pulmonary disease plus chronic heart failure (n = 1; 10%).

Individual study RRs ranged from 0.20 (95% CI, 0.04-0.88) (Benzo et al., 2016) to 1.2 (95% CI, 0.38–3.77) (Marusic et al., 2013). The continuity of care interventions were associated with a lower readmission rate in 207 of 1595 patients in the experimental group (12.9%), versus 264 of 1645 patients in the control group (16%) (RR, 0.84 [95% CI, 0.71-0.99] p = 0.04; Cochran Q χ^2, 9.32, p = 0.41; I^2, 3%). No publication bias was detected.

Meta-analyses of subgroup showed a statistically significant effect if the interventions addressed the three continuity dimensions (relational, management and relational) (RR, 0.77 [95% CI, 0.63-0.93] p = 0.006; I^2, 19.4%, p = 0.28) (Table 3).

3.5.2. < Months $\leq$3 readmission

Data for readmission rates at 1–3 months were reported in eleven studies, 1 of which evaluated readmission rates at 2 months, while the others considered 3-month readmission rates.

Table 2
Characteristics of included studies.

Author/year	Country	Disease	Sample size (N)	COC dimension			Intervention Type	Provider
				Informational	Relational	Management		
Barker et al., 2012	Australia	CHF	114	X	X	X	Medication reconciliation Home visits	Pharmacist
Benzo et al., 2016	USA	COPD	215	X	X	X	Written Emergency Plan Self-management Daily exercises Home visit Telephone follow up Patient hotline	Nurse Physiotherapist
Blue et al., 2001	UK	CHF	165	X		X	Home visits Liaison with healthcare provider Self-management Telephone follow up Informational booklet	Specialist nurse
Braun et al., 2009	Israel	MCD	209	X	X	X	Discharge planning Telephone follow up	Missing
Chow and Wong, 2014	China	MCD	185	X	X	X	Comprehensive patient assessment Home visit Self-management Telephone follow up	Nurse
Cleland et al., 2005	Germany, UK, Netherlands	CHF	255	X		X	Liaison with healthcare provider Home tele-monitoring Patient hotline	Nurse
Coleman et al., 2006	USA	MCD	750	X	X	X	Transitional care model Self-management	Nurse
Collinsworth et al., 2018	USA	COPD	308	X	X		Patient education Self-management Telephone follow up Liaison with healthcare provider	Respiratory therapist
Courtney et al., 2009	Australia	MCD	122		X	X	Transitional care model (with liaison with social service) Self-management Exercise intervention	Nurse Physiotherapist Social worker
DeBusk et al., 2004	USA	CHF	462			X	Informational booklet Telephone follow up Self management Coordination of care services	Nurse
Doughty et al., 2002	New Zealand	CHF	197	X		X	Clinic visit Discharge planning Liaison with healthcare provider Educational booklet Home visit	Cardiologist General practitioner Nurse
Dunn et al., 1994	UK	MCD	204			X	Home visit	Chiropody General practitioner Nurse
Ekman et al., 1998	Sweden	CHF	158	X	X	X	Patient hotline Liaison with healthcare provider Self-management Clinic visit, Home visit	Nurse
González-Guerrero et al., 2014	Spain	CHF	117		X	X	Patient education Telephone follow up, Social services	Nurse Geriatrician Social worker
Harrison et al., 2002	Canada	CHF	192	X	X	X	Transitional Care Model	Nurse
Hermiz et al., 2002	Australia	COPD	147	X		X	Home visit Self-management Patient education Liaison with healthcare provider Telephone follow up	Nurse
Hughes et al., 2000	USA	CHF, COPD	1966		X	X	Home visit Management of patients across organizational boundaries (social services)	Nurse Social worker Physician
Jaarsma et al., 1999	USA	CHF	179	X	X	X	Patient education Home visit Telephone follow up Self-management	Nurse
Krumholz et al., 2002	USA	CHF	88			X	Informational booklet Home visit Telephone follow up Telemonitoring	Nurse
Kwok et al., 2004	China	CLD	149	X		X	Comprehensive patient assessment Patient hotline Home visit Liaison with healthcare provider	Nurse
Kwok et al., 2008	China	CHF	105	X		X	Comprehensive patient assessment Home visit Patient hotline Liaison with healthcare provider	Nurse
Leventhal et al., 2011	Switzerland	CHF	42		X	X	Informational booklet Home visit Self-management Telephone follow up	Nurse
Lopez Cabezas et al., 2006	Spain	CHF	134	X		X	Patient education Telephone follow up Home visit	Pharmacists Cardiologists
Marusic et al., 2013	Croatia	MCD	160			X	Medication reconciliation and management Home visit	Pharmacist
Rainville, 1999	USA	CHF	34			X	Informational booklet Telephone follow up	Pharmacist Nurse
Rich et al., 1995	USA	CHF	282		X	X	Home visit Telephone follow up	Nurse Dietician Cardiologist
Ritchie et al., 2016	USA	CHF, COPD	478		X	X	Transitional Care Model Self-management	Nurse
Wong et al., 2014	China	MCD	406	X	X	X	Transitional Care Model Home visit Telephone follow up Self-management	Nurse
Wong et al., 2008	China	MCD	354	X	X	X	Transitional Care Model Home visit Telephone follow up Self-management	Nurse
Yu et al., 2015	Japan	CHF	178	X	X	X	Transitional Care Model Self-management	Nurse

Key: COC = Continuity Of Care; CHF = chronic heart failure; MCD = multi-chronic disease; COPD = chronic obstructive pulmonary disease; CLD = chronic lung disease.

The control and experimental groups included 3003 patients diagnosed with multi chronic diseases (n = 5; 45.4%), chronic obstructive pulmonary disease (n = 2; 18.1%), and chronic heart failure (n = 4; 36.3%).

Individual study RRs ranged from 0.46 (95% CI, 0.21–1.00) (Benzo et al., 2016) to 1.36 (95% CI, 0.72–2.59) (Hermiz et al., 2002). The continuity of care interventions were associated with a lower readmission rate in 325 of 1480 patients in the experimental group

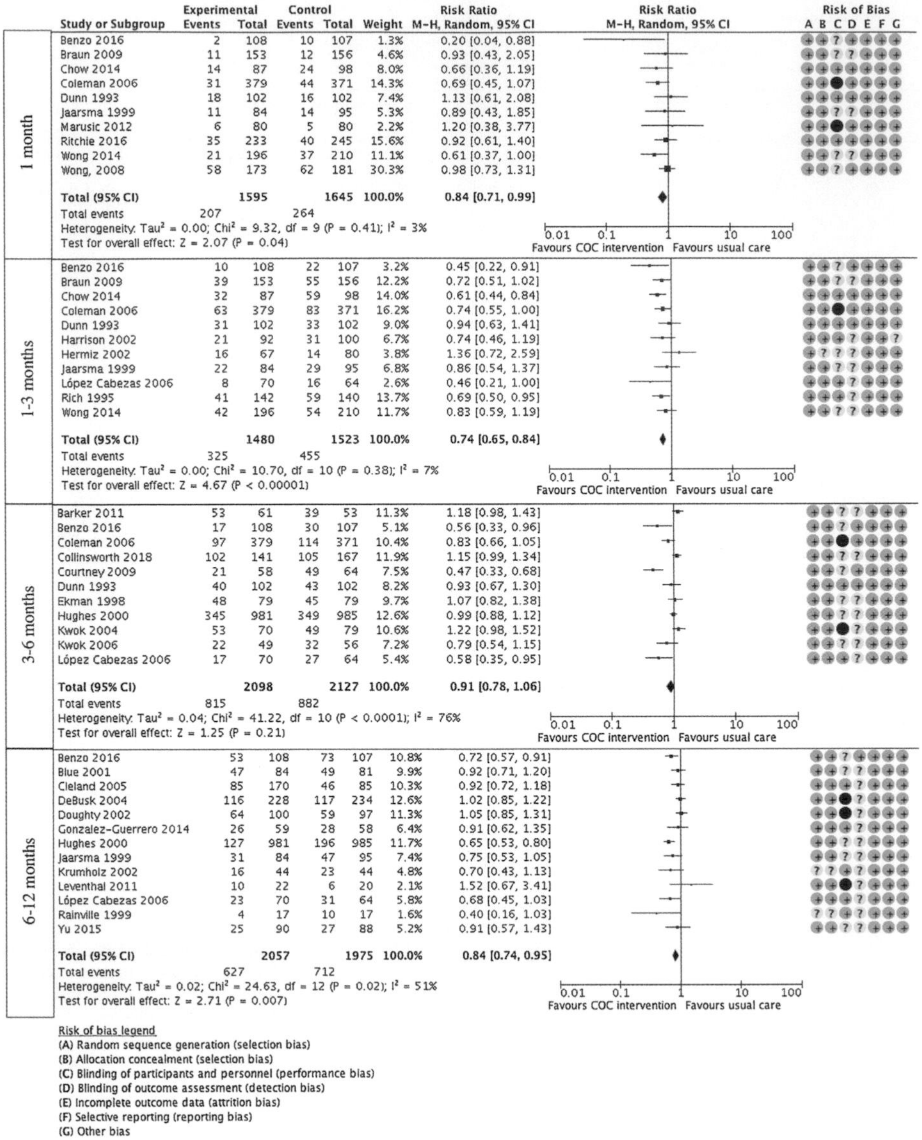

6   G. Facchinetti et al./International Journal of Nursing Studies 101 (2020) 103396

Fig. 2. Forest plot: effect of continuity of care interventions on readmission rate at 1 month, from 1 to 3 months, from 3 to 6 months, and from 6 to 12 months after hospital discharge.

(21.9%), versus 455 of 1523 patients in the control group (29.8%) (RR, 0.74 [95% CI, 0.65–0.84] p < 0.001; Cochran Q χ^2, 10.7, p = 0.38; I^2, 7%). No publication bias was detected.

A positive association for studies that addressed the three continuity dimensions (RR, 0.72 [95% CI, 0.62–0.83] p = 0.000; I^2 0.0%, p = 0.67) was found (Table 3).

3.6. Long term readmission

In this group 17 different and concurrent types of interventions were identified. Of these the most frequent interventions were: home visit (65%), self-management (45%), informational booklet (30%), patient hotline (25%), and liaison with healthcare provider (25%).

G. Facchinetti et al. / International Journal of Nursing Studies 101 (2020) 103396   7

Table 3
Meta-analysis of the risk of hospital readmission stratified by continuity of care dimensions.

SUBGROUPS	Readmission	Studies (N)	RR (95% CI)	I^2 (%)	p^*
ALL CONTINUITY OF CARE DIMENSIONS	1 month	7	0.77 (0.63-0.93)	19.40	0.28
	1< months ≤3	7	0.72 (0.62-0.83)	0.00	0.67
	3< month ≤6	4	0.91(0.79-1.04)	76.5	0.00
	6< month ≤12	3	0.76 (0.64-0.91)	0.00	0.67
ANY CONTINUITY OF CARE DIMENSIONS	1 month	3	1.00 (0.72-1.39)	0.00	0.82
	1< months ≤3	4	0.79 (0.63-0.99)	51.2	0.10
	3< month ≤6	6	0.93 (0.85-1.02)	79.5	0.00
	6< month ≤12	10	0.84 (0.76-0.92)	58.7	0.01

Key: * p value for heterogeneity.

3.6.1. < Month ≤6 readmission

Eleven studies evaluated 6-month readmission rates. The control and experimental groups included 4225 patients diagnosed with multi chronic diseases (n = 3; 27%), chronic obstructive pulmonary disease (n = 2; 18%), chronic heart failure (n = 4; 36%), chronic obstructive pulmonary disease plus chronic heart failure (n = 1; 9%) and chronic lung disease (n = 1; 9%).

Individual study RRs ranged from 0.47 (95% CI, 0.33-0.68) (Courtney et al., 2009) to 1.22 (95% CI, 0.98–1.52) (Kwok et al., 2004). There appeared to be a reduction in hospital readmission with continuity interventions (RR, 0.91 [95% CI, 0.78–1.06]; p = 0.21). However, both approaches for heterogeneity indicated considerable heterogeneity ($Q\chi^2$ 41.22, p < 0.001; I^2 = 76%) for this outcome, with the presence of publication bias on the test for asymmetry of the funnel plot, and a borderline small size effect (p = 0.075).

Null association with high heterogeneity was noted for studies that addressed either three continuity dimensions (RR, 0.91 [95% CI, 0.79–1.04] p = 0.1; I^2 76.5%, p = 0.005) or any continuity dimension (RR, 0.93 [95% CI, 0.85–1.02] p = 0.12; I^2 79.5%, p = 0.000) (Table 3).

3.6.2. < Month ≤12 months readmission

A total of 13 studies are included in this timeframe, 1 of which considered 8 months, 3 studies considered 9 months, while the others considered 12 months readmission rate.

The control and experimental groups included 4032 patients diagnosed with chronic obstructive pulmonary disease (n = 1; 7.69%), chronic heart failure (n = 11; 84.6%), and chronic obstructive pulmonary disease plus chronic heart failure (n = 1; 7.69%).

Individual study RRs ranged from 0.40 (95% CI, 0.16–1.03) (Rainville, 1999) to 1.52 (95% CI, 0.67–3.41) (Leventhal et al., 2011). Although the pooled data on hospital readmission are in favour of intervention (RR, 0.84 [95% CI, 0.74-0.95]), the Cochran Q χ^2 of 24.63 (p = 0.02), and the I^2 of 51% suggested the presence of a moderate study variability. Moreover, publication bias was detected among studies (p = 0.49).

We observed a positive association for studies that addressed three continuity dimensions (RR, 0.76 [95% CI, 0.64–0.91] p = 0.003; I^2 0.0%, p = 0.67) (Table 3), but an important heterogeneity between studies (RR, 0.84 [95% CI, 0.76–0.92] p = 0.000; I^2 58.7%, p = 0.01) that addressed any continuity dimensions precludes any conclusion on the effectiveness of such interventions.

3.7. Sensitivity analysis

The recalculation of the pooled estimates RR did not significantly alter the effect of the continuity interventions on all-cause readmission.

4. Discussion

To our knowledge, this is the first systematic review and metanalysis specifically evaluating the effectiveness of continuity of care interventions in older people with chronic diseases in reducing hospital readmission in the short and long term after hospital discharge.

Continuity of care interventions in the short term are associated with lower readmission rates. In the long term from discharge the impact on readmission rates becomes inconclusive, with high/moderate statistical heterogeneity (I^2 = 76%, 51%). This means that as the follow-up time becomes longer, the effect of continuity of care interventions becomes unclear.

Although a recent Cochrane review did not focus specifically on continuity interventions in chronically ill older people, but on discharge planning elements in a broader population, their results showing a lower readmission rate at three months from discharge are consistent with our findings (Goncalves-Bradley et al., 2016).

A meta-analysis of 42 RCTs targeting 30-day readmissions (Leppin et al., 2014), found a pooled risk ratio of 0.82 (95% CI, 0.73-0.91) that is very similar to our results at the same time frame (RR, 0.84 [95% CI, 0.71-0.99]). However, while Leppin et al. (2014) failed to find an interaction between their results and the age of participants, our analysis shows the consistent and beneficial effect of continuity of care intervention in reducing 30-day readmissions in older people. This finding is important for clinical practice because historically about a quarter of older people are readmitted to hospital within the first three months of discharge (Nuckols et al., 2017).

No clear evidence of continuity of care interventions on hospital readmissions in the long term was shown, mainly due to heterogeneity of the studies that biased the analyses. This is consistent with a study on the effectiveness of strategies to promote safe transition of older people that showed how multi-competent continuity interventions were effective in reducing readmissions within 3 months, but found no evidence for their benefit in the longer term (Mansah et al., 2009).

Older people with chronic diseases usually require frequent hospitalization to manage the exacerbations of their chronic disorders. When they enter the hospital setting the focus of care shifts from chronic to acute management to stabilize it (Vashi et al., 2013). As a consequence, early readmissions are attributed to the hospital's insufficient recognition of care needs, closely connected with the underlying diseases that have determined the admission, and to a poor discharge process (Zuckerman et al., 2016). Conversely, readmissions after a longer time are more likely to be due to events related to patient self-management, outpatient care, socio-economic issues, and community resources, rather than to the underlying disease (Kripalani et al., 2014).

8   G. Facchinetti et al./International Journal of Nursing Studies 101 (2020) 103396

Our results outline the effectiveness of continuity interventions in reducing only short-term readmission and urge hospitals to focus their efforts on the management of chronicity, looking for longitudinal strategies (Dharmarajan et al., 2013; Sheingold et al., 2016) to reduce also long-term readmissions.

In addition, the subgroup analyses showed that the continuity dimensions addressed by the interventions did interact with measure effectiveness. In particular, this effect is clearer when the interventions addressed all three continuity dimensions (informational, management and relational). Our findings confirm previous evidence in which the number of dimensions of continuity interventions were significantly related to their effectiveness (Bradley et al., 2013; Burke et al., 2014, Kripalani et al., 2014), and confirm the necessity to plan multimodal interventions that include as many continuity of care dimensions as possible (van Walraven et al., 2010v). It should be noted that management continuity is present in almost all of the RCTs analysed. This confirms the study by van Servellen et al. (2006), where management continuity is viewed as an integral part of any form of continuity without which neither informational nor relational continuity would be possible.

Finally, our review identified that the most used interventions were telephone follow-up and home visits in the short and long term group respectively. Literature confirms that telephone follow-up is the most frequently used 30-day post-discharge intervention, but also highlights inconclusive evidence about its effect (Mistiaen and Poot, 2006). As regards home visiting in the long term, it demonstrated a small relative effect that may not be clinically important (Mayo-Wilson et al., 2014).

Our review provides much needed evidence that continuity of care reduces short term hospital readmission, and may thus provide added value in the care of older people with chronic conditions. Clear recommendations have emerged from this review for primary care to improve continuity of care. Our research supports the importance of the *synchronization* of the three continuity dimensions during healthcare delivery. In fact, despite previous constant efforts to find the most effective interventions to reduce readmission, the key challenge is to provide different interventions addressing all of the continuity dimensions synchronously. Undoubtedly, any effective intervention will need to be implemented using a robust infrastructure of community services to provide ongoing assistance over time.

Moreover, the inconsistent effectiveness of continuity interventions in reducing long term readmission suggests that healthcare systems should be designed to support long term care of chronicity. With this aim it would also be necessary to plan wider and longer term interventions with reinforcement contacts able to modify patient behaviours (Cakir et al., 2017; Gupta and Fonarow, 2018). Besides, health policies should monitor long term readmissions by introducing strategies that force hospitals to pay attention to this outcome also, similar to the penalties for 30 day readmissions.

Finally, policymakers should recognize the need to reduce undesirable readmissions due to discontinuity of care and to promote continuity while improving the quality of care, thus increasing the value of the healthcare system by reducing cost without worsening quality.

Our study has several limitations. First, although we implemented comprehensive search strategies, we may not have identified all RCTs. Second, to enhance study homogeneity, we considered only studies measuring readmission rates as number of patients readmitted and with congruence between intervention and follow-up time.

The studies included comprised some multicomponent interventions differing substantially in their approach, thus it was nearly impossible to analyse which components of these made a difference to any of the outcomes assessed. Moreover, when labelling the types of continuity, some dimensions could not be clearly described or were difficult to extract, leading to an underestimation of the continuity accounted for. Finally, this review focused only on the hospital readmission outcome, and did not address other relevant health- or cost-related outcomes. Further research is needed to address the latter issues.

5. Conclusions

Continuity of care interventions prevent hospital readmissions in the short term in older people with chronic diseases. The evidence about the effectiveness of continuity interventions aiming to reduce long term readmissions, is inconclusive, suggesting the need to focus on it more strongly.

In particular, since long term readmissions are related to both clinical and socioeconomic factors, they could be prevented by closer cooperation and integration across different contextual boundaries (social, clinical, cultural), formal partnerships between acute-care hospitals and community-based organizations (Linertova et al., 2011).

Larger, well-conducted studies should continue to collect data on the effectiveness of continuity of care interventions in the long term.

Declaration of Competing Interest

The authors have no conflicts in the cover letter as well as in the manuscript, as noted above.

Acknowledgments

This research did not receive any specific grant from funding agencies in the public, commercial, or not-for-profit sectors.

Appendix A. Supplementary data

Supplementary material related to this article can be found, in the online version, at doi:https://doi.org/10.1016/j.ijnurstu.2019.103396.

References

Barker, A.L., Barlis, P., Berlowitz, D.J., Page, K., Jackson, B.L., Lim, W.K., 2012. Pharmacist directed home medication reviews in patients with chronic heart failure: a randomised clinical trial. Int. J. Cardiol. 159 (2), 139–143.

Benzo, R., Vickers, K., Novotny, P.J., Tucker, S., Hoult, J., Neuenfeldt, P., Connett, J., Lorig, K., McEvoy, C., 2016. Health coaching and chronic obstructive pulmonary disease rehospitalization. A Randomized Study. Am J Respir Crit Care Med 194 (6), 672–680.

Berry, J.G., Gay, J.C., Joynt Maddox, K., Coleman, E.A., Bucholz, E.M., O'Neill, M.R., Blaine, K., Hall, M., 2018. Age trends in 30 day hospital readmissions: US national retrospective analysis. BMJ 360, k497.

Blakey, E.P., Jackson, D., Walthall, H., Aveyard, H., 2017. What is the experience of being readmitted to hospital for people 65 years and over? A review of the literature. Contemp. Nurse 53 (6), 698–712.

Blue, L., Lang, E., McMurray, J.J., Davie, A.P., McDonagh, T.A., Murdoch, D.R., Petrie, M. C., Connolly, E., Norrie, J., Round, C.E., Ford, I., Morrison, C.E., 2001. Randomised controlled trial of specialist nurse intervention in heart failure. BMJ 323 (7315), 715–718.

Bradley, E.H., Curry, L., Horwitz, L.I., Sipsma, H., Wang, Y., Walsh, M.N., Goldmann, D., White, N., Pina, I.L., Krumholz, H.M., 2013. Hospital strategies associated with 30-day readmission rates for patients with heart failure. Circ. Cardiovasc. Qual. Outcomes 6 (4), 444–450.

Braun, E., Baidusi, A., Alroy, G., Azzam, Z.S., 2009. Telephone follow-up improves patients satisfaction following hospital discharge. Eur. J. Intern. Med. 20 (2), 221–225.

Burke, R.E., Guo, R., Prochazka, A.V., Misky, G.J., 2014. Identifying keys to success in reducing readmissions using the ideal transitions in care framework. BMC Health Serv. Res. 14, 423.

Cakir, B., Kaltsounis, S.K.D.J., Kopf, S., Steiner, J., 2017. Hospital readmissions from patients' perspectives. South. Med. J. 110 (5), 353–358.

Chow, S.K., Wong, F.K., 2014. A randomized controlled trial of a nurse-led case management programme for hospital-discharged older adults with co-morbidities. J. Adv. Nurs. 70 (10), 2257–2271.

APPENDIX A 455

G. Facchinetti et al. / International Journal of Nursing Studies 101 (2020) 103396 9

Cleland, J.G., Louis, A.A., Rigby, A.S., Janssens, U., Balk, A.H., Investigators, T.-H., 2005. Noninvasive home telemonitoring for patients with heart failure at high risk of recurrent admission and death: the Trans-European Network-Home-Care Management System (TEN-HMS) study. J. Am. Coll. Cardiol. 45 (10), 1654–1664.

Cochran, W.G., 1954. Some methods for strengthening the common χ 2 tests. Biometrics 10 (4), 417–451.

Coleman, E.A., 2003. Falling through the cracks: challenges and opportunities for improving transitional care for persons with continuous complex care needs. J. Am. Geriatr. Soc. 51 (4), 549–555.

Coleman, E.A., Parry, C., Chalmers, S., Min, S.J., 2006. The care transitions intervention: results of a randomized controlled trial. Arch. Intern. Med. 166 (17), 1822–1828.

Collinsworth, A.W., Brown, R.M., James, C.S., Stanford, R.H., Alemayehu, D., Priest, E.L., 2018. The impact of patient education and shared decision making on hospital readmissions for COPD. Int. J. Chron. Obstruct. Pulmon. Dis. 13, 1325–1332.

Courtney, M., Edwards, H., Chang, A., Parker, A., Finlayson, K., Hamilton, K., 2009. Fewer emergency readmissions and better quality of life for older adults at risk of hospital readmission: a randomized controlled trial to determine the effectiveness of a 24-week exercise and telephone follow-up program. J. Am. Geriatr. Soc. 57 (3), 395–402.

DeBusk, R.F., Miller, N.H., Parker, K.M., Bandura, A., Kraemer, H.C., Cher, D.J., West, J. A., Fowler, M.B., Greenwald, G., 2004. Care management for low-risk patients with heart failure: a randomized, controlled trial. Ann. Intern. Med. 141 (8), 606–613.

Dharmarajan, K., Hsieh, A.F., Lin, Z., Bueno, H., Ross, J.S., Horwitz, L.I., Barreto-Filho, J. A., Kim, N., Suter, L.G., Bernheim, S.M., Drye, E.E., Krumholz, H.M., 2013. Hospital readmission performance and patterns of readmission: retrospective cohort study of Medicare admissions. BMJ 347, f6571.

Doughty, R.N., Wright, S.P., Pearl, A., Walsh, H.J., Muncaster, S., Whalley, G.A., Gamble, G., Sharpe, N., 2002. Randomized, controlled trial of integrated heart failure management: the auckland heart failure management study. Eur. Heart J. 23 (2), 139–146.

Dunn, R.B., Lewis, P.A., Vetter, N.J., Guy, P.M., Hardman, C.S., Jones, R.W., 1994. Health visitor intervention to reduce days of unplanned hospital re-admission in patients recently discharged from geriatric wards: the results of a randomised controlled study. Arch. Gerontol. Geriatr. 18 (1), 15–23.

Dye, C., Willoughby, D., Aybar-Damali, B., Grady, C., Oran, R., Knudson, A., 2018. Improving chronic disease self-management by older home health patients through community health coaching. Int. J. Environ. Res. Public Health 15 (4) .

Ekman, I., Andersson, B., Ehnfors, M., Matejka, G., Persson, B., Fagerberg, B., 1998. Feasibility of a nurse-monitored, outpatient-care programme for elderly patients with moderate-to-severe, chronic heart failure. Eur. Heart J. 19 (8), 1254–1260.

Gerhardt, G., Yemane, A., Hickman, P., Oelschlaeger, A., Rollins, E., Brennan, N., 2013. Medicare readmission rates showed meaningful decline in 2012. Medicare Medicaid Res. Rev. 3 (2) .

Goncalves-Bradley, D.C., Lannin, N.A., Clemson, L.M., Cameron, I.D., Shepperd, S., 2016. Discharge planning from hospital. Cochrane Database Syst. Rev. 1 CD000313.

González-Guerrero, J.L., Alonso-Fernández, T., García-Mayolín, N., Gusi, N., Ribera-Casado, J.M., 2014. Effectiveness of a follow-up program for elderly heart failure patients after hospital discharge. A randomized controlled trial. Eur. Geriatr. Med. 5 (4), 252–257.

Gupta, A., Fonarow, G.C., 2018. The Hospital Readmissions Reduction Program-learning from failure of a healthcare policy. Eur. J. Heart Fail..

Guthrie, B., Saultz, J.W., Freeman, G.K., Haggerty, J.L., 2008. Continuity of care matters. BMJ 337, a867.

Haggerty, J.L., Reid, R.J., Freeman, G.K., Starfield, B.H., Adair, C.E., McKendry, R., 2003. Continuity of care: a multidisciplinary review. BMJ 327 (7425), 1219–1221.

Hansen, L.O., Young, R.S., Hinami, K., Leung, A., Williams, M.V., 2011. Interventions to reduce 30-day rehospitalization: a systematic review. Ann. Intern. Med. 155 (8), 520–528.

Harrison, M.B., Browne, G.B., Roberts, J., Tugwell, P., Gafni, A., Graham, I.D., 2002. Quality of life of individuals with heart failure: a randomized trial of the effectiveness of two models of hospital-to-home transition. Med. Care 40 (4), 271–282.

Hermiz, O., Comino, E., Marks, G., Daffurn, K., Wilson, S., Harris, M., 2002. Randomised controlled trial of home based care of patients with chronic obstructive pulmonary disease. BMJ 325 (7370), 938.

Higgins, J.G.S., 2011. Cochrane Handbook for Systematic Reviews of Interventions Version 5.1.0 [updated March 2011] Available from. The Cochrane Collaboration. http://handbook.cochrane.org.

Higgins, J.P., Altman, D.G., Gotzsche, P.C., Juni, P., Moher, D., Oxman, A.D., Savovic, J., Schulz, K.F., Weeks, L., Sterne, J.A., 2011. Cochrane Bias methods, G., cochrane statistical methods, G. The Cochrane Collaboration's tool for assessing risk of bias in randomised trials. BMJ 343, d5928.

Higgins, J.P., Thompson, S.G., Deeks, J.J., Altman, D.G., 2003. Measuring inconsistency in meta-analyses. BMJ 327 (7414), 557–560.

Hughes, S.L., Weaver, F.M., Giobbie-Hurder, A., Manheim, L., Henderson, W., Kubal, J. D., Ulasevich, A., Cummings, J., Department of Veterans Affairs Cooperative Study Group on Home-Based Primary, C, 2000. Effectiveness of team-managed home-based primary care: a randomized multicenter trial. JAMA 284 (22), 2877–2885.

Jaarsma, T., Halfens, R., Huijer Abu-Saad, H., Dracup, K., Gorgels, T., van Ree, J., Stappers, J., 1999. Effects of education and support on self-care and resource utilization in patients with heart failure. Eur. Heart J. 20 (9), 673–682.

Kripalani, S., Theobald, C.N., Anctil, B., Vasilevskis, E.E., 2014. Reducing hospital readmission rates: current strategies and future directions. Annu. Rev. Med. 65, 471–485.

Kristensen, S.R., Bech, M., Quentin, W., 2015. A roadmap for comparing readmission policies with application to Denmark, England, Germany and the United States. Health Policy (New York) 119 (3), 264–273.

Krumholz, H.M., Amatruda, J., Smith, G.L., Mattera, J.A., Roumanis, S.A., Radford, M.J., Crombie, P., Vaccarino, V., 2002. Randomized trial of an education and support intervention to prevent readmission of patients with heart failure. J. Am. Coll. Cardiol. 39 (1), 83–89.

Kwok, T., Lee, J., Woo, J., Lee, D.T., Griffith, S., 2008. A randomized controlled trial of a community nurse-supported hospital discharge programme in older patients with chronic heart failure. J. Clin. Nurs. 17 (1), 109–117.

Kwok, T., Lum, C.M., Chan, H.S., Ma, H.M., Lee, D., Woo, J., 2004. A randomized, controlled trial of an intensive community nurse-supported discharge program in preventing hospital readmissions of older patients with chronic lung disease. J. Am. Geriatr. Soc. 52 (8), 1240–1246.

Lalkhen, H., Mash, R., 2015. Multimorbidity in non-communicable diseases in South African primary healthcare. S. Afr. Med. J. 105 (2), 134–138.

Leppin, A.L., Gionfriddo, M.R., Kessler, M., Brito, J.P., Mair, F.S., Gallacher, K., Wang, Z., Erwin, P.J., Sylvester, T., Boehmer, K., Ting, H.H., Murad, M.H., Shippee, N.D., Montori, V.M., 2014. Preventing 30-day hospital readmissions: a systematic review and meta-analysis of randomized trials. JAMA Intern. Med. 174 (7), 1095–1107.

Leventhal, M.E., Denhaerynck, K., Brunner-La Rocca, H.P., Burnand, B., Conca-Zeller, A., Bernasconi, A.T., Mahrer-Imhof, R., Froelicher, E.S., De Geest, S., 2011. Swiss Interdisciplinary Management Programme for Heart Failure (SWIM-HF): a randomised controlled trial study of an outpatient inter-professional management programme for heart failure patients in Switzerland. Swiss Med. 141, w13171.

Liberati, A., Altman, D.G., Tetzlaff, J., Mulrow, C., Gotzsche, P.C., Ioannidis, J.P., Clarke, M., Devereaux, P.J., Kleijnen, J., Moher, D., 2009. The PRISMA statement for reporting systematic reviews and meta-analyses of studies that evaluate health care interventions: explanation and elaboration. PLoS Med. 6 (7), e1000100.

Linertova, R., Garcia-Perez, L., Vazquez-Diaz, J.R., Lorenzo-Riera, A., Sarria-Santamera, A., 2011. Interventions to reduce hospital readmissions in the elderly: in-hospital or home care. A systematic review. J. Eval. Clin. Pract. 17 (6), 1167–1175.

Lopez Cabezas, C., Falces Salvador, C., Cubi Quadrada, D., Arnau Bartes, A., Ylla Bore, M., Muro Perea, N., Homs Peipoch, E., 2006. Randomized clinical trial of a postdischarge pharmaceutical care program vs regular follow-up in patients with heart failure. Farm. Hosp. 30 (6), 328–342.

Mansah, M., Fernandez, R., Griffiths, R., Chang, E., 2009. Effectiveness of strategies to promote safe transition of elderly people across care settings. JBI Libr. Syst. Rev. 7 (24), 1036–1090.

Mantel, N., Haenszel, W., 1959. Statistical aspects of the analysis of data from retrospective studies of disease. J. Natl. Cancer Inst. 22 (4), 719–748.

Marusic, S., Gojo-Tomic, N., Erdeljic, V., Bacic-Vrca, V., Franic, M., Kirin, M., Bozikov, V., 2013. The effect of pharmacotherapeutic counseling on readmissions and emergency department visits. Int. J. Clin. Pharm. 35 (1), 37–44.

Massimi, A., De Vito, C., Brufola, I., Corsaro, A., Marzuillo, C., Migliara, G., Rega, M.L., Ricciardi, W., Villari, P., Damiani, G., 2017. Are community-based nurse-led self-management support interventions effective in chronic patients? Results of a systematic review and meta-analysis. PLoS One 12 (3), e0173617.

Mayo-Wilson, E., Grant, S., Burton, J., Parsons, A., Underhill, K., Montgomery, P., 2014. Preventive home visits for mortality, morbidity, and institutionalization in older adults: a systematic review and meta-analysis. PLoS One 9 (3), e89257.

Mistiaen, P., Poot, E., 2006. Telephone follow-up, initiated by a hospital-based health professional, for postdischarge problems in patients discharged from hospital to home. Cochrane Database Syst. Rev.(4) CD004510.

Naylor, M.D., 2012. Advancing high value transitional care: the central role of nursing and its leadership. Nurs. Adm. Q. 36 (2), 115–126.

Nuckols, T.K., Keeler, E., Morton, S., Anderson, L., Doyle, B.J., Pevnick, J., Booth, M., Shanman, R., Arifkhanova, A., Shekelle, P., 2017. Economic evaluation of quality improvement interventions designed to prevent hospital readmission: a systematic review and meta-analysis. JAMA Intern. Med. 177 (7), 975–985.

Pacho, C., Domingo, M., Nunez, R., Lupon, J., Moliner, P., de Antonio, M., Gonzalez, B., Santesmases, J., Vela, E., Tor, J., Bayes-Genis, A., 2017. Early postdischarge STOP-HF-Clinic reduces 30-day readmissions in old and frail patients with heart failure. Rev. Esp. Cardiol. Engl. Ed (Engl Ed) 70 (8), 631–638.

Pengpid, S., Peltzer, K., 2017. Multimorbidity in chronic conditions: public primary care patients in four greater mekong countries. Int. J. Environ. Res. Public Health 14 (9) .

Rainville, E.C., 1999. Impact of pharmacist interventions on hospital readmissions for heart failure. Am. J. Health. Syst. Pharm. 56 (13), 1339–1342.

Reid, R., Haggerty, J., McKendry, R., 2002. Defusing the Confusion: Concepts and Measures of Continuity of Healthcare. .

Rich, M.W., Beckham, V., Wittenberg, C., Leven, C.L., Freedland, K.E., Carney, R.M., 1995. A multidisciplinary intervention to prevent the readmission of elderly patients with congestive heart failure. N. Engl. J. Med. 333 (18), 1190–1195.

Ritchie, C.S., Houston, T.K., Richman, J.S., Sobko, H.J., Berner, E.S., Taylor, B.B., Salanitro, A.H., Locher, J.L., 2016. The E-Coach technology-assisted care transition system: a pragmatic randomized trial. Transl. Behav. Med. 6 (3), 428–437.

Russell, D., Rosati, R.J., Rosenfeld, P., Marren, J.M., 2011. Continuity in home health care: is consistency in nursing personnel associated with better patient outcomes? J. Healthc. Qual. 33 (6), 33–39.

10   G. Facchinetti et al. / International Journal of Nursing Studies 101 (2020) 103396

Sheingold, S.H., Zuckerman, R., Shartzer, A., 2016. Understanding medicare hospital readmission rates and differing penalties between safety-net and other hospitals. Health Aff. (Millwood) 35 (1), 124–131.

Unruh, M.A., Jung, H.Y., Vest, J.R., Casalino, L.P., Kaushal, R., Investigators, H., 2017. Meaningful use of electronic health records by outpatient physicians and readmissions of medicare fee-for-Service beneficiaries. Med. Care 55 (5), 493–499.

van Servellen, G., Fongwa, M., Mockus D'Errico, E., 2006. Continuity of care and quality care outcomes for people experiencing chronic conditions: a literature review. Nurs. Health Sci. 8 (3), 185–195.

van Walraven, C., Oake, N., Jennings, A., Forster, A.J., 2010v. The association between continuity of care and outcomes: a systematic and critical review. J. Eval. Clin. Pract. 16 (5), 947–956.

Vashi, A.A., Fox, J.P., Carr, B.G., D'Onofrio, G., Pines, J.M., Ross, J.S., Gross, C.P., 2013. Use of hospital-based acute care among patients recently discharged from the hospital. JAMA 309 (4), 364–371.

Wong, F.K., Chow, S., Chung, L., Chang, K., Chan, T., Lee, W.M., Lee, R., 2008. Can home visits help reduce hospital readmissions? Randomized controlled trial. J. Adv. Nurs. 62 (5), 585–595.

Wong, F.K., Chow, S.K., Chan, T.M., Tam, S.K., 2014. Comparison of effects between home visits with telephone calls and telephone calls only for transitional discharge support: a randomised controlled trial. Age Ageing 43 (1), 91–97.

World Health Organization, 2014. Global Status Report on Noncommunicable Diseases. World Health Organization, Switzerland.

Yang, F., Xiong, Z.F., Yang, C., Li, L., Qiao, G., Wang, Y., Zheng, T., He, H., Hu, H., 2017. Continuity of care to prevent readmissions for patients with chronic obstructive pulmonary disease: a systematic review and meta-analysis. COPD 14 (2), 251–261.

Yu, D.S., Lee, D.T., Stewart, S., Thompson, D.R., Choi, K.C., Yu, C.M., 2015. Effect of nurse-implemented transitional care for chinese individuals with chronic heart failure in Hong Kong: a randomized controlled trial. J. Am. Geriatr. Soc. 63 (8), 1583–1593.

Zuckerman, R.B., Sheingold, S.H., Orav, E.J., Ruhter, J., Epstein, A.M., 2016. Readmissions, observation, and the hospital readmissions reduction program. N. Engl. J. Med. 374 (16), 1543–1551.

International Journal of Nursing Studies 101 (2020) 103417

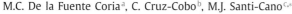

Contents lists available at ScienceDirect

International Journal of Nursing Studies

journal homepage: www.elsevier.com/ijns

Effectiveness of a primary care nurse delivered educational intervention for patients with type 2 diabetes mellitus in promoting metabolic control and compliance with long-term therapeutic targets: Randomised controlled trial

M.C. De la Fuente Coria[a], C. Cruz-Cobo[b], M.J. Santi-Cano[c,*]

[a] Primary Health Care District of Bay of Cádiz-La Janda, Andalucía, Spain
[b] Faculty of Nursing and Physiotherapy, University of Cádiz, Spain
[c] Research Group on Nutrition: Molecular, Pathophysiological and Social Issues, University of Cádiz, Avda. Ana de Viya, 52, 11009 Cádiz, Spain

ARTICLE INFO

Article history:
Received 9 April 2019
Received in revised form 29 August 2019
Accepted 1 September 2019

Keywords:
Clinical trial
Diabetes mellitus type 2
Education
Health promotion
Nurse
Self-management

ABSTRACT

Background: Systematic reviews and meta-analyses have shown very different values for the effectiveness of education in type 2 diabetes mellitus. However, the achievement of therapeutic targets after educational programs has been poorly evaluated.
Objective: Evaluate the effectiveness of a structured and individualised education program for type 2 diabetes, provided by a primary care nurse, which featured educational reinforcements and family support to achieve metabolic control, and long-term therapeutic targets.
Methods: Randomised controlled clinical trial with two arms: Intervention and control group. The intervention consisted of six face-to-face sessions of 30 min and follow-ups after 12 and 24 months for 236 participants with type 2 diabetes mellitus in a primary care setting in Andalusia (Spain). The primary outcome variables were the values and achievement of the type 2 diabetes mellitus control targets established by the American Diabetes Association: Glycated haemoglobin, fasting blood glucose, total cholesterol, low-density lipoprotein-cholesterol, high-density lipoprotein-cholesterol, triglycerides, systolic and diastolic blood pressure. The secondary outcome variable was body mass index.
Results: From an overall total of 236 participants, 54.2% were male and the average age was 65.1 ± 9.5. After 12 months, the glycated haemoglobin level and systolic blood pressure decreased in the intervention group. After 24 months, the following variables significantly improved among the intervention group participants: basal glycemia, glycated haemoglobin, total cholesterol low-density lipoprotein cholesterol, and diastolic blood pressure. The glycated haemoglobin target ($<7\%$) was better achieved in the intervention group than in the control group (35.2% vs 24.7%, $p < 0.003$). The rest of the targets were not met.
Conclusion: Continual diabetes education with reinforcement sessions provided by a nurse achieved reductions in glycated haemoglobin, basal glycaemia, total cholesterol, low-density lipoprotein-cholesterol and systolic blood pressure in both the medium and long term. It also increased the proportion of participants who achieved the therapeutic target of glycated haemoglobin.

© 2019 Elsevier Ltd. All rights reserved.

What is already known about the topic?

- Evidence-based guidelines have established quality standards for diabetes education programs.

- The effectiveness of diabetes education in terms of improvements in glycated haemoglobin and other cardiovascular risk factors has shown very different values.

What this paper adds

- The structured and individualised, education intervention, delivered by an expert nurse, has been effective in reducing biochemical parameters in the medium and long term.

* Corresponding author.
E-mail addresses: delafuentecoriam@yahoo.es (M.C. De la Fuente Coria), celia.cruz@uca.es (C. Cruz-Cobo), mariajose.santi@uca.es (M.J. Santi-Cano).

https://doi.org/10.1016/j.ijnurstu.2019.103417
0020-7489/© 2019 Elsevier Ltd. All rights reserved.

2 *M.C. De la Fuente Coria, C. Cruz-Cobo and M.J. Santi-Cano/International Journal of Nursing Studies 101 (2020) 103417*

- Glycated haemoglobin was the therapeutic target that showed significant long-term improvements.
- Innovative strategies such as educational reinforcements and involving family members could increase glycemic control.

1. Introduction

Diabetes mellitus has now reached global epidemic proportions, with a worldwide prevalence of 8.5% in the adult population. Within the European Union, the prevalence varies between countries: 6% in Austria; 7.4% in Germany; 8% in France; 9.4% in Spain; 9.5% in Poland; 9.6% in the Czech Republic; 10% in Hungary; and 10.3% in Bulgaria (World Health Organization, 2016).

Globally, in 2017, the North America and Caribbean region had the highest prevalence of diabetes mellitus (11.0%). The South-East Asia region had intermediate prevalence (10.1%) and the Africa region had the lowest prevalence (4.4%) likely due to lower levels of urbanisation, lower prevalence of obesity and higher rates of communicable diseases (International Diabetes Federation, 2017a).

The type 2 diabetes epidemic has been attributed to urbanisation and environmental transitions (work and diet pattern changes) which favour sedentary occupations and a rise in caloric consumption (Ley et al., 2014).

There is scientific evidence that type 2 diabetes mellitus prevalence in children and young people is increasing in some countries. It is strongly associated to the dramatic rise in obesity prevalence and physical inactivity among children and adolescents. Type 2 diabetes mellitus in childhood could become a real public health issue in some countries (Al-Saeed et al., 2016).

Diabetes is a major cause of morbidity and mortality because it can cause blindness, kidney failure, myocardial infarction, stroke, and lower limb amputation. Diabetes is thought to have been the direct cause of 1.6 million deaths in 2015. In addition, 2.2 million people died from cardiovascular disease, attributable to hyperglycaemia, of which 43% occurred in people younger than 70 years old (Sarwar et al., 2010; Bourne et al., 2013; Saran et al., 2015; World Health Organization, 2016).

Moreover, the economic costs related to diabetes in the form of loss of work and income, medication, hospitalisation and ambulatory care are very high, both for patients and health systems. Furthermore World Health Organization projections predict that diabetes will be the seventh cause of mortality in 2030 (Mathers and Loncar, 2006; World Health Organization, 2016).

Nowadays, cost-effective interventions are available to control diabetes through diet, physical activity, medication, measuring blood pressure and blood lipids, and periodic examinations to detect any injury to eyes, kidneys or feet. All these measures can prevent or delay the complications of diabetes. Comprehensive diabetes care requires that action is taken through diabetes education programs, aimed at improving people knowledge and behaviour regarding the self-management of diabetes (Powers et al., 2015).

Evidence-based guidelines consider diabetes education to be one of the keys in managing diabetes (Guideline NICE, 2015). Quality standards for diabetes education programs have been established (International Diabetes Federation, 2017b). Likewise, American Diabetes Association advises compliance with therapeutic targets of glycated haemoglobin <7%, fasting blood glucose between 80 and 130 mg/dL, blood pressure <140/90 mmHg and low-density lipoprotein-cholesterol <100 mg/dL, in order to reduce or delay the micro and macro-vascular complications of diabetes (American Diabetes Association, 2018).

The effectiveness of education in terms of seeing an improvement in glycated haemoglobin and other cardiovascular risk factors has shown very different values in systematic reviews and meta-analyses with average reductions in glycated haemoglobin of −0.74%, ranging from −2.5% to 0.6% vs. −0.17%, ranging from −1.7% to 1.5% in control groups, depending on the intervention's characteristics (individualised or group, duration, frequency and evaluation of follow-up, short-term or long-term) (Chrvala et al., 2016; Odgers et al., 2017). Nevertheless, the achievement of the therapeutic targets following educational programs has been poorly evaluated.

The main objective of this study was to evaluate the effectiveness of using a structured, individualised type 2 diabetes education program, provided by a primary care nurse, to control type 2 diabetes mellitus patients, evaluated through the participant's glycated haemoglobin, blood pressure, body mass index measurements and their lipid profile as well as whether or not they achieve, the therapeutic targets of long-term control.

2. Methods

2.1. Design

A randomized controlled clinical trial with two arms: an intervention group (carried out by a nurse), and a control group (usual care), with a follow-up after 12 and 24 months.

The sample size was calculated to obtain a confidence level of 95%, a statistical power of 90%, a minimum difference to be detected regarding glycosylated haemoglobin of 1% and, a variance of 4% (Khunti et al., 2012). A sample size of 69 participants was obtained in both the intervention and control group.

The inclusion criteria were: Patients with type 2 diabetes mellitus, between 18 and 80 years of age, who agreed to participate in the study and signed the informed consent. The exclusion criteria were: cognitive impairment, significant alteration of physical mobility, not accepting the educational advice, type 1 diabetes mellitus, gestational diabetes.

2.2. Recruitment of the participants

Participants were recruited from a primary care centre in the Bahía de Cádiz-La Janda district, Andalusia (Spain), identified through electronic medical records. Four hundred patients of both genders with type 2 diabetes mellitus were eligible between June 2014 and June 2017.

During the first month, all patients diagnosed with type 2 diabetes mellitus were invited to participate in the study through nursing consultations, or telephone calls. Out of the 400 patients, 53 refused to participate, and 65 were excluded. The rest of the patients were individually met in the consulting room to inform them about the study. In the end, 236 participants completed the study: 97 participants in the intervention group and 139 in the usual care group (Fig. 1). The loss of follow-up in the intervention group was 30% (n = 43). Reasons for loss to follow-up were death (n = 2), moved to another city (n = 1) and declined (n = 40, due to too busy, lack of time or out of contact). The sample loss in the usual care was 0.7% (1 death).

2.3. Intervention

The intervention consisted of 6 face-to-face sessions lasting 30 min. They consisted of structured, individualised education, carried out by one trained nurse with more than 10 years of experience in type 2 diabetes mellitus education. The educational sessions were delivered over a period of 6 months, with educational reinforcements after 12 and 18 months. The participant had to attend the sessions accompanied by a family member/caregiver. The contents were based on those proposed by American Association of Diabetes Educator (2018): basic knowledge of diabetes, healthy eating, physical activity, self-monitoring of blood glucose, medication, risk reduction, problem solving, and effective coping.

M.C. De la Fuente Coria, C. Cruz-Cobo and M.J. Santi-Cano / International Journal of Nursing Studies 101 (2020) 103417   3

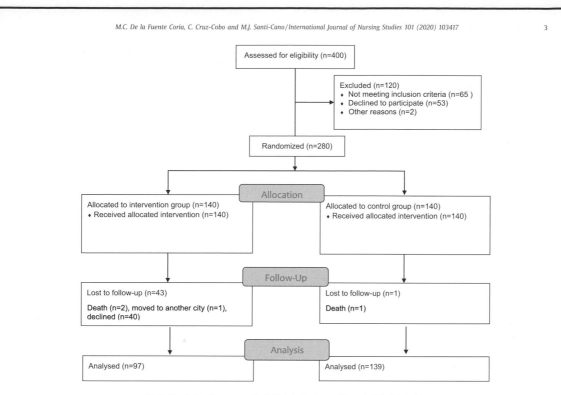

Fig. 1. Flowchart of the progress of individuals in the phases of the controlled clinical trial.
CONSORT 2010 flow diagram.

A brochure containing educational contents, control objectives, and a self-management booklet were provided to the participants. Goal setting and motivational interviewing techniques were used. The educational model was based on the model of empowerment: promoting participation and strengthening the person's autonomy (Asimakopoulou et al., 2012; Inzucchi et al., 2012). Active recruitment of diabetic participants who did not attend voluntarily was performed by telephone when necessary. Telephone calls were made when participants were absent from any scheduled appointments, as indicated in the protocol, in order to encourage them to participate. A date was proposed. Participants who attended at least three sessions during the first 12 months were eligible for follow up.

The control group received usual medical care at the health centre. The usual care consisted of advice on healthy lifestyle choices carried out by nurses at the health centre during the routine appointments with control group participants for clinical and analytical assessment (at least twice a year) as per the Primary Care protocol, but no structured diabetes education was provided.

2.4. Outcome measures and data collection

The primary outcome variables were the values and achievement of type 2 diabetes mellitus control targets established by the American Diabetes Association (2011): Glycated haemoglobin concentration (<7%), fasting blood glucose (<130 mg/dL), plasma concentration of total cholesterol (<200 mg/dL), low-density lipoprotein cholesterol (<100 mg/dL), high-density lipoprotein cholesterol (>40 mg/dL in males and >50 mg/dL in women),

triglycerides (<150 mg/dL). The blood samples were collected by health centre nurses early in the morning after fasting overnight (at least 10 h), for glycated haemoglobin and lipid measurements. All determinations were performed at the same laboratory at the reference hospital (University Hospital of Puerto Real). Glycated haemoglobin levels were measured using high-performance liquid chromatography (AKRAY HA 8180V, Menarini Diagnostics) and lipid levels were measured using enzymatic colorimetric assay.

Systolic blood pressure (<130 mmHg) and diastolic blood pressure (<80 mmHg) were also primary variables. Blood pressure was measured by a nurse in the consulting room using a professional digital sphygmomanometer, applying accepted methods (Chobanian et al., 2003). The secondary outcome variable was body mass index calculated as [weight (kg)/height^2 (m)]. Weight was measured by a nurse with participants removing shoes or heavy clothing, using standard calibrated scales (Seca 711, Hamburg, Germany) to the nearest 0.1 kg. Height was measured by a nurse using a portable stadiometer (Seca 264 height rod) to the nearest 0.1 cm. The variables were measured before the intervention, and after the intervention: after 12 months, and after 24 months. Blinding was used in the database registry and results analysis.

2.5. Statistical analysis

For the statistical analysis, the IBM SPSS (version 24.0) program was used. Quantitative and qualitative descriptive statistics were carried out on the results using the mean ± standard deviation and frequencies. For the comparison of means, the Student's t-test was used when the variables presented normal distribution, and

4   M.C. De la Fuente Coria, C. Cruz-Cobo and M.J. Santi-Cano / International Journal of Nursing Studies 101 (2020) 103417

Table 1
Baseline data for intervention and control groups.

Variables	TG $n=236$	IG $n=97$	CG $n=139$	P
Age (years)	65.1 ± 9.5	64.5 ± 9.6	65.5 ± 9.5	0.434
Males %(n)	54.2 (128)	54.6 (53)	54.0 (75)	1.000
Diabetes years	7.6 ± 4.1	8.8 ± 4.4	6,7 ± 3,6	0.000[a]
BMI (kg/m²)	30.8 ± 4.3	31.4 ± 4.5	29.3 ± 3.6	0.022
SBP (mmHg)	135.91 ± 17.28	133.47 ± 16.79	138.22 ± 17.50	0.112
DBP (mmHg)	77.19 ± 10.20	76.79 ± 9.10	77.57 ± 11.14	0.941
FBG (mg/dl)	145.0 ± 45.0	140.5 ± 35.3	148.2 ± 50.6	0.255
HbA1c 1 (%)	7.5 ± 1.4	7.6 ± 1.4	7.4 ± 1.5	0.532
TC (mg/dl)	204.2 ± 40.0	199.0 ± 38.8	208.9 ± 40.7	0.109
LDL-c (mg/dl)	121.3 ± 34.3	115.4 ± 32.9	125.9 ± 34.8	0.077
HDL-c (mg/dl)	49.3 ± 13.1	48.0 ± 12.9	50.3 ± 13.2	0.270
TG (mg/dl)	159.6 ± 84.8	146.2 ± 62.4	169.0 ± 96.5	0.075
Diet/exercise treatment	6.8 (15)	7.3 (7)	6.5 (8)	0.795
OADs treatment	67.7 (149)	67.7 (65)	67.6 (84)	1.000
Insulin treatment %	25.5 (56)	25.0 (24)	25.8 (32)	1.000

TG: Total Group. IG: Intervention Group. CG: Control Group.
[a] Mann–Whitney U test. BMI 1: body mass index at the beginning of the study. SBP 1: systolic blood pressure at the beginning of the study. DBP 1: diastolic blood pressure at the beginning of the study. FBG: fasting blood glucose. HbA1c 1: glycated haemoglobin at the beginning of the study. TC 1: total cholesterol at the beginning of the study. LDL-c: cholesterol bound to low density lipoprotein at the beginning of the study. HDL-c: cholesterol bound to high density lipoprotein at the beginning of the study. TG: triglycerides. OADs: oral antidiabetics.

the Mann–Whitney U and Wilcoxon tests were applied if the variables were not normally distributed. For the comparison of proportions, the Pearson Chi-square test was used. A value of $p < 0.05$ was considered statistically significant.

2.6. Ethical considerations

The study was conducted under the standards and ethical criteria of the Helsinki declaration, and was submitted to the approval of the Ethics and Research Committee of the Bahía de Cádiz-La Janda Health District. All participants were informed about the nature of the study and their consent to participate in it was requested.

3. Results

The baseline characteristics of the participants are shown in Table 1. Among these participants, 54.2% were male, and the mean age was similar in both groups 65.1 ± 9.5. The mean number of years of onset of type 2 diabetes mellitus was 7.6 years ± 4.1 years, somewhat lower in the control group. At the beginning of the study, both groups were comparable since no statistically significant differences were observed in the outcome variables between the intervention and control groups, except for lower body mass index in the control group. The baseline glycated haemoglobin levels in the intervention and control groups were moderately elevated and similar in both groups. (7.6% vs 7.4, $p = 0.532$).

Table 2 shows the mean values ± standard deviation and the difference of means, 95% CI, of the outcome variables after 12 and 24 months of follow-up. After 12 months of follow-up, a decrease in glycated haemoglobin was observed in the intervention group, but not in the control group (−0.55, 95% CI −0.20, −0.90, $p < 0.001$ vs +0.06, −0.14, +0.28, $p = 0.530$). However, the difference between the groups was not statistically significant at this stage of follow-up. Systolic blood pressure was statistically lower after 12 months in the intervention group (−1.7, 95% CI −5.2, +1.8 vs +0.9, 95% CI −3.6, +5.5, $p < 0.024$).

After 24 months of follow-up, a significant decrease in fasting blood glucose was detected in the intervention group (−8.1 mg/dL, 95% CI −19.8, +3.4 $p < 0.015$). Decreases were also detected in glycated haemoglobin (−0.82%, 95% CI −0.50, −1.14, vs +0.08, −0.20, +0.37, $p = 0.003$), total cholesterol (−17.7 mg/dL, 95% CI −26.7, −8.7 vs −2.3, 95% CI −12.5, +7.8, $p < 0.008$), low-density lipoprotein cholesterol (−12.1 mg/dL, 95% CI −21.0,

−3.1 vs −1.2, 95% CI −11.8, +9.3, $p < 0.040$), and systolic blood pressure (−3.5 mmHg, 95% CI −7.7, +0.5 vs +2.6, 95% CI −1.3, +6.7, $p < 0.000$). High-density lipoprotein cholesterol, triglycerides, diastolic blood pressure and body mass index values were not modified.

With regard to the achievement of therapeutic objectives (Table 3), attaining the glycated haemoglobin target (<7%) was statistically higher after 24 months in the intervention group: 35.2% vs 24.7%, $p < 0.003$. There was no improvement of the control goal in other variables: fasting blood glucose, total cholesterol, low-density lipoprotein cholesterol, high-density lipoprotein cholesterol, triglycerides, or blood pressure.

4. Discussion

Our study found that the educational intervention had favourable effects in the medium and long term on fasting blood glucose, glycated haemoglobin, total cholesterol, low-density lipoprotein cholesterol and systolic blood pressure. Likewise, the therapeutic objective that showed significant long-term improvements with the educational intervention was glycated haemoglobin.

At the beginning of the study, both intervention and control groups were comparable as shown by the similar figures in the outcome variables (Table 1). Baseline glycated haemoglobin levels were not excessively high (7.6% vs 7.4, $p = 0.532$). In general, studies that include participants with higher baseline glycated haemoglobin levels (8–9%) tend to experience more significant differences than those with lower levels (Chrvala et al., 2016).

Response rates of our study were high after two years of follow-up: 70% of participants in the intervention group and 99% in the control group. This compares positively with other self-management education interventions that obtained long term follow up data in the intervention group from 51% (Mohamed et al., 2013) to 60% (Eakin et al., 2014) of the original participants. Overall, interventions and follow up periods of shorter duration have shown lower loss of follow up (Kim et al., 2015; Merakou et al., 2015). However, some of these programmes have found no difference in biomedical outcomes at long term (Khunti et al., 2012; Mash et al., 2014). The optimal dose of intervention would have to be examined in further studies. The attendance of participants at educational sessions and therefore exposure to the intervention is also considered as an important factor in the success of the educational programme.

M.C. De la Fuente Coria, C. Cruz-Cobo and M.J. Santi-Cano/International Journal of Nursing Studies 101 (2020) 103417

Table 2
Change in outcomes at 12 and 24 months.

	IG mean ± SD difference of means (CI 95%)	p	CG mean ± SD difference of means (CI 95%)	p	P (IG)/(CG)
FBG					
12 months	135 ± 42	0.141	144.2 ± 51.4	0.446	0.154
	−6.8 (−15.9, +2.3)		−3.2 (−11.5, +5.1)		
24 months	132.3 ± 42.3	**0.015**[a]	139.7 ± 41.8	0.234	0.214
	−8.1 (−19.8, +3.4)		−6.2 (−16.6, +4.1)		
HbA1c%					
12 months	7.06 ± 1.26	**0.001**[a]	7.42 ± 1.36	0.530	0.105
	−0.55 (−0.20, −0.90)		+0.06 (−0.14, +0.28)		
24 months	6.82 ± 0.96	**0.000**[a]	7.37 ± 1.25	0.565	**0.003**[a]
	−0.82 (−0.50, −1.14)		+0.08 (−0.20, +0.37)		
TC					
12 months	201.5 ± 40.2	0.593	209.8 ± 38.5	0.139	0.449
	+2.3 (−6.4, +11.1)		+6.6 (−2.2, +15.4)		
24 months	183.0 ± 31.1	**0.000**	201.9 ± 40.2	0.644	**0.008**
	−17.7 (−26.7, −8.7)		−2.3 (−12.5, +7.8)		
LDL-c					
12 months	120.6 ± 35.1	0.168	127.4 ± 30.8	0.065	0.989
	+5.3 (−2.2, +12.9)		+7.6 (−0.4, +15.8)		
24 months	104.9 ± 27.2	**0.009**	120.9 ± 34.0	0.816	**0.040**
	−12.1 (−21.0, −3.1)		−1.2 (−11.8, +9.3)		
HDL-c					
12 months	47.8 ± 12.0	0.935	49.3 ± 12.9	0.642	0.999
	0.08 (−2.0, −2.2)		−0.44 (−2.34, +1.45)		
24 months	47.9 ± 11.5	0.572	53.3 ± 16.8	0.337	0.428
	−0.6 (−2.7, +1.5)		+1.92 (−2.04, +5.88)		
TG					
12 months	146.3 ± 57.9	0.703	164.2 ± 76.5	0.705	0.285
	−2.8 (−17.7, +12.0)		−3.2 (−20.0, +13.6)		
24 months	147.9 ± 59.4	0.863	155.2 ± 82.9	0.255	0.598
	−1.3 (−16.5, +13.9)		−11.0 (−30.3, +8.1)		
SBP					
12 months	131.7 ± 14.4	0.336	139.5 ± 18.6	0.670	**0.024**[a]
	−1.7 (−5.2, +1.8)		+0.9 (−3.6, +5.5)		
24 months	129.8 ± 13.8	0.086	141.4 ± 19.4	0.188	**0.000**
	−3.5 (−7.7, +0.5)		+2.6 (−1.3, +6.7)		
DBP					
12 months	75.5 ± 7.5	0.233	77.0 ± 10.5	0.669	0.899
	−1.2 (−3.3, +0.8)		−0.60 (−3.39, +2.19)		
24 months	73.9 ± 8.7	0.057	76.5 ± 12.2	0.448	0.285
	−2.5 (−4.9, −0.05)		−1.2 (−4.3, +1.9)		
BMI					
12 months	30.7 ± 3.7	0.074	29.3 ± 3.7	0.402	0.691
	−0.4 (−0.9, +0.04)		−0.2 (−0.8, +0.3)		
24 months	31.1 ± 4.0	0.853	29.1 ± 3.1	0.937	0.279
	+0.04 (−0.4, +0.5)		−0.02 (−0.58, +0.53)		

IG: Intervention Group. CG: Control Group. BMI: body mass index. SBP: systolic blood pressure. DBP: diastolic blood pressure. FBG: fasting blood glucose. HbA1c 1: glycated haemoglobin. TC: total cholesterol. LDL-c: cholesterol bound to low density lipoprotein. HDL-c: cholesterol bound to high density. TG: triglycerides.
[a] Wilcoxon.

In our study, we observed a statistically significant average decrease in glycated haemoglobin in the intervention group compared to the control group after 12 months (−0.55 vs +0.06, $p = 0.530$) and after 24 months (−0.82%, vs +0.08, $p = 0.003$) (Table 2). These results may be clinically relevant since in accordance with the UK Prospective Diabetes Study (UKPDS,1998), a 0.9% decrease in glycated haemoglobin is associated with a 25% reduction in microvascular complications, a 10% decrease in mortality related to diabetes and a 6% reduction in all causes of mortality. After 24 months of education, glycated haemoglobin decreased by 0.8%, revealing that our participants could benefit from these improvements.

However, there are unanswered questions concerning the ideal way to provide type 2 diabetes mellitus education, such as the type of education (individual or group; face-to-face or distance), frequency and number of sessions, contact time between the educator and the participant, type of educator (nurse, health worker, diabetes mellitus type 2 patients), training, educator experience, use of new technologies and barriers to self-management (Coppola et al., 2016).

The type of education used in our study was individual. Whether to use individual or group education, is a controversial issue. The main advantage of individual education is that it enables personalised intervention and creates mutual trust and strong interaction between the participant and educator. The biggest advantage of group education is its greater cost-effectiveness, since it is possible to group more participants with a single educator. However, it can be difficult to implement group education due to logistical and organisational problems. (Coppola et al., 2016).

A recent systematic review with meta-analysis that included 47 studies with 8533 type 2 diabetes mellitus participants found that group education was more effective in improving clinical outcomes than usual care and individual education (Odgers et al., 2017). The greatest reductions in glycated haemoglobin were obtained with group education compared to the control group after 12–14 months and 24 months, with an average difference of −0.33%. After 36–48 months there was a difference of −0.93%, but no difference was found after 24 months. As we can observe, the effects of the intervention also vary depending on the time at which it is followed up. The evaluations in our study were

6   M.C. De la Fuente Coria, C. Cruz-Cobo and M.J. Santi-Cano / International Journal of Nursing Studies 101 (2020) 103417

Table 3
Compliance with targets at 12 and 24 months.

Variables % (n)	Total $n = 236$	IG $n = 97$	p within the IG[a]	CG $n = 139$	p within the CG[a]	p IG/CG
FBG baseline	41.6 (77)	38.2 (29)		44.0 (48)		0.452
12 months	48.3 (98)	53.4 (47)	**0.031**	44.3 (51)	1.000	0.206
24 meses	51.5 (103)	25,5 (51)	**0.008**	26.0 (52)	0.424	0.203
HbA1c baseline	44.6 (75)	40.7 (33)		48.3 (42)		0.354
12 months	53.3 (104)	59.1 (55)	**0.011**	48.0 (49)	0.481	0.151
24 months	59.9 (109)	35.2 (64)	**0.001**	24.7 (45)	0.383	**0.003**
TC baseline	50.9 (85)	55.7 (44)		46.6 (41)		0.279
12 months	44.0 (81)	45.7 (42)	0.263	42.4 (39)	0.238	0.767
24 months	55.8 (106)	28.4 (54)	0.078	27.4 (52)	1.000	0.142
LDL-c baseline	27.4 (37)	32.2 (19)		23.7 (18)		0.332
12 months	22.3 (39)	23.9 (21)	0.503	20.7 (18)	0.109	0.717
24 months	30.9 (54)	14.9 (26)	0.267	16.0 (28)	0.267	0.746
HDL-c baseline	63.2 (98)	64.8 (46)		61.9 (52)		0.741
12 months	60.6 (106)	59.1 (52)	0.227	62.1 (54)	1.000	0.758
24 months	65.0 (115)	31.1 (55)	0.553	33.9 (60)	1.000	0.755
TG baseline	56.7 (102)	60.8 (45)		53.8 (57)		0.364
12 months	56.9 (99)	61.2 (52)	1.000	52.8 (47)	0.571	0.287
24 months	62.8 (120)	30.4 (58)	0.134	32.5 (62)	0.265	0.552
BP baseline	17.2 (30)	17.6 (15)		16.9 (15)		0.615
12 months	20.0 (39)	23.4 (22)	0.344	16.8 (17)	0.617	0.285
24 months	23.3 (44)	11.6 (22)	0.307	11.6 (22)	0.371	0.604

IG: Intervention Group. CG: Control Group. BMI: body mass index. BP: blood pressure. FBG: fasting blood glucose. HbA1c 1: glycated haemoglobin. TC: total cholesterol. LDL-c: cholesterol bound to low density lipoprotein. HDL-c: cholesterol bound to high density. TG: triglycerides.

[a] McNemar. Target of BG $\leq$ 130 mg/dl%, Target of HbA1c < 7%, Target of TC $\leq$ 200 mg/dL, target of LDL-c < 100 mg/dL, target of HDL-c males > 40 mg/dL women > 50 mg/dL, target of TG < 150 mg/dl, target of BP < 130/80 mmHg.

performed for medium term (after 12 months) and long term (after 24 months) outcomes. In both, beneficial effects were observed in the variables studied.

Chrvala et al. (2016) performed a systematic review of 118 studies, in which they observed an average reduction in glycated haemoglobin of 0.74% in the intervention group and 0.17% in the control group. They state that the programs that used a combination of individual and group methods obtained the best results in decreasing of glycated haemoglobin (−1.10%) compared with only group (−0.62%) or individual education (−0.78%).

The number and frequency of education sessions, as well as the ideal total contact time between the educator and the patient are also controversial issues. In the aforementioned meta-analysis by Odgers et al. (2017), the greatest reduction in glycated haemoglobin was obtained in longer intervention periods (13–60 months) (−0.66%), compared to shorter interventions (<1 month, 1–3 months, 4–6 months, 7–12 months); <5 sessions (−0.46%) compared to more numerous ones (6–10 sessions, 11–20 sessions and > 21 sessions); $\leq$ 8 h contact time (−0.45%) compared to those with a higher number of hours (9–12 h, 13–18 h, 19–30 h, $\geq$31 h); and with the participation of a family member (−0.36%). The intervention in our study consisted of six educational sessions of 20–30 min over 18 months. Four of the sessions took place in the first 6 months with reinforcements after 12 and 18 months. The total contact time was 2–3 h. The participant agreed that they would attend the diabetes education sessions with a family member. Family involvement and support is important to achieve the objectives that are proposed.

In contrast, in the aforementioned systematic review by Chrvala et al. (2016), several studies that obtained a significant reduction in glycated haemoglobin emphasized a higher number of contact hours. Furthermore, in patients with high glycated haemoglobin values (>9%), a significant decrease was also observed. The authors concluded that the way education is provided, its contact hours and the baseline glycated haemoglobin influence improvements in glycated haemoglobin.

Another study conducted in the USA, examined a mixed intervention (group and later individual telephone advice once a month) over 12 months. It achieved a reduction of 1–1.3%

glycated haemoglobin (Kim et al., 2015). On the contrary, in a study carried out in Australia, in which the intervention consisted only of telephone calls over a period of 18 months, evaluated after 24 months, no changes were obtained in metabolic markers (Eakin et al., 2014).

In our study, as well as the initial 6 months of diabetes education, we performed reinforcement sessions after 12 and 18 months. There is evidence that educators who contact their diabetes mellitus patients more regularly have better results (Chrvala et al., 2016). The importance of continuing education is evident in short studies (4 months) that do not observe metabolic changes one year after the intervention (Mash et al., 2014). The results obtained from the educational intervention generally drop over time. Therefore, it is important to reinforce education through regular sessions. In a recent systematic review of the effectiveness of diabetes education in Chinese adults, the authors concluded that glycemic control was better in studies that used continuous education with information reinforcement strategies (Choi et al., 2016).

As for the type of educator, in our study, the diabetes education was provided by a primary care nurse. Different studies have shown the effectiveness of diabetes education DE provided by different types of educators and levels of training: nurses, doctors, dieticians or nutritionists, health teams, health workers or diabetes mellitus patients. However, nurses are the most common educators (Coppola et al., 2016).

Regarding the other outcome variables, fasting blood glucose in the meta-analysis of Odgers et al. (2017) 0.68 mmol/L (12 mg/dL) decreased, only after 12–14 months, but not at the other time intervals. The fasting blood glucose figure should be maintained <130 mg/dL in individuals with type 2 diabetes mellitus (American Diabetes Association, 2018) to reduce the progression of microvascular complications. In our study, fasting blood glucose decreased significantly by 8 mg/dL in the intervention group after 24 months, but not in the control group. However, the data suggest that the improvements in fasting blood glucose appear to be less clinically important than those of glycated haemoglobin.

With regard to body mass index, our results show no significant decreases after the intervention. It is known that sustained weight loss (>12 months) of 5 kg in patients with diabetes melli-

M.C. De la Fuente Coria, C. Cruz-Cobo and M.J. Santi-Cano / International Journal of Nursing Studies 101 (2020) 103417   7

tus type 2 improves fasting blood glucose, lipid profile, and blood pressure. These results coincide with previous systematic reviews. In the study by Odgers et al. (2017) body mass index was not significantly modified either.

Our results show significant improvements after the 24 months interventions, both in total cholesterol and low-density-lipoprotein cholesterol and after 12 and 24 months in the systolic blood pressure. The clinical significance of these results is highlighted, since improving lipids and controlling of blood pressure in diabetes mellitus type 2 patients can reduce the risk of micro and macrovascular complications (Stratton et al., 2000). Nevertheless, Odgers et al. (2017) did not observe significant changes in systolic blood pressure, total cholesterol, low-density lipoprotein cholesterol, or high-density lipoprotein cholesterol.

A study conducted in Sweden, featuring education over 6 months and a 12 month follow-up, showed that both group and individual education were similar in terms of reducing glycated haemoglobin (−0.5% and −0.4%) after 12 months. However, the rest of the anthropometric and lipid variables were not modified (Jutterstrom et al., 2016). Unlike these studies, in Greece, a brief 3-week group intervention using conversational mapping saw improvements in glycated haemoglobin, lipids, and body mass index, after 6 months (Merakou et al., 2015).

Another group study (4 sessions: 4 h) developed in Qatar, found a decrease in glycated haemoglobin and body mass index after 12 months, but not in the lipid profile (Mohamed et al., 2013). A Belgian study, using telephone telecoaching, managed to reduce glycated haemoglobin, lipids and body mass index (Odnoletkova et al., 2016). Pérez et al. (2015) also observed with their diabetes education program that they had a positive impact on glycated haemoglobin, but not on lipids or body mass index. Similarly, in a study carried out by health workers in the US, with a 12-month, 7-h individual education program, glycated haemoglobin decreased, but not blood pressure BP, body mass index BMI, or lipids (Prezio et al., 2013). A recent meta-analysis that included 28 studies, showed that culturally adapted education resulted in a reduction in glycated haemoglobin over a 24-month period. However, it did not obtain benefits in other variables such as blood pressure and lipids (Creamer et al., 2016). Therefore, the variable that decrease most frequently is glycated haemoglobin. Body mass index, blood pressure and plasma lipids do not usually benefit from the intervention in the same way.

With regard to achieving therapeutic objectives, our study found that achieving glycated haemoglobin <7% target was significantly higher in the intervention group than in the control group (35.2% vs. 24.7%, $p = 0.003$), while the rest of the objectives (fasting blood glucose, lipids and blood pressure) were not improved. Due to scientific evidence showing that the control of these factors helps to reduce type 2 diabetes mellitus complications, the American Diabetes Association advises to achieve the therapeutic objectives for these patients (American Diabetes Association, 2018). However, there are studies that show that achieving of the three therapeutic targets (glycated haemoglobin <7%, low-density lipoprotein-cholesterol <100 mg/dL and blood pressure <130-80 mmHg) happens in only 18.8% of American diabetic patients (Stark et al., 2013). In addition, in most diabetes education trials, the reduction in the figures of each variable after the intervention is analysed, but target achievements is not.

There are many barriers to self-managing diabetes mellitus type 2 including cultural, motivational and, cognitive as well as poor self-management skills. These must be identified by educators. For this purpose, individual sessions may be more useful than group sessions. Individual sessions can also be episodically used even when the education program is based on group sessions (Coppola et al., 2016). A recent systematic review has shown that the cost of education programs for diabetes self-management is modest and probably cost-effective in the long term (Lian et al., 2017).

The strengths of the present trial include the recruitment of a representative sample of patients with diabetes mellitus type 2 in primary care, long-term follow-up (24 months), the goal of evaluating the achievement of therapeutic targets, and the homogeneity of baseline figures in the intervention and control group. All these signal that the intervention carried out produced a favourable response in the clinical parameters.

4.1. Limitations

Among the limitations of the trial, it should be noted that no blinding was used regarding group allocation, which is difficult in this type of study. Secondly, changes in medication were not taken into account. Medication adjustments in these participants are inevitable, and they may have an influence both on the intervention and control group. Finally, the sample came from a single health centre. Therefore, the results cannot be generalised for the entire population. However, as we can see, the figures of the outcome variables are similar to those observed in the different reviews and meta-analyses, which support the representativeness of the sample.

4.2. Implications for practice

The present study has clinical and research implications. Education in diabetes can optimise glycemic control in patients, and ongoing diabetes education intervention can achieve favourable long-term results. Thus, innovative strategies such as educational reinforcements and family involvement could increase glycemic control. The educator's level of qualification and continual training; the availability of material and human resources; and the planning and continuous evaluation of the diabetes education programs are necessary to strengthen this program.

5. Conclusion

In conclusion, this study shows that our educational intervention in diabetes provided by a primary care nurse over six months, with reinforcement sessions after 12 and 18 months, together with family support can achieve reductions in glycated haemoglobin, fasting blood glucose, total cholesterol, low-density lipoprotein cholesterol and systolic blood pressure in the medium and long term. It also causes an increase in the number of participants who meet the therapeutic target of glycated haemoglobin. Our intervention could be interpreted as a way of delaying the progression of the disease.

Conflict of interest

None.

Funding

University of Cádiz and Public Health Care of Andalucía (Spain) have supported the project.

References

Al-Saeed, A.H., Constantino, M.I., Molyneaux, L., D'Souza, M., Limacher-Gisler, F., Luo, C., Wu, T., Twigg, S.M., Yue, D.K., Wong, J., 2016. An inverse relationship between age of type 2 diabetes onset and complication risk and mortality: the impact of youth-onset type 2 diabetes. Diabet. Care 39 (5), 823–829. doi: 10.2337/dc15-0991.

8 M.C. De la Fuente Coria, C. Cruz-Cobo and M.J. Santi-Cano/International Journal of Nursing Studies 101 (2020) 103417

American Association of Diabetes Educator, 2018. AADE7 Self-care Behaviors. https://www.diabeteseducator.org/living-with-diabetes/aade7-self-care-behaviors (Accessed 4 January 2019).

American Diabetes Association, 2018. Standars of Medical Care in Diabetes. Diabet. Care 41 (1). S55–S64, S86–S104 http://care.diabetesjournals.org/content/41/Supplement_1.cover-expansion .

American Diabetes Association, 2011. Standards of medical care in diabetes-2011. Diabet. Care 34 (l), 11–61. doi:10.2337/dc11-S011.

Asimakopoulou, K., Gilbert, D., Newton, P., Scambler, S., 2012. Back to basics: re-examining the role of patient empowerment in diabetes. Patient Educ. Couns. 86 (3), 281–283. doi:10.1016/j.pec.2011.03.017.

Bourne, R.R.A., Stevens, G.A., White, R.A., Smith, J.L., Flaxman, S.R., Price, H., Jonas, J.B., Keeffe, J., Leasher, J., Naidoo, K., Pesudovs, K., Resnikoff, S., Taylor, H.R., Vision Loss Expert Group, 2013. Causes of vision loss worldwide, 1990–2010: a systematic analysis. Lancet Glob. Heal. 1 (6), 339–349. doi:10.1016/S2214-109X(13)70113-X.

Chobanian, A.V., Bakris, G.L., Black, H.R., Cushman, W.C., Green, L.A., Izzo, J.L., Jones, D.W., Materson, B.J., Oparil, S., Wright, J.T., Roccella, E.J., Joint National Committee on Prevention, Detection, Evaluation, and Treatment of High Blood Pressure. National Heart, Lung, and Blood Institute, National High Blood Pressure Education Program Coordinating Committee, 2003. Seventh report of the joint national committee on prevention, detection, evaluation, and treatment of high blood pressure. Hypertension 42, 1206–1252. doi:10.1161/01.HYP.0000107251.49515.c2.

Choi, T.S.T., Davidson, Z.E., Walker, K.Z., Lee, J.H., Palermo, C., 2016. Diabetes education for chinese adults with type 2 diabetes: a systematic review and meta-analysis of the effect on glycemic control. Diabet. Res. Clin. Pract. 116, 218–229. doi:10.1016/j.diabres.2016.04.001.

Chrvala, C.A., Sherr, D., Lipman, R.D., 2016. Diabetes self-management education for adults with type 2 diabetes mellitus: a systematic review of the effect on glycemic control. Patient Educ. Couns. 99 (6), 926–943. doi:10.1016/J.PEC.2015.11.003.

Coppola, A., Sasso, L., Bagnasco, A., Giustina, A., Gazzaruso, C., 2016. The role of patient education in the prevention and management of type 2 diabetes: an overview. Endocrine 53 (1), 18–27. doi:10.1007/s12020-015-0775-7.

Creamer, J., Attridge, M., Ramsden, M., Cannings-John, R., Hawthorne, K., 2016. Culturally appropriate health education for type 2 diabetes in ethnic minority groups: an updated cochrane review of randomized controlled trials. Diabet. Med. 33 (2), 169–183. doi:10.1111/dme.12865.

Eakin, E.G., Winkler, E.A., Dunstan, D.W., Healy, G.N., Owen, N., Marshall, A.M., Graves, N., Reeves, M.M., 2014. Living well with diabetes: 24-month outcomes from a randomized trial of telephone-delivered weight loss and physical activity intervention to improve glycemic control. Diabet. Care 37 (8), 2177–2185. doi:10.2337/dc13-2427.

Guideline NICE, 2015. Type 2 Diabetes in Adults: Management. https://www.nice.org.uk/guidance/ng28 (Accessed 2 January 2019).

International Diabetes Federation. Diabetes Atlas. eighth ed., 2017a. www.diabetesatlas.org (Accessed 1 July 2019).

International Diabetes Federation. Recommendations for Managing Type 2 Diabetes in Primary Care, 2017b. www.idf.org/managing-type2-diabetes (Accessed 13 March 2019).

Inzucchi, S.E., Bergenstal, R.M., Buse, J.B., Diamant, M., Ferrannini, E., Nauck, M., Peters, A.L., Tsapas, A., Wender, R., Matthews, D.R., European association for the study of diabetes (EASD), 2012. Management of hyperglycaemia in Type 2 diabetes: a patient-centered approach: position statement of the American Diabetes Association (ADA) and the European Association for the Study of Diabetes (EASD). Diabet. Care 35 (6), 1364–1379. doi:10.2337/dc12-0413.

Jutterström, L., Hörnsten, Å., Sandström, H., Stenlund, H., Isaksson, U., 2016. Nurse-led patient-centered self-management support improves hba1c in patients with type 2 diabetes—a randomized study. Patient Educ. Couns. 99 (11), 1821–1829. doi:10.1016/j.pec.2016.06.016.

Khunti, K., Gray, L.J., Skinner, T., Carey, M.E., Realf, K., Dallosso, H., Fisher, H., Campbell, M., Heller, S., Davies, M.J., 2012. Effectiveness of a diabetes education and self-management programme (DESMOND) for people with newly diagnosed type 2 diabetes mellitus: three-year follow-up of a cluster randomized controlled trial in primary care. BMJ 344, 2333. doi:10.1136/bmj.e2333.

Kim, M.T., Kim, K.B., Huh, B., Nguyen, T., Han, H.-R., Bone, L.R., Levine, D., 2015. The effect of a community-based self-help intervention. Am. J. Prev. Med. 49 (5), 726–737. doi:10.1016/j.amepre.2015.04.033.

Ley, S.H., Hamdy, O., Mohan, V., Hu, F.B., 2014. Prevention and management of type 2 diabetes: dietary components and nutritional strategies. Lancet 383, 1999–2007. doi:10.1016/S0140-6736(14)60613-9.

Lian, J.X., McGhee, S.M., Chau, J., Wong, C.K.H., Lam, C.L.K., Wong, W.C.W., 2017. Systematic review on the cost-effectiveness of self-management education programme for type 2 diabetes mellitus. Diabet. Res. Clin. Pract. 127, 21–34. doi:10.1016/j.diabres.2017.02.021.

Mash, R.J., Rhode, H., Zwarenstein, M., Rollnick, S., Lombard, C., Steyn, K., Levitt, N., 2014. Effectiveness of a group diabetes education programme in under-served communities in South Africa: a pragmatic cluster randomized controlled trial. Diabet. Med. 31 (8), 987–993. doi:10.1111/dme.12475.

Mathers, C.D., Loncar, D., 2006. Projections of global mortality and burden of disease from 2002 to 2030. PLoS Med. 3 (11), 442. doi:10.1371/journal.pmed.0030442.

Merakou, K., Knithaki, A., Karageorgos, G., Theodoridis, D., Barbouni, A., 2015. Group patient education: effectiveness of a brief intervention in people with type 2 diabetes mellitus in primary health care in Greece: a clinically controlled trial. Health Educ. Res. 30 (2), 223–232. doi:10.1093/her/cyv001.

Mohamed, H., Al-Lenjawi, B., Amuna, P., Zotor, F., Elmahdi, H., 2013. Culturally sensitive patient-centred educational programme for self-management of type 2 diabetes: a randomized controlled trial. Prim. Care Diabetes 7 (3), 199–206. doi:10.1016/j.pcd.2013.05.002.

Odgers-Jewell, K., Ball, L.E., Kelly, J.T., Isenring, E.A., Reidlinger, D.P., Thomas, R., 2017. Effectiveness of group-based self-management education for individuals with type 2 diabetes: a systematic review with meta-analyses and meta-regression. Diabet. Med. 34 (8), 1027–1039. doi:10.1111/dme.13340.

Odnoletkova, I., Goderis, G., Nobels, F., Fieuws, S., Aertgeerts, B., Annemans, L., Ramaekers, D., 2016. Optimizing diabetes control in people with type 2 diabetes through nurse-led telecoaching. Diabet. Med. 33 (6), 777–785. doi:10.1111/dme.13092.

Pérez-Escamilla, R., Damio, G., Chhabra, J., Fernandez, M.L., Segura-Pérez, S., Vega-López, S., Kollannor-Samuel, G., Calle, M., Shebl, F.M., D'Agostino, D., 2015. Impact of a community health workers-led structured program on blood glucose control among Latinos with type 2 diabetes: the Dialbest trial. Diabetes Care 38 (2), 197–205. doi:10.2337/dc14-0327.

Powers, M.A., Bardsley, J., Cypress, M., Duker, P., Funnell, M.M., Hess Fischl, A., Maryniuk, M.D., Siminerio, L., Vivian, E., 2015. Diabetes self-management education and support in type 2 diabetes: a joint position statement of the American Diabetes Association, the American Association of Diabetes Educators, and the academy of nutrition and dietetics. J. Acad. Nutr. Diet. 115 (8), 1323–1334. doi:10.1016/j.jand.2015.05.012.

Prezio, E.A., Cheng, D., Balasubramanian, B.A., Shuval, K., Kendzor, D.E., Culica, D., 2013. Community diabetes education (CoDE) for uninsured Mexican Americans: a randomized controlled trial of a culturally tailored diabetes education and management program led by a community health worker. Diabetes Res. Clin. Pract. 100 (1), 19–28. doi:10.1016/j.diabres.2013.01.027.

Saran, R., Li, Y., Robinson, B., Ayanian, J., Balkrishnan, R., Bragg-Gresham, J., Chen, J.T.L., Cope, E., Gipson, D., He, K., Herman, W., Heung, M., Hirth, R.A., Jacobsen, S.S., Kalantar-Zadeh, K., Kovesdy, C.P., Leichtman, A.B., Lu, Y., Molnar, M.Z., Morgenstern, H., Nallamothu, B., O'Hare, A.M., Pisoni, R., Plattner, B., Port, F.K., Rao, P., Rhee, C.M., Schaubel, D.E., Selewski, D.T., Shahinian, V., Sim, J.J., Song, P., Streja, E., Kurella Tamura, M., Tentori, F., Eggers, P.W., Agodoa, L.Y.C., Abbott, K.C., 2015. US renal data system 2014 annual data report: epidemiology of kidney disease in the United States. Am. J. Kidney Dis. 66 (3), A7. doi:10.1053/j.ajkd.2015.05.001.

Stark Casagrande, S., Fradkin, J.E., Saydah, S.H., Rust, K.F., Cowie, C.C., 2013. The prevalence of meeting A1C, blood pressure, and ldl goals among people with diabetes, 1988–2010. Diabet. Care 36 (8), 2271–2279. doi:10.2337/dc12-2258.

Stratton, I.M., Adler, A.I., Neil, H.A., Matthews, D.R., Manley, S.E., Cull, C.A., Hadden, D., Turner, R.C., Holman, R.R., 2000. Association of glycaemia with macrovascular and microvascular complications of type 2 diabetes (UKPDS 35): prospective observational study. BMJ 321, 405–412.

Sarwar, N., Gao, P., Seshasai, S.R.K., Gobin, R., Kaptoge, S., Di Angelantonio, E., Ingelsson, E., Lawlor, D.A., Selvin, E., Stampfer, M., Stehouwer, C.D.A., Lewington, S., Pennells, L., Thompson, A., Sattar, N., White, I.R., Ray, K.K., Danesh, J., The Emerging Risk Factors Collaboration, 2010. Diabetes mellitus, fasting blood glucose concentration, and risk of vascular disease: a collaborative meta-analysis of 102 prospective studies. Lancet 375, 2215–2222. doi:10.1016/S0140-6736(10)60484-9.

UK Prospective Diabetes Study (UKPDS) Group, 1998. Effect of intensive blood-glucose control with metformin on complications in overweight patients with type 2 diabetes (UKPDS 34). Lancet 352, 854–865. doi:10.1016/S0140-6736(98)07037-8.

World Health Organization, 2016. Global Report on Diabetes. World Health Organization http://www.who.int/iris/handle/10665/204871.

Journal of Pediatric Nursing 50 (2020) 1–4

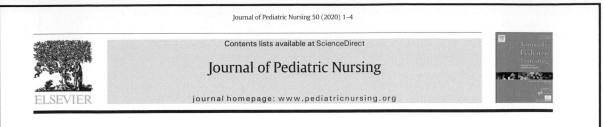

Contents lists available at ScienceDirect

Journal of Pediatric Nursing

journal homepage: www.pediatricnursing.org

Effectiveness of a Staff Resilience Program in a Pediatric Intensive Care Unit

Stacy Flanders [a],*, Debra Hampton [b], Pam Missi [c], Charlotte Ipsan [c], Cis Gruebbel [d]

[a] Cardiac Intensive Care Unit at Norton Children's Hospital, Louisville, KY, United States of America
[b] University of Kentucky College of Nursing, Lexington, KY, United States of America
[c] Women's and Children's Hospital, Norton Healthcare, Louisville, KY, United States of America
[d] Norton Children's Hospital, Norton Healthcare, Louisville, KY, United States of America

ARTICLE INFO

Article history:
Received 27 August 2019
Revised 4 October 2019
Accepted 4 October 2019

Keywords:
Pediatrics
Intensive care nurses
Resilience
Turnover
Burnout

ABSTRACT

Background: Compassion fatigue (CF) and secondary traumatic stress (STS) is prevalent in intensive care nurses, especially in pediatric intensive care nurses (PICU). CF, which includes STS and burnout, leads to reduced employee engagement and nursing turnover.

Purpose: The purpose of this project was to evaluate the impact of a staff resilience program on nursing turnover, employee engagement and compassion satisfaction among nurses in a PICU.

Design and methods: A retrospective pre-test and post-test design was used to evaluate the impact of a staff resilience program on turnover, engagement, and Professional Quality of Life (ProQOL), which measured compassion satisfaction and compassion fatigue.

Results: RN turnover was reduced and employee engagement was improved, although the differences were not statistically significant. The aggregate scores of the ProQOL indicated the RN's had low levels of CF with high levels of compassion satisfaction post implementation of the resilience program. Years of work experience was positively associated with compassion satisfaction and work engagement.

Conclusions: Education regarding the prevention of CF and burnout coupled with interventions designed to promote resilience can be effective in reducing CF and in building compassion satisfaction.

Practice implications: Doing an assessment of compassion fatigue and following up with the implementation of interventions to build staff resilience and promote psychological health can lead to positive outcomes, as demonstrated by the increase in work engagement and compassion satisfaction when burnout and CF decreased.

© 2018 Published by Elsevier Inc.

Introduction

As the healthcare environment continues to change and become more complex, nurses are faced with environmental and emotional challenges. Some areas are more stressful to work in than others. A Pediatric Intensive Care Unit (PICU) can be a stimulating and rewarding place to work, but this setting also can be very emotionally difficult (Meadors & Lamson, 2008). Nurses who work in intensive care settings are at high risk for compassion fatigue (CF), secondary traumatic stress (STS), and ultimately nursing burnout (Meadors & Lamson, 2008). CF, STS and burnout can cause decreased productivity, decreased job satisfaction, and increased turnover for nurses resulting in increased healthcare costs and negative patient outcomes (Adwan, 2014).

* Corresponding author at: 231 East Chestnut Street, Louisville, KY 40202, United States of America.

E-mail addresses: stacy.flanders@nortonhealthcare.org (S. Flanders),
debra.hampton@uky.edu (D. Hampton), pam.missi@nortonhealthcare.org (P. Missi),
charlotte.ipsan@nortonhealthcare.org (C. Ipsan).

Research suggests interventions aimed at building resilience can mitigate the effects of CF, STS and burnout (Cocker & Joss, 2016).

CF is often described as the cost of caring. The term CF is frequently used synonymously with STS, which is described as the stress one experiences from caring for a person who has suffered from a traumatic event (Sorenson, Bolick, Wright, & Hamilton, 2016). Stamm (2010) notes that compassion fatigue has two aspects, burnout (exhaustion, anger, frustration, depression) and STS. STS occurs when healthcare providers are repeatedly exposed to patients' suffering from trauma or devastating illnesses and can ultimately lead to nursing burnout. Nurses who work in a PICU may be at an even higher risk for CF as advances in medical technology have allowed children to live longer and with more complex chronic conditions (Meadors & Lamson, 2008). Pediatric nurses are exposed to repeated patient suffering and death and experience the emotional responses from parents to their children's illness (Berger, Polivka, Smoot, & Owens, 2015).

CF can cause physical health issues for nurses including lack of energy, anxiety, inability to sleep, depression, and burnout. CF may also result in decreased productivity, decreased employee engagement, and

https://doi.org/10.1016/j.pedn.2019.10.007
0882-5963/© 2018 Published by Elsevier Inc.

2 *S. Flanders et al. / Journal of Pediatric Nursing 50 (2020) 1–4*

increased turnover for nurses (**Berger et al., 2015**). Nurses suffering from CF often lack empathy for their patients and find it difficult to find satisfaction in their job (**Adwan, 2014**).

Understanding how CF contributes to nursing burnout and developing interventions to improve compassion satisfaction, build resilience, and reduce nursing burnout and turnover is important. Compassion satisfaction is "about the pleasure you derive from being able to do your work well" (**Stamm, 2010**, p. 12). Resilience is "a concept that proposes a recurrent human need to weather periods of stress and change successfully throughout life. The ability to weather each period of disruption and reintegration leaves the person better able to deal with the next change" (**Resilience, 2009**). Individuals with high compassion satisfaction and resilience are less likely to suffer from CF and burnout (**Stamm, 2010**).

The literature supports strategies aimed at promoting compassion satisfaction and resilience. CF education can have a positive effect on reducing CF. A systematic review of CF interventions targeted towards healthcare workers illustrated that interventions focused on providing education and improving resilience appeared to have the most impact on reducing CF (**Cocker & Joss, 2016**). **Zadeh, Gamba, Hudson, and Wiener (2012)** performed a quality improvement study evaluating the effectiveness of a wellness program for pediatric nurses. The researchers found that a 10 session wellness program was identified as very helpful and >75% of the participants noted that the education would positively change the way they performed their current job.

According to current literature, education on CF, burnout and compassion satisfaction can reduce CF and burnout and improve compassion satisfaction. This can result in higher levels of job satisfaction and less burnout (**Cocker & Joss, 2016**). Participants who reported higher compassion satisfaction were less at risk for CF and burnout (**Meyer, Li, Klaristenfeld, & Gold, 2015; Stamm, 2010**). **Adwan (2014)** suggested that interventions aimed at helping pediatric nurses identify and deal with grief could mitigate the grief nurses suffer from a patient death and improve job satisfaction. Pediatric providers who participated in an educational seminar on CF reported improved knowledge of stress reduction techniques and more feelings of peace and calmness (**Meadors & Lamson, 2008**). The purpose of this study was to evaluate the impact of a staff resilience program that included some educational components, in a PICU on Professional Quality of Life (ProQOL), to include CF, burnout, and compassion satisfaction, in addition to the impact on employee engagement and nursing turnover. The resilience program was developed and implemented by an interdisciplinary team, to include the Nurse Manager, Assistant Nurse Manager, Unit Educator, Chaplain, Child Life Therapist, and specific unit registered nurses.

Methods

Resilience program

A retrospective pre-test and post-test design was used in this study. The Pediatric ICU staff resilience program consisted of education to every RN in the PICU regarding CF, STS, burnout, and staff resilience. In addition, training was provided based on the American Association of Critical Care Nurses (AACN) six standards for a healthy working environment (skilled communication, meaningful recognition, appropriate staffing, true collaboration, effective decision making, and authentic leadership) (**AACN, 2016**). Staff resilience strategies included formal and informal debriefings, art, music, and pet therapy. Informal debriefings were offered every other month through breakfast with the chaplain. Twice a year, a formal ethical debriefing led by a trained pediatric ethicist was offered. Art and music therapy interventions were alternated every other month. Art therapy interventions included a variety of crafting options, making sugar scrubs and bath bombs. Music therapy was led by staff volunteers and included singing and playing of instruments in the nursing stations. Pet therapy was provided to the staff by child life once a week. A private Facebook page was developed for the staff on the unit. The Facebook page was used for communication, celebrations, and information on upcoming staff resilience activities. Lastly, monthly celebrations occurred during heart month (February) and critical care awareness month (May). Unit t-shirts were designed and available for staff to purchase. In addition, a wide variety of activities were offered throughout the months including contests, photo booths, and ice cream socials. Prior to the implementation of the staff resilience program, there were no formal methods in the department addressing burnout and resilience.

Setting and sample

The study was based in a 34 bed PICU in a children's hospital located within the south central part of the United States. The hospital offers specialized care in cardiac surgery, cardiology, oncology, neurology, neurosurgery, and is a level one trauma center. Inclusion criteria for the study included all RN's who worked in the PICU as of January 2018 who had been working in the PICU for a minimum of three months ($N = 150$).

Procedures

Approval for this study was obtained through an affiliated university Institutional Review Board and the organization's Office of Research. Employee engagement, using six Press Ganey employee engagement items, was measured in 2016 prior to implementation of the resilience program and again during the first 3 months of 2018. The scale consisted of the six Likert scale items (1–5) with higher numbers indicating a positive response. An example was: "I am proud to tell people I work for this organization". RN turnover results from 2016 were compared to RN turnover for 2017. In addition, an evaluation of CF (STS and burnout) and compassion satisfaction was assessed post implementation during the first 3 months of 2018 using the Professional Quality of Life (ProQOL) Scale (**Stamm, 2010**). The ProQOL is commonly used to measure the impact of helping individuals who experience suffering and trauma and has demonstrated reliability and validity in multiple published studies. The instrument has subscales for compassion satisfaction and compassion fatigue which includes two components, STS and burnout (**ProQOL.org, 2012; Stamm, 2010**).

Data collection

Data for this study was obtained either electronically using an employee survey or from Human Resources. RN turnover data and 2016 employee engagement scores were requested and provided by the organization's Human Resources Department. Research electronic data capture (**Harris et al., 2009; REDCap, 2004**) was used to administer the ProQOL and the 2018 employee engagement survey.

Data analysis

Descriptive statistics, including frequency distributions and means were used to describe the demographic characteristics of the participating RN's. All analyses were conducted using SPSS version 22; an alpha level of 0.05 was used to determine statistical significance. Correlations between education level and experience were assessed for impact on CF, STS, burnout, compassion satisfaction and engagement using Spearman's Rho. Pearson's correlation was used to evaluate relationships between CF, STS, burnout, and compassion satisfaction. A t-test was used to determine statistical significance of impact of program on RN turnover and engagement.

Results

Over 90% of the nurses held a Bachelor's degree in Nursing or higher (9% Associate; 87% BSN; 4% MSN). Approximately two-thirds of

S. Flanders et al. / Journal of Pediatric Nursing 50 (2020) 1–4

3

respondents (68%) had five years or less experience as a nurse (<1, 30%; 1–5, 38%; 5–10, 7%; >10, 25%).

RN turnover and employee engagement scores improved as an outcome of the resiliency program. RN turnover was reduced during the implementation year of the staff resilience program by 6%, although the decrease in turnover was not statistically significant ($p = .22$). In addition, employee engagement scores ($n = 82$ pre-intervention compared to $n = 75$ post-intervention) increased from a mean score of 4.15 to 4.18, but that change was not a statistically significant improvement ($p = .67$).

Evaluation of the aggregate ProQOL scores ($n = 70$) were encouraging. CF (STS and burnout aggregate scores) were low, while compassion satisfaction scores were high. The average STS score was 20.4 (see Table 1). Burnout scores averaged 21.7. Inversely, the average score among participants for compassion satisfaction was 42.6. There was a statistically significant positive correlation between compassion satisfaction and engagement ($r = 0.45$; $p < .001$). Additionally, there was a statistically significant positive correlation between years of experience and engagement ($r = 0.27$; $p = .018$) and years of experience and compassion satisfaction ($r = 0.29$; $p = .015$), suggesting that as years of experience increased so did compassion satisfaction and engagement (Table 2). A statistically significant negative correlation was found between engagement and burnout ($r = -0.44$; $p < .001$), indicating that as burnout increased engagement decreased. The same was true for engagement and STS ($r = -0.34$; $p = .004$); as STS increased, engagement decreased. There was also a statistically significant negative correlation between compassion satisfaction in comparison to STS ($p = .024$) and burnout ($r = -0.62$; $p < .001$) indicating that as compassion satisfaction increased, burnout and STS decreased. Finally, there was a statistically significant positive correlation between STS and burnout ($r = 0.50$; $p < .001$) suggesting that as STS increased so did burnout.

Discussion

The results of this evaluation suggested that a staff resilience program can be an effective intervention to mitigate compassion fatigue, STS and reduce burnout in PICU nurses. Reducing compassion fatigue is important to prevent nursing turnover and improve employee engagement. Nursing turnover is costly to organizations and disengaged employees can have a negative impact on the delivery of quality care and patient satisfaction. Compassion satisfaction can mitigate the effects of CF resulting in reduced burnout (Stamm, 2010). A 6% reduction in RN turnover and an increase in employee engagement was noted as an outcome of the resilience program, but the results were not statistically significant. However, when comparing the aggregate results of the ProQOL, the RN's scored low in STS (20.4) and burnout (21.7) and high for compassion satisfaction (42.6). STS and burnout scores totaling <22 indicate low levels of STS and burnout respectively. Compassion satisfaction scores >42 equal high levels of compassion satisfaction, while scores between 23 and 41 are average (Stamm, 2010). Reducing burnout and improving compassion satisfaction are important for the organization, as well as the mental health of the nurses (Berger et al., 2015). These results supported past studies that have shown staff resilience education/strategies can result in less CF and burnout and improve compassion satisfaction (Cocker & Joss, 2016).

There was a statistically significant, moderately high negative correlation between compassion satisfaction and burnout, suggesting that as compassion satisfaction increased burnout was reduced. There was also

Table 1
Aggregate ProQOL scores ($N = 70$).

	Mean	SD	Interpretation of results
Secondary traumatic stress	20.4	5.2	Low
Burnout	21.7	4.4	Low
Compassion satisfaction	42.6	3.9	High

Table 2
Correlations ($N = 70$).

	Engagement	Compassion satisfaction	Burnout	STS
Years of experience	0.27*	0.29*	−0.22	−0.03
	0.018	0.015	0.074	0.807
Engagement		0.45**	−0.44**	−0.34*
		<0.001	<0.001	0.004
Compassion			−0.62**	−0.27*
Satisfaction			<0.001	0.024
Burnout				0.50**
				<0.001

Note: Cells contain correlation coefficient in the top row and associated p-value $r (p)$ on the second row.
* Indicates statistical significance $p < .05$.
** Indicates statistical significance $p < .001$.

a statistically significant positive correlation between compassion satisfaction and engagement indicating those employees who have high compassion satisfaction also appear to be more engaged employees. The positive correlation between years of experience and higher levels of engagement and compassion satisfaction may indicate that employees with high compassion satisfaction are more likely to stay; employees with low levels of compassion satisfaction likely suffer from more STS and burnout and therefore may be more likely to leave the organization.

These results are important for organizations to consider when implementing interventions to support PICU nurses and reduce RN turnover. The results from the ProQOL indicate a staff resilience program can have a positive impact on pediatric intensive care nurses and support other clinical studies that have shown as compassion satisfaction increase, CF and burnout decrease (Stamm, 2010). Additionally, education on CF, STS and burnout can be an effective method to reduce these feelings (Zadeh et al., 2012).

Limitations

Limitations to this study include the time frame of evaluation. The program was implemented in 2017, and the evaluation of engagement, CF and compassion satisfaction occurred in early 2018. It would have been helpful to have a pre and post comparison of the ProQOL scores, rather than only the post evaluation. In addition, this was a single center study with convenience sampling. Employee engagement scores for this department were already above the national average before the implementation of the program. Lastly, RN turnover was evaluated during the intervention period; therefore, it is unclear if the program had a sustained impact on turnover.

Conclusion and implications for practice

CF and burnout are prevalent in ICU nurses, as well as pediatric nurses. While there seems to be strong agreement in the literature that compassion fatigue and burnout exist in intensive care nurses (Cocker & Joss, 2016), there are very few studies specific to the pediatric environment. The literature supports education on compassion fatigue (Meadors & Lamson, 2008), but it is unclear which resilience building interventions make a difference. There were no reported negative consequences to the implementation of the staff resilience program in the setting for this study, and the results indicated that education and interventions were helpful in reducing CF and improving compassion satisfaction. It seems prudent that organizations and nursing leaders should provide education and interventions to pediatric intensive care nurses regarding CF/STS, burnout, and compassion satisfaction/resilience. This includes the definitions of each, symptoms, and interventions that promote compassion satisfaction/resilience.

CF and burnout can have negative consequences for the nurse, the patients they are caring for, and the organization leading to negative

4   *S. Flanders et al. / Journal of Pediatric Nursing 50 (2020) 1–4*

physical symptoms for the nurse, decreased job productivity, decreased employee engagement, increased turnover, and burnout. The results of this study illustrated that years of experience was associated with compassion satisfaction, or joy in your work, and higher work engagement. This was a positive finding in relation to the nursing workforce, since nurses who are happy are more likely to work more years. Additionally, we know that environments where nurses are more satisfied and engaged have improved patient satisfaction. Future research needs to be focused around using standardized tools to measure CF, compassion satisfaction, and resilience as well as specific interventions for pediatric intensive care nurses. Longitudinal studies would be helpful to determine the sustainability of the results over time. An assessment of the emotional health of nurses in the work environment, using an instrument such as the ProQOL scale, would offer important information for healthcare leaders. Healthcare organizations should focus on providing resilience building interventions in high stress environments like the PICU, to promote compassion satisfaction and decrease CF among nurses what work in the environments.

Funding

No grants for this project. This project work was fully funded through the University of Kentucky College of Nursing and Norton Healthcare academic partnership.

CRediT authorship contribution statement

Stacy Flanders: Conceptualization, Methodology, Writing - original draft, Writing - review & editing, Visualization, Project administration. **Debra Hampton:** Methodology, Writing - review & editing, Visualization, Supervision. **Pam Missi:** Writing - review & editing. **Charlotte Ipsan:** Writing - review & editing. **Cis Gruebbel:** Writing - review & editing.

References

Adwan, J. Z. (2014). Pediatric nurses' grief experience, burnout, and job satisfaction. *Journal of Pediatric Nursing, 29*, 329–336.

American Association of Critical Care Nurses (2016). *AACN standards for establishing and sustaining healthy work environments: A journey to excellence* (2nd ed.) Retrieved from www.aacn.org (on April 4th 2018).

Berger, J., Polivka, B., Smoot, E. A., & Owens, H. (2015). Compassion fatigue in pediatric nurses. *Journal of Pediatric Nursing, 30*, 11–17.

Cocker, F., & Joss, N. (2016). Compassion fatigue among healthcare, emergency, and community service workers: A systematic review. *International Journal of Environmental Research and Public Health, 13*(618), 1–18.

Harris, P. A., Taylor, R., Thielke, R., Payne, J., Gonzalez, N., & Conde, J. G. (2009). Research electronic data capture (REDCap)—A metadata-driven methodology and workflow process for providing translational research informatics support. *Journal of Biomedical Informatics, 42*(2), 377–381.

Meadors, P., & Lamson, A. (2008). Compassion fatigue and secondary traumatization: Provider self care on intensive care units for children. *Journal of Pediatric Health Care, 22*, 24–34.

Meyer, R. M., Li, A., Klaristenfeld, J., & Gold, J. I. (2015). Pediatric novice nurses: Examining compassion fatigue as a mediator between stress exposure and compassion satisfaction, burnout, and job satisfaction. *Journal of Pediatric Nursing, 30*, 174–183.

ProQOL.org. The Center for Victims of Torture (2012). Professional quality of life measure. https://proqol.org/ProQol_Test.html.

Research Electronic Data Capture (REDCap) (2004). Retrieved from http://projectredcap.org (on January 15th, 2018).

Resilience (2009). Mosby's Medical Dictionary (8th ed.) Retrieved July 16, 2019 from https://medical-dictionary.thefreedictionary.com/resilience.

Sorenson, C., Bolick, B., Wright, K., & Hamilton, R. (2016). Understanding compassion fatigue in healthcare providers: A review of current literature. *Journal of Nursing Scholarship, 48*, 456–465.

Stamm, B. H. (2010). *The concise ProQOL manual* (2nd ed.) Retrieved from http://www.proqol.org/uploads/ProQOL_Concise_2ndEd_12-2010.pdf.

Zadeh, S., Gamba, N., Hudson, C., & Wiener, L. (2012). Taking care of care providers: A wellness program for pediatric nurses. *Journal of Pediatric Oncology Nursing, 29*, 294–299.

Applied Nursing Research 51 (2020) 151186

Contents lists available at ScienceDirect

Applied Nursing Research

journal homepage: www.elsevier.com/locate/apnr

ELSEVIER

Stress-related vulnerability and usefulness of healthcare education in Parkinson's disease: The perception of a group of family caregivers, a cross-sectional study

Di Stasio Enrico[a], Di Simone Emanuele[b], Galeti Arianna[c], Donati Daniele[b], Guidotti Chiara[d], Tartaglini Daniela[d], Chiarini Massimiliano[e], Marano Massimo[f], Di Muzio Marco[g], Cianfrocca Claudia[b,*]

[a] Institute of Biochemistry and Clinical Biochemistry, Università Cattolica del Sacro Cuore, Rome, Italy
[b] Department of Biomedicine and Prevention, University of Rome Tor Vergata, Italy
[c] Nursing Department, Sapienza University of Rome, Italy
[d] DAPS Università Campus Bio-Medico of Rome, Italy
[e] Department of Public Health and Infectious Diseases, Sapienza University of Rome, Italy
[f] Unit of Neurology, Neurophysiology, Department of Medicine, University Campus Bio-Medico of Rome, Italy
[g] Department of Clinical and Molecular Medicine, Sapienza University of Rome, Italy

ARTICLE INFO

Keywords:
Caregiver burden
Chronic disease
Healthcare education
Caregiver need

ABSTRACT

Parkinson's disease is associated with a high assistive complexity, thus generating in caregivers a burden proportional to the intensity of the care provided. This study aims to evaluate whether the stress-related level of caregivers is related to their perception of the need for healthcare education. A cross-sectional study was conducted on 69 family caregivers that completed the Stress-related Vulnerability Scale (SVS scale) with a tool of proposed interventions stratified according to caregivers' need as "nothing", "somewhat", "moderately" and "extremely". A direct association between the SVS scale and the perception of the usefulness of interventions was detected, and significant differences were observed for "Caregivers tele-support group" and "Peer-led support group" interventions, thus suggesting an important role for caregivers' emotional status in considering of training courses. Caregivers are split between low vulnerability, with minimal perception of training need, and high burden state with the acute necessity of support to manage patients.

1. Background

Parkinson's disease (PD) is a neurodegenerative, chronic and progressive illness that mainly involves the control of movement and balance. It is the most frequent of the movement disorder diseases and is characterized by tremor (Obeso et al., 2017). Moreover, it is the second most common neurodegenerative disease after Alzheimer's. The incidence rate varies between 8 and 18 new cases out of every 100,000 people a year, and the mortality rate is 2/6 new cases out of every 100,000 people a year. Nowadays, 3‰ of world population is affected by PD, the average age of onset is 58–60 years (Dorsey et al., 2007). People affected by PD, like other chronic diseases, need to have access to integrated clinical care supplied by healthcare providers like physiotherapists, speech therapists, nutritionists and occupational therapists to overcome everyday problems that cannot be managed through

medications or surgical interventions. In the advanced stages, PD is associated with a high assistive complexity, related to a drastic reduction of patient's independence in performing activities of daily living. This causes the need to be helped and supported, especially at home (Adler & Mehta, 2014). Informal caregivers called "family caregivers", whose role is of utmost importance, are involved in the care process and often guarantee the greatest part of the assistance at domicile. They take care of their loved ones by managing common difficulties and facing the progressive deterioration of patients' conditions (Brulletti et al., 2015).

The continuous involvement in caregiving could lead to the "caregiver burden", an extreme sense of vulnerability caused by the perception that caregiving negatively affects the caregiver's life. This condition, which is associated with the lack of technical skills and information about medical treatment and clinical care processes, leads

---

* Corresponding author.
 E-mail addresses: c2211@inwind.it, claudia.cianfrocca@policlinicoumberto1.it (C. Cianfrocca).

https://doi.org/10.1016/j.apnr.2019.151186
Received 12 May 2019; Received in revised form 7 August 2019; Accepted 2 September 2019

E. Di Stasio, et al.

Applied Nursing Research 51 (2020) 151186

the caregivers to perceive some needs (Zarit, Todd, & Zarit, 1986). Moreover, as stated in the literature, there is a link between the needs perceived by caregivers of PD patients and the unpredictability of the motor and non-motor symptoms of the disease, the care-receiver's degree 50 of disability, the progress of the disease, the number of hours of assistance a day and the duration of the illness. The most mentioned need by caregivers is acquiring adequate training about the evolution of the disease and the management of the symptoms and emotions at home (Grun, Pieri, Vaillant, & Diederich, 2016; Ashrafian, Feizollahzadeh, Rahmani, & Davoodi, 2018; Chiarini et al., 2017; Eluvathingol Jose & Portillo, 2013; Boersma et al., 2017).

A study conducted in 2015 by Lageman et al. showed that the global distress of PD caregivers does not correlate with patient's disability and the need for support is always perceived from the moment of diagnosis onwards (Lageman, Mickens, & Cash, 2015).

On the other hand, a review conducted in 2014 focused on caregivers of people affected by PD and highlighted that the burden is directly proportional to the intensity of the assistance provided (hours a day) (Bhimani, 2014). Having the possibility of taking part in training classes to manage PD symptoms at home or giving this opportunity to the patient could decrease the burden level of both caregivers and care-receivers, and a sound training might prevent the sense of incompetence, anxiety, depression and insomnia, which negatively affect caregivers' quality of life and health (Bhimani, 2014; Boersma et al., 2017; Udow et al., 2017).

Together with all the healthcare professionals who work in favour of patients affected by PD and their caregivers, nurses play a pivotal role in the daily management of patients as they are the agents of change and improvement in care pathway. Nursing staff spends most of the time at patients' side during hospitalization, and the attitude of these professionals to empathy encourages patients and familial caregivers to express their needs on which are based personalized healthcare plans. Moreover, their support and training awake caregivers' educational needs, improve their confidence and help them in understanding the importance of their role (Fernandes & Angelo, 2016).

The key role of family caregivers and the importance of their training is a topic treated in literature. Some studies showed the importance of the individualized training done by nurses specialized in Parkinson' disease. They highlighted both the ability in understanding the disease and all the fundamental aspects that impact on the patient's daily life, and in acquiring the competencies to manage the patient at home properly (Hellqvist & Berterö, 2015; Kuo et al., 2017).

Others highlighted the positive support that online and telematics training courses can give to caregivers, reducing anxiety and depression. Educational instantaneous interventions done through electronic devices gave the opportunity to create a strong collaborative relationship with healthcare professionals and simultaneous classes helped caregivers that could share their emotions (Blom, Zarit, Groot Zwaaftink, Cuijpers, & Pot, 2015; Shah et al., 2015).

Finally, other researches pointed out the effectiveness of training in theoretical and practical courses during which caregivers could learn and acquire technical skills and even share their opinions and experiences of caregiving, thus generating a decrease of burden levels (Abendroth, Greenblum, & Gray, 2014; Cianfrocca et al., 2018; Habermann & Davis, 2006; Katsuki et al., 2011; Zingaretti, 2011).

However, even though the topic of caregiver's training is widely explored in literature, the role of stress vulnerability on PD patients' caregivers' perceptions regarding the usefulness of training courses and the advantages of such interventions on their quality of life have not been explored yet.

2. Aim

This study aims to evaluate whether the stress level of familial caregivers of Parkinson's disease patients is related to their perception of the need and usefulness of healthcare education.

3. Materials and methods

3.1. Design

A cross-sectional study involving familial caregivers of patients affected by Parkinson's disease was conducted from July to September 2017.

3.2. Study sample and inclusion and exclusion criteria

69 family caregivers were voluntarily enrolled during the bi-monthly visits with the neurologist at the neurologist office into an Italian Polyclinc. Inclusion criteria were: a) age higher than 18 years old and b) being the familial caregiver of Parkinson's disease patients suffering from Parkinson's disease at stage 2.5 / 3, with Montreal Cognitive Scale (MoCA) > 24.

3.3. Tools and data collection

The study was conducted and then reported according to the STROBE checklist. Sociodemographic data were assessed through a questionnaire. Moreover, each participant was asked to answer two different questionnaires. The first is the Stress-related Vulnerability Scale (SVS scale) an Italian tool, created and validated in Italy in 2010 and used to measure the vulnerability related to stressful events and situations, like being a familial caregiver and the lack of support received (Tarsitani, Battisti, Biondi, & Picardi, 2010).

The SVS Scale is a self-completed questionnaire that considers "the last month" as a reference period and gives an overall score that indicates a growing measure of stress-related vulnerability. The overall score is obtained from the sum of the scores extracted from the answers given to each single item of the scale. The tool was built on the basis of the scientific literature concerning the measurement of stress and social support. The version used in this study was obtained from a selection of the items of other previous versions, chosen according to the psychometric characteristics. During the process of validation the SVS was administered twice to a non-clinical sample of 202 subjects together with validated tools for stress and social support measurement as the Perceived Stress Scale created by Cohen, Kamarck, and Mermelstein (1983)), and the Multidimensional Scale of Perceived Social Support created by Zimet, Dahlem, Zimet, and Farley (1988). The homogeneity and reliability of the SVS re-test test were satisfactory, the subscales have shown a good convergent validity with the other scales mentioned above and already validated for the measurement of subjective stress and social support. Moreover, the SVS showed a sensitivity to change, with a significant association between changes in the total score and life events occurring in a six-month interval between two evaluations (Tarsitani et al., 2010). The scale consists of 9 items scored on a 4-point Likert scale. Three score ranges have been fixed according to the three different vulnerability levels:

From 0 to 10 points: normal vulnerability level (Normal SVS); it indicates a stress-related vulnerability that falls within the normal range or in any case does not seem to represent a significant risk factor for the state of health.

From 11 to 18 points: significative vulnerability level (Significative SVS); it indicates a level of vulnerability above the average that may pose a significant risk of future health problems.

From 18 to 27 points: high vulnerability level (High SVS); it indicates significant levels of tension and demoralization, often associated with poor interpersonal support. This score allows to identify people who could benefit from targeted supportive interventions.

The second tool is a self-assessed questionnaire created "ad hoc" according to the existing literature that proposes five specific nursing educational interventions aimed at caregiver training and support. During the survey the opinion of the participants about the usefulness of these proposed interventions was asked to understand whether a

E. Di Stasio, et al.   Applied Nursing Research 51 (2020) 151186

higher level of stress is related to a higher consideration of the usefulness of the proposed interventions.

The tool is composed of the five proposed interventions:

- Intervention n°1: Supporting and training interventions provided by nurses specializing in Parkinson's disease (Hellqvist & Berterö, 2015); (Int. 1: S&T).

- Intervention n°2: Psychoeducational and skill training (how to preserve health, how to take care of the care-receiver, how to get information about the disease) interventions for caregivers provided by qualified nurses (Habermann & Davis, 2006); (Int.2: PST).

- Intervention n°3: Caregivers tele-support groups led by nurses specializing in caregiver education (Shah et al., 2015); (Int.3: TSG).

- Intervention n°4: Peer-led support groups among caregivers of people with Parkinson's disease aimed at sharing mutually personal experiences, socializing and exchanging advice (Abendroth et al., 2014); (Int.4: PLG).

- Intervention n°5: Multidisciplinary classes led by medical and nursing staff aimed at providing caregivers with a practical aid to improve their care activity (Zingaretti, 2011); (Int.5: MCS).

For each intervention, the possible answers were scored on a 4-point Likert scale and a "total interventions score" parameter, ranging from 0 (each intervention answer as "Nothing") to 15 (each intervention answer as "Extremely") was created, adding together the scores of each intervention.

3.4. Statistical analysis

Statistical analysis was performed by using the Statistical Package for Social Science (SPSS), release 15.0. Categorical variables were expressed as frequencies and the X2-test was used to assess the significance of the differences between subgroups; standardized residual analysis was performed to locate the significant different subgroup frequency. Moreover, to determine the relevance of the observed frequency differences, the effect size (w) of each comparison was calculated. A probability of < 0.05 was considered statistically significant.

Ethical approval

The aim of the study was explained during the enrolment by the neurologist and was even written upon informed consent. Each participant could answer the questionnaires anonymously.

4. Results

In Table 1, the demographical parameters of the population under study stratified according to SVS classes are reported. Seventy-one percent of the sample is composed of females and 72% is over the age of 60. No significant differences were detected in the frequency distribution of gender, age, kinship, education and marital status among SVS subgroups. Concerning the proposed interventions, specific profiles of distribution were observed for total addressed intervention priority (total interventions score) as a function of SVS classes (p = 0.060, w = 0.30 corresponding to a "medium" effect). A high frequency of low score answers is evident in Normal and Significative SVS subgroups

(39% and 56% of score 0–3, respectively). The proportions constantly decrease as the total score increases down to 19% and 25% at 12–15 total score, respectively. On the other hand, the frequency of High SVS subgroup progressively rises from 6% at 0–3 to 56% at 12–15 total score (Fig. 1). Table 2 reports the distribution of each proposed intervention (Int. 1: S&T; Int.2: PST; Int.3: TSG; Int.4: PLG; Int.5: MCS) in SVS subgroups. Significant differences in class frequency were observed for "Int.3: TSG" and "Int.4: PLG" (p = 0.034, w = 0.31-"medium", and p = 0.048, w = 0.30-"medium", respectively) and located in "Extremely" answers in High SVS subgroup for intervention 3 and in "Extremely" and "Nothing" answers in High and Normal SVS subgroups, respectively, for intervention 4. A significance of 0.134 (w = 0.27-small), 0.064 (w = 0.29-small) and 0.095 (w = 0.28-small) was measured for interventions 1, 2 and 5, respectively.

Finally, considering the answer profiles according to SVS classes, a recurrent decrease and increase between Normal and High SVS (in total and each specific intervention) were observed of "Nothing" and "Extremely", respectively. A mixed pattern was detected for "Somewhat" and "Moderately" answers.

5. Discussion

Supporting PD patients' familial caregivers represents an important task for the nursing profession. Parkinson's disease negatively affects both patients' and caregivers' lives. Familial caregivers assure almost 80% of the care provided to chronic patients, and high levels of caregiving can cause discomfort symptoms like depression, anxiety and sleep disturbances, leading to the caregiver burden (Naiditch, Triantafillou, Di Santo, et al., 2013; Nobili, Massaia, Isaia, et al., 2011; Torny, Videaud, Chatainier, Tarrade, & Meissner, 2018).

One of the main causes of burden is that family caregivers feel insufficiently trained even in the basic activities of daily living and, therefore, unprepared to undertake the tasks of caregiving (Grün, Pieri, Vaillant, & Diederich, 2016; Morley et al., 2012; Raccichini et al., 2015). The most mentioned need expressed by caregivers is to acquire adequate training about the evolution of the disease and the management of the symptoms at home (Eluvathingol Jose & Portillo, 2013). Even though training is considered one of the most important interventions to help caregivers, only a few studies have treated this theme by considering the PD patient caregivers' perception, the role of caregiver stress-related vulnerability, and their assessment of the effectiveness of healthcare educational programs. In the present manuscript, the perception of the usefulness of the five specific proposed interventions has been studied considering the SVS scale levels. A direct association between SVS scale levels and the perception of the usefulness of the nursing interventions can be detected, thus suggesting an important role of caregivers' emotional status in considering training courses. "Extremely" answers are always higher than 43% in the subjects belonging to High SVS subgroup. On the other hand, the mean frequency of "Nothing" answers is 40% in Normal SVS subjects; a mixed profile is observed in the Significant SVS subgroup. Moreover, even though the recruited subjects are equally split into SVS subgroups (31, 36 and 33%, respectively), "Nothing" and "Extremely" options represent 35% and 28%, whereas "Somewhat" and "Moderately" answers

Table 1
Demographical parameters of the population under study.

	Population under study (n = 69)	Normal SVS	Significative SVS	High SVS	p
Gender (male/female) (%)	29 / 71	38 / 62	28 / 72	22 / 78	0.485
Age (30–60/ > 60 yrs)	28 / 72	29 / 71	40 / 60	13 / 87	
Kinship (cs/pr/sn/br)	78/7/12/3	81/5/10/5	80/8/12/−	74/9/13/4	
Education (el/sc/hs/g)	7/32/73/13	5/33/43/19	8/28/52/12	9/35/48/9	
Marital status (um/mr/ch/dv/wd)	15 /71/4/4/4	10/76/−/5/10	16/72/4/−/8	17/65/9/9/−	

Legend: cs = consort, pr = partner, sn = son, br = brother, el = elementary, sc = secondary, hs = high school, gr = gradutation, um = unmarried, mr = married, ch = cohabitant, dv = divorced, wd = widower.

E. Di Stasio, et al.

Applied Nursing Research 51 (2020) 151186

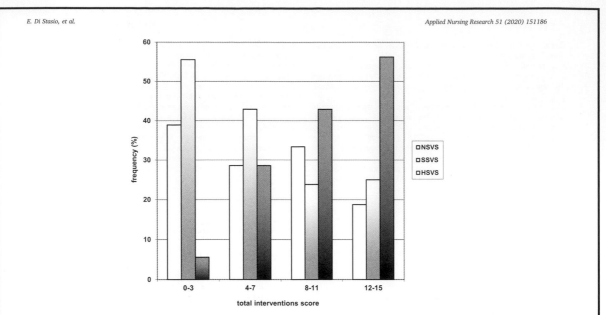

Fig. 1. SVS classes' frequency (%) distribution in quartiles total intervention score. A decrease of Normal/Significative and an increase of High SVS class frequency can be observed as the total score raises. (p = 0.060.)

Table 2
Frequency distribution (%) of responses to each specific intervention in different SVS subgroups.

	Normal SVS (%)	Significative SVS (%)	High SVS (%)	p
Supporting and training interventions				
Nothing	52.4	36.0	17.4	0.134
Somewhat	14.3	20.0	21.7	
Moderately	9.5	28.0	17.4	
Extremely	23.8	16.0	43.5	
Psychoeducational and skill training				
Nothing	23.8	36.0	13.0	0.064
Somewhat	23.8	32.0	21.7	
Moderately	19.0	16.0	4.3	
Extremely	33.3	16.0	60.9	
Caregivers tele-support groups				
Nothing	42.9	56.0	34.8	0.034
Somewhat	19.0	24.0	8.7	
Moderately	28.6	8.0	13.0	
Extremely	9.5	12.0	43.5	
Peer-Led support groups				
Nothing	42.9	28.0	4.3	0.048
Somewhat	9.5	20.0	21.7	
Moderately	19.0	32.0	21.7	
Extremely	28.6	20.0	52.2	
Multidisciplinary classes				
Nothing	38.1	32.0	21.7	0.095
Somewhat	14.3	20.0	17.4	
Moderately	23.8	28.0	4.3	
Extremely	23.8	20.0	56.5	

reach only 19% each of total answers, respectively.

Therefore, caregivers seem to switch between two major conditions: low vulnerability level, with the minimal perception of training need and high burden state with the impending necessity of support to manage PD patients. Therefore, in the population under study, caregivers' vulnerability seems to be equally distributed in the three SVS levels, and the perception of receiving nursing educational interventions as very useful is directly related to the increase of burden level. Moreover, what clearly emerges from the study is the need of sharing experiences that is associated to the stress levels of caregivers. In fact significant differences were detected in the estimated usefulness of the interventions 3 "Caregivers tele-support groups" and 4 "Peer-led support groups among" according to the stress levels of caregivers and these interventions are referred to the opportunity to share experiences and emotions.

6. Limits

This study has some limitations. The first limit is represented by the small number of the population under study (n = 69). Moreover, the survey could help in understanding the perception of the usefulness of the proposed interventions, but no question investigated whether caregivers had ever attended courses like the ones proposed. Furthermore, a timing evolution of caregiver's burden level and training need should be traced to detect the incidence of increasing periods of stressing condition on the perception of assistance and help requirement. Another limit is that it is not possible to correlate the results with the severity of the patient's illness, as there is no available data.

Another data missing is about both patients' and caregivers' illnesses and comorbidities. The tool used to assess caregiver vulnerability represents another limit. The SVS scale is not created and based on caregivers of PD patients; no tool like this exists as of now. So it is necessary to adapt the existing tools to this particular category of caregivers.

7. Conclusion

The usefulness of healthcare education addressed to familial caregivers in Parkinson's disease cases emerges from the existing literature. It could lead to an enhancement of the quality of life of both patients and caregivers. However, this article deals with a broad issue that needs to be further deepened through additional focused research as it treats a theme not sufficiently explored.

E. Di Stasio, et al. *Applied Nursing Research 51 (2020) 151186*

The stress-related vulnerability seems to be related to the perception of the usefulness of the interventions proposed. What emerges is that, probably, the more you are stressed and involved in care management at home, the more you need to be helped.

Moreover, it could be supposed that the lack of positive perception about educational support is due to a lack of awareness of the progression of the pathology or to a partial involvement in the care process. However, further studies about this topic should be conducted, first by increasing the sample size and even by correlating the stress-related vulnerability with the perception of the usefulness of the educational support, patients' clinical conditions and the number of hours of care actually delivered by the caregiver at home. Finally, the importance of the evolution of help-need perception related to the progress in time of the caregiver's burden and the care-receiver's disease progression should be pointed out.

Funding

No specific grant from any funding agency in the public, commercial, or not-for-profit sectors was received for this research.

Declaration of competing interest

The author(s) declare no potential conflict of interest concerning the research, authorship, or publication of this article.

References

Abendroth, M., Greenblum, C. A., & Gray, J. A. (2014). The value of peer-led support groups among caregivers of persons with Parkinson's disease. *Holistic Nursing Practice, 28*(1), 48–54. https://doi.org/10.1097/HNP.0000000000000004.

Adler, R., & Mehta, R. (2014). *Catalyzing technology to support family caregiving.* National Alliance for Caregiving 1–18.

Ashrafian, S., Feizollahzadeh, H., Rahmani, A., & Davoodi, A. (2018). The unmet needs of the family caregivers of patients with Cancer visiting referral Hospital in Iran. *Asia-Pacific Journal of Oncology Nursing, 5.* https://doi.org/10.4103/apjon.apjon_7_18.

Bhimani, R. (2014). Understanding the burden on caregivers of people with Parkinson's: A scoping review of the literature. *Rehabilitation Research and Practice, 2014*, 718527. https://doi.org/10.1155/2014/718527.

Blom, M. M., Zarit, S. H., Groot Zwaaftink, R. B. M., Cuijpers, P., & Pot, A. M. (2015). Effectiveness of an Internet intervention for family caregivers of people with dementia: Results of a randomized controlled trial. *PLoS One, 10*(2), e0116622. https://doi.org/10.1371/journal.pone.0116622.

Boersma, I., Jones, J., Coughlan, C., Carter, J., Bekelman, D., Miyasaki, J., & Kluger, B. (2017). Palliative care and Parkinson's disease: Caregiver perspectives. *Journal of Palliative Medicine, 20*(9), https://doi.org/10.1089/jpm.2016.0325.

Brulletti, G., Comini, L., Scalvini, S., Morini, R., Luisa, A., Paneroni, M., & Vitacca, M. (2015). A two-year longitudinal study on strain and needs in caregivers of advanced ALS patients. *Amyotrophic lateral sclerosis & frontotemporal degeneration, 16*(3–4), 187–195. https://doi.org/10.3109/21678421.2014.974616.

Chiarini, M., Di Simone, E., Scafuro, C., Auddino, F., Fabbri, M., Delli Poggi, A., … Di Muzio, M. (2017). Health self-perception in patient with Crohn's disease: A web survey. La Clinica Terapeutica, 168(6), e401–e405.

Cianfrocca, C., Caponnetto, V., Donati, D., Lancia, L., Tartaglini, D., & Di Stasio, E. (2018). The effects of a multidisciplinary education course on the burden, health literacy and needs of family caregivers. *Applied Nursing Research, 44*(2018), 100–106. https://doi.org/10.1016/j.apnr.2018.10.004.

Cohen, S., Kamarck, T., & Mermelstein, R. (1983). A global measure of perceived stress. *Journal of Health and Social Behavior, 24*, 385–396.

Dorsey, E. R., Constantinescu, R., Thompson, J. P., Biglan, K. M., Holloway, R. G., Kieburtz, K., & Tanner, C. M. (2007). Projected number of people with Parkinson

disease in the most populous nations, 2005 through 2030. *Neurology, 68*(5), 384–386. https://doi.org/10.1212/01.wnl.0000247740.47667.03.

Eluvathingol Jose, G., & Portillo, M. C. (2013). Needs and support networks of informal caregivers of people with Parkinson's disease: A literature review. *Revista De Enfermeria (Barcelona, Spain), 36*(7–8), 52–60.

Fernandes, C. S., & Angelo, M. (2016). Family caregivers: What do they need? An integrative review. *Revista Da Escola De Enfermagem Da U S P, 50*(4), 675–682. https://doi.org/10.1590/S0080-623420160000500019.

Grün, D., Pieri, V., Vaillant, M., & Diederich, N. J. (2016). Contributory factors to caregiver burden in Parkinson disease. *Journal of the American Medical Directors Association, 17*(7), 626–632. https://doi.org/10.1016/j.jamda.2016.03.004.

Habermann, B., & Davis, L. L. (2006). Lessons learned from a Parkinson's disease caregiver intervention pilot study. *Applied Nursing Research: ANR, 19*(4), 212–215. https://doi.org/10.1016/j.apnr.2005.12.003.

Hellqvist, C., & Berterö, C. (2015). Support supplied by Parkinson's disease specialist nurses to Parkinson's disease patients and their spouses. *Applied Nursing Research: ANR, 28*(2), 86–91. https://doi.org/10.1016/j.apnr.2014.12.008.

Katsuki, F., Takeuchi, H., Konishi, M., Sasaki, M., Murase, Y., Naito, A., & Furukawa, T. A. (2011). Pre-post changes in psychosocial functioning among relatives of patients with depressive disorders after Brief Multifamily Psychoeducation: A pilot study. *BMC Psychiatry, 11*, 56. https://doi.org/10.1186/1471-244X-11-56.

Kuo, L.-M., Huang, H.-L., Liang, J., Kwok, Y.-T., Hsu, W.-C., Liu, C.-Y., & Shyu, Y.-I. L. (2017). Trajectories of health-related quality of life among family caregivers of individuals with dementia: A home-based caregiver-training program matters. *Geriatric Nursing (New York, N.Y.), 38*(2), 124–132. https://doi.org/10.1016/j.gerinurse.2016.08.017.

Lageman, S. K., Mickens, M. N., & Cash, T. V. (2015). Caregiver-identified needs and barriers to care in Parkinson's disease. *Geriatric Nursing (New York, N.Y.), 36*(3), 197–201. https://doi.org/10.1016/j.gerinurse.2015.01.002.

Morley, D., Dummett, S., Peters, M., Kelly, L., Hewitson, P., Dawson, J., & Jenkinson, C. (2012). Factors influencing quality of life in caregivers of people with Parkinson's disease and implications for clinical guidelines. *Parkinson's Disease, 2012*, 190901. https://doi.org/10.1155/2012/190901.

Naiditch, M., Triantafillou, J., Di Santo, P., et al. (2013). User perspectives in long term care and role of informal carers. In K. Leichsenring, J. Billings, & H. Nies (Eds.). *Long term care in Europe: Improving policy and practice* (pp. 45–80). Basingstoke, UK: Palgrave Macmillan.

Nobili, G., Massaia, M., Isaia, G., et al. (2011). Valutazione dei bisogni del caregiver di pazienti affetti da demenza: esperienza in una unità di valutazione Alzheimer. *Giornale di Gerontologia, 343*(59), 71–74.

Obeso, J. A., Stamelou, M., Goetz, C. G., Poewe, W., Lang, A. E., Weintraub, D., & Stoessl, A. J. (2017). Past, present, and future of Parkinson's disease: A special essay on the 200th Anniversary of the Shaking Palsy. *Movement Disorders: Official Journal of the Movement Disorder Society, 32*(9), 1264–1310. https://doi.org/10.1002/mds.27115.

Raccichini, A., Spazzafumo, L., Castellani, S., Civerchia, P., Pelliccioni, G., & Scarpino, O. (2015). Living with mild to moderate Alzheimer patients increases the caregiver's burden at 6 months. *American Journal of Alzheimer's Disease and Other Dementias, 30*(5), 463–467. https://doi.org/10.1177/1533317514568339.

Shah, S. P., Glenn, G. L., Hummel, E. M., Hamilton, J. M., Martine, R. R., Duda, J. E., & Wilkinson, J. R. (2015). Caregiver tele-support group for Parkinson's disease: A pilot study. *Geriatric Nursing (New York, N.Y.), 36*(3), 207–211. https://doi.org/10.1016/j.gerinurse.2015.02.002.

Tarsitani, L., Battisti, F., Biondi, M., & Picardi, A. (2010). Development and validation of a stress related vulnerability scale. *Epidemiologia e Psichiatria Sociale, 19*(2), 178–182.

Torny, F., Videaud, H., Chatainier, P., Tarrade, C., Meissner, W., G., Couratier, P. (2018). Factors associated with spousal burden in Parkinson's disease. Revue Neurologique, 19. pii: S0035-3787(17)30697-5. doi: https://doi.org/10.1016/j.neurol.2018.01.372.

Udow, S. J., Hobson, D. E., Kleiner, G., Masellis, M., Fox, S. H., Lang, A. E., & Marras, C. (2017). Educational needs and considerations for a visual educational tool to discuss Parkinson's disease. *Movement Disorders Clinical Practice, 5*(1), 66–74 (doi: 364 10.1002/mdc3.12563).

Zarit, S. H., Todd, P. A., & Zarit, J. M. (1986). Subjective 365 burden of husbands and wives as caregivers: A longitudinal study. *Gerontologist, 26*(3), 260–266.

Zimet, G., Dahlem, N. W., Zimet, S. G., & Farley, G. K. (1988). The multidimensional scale of perceived social support. *Journal of Personality Assessment, 52*(1), 30–41. https://doi.org/10.1207/s15327752jpa5201_2.

Zingaretti, M. (2011). *Familiari-Caregiver: una presenza in attesa di visibilità. 30*, Assistenza Infermieristica e Ricerca 1.

International Journal of Nursing Studies 101 (2020) 103416

Contents lists available at ScienceDirect

International Journal of Nursing Studies

journal homepage: www.elsevier.com/ijns

"It's up to me with a little support" – Adherence after myocardial infarction: A qualitative study

Admi Hanna [a,b,*], Eilon-Moshe Yael [b], Levy Hadassa [b], Eisen Iris [c], Nikolsky Eugenia [d,e], Gepstein Lior [c,e,f], Satran Carmit [a], Ore Liora [g]

[a] Nursing Department, Yezreel Valley College, Israel
[b] Rambam Health Care Campus, Haifa, Israel
[c] Cardiology Department, Rambam Health Care Campus, Haifa, Israel
[d] Cardiovascular Research Unit, Rambam Health Care Campus, Israel
[e] Technion-Israel Institute of Technology, Haifa, Israel
[f] The Rappaport Faculty of Medicine and Research Institute, Israel
[g] Health Systems Management, Yezreel Valley College, Israel

ARTICLE INFO

Article history:
Received 19 January 2019
Received in revised form 25 August 2019
Accepted 29 August 2019

Keywords:
Myocardial infarction
Adherence
Health-related behaviors
Motivational theory
Cardiac rehabilitation
Healthy lifestyle
Self-care

ABSTRACT

Background: Ischemic heart disease and stroke remain the leading causes of death globally. Poor adherence to treatment amongst patients with chronic health conditions is a global unresolved problem of enormous magnitude. Despite extensive research in the field of adherence behaviors, few studies have focused on motivational aspects that can enhance adherence from the patients' points of view post myocardial infarction.

Aim: To gain insights into the perceptions that underline health-related adherence behaviors, from the perspective of patients who experienced a heart attack.

Design: A phenomenological approach.

Methods: The study used a content analysis method, with qualitative criteria to establish trustworthiness. Interviews were conducted with a purposive sample of 22 participants post myocardial infarction, recruited from a hospital cardiac rehabilitation program and communities in Northern Israel.

Results: The abstraction process generated two main categories and six sub-categories imbedded in the Self Determination Theory framework. While inner self determination or willpower, as expressed by the participants, was perceived as the most crucial motivator, it was insufficient. A sense of self competency and the ability to tailor life changes, according to personal preferences, is needed to turn willpower into practice. Extrinsic motivators such as family members, especially spouses and health professionals, are important to strengthen intrinsic motivation. Attitudes of caring, respect for values, and autonomy as opposed to patronization were perceived as helpful. The benefits of a cardiac rehabilitation program were articulated by attendees of the program in contrast to excuses by non-attendees

Conclusion: Understanding adherence as a complex holistic phenomenon could advance theoretical insights and enhance adherence to therapies and healthy lifestyle among people post myocardial infarction.

Impact: Study findings may advance the self-care of people with long-term health conditions, and assist professionals to conduct interventions that strengthen adherence. Increased adherence can impact life expectancy, quality of life, and reduce the economic burden on health care systems and societies.

© 2019 Published by Elsevier Ltd.

* Corresponding author at: Head of Nursing Department, Yezreel Valley College, Israel.
E-mail addresses: hannaa@yvc.ac.il, h_admi@rmc.gov.il (A. Hanna).

https://doi.org/10.1016/j.ijnurstu.2019.103416
0020-7489/© 2019 Published by Elsevier Ltd.

2   A. Hanna, E.-M. Yael and L. Hadassa et al./International Journal of Nursing Studies 101 (2020) 103416

What is already known about the topic?

- Adherence to long-term therapies is approximately 50% in developed countries and lower in low and middle-income countries.
- Poor adherence of people with chronic diseases leads to mortality, morbidity, poor quality of life and increased economic burden on health care systems.
- Despite the large number of variables that were identified as related to adherence, not much has been understood that increases adherence behaviors.

What this paper adds

- Non-adherence is a complex holistic phenomenon that cannot be resolved by addressing single attributes such as increasing health literacy.
- Families and healthcare providers can strengthen motivation, willpower and self-competency by respecting personal preferences and autonomy.
- Health care practitioners should establish tailored plans of care, in cooperation with patients, rather than dictate medical instructions for patients.

1. Introduction

Poor adherence to treatment amongst patients with chronic health conditions is a global unresolved problem of enormous magnitude. Adherence is defined by the WHO (World Health Organization) report as "the extent to which a person's behavior – taking medication, following a diet, and/or executing lifestyle changes, corresponds with agreed recommendations from a health care provider." (Sabaté et al., 2003, p. 3). The report estimates adherence to long-term therapies is approximately 50% in developed countries, assuming much lower adherence in low and middle-income countries.

A recent US study on five lifestyle risk factors (smoking, BMI, physical activity, diet and alcohol intake) revealed a significantly prolonged life expectancy at age 50 (14 years for men and 12.2 years for women) among those with healthy lifestyle habits (Li et al., 2018). Worldwide, poor adherence in growing populations with chronic diseases leads to mortality, morbidity, poor quality of life, and creates an immense economic burden on health care systems and societies (Bansilal et al., 2016; Kotseva et al., 2017; Sabaté et al., 2003).

Ischemic heart disease and stroke are the world's biggest killers, accounting for a combined 15.2 million deaths in 2016. These diseases have remained the leading causes of death globally in the past 15 years (World Health Organization, 2018). Mortality rates for acute myocardial infarction (MI) decreased substantially during the last four decades, due to significant advances in prevention and interventions (Wilson and Douglas, 2013). For example, most patients receive health behavior guidance after a cardiac event and referral to cardiac rehabilitation programs. Cardiac rehabilitation programs involve interventions such as physical activity counseling, exercise training, nutritional counseling, weight control management, lipid management, blood pressure monitoring, smoking cessation, and psychosocial management (Piepoli et al., 2010). In spite of guidance and rehabilitation programs, the tendency is for short-term adherence, diminishing in the subsequent 1–2 years to approximately 50% adherence (Crowley et al., 2015).

In Israel, MI is the second most common cause of death, accounting for 15% of mortality (Israeli Ministry of Health, 2018). In 2018, 79% of the Israeli population were Jews and 21% Arabs (85% of the Arabs were Muslims and the remainder Christians and Druze). There is still evidence of inequalities in health care in Israel among three population groups: non-Jews, people living in the periphery and among people with poor socioeconomic status. These characteristics are often correlated. Arabs have worse health status than Jews on many indicators, including heart diseases. North and south districts have higher mortality rates than central Israel. Regardless of ethnic origin, poor socioeconomic status is associated with poor adherence to treatment protocols and worse health outcomes (Colombo, 2012).

A health literacy survey was conducted in Israel among 600 adults randomly selected from a national database. Home interviews were conducted in Hebrew, Russian, and Arabic. Results indicated that income and years of education were significantly associated with health literacy, playing a key role in determining self-assessed health, beyond sociodemographic variables (Levin-Zamir et al., 2016). Identifying indicators that play a significant role in health disparities contribute to a better understanding of the problem and a basis for health promotion actions, further research, and health policy.

Numerous studies have investigated factors that facilitate or inhibit adherence among patients post MI. The different methodological approaches and methods make it difficult to compare findings. However, many attributes are known to be related to the phenomenon of adherence among people post MI, such as personal attributes, the role of family, and the role of health care providers.

1.1. Personal attributes and adherence

Middle aged (50–69 years) patients had higher adherence than oldest (≥70 years) and youngest (<50 years) patients (Crowley et al., 2015; Kronish and Ye, 2013). Adherence is worse in patients with low education levels (<12 years of school) and health literacy (Crowley et al., 2015). Low socioeconomic status was also found to increase non-adherence to medication and smoking cessation (Campbell et al., 2014; Crowley et al., 2015; Jackevicius et al., 2008; Kronish and Ye, 2013).

Illness perceptions and health beliefs were found to play a role in patient self-care in qualitative studies, from being well, fully recovered and having a zest for life; to being ill with constant concerns, and uncertainty about the future (Bergman et al., 2009; Gregory et al., 2006). Feelings of anxiety, depression and threat of complications (e.g., recurrent MI or stroke) were found to be triggers for both adherence and non-adherence (Choudhry et al., 2014; Johansson et al., 2007).

Several studies identified variability in adherence in different ethnic and cultural groups (Fernandez et al., 2015; Groleau et al., 2010; Zhang et al., 2014). Zhang et al. (2014) found racial/ethnic differences in medication adherence among five American groups, with poorer adherence in minorities. The influence of culture was found in French Canadians who attributed spiritual meaning to the heart that shaped their myocardial infarction experience (Groleau et al., 2010).

1.2. The role of the family in adherence

Family relationships and support were identified as important driving forces, especially if family members shared the change in lifestyle. Patients without family, or who live alone or are socially isolated, are highly vulnerable to poor self-care. For example, dietary adherence was found to be poor among patients without supportive family and medication (Dunbar et al., 2008; Fernandez et al., 2015). On the other hand, relationships with family and friends can become strained after a myocardial event. For example, over-protective families and friends can prevent patients from performing important activities such as mild exercise (Roebuck et al., 2001), while more than one social gathering per week is a significant statistical predictor of non-adherence to diet (Ali et al., 2017).

A. Hanna, E.-M. Yael and L. Hadassa et al./International Journal of Nursing Studies 101 (2020) 103416   3

1.3. The role of health care providers in adherence

A qualitative study with 35 participants recovering from MI explored which experiences would have helped them to adhere to a healthy lifestyle. A major finding was the desire for long-term follow up and support from health care practitioners. Participants emphasized the need for regular professional supervision, obtaining support and reassurance for themselves and their families, and cardiac rehabilitation classes with people who shared similar experiences (Gregory et al., 2006). Awareness of healthy lifestyle can be also raised in the public and community arena, including changes in food products at stores and restaurants, and using the media as change agents (Fernandez et al., 2015; Kronish and Ye, 2013).

Despite the proven effectiveness of self-care interventions, patient participation after MI is poor (Al-Mallah et al., 2016; Barnason et al., 2012; Giannuzzi et al., 2008). A randomized control trial on the effect of a supportive educational intervention found higher levels of self-care knowledge, motivation, and skills among patients after MI, compared to a baseline and control group (Mohammadpour et al., 2015). Barriers predicting poor participation in cardiac rehabilitation programs can be classified into person-related and program related. Personal factors included elderly, single, women, people with comorbidities, unemployed, less educated, lower income, and lack of motivation. Program related factors included accessibility barriers, such as distance from cardiac rehabilitation facilities, inconvenient scheduling, and transportation difficulties. These barriers were similar in Europe and the USA (Jones et al., 2007; Ruano-Ravina et al., 2016).

Despite extensive research in the field of adherence, most previous studies focused on identifying discrete factors that correlate with poor adherence such as age, socioeconomic and cultural attributes, health beliefs, the role of the family, and impact of health care providers. However, there is still a gap in understanding why adherence is poor internationally. Few studies have tried to gain a more holistic approach on motivational aspects from the point of view of patients who experienced a heart attack event.

1.3.1. Theoretical framework

The phenomenon of adherence, as defined by the World Health Organization, is related to people's health behaviors (Sabaté et al., 2003). The reasons people behave in one way or another reflects their beliefs and the way they feel and think. Motivational theories provide conceptual underpinnings of this complex phenomenon. The self-determination theory is a motivational theory that addresses the reasons or goals promoting a behavior. There are two different types of motivation: intrinsic and extrinsic. Intrinsic motivation is "doing something because it is inherently interesting or enjoyable" and extrinsic motivation is "doing something because it leads to a separable outcome" (Ryan and Deci, 2000, p. 55).

Intrinsic motivation can be enhanced when people experience feelings of self-competence and autonomy. Whereas extrinsic motivation is characterized by feelings of being pressured or controlled. However, in general, some adult behaviors are not driven by intrinsic motivations. Social rules and demands often require taking responsibility for actions and tasks that are not necessarily rewarding in terms of interest or pleasure. According to the self-determination theory, processes of internalizing and integrating extrinsic motivations can transform them into intrinsic motivations. These processes are enhanced by adopting external values and regulations, and incorporating them as part of a sense of self (Ryan and Deci, 2000).

Another theory that contributes to a better understanding of the underlying reasoning of human functioning is the self-efficacy theory. Self-efficacy is defined by Bandura (2010) as peoples' beliefs about their competencies to perform during events that affect their lives. A strong sense of self-efficacy enhances people's functioning (i.e., how they feel, think and behave) and their personal well-being. People with strong self-efficacy approach difficult tasks as challenges to be mastered, rather than threats to be avoided. Lack of motivation can result from a personal perception that the cause is not valued; lack of self-efficacy to carry out a behavior; or disbelief that the action will lead to the expected consequences. Competence, autonomy, and relatedness were found to increase intrinsic motivation and support the internalization and integration of extrinsic motivation (Bandura, 2010, 2001; Ryan and Deci, 2000).

The self-determination theory and self-efficacy theory serve as an organizing theoretical framework to better understand the complexity of the phenomenon of adherence. Health care consumers can benefit from health care professionals who increase their motivation for adherence, strengthen their self-efficacy and respect their autonomy. In the context of post MI, empirical studies support this theory, indicating that poor adherence is related to a lack of self-efficacy and motivation. Non-adherence among people post MI was found to be characteristic of people who do not believe efforts to change their lifestyle would result in better health, or did not feel competent to carry out the required changes (Ruano-Ravina et al., 2016). Health care providers should have expertise about human motivation in addition to their clinical expertise, in order to foster among their patients a healthy lifestyle and adherence to medical recommendations.

The aim of this study is to gain deeper insights into perceptions and interpretations that underlie health-related adherence behaviors, from the perspectives of people who have experienced heart attack. The focus of this study is to identify factors that facilitate or inhibit adherence to therapies and healthy lifestyle.

2. Method

2.1. Design

This study used a phenomenological inductive approach and the content analysis method to gain understanding of the adherence phenomenon from the perspectives of people who had experienced MI (Graneheim et al., 2017).

2.2. Participants

A purposive sample of 22 participants post MI were recruited from a hospital cardiac rehabilitation unit and from two different communities in Northern Israel (Table 1). The socio-demographic and cultural characteristics of the participants reflect Israel's population who experienced MI in the past. The participants were chosen from different cultures to obtain a diversity of experiences from different perspectives. The socioeconomic status of the eight Arab respondents was lower, and their level of academic education higher (3/8 Arab participants held bachelor's degrees compared to 3/14 Jewish participants). The majority of Arabs lived in large cities and only two in villages, while eight Jews also lived in cities and six in a kibbutz (i.e., a collective community in Israel traditionally based on agriculture, and today includes industry and high-tech).

2.3. Data collection

A semi-structured in-depth interview guide was developed based on scientific literature, expert peer review by two cardiologist physicians, two cardiology nurses, and three qualitative researchers. The interview guide included a set of 44 predetermined, open-ended questions including prompts, in a way that encouraged participants to convey their viewpoints. In addition, other questions emerged from the dialog. The guide was organized around seven topics: demographics; initial experiences around

4   A. Hanna, E.-M. Yael and L. Hadassa et al. / International Journal of Nursing Studies 101 (2020) 103416

Table 1
Characteristics of interviewed participants[a].

Characteristics	Hospital Cardiac Rehabilitation (CR) program	Community	
		Kibbutz	Arab Community (AC)[b]
Total = 22	9	7	**6**
Age (years)			
Mean ± SD (range)	68.8 ± 9.7 (58–83)	61.9 ± 5.5 (55–71)	64.3 ± 12.8 (50–79)
50–59	2	3	3
60–69	3	3	–
70+	4	1	3
Gender:			
Male	9	5	6
Female	–	2	–
Religion			
Jewish	7	7	–
Muslim	1		4
Christian	1		2
Family status			
Single	1	–	–
Married	5	6	5
Widower	1	–	1
Divorced	2	1	–
Socioeconomic status			
Low	1	–	3
Average	7	7	3
Above average	1	–	–
Education			
Elementary/high school	7	3	3
Diploma	1	2	–
Bachelor's degree	1	2	3
Years from first MI			
	10.8 ± 6.8 (0.5–21)	7.8 ± 4.4 (0.5–15)	15.7 ± 6.4 (2–21)
Mean ± SD (range) up to 5	2	2	1
6–10	3	3	–
11–15	1	2	1
16+	3	–	4

[a] The participants are identified in the text by their age and place of interview (CR, Kibbutz or AC).
[b] Arab community (AC) refers to a city or village.

diagnosis; perceptions of self with the disease; health literacy; health care system and healthcare providers; adherence to medical regimen and lifestyle changes; long term outlook and tips for others in similar situations. Examples of questions: What in your opinion helps people preserve their health? From your experience, what works best for you? (Prompts: what kind of help is most meaningful, who plays a significant role? who else?). What of all the things you want to do for your health is more difficult for you to do? (Prompts: What else? Why? How do you explain it?

The hospital interviews took place in the cardiac rehabilitation unit, before or after participants' scheduled follow-up visits. The cardiac rehabilitation nurse contacted the participants by telephone, prior to their scheduled clinic visit, and asked their permission to participate in the study interview. The community interviews were scheduled by phone calls or face to face, at a time and place of convenience to the participants (i.e., home or coffee shop). Interviews lasted approximately 45–60 min.

The primary investigator conducted ten interviews, and supervised four nursing students, who conducted twelve more interviews as partial requirement of a qualitative seminar. Six interviews were conducted in Arabic, then translated into Hebrew by two Arabic-speaking nursing students who were also proficient in Hebrew; Hebrew is required for advanced nursing students in higher education. The remaining interviews were conducted in Hebrew. All the participants' quotations were translated into English by the primary investigator, and back translated by one of the bilingual co-researchers to ensure that meaning was retained. All translations were edited by a professional Israeli-American editor. Field notes were collected and all interviews recorded and transcribed.

2.4. Ethical considerations

Approval was granted by the hospital's Helsinki human subjects committee and a college based ethical committee. The study objectives and voluntary nature of the study were explained to participants, who were told they have the right to withdraw from the study at any time. Written informed consent was obtained. Confidentiality was assured by not revealing the identity of the participants.

2.5. Data analysis

All the interview transcripts and the field notes were analyzed by the primary investigator. The co-researchers, not directly connected to the interview process, independently analyzed half of the transcripts. The 22 interview transcripts were randomly divided into two groups (i.e., even and odd) and each group included five interviews with cardiac rehabilitation participants and six with community participants. Findings were compared and discussed by the research team during organized meetings until consensus was reached.

A content analysis method was used, starting with systematic coding by four independent researchers. The initial coding tree was modified during the analysis process. By comparing and contrasting similar categories across all interviews, emerging themes were inductively derived from the raw data. Finally, categories and sub-categories were organized based on the raw data and theoretical framework (Tong et al., 2007).

The interpretation and abstraction process included identifying patterns and meanings of the themes. The relationships between

A. Hanna, E.-M. Yael and L. Hadassa et al./International Journal of Nursing Studies 101 (2020) 103416   5

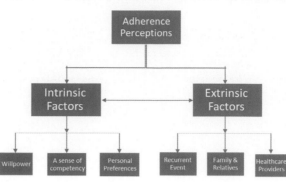

Fig. 1. Adherence to medical recommendations and healthy lifestyle after myocardial infarction: schematic diagram of the study's central category, main categories, sub-categories and the relationships among them.

the core category, main categories, and sub-categories were identified and described. Theoretical saturation was achieved when no new insights were identified from the data. Saturation was reached after eight interviews with cardiac rehabilitation participants and ten interviews with community participants. Four more interviews (two in each group) were conducted to ensure saturation. Finally, the findings were discussed and compared to existing literature (Graneheim et al., 2017).

2.6. Trustworthiness

Criteria of credibility, transferability, dependability, and confirmability were used to establish study trustworthiness (Guba and Lincoln, 1989). Credibility was achieved by in-depth interviews with participants followed by peer debriefing. The primary investigator performed coding, categorization, and analysis of all the data.

Dependability was reached by process audit, i.e., documentation of every step in the analysis process was maintained for evaluation by peer researchers. Confirmability was established by providing a description and rationale for the decisions made based on the findings, helping to ensure they accurately portrayed participants' responses. Transferability was established by extensive descriptions collected through in-depth interviews. The descriptions provide the basis for outside reviewers to judge transferability (Guba and Lincoln, 1989).

3. Findings

In accordance with the study aim, the central focus was the experience of adherence to medical recommendations and healthy lifestyle from the perspective of patients who underwent MI. The abstraction process generated two main categories and six sub-categories embedded in the self-determination theory framework. Fig. 1 demonstrates the formulation of concepts and the relationships among them. In order to understand what motivates people to adhere, the participants were asked to share their experiences of facilitators and barriers to adherence.

3.1. Adherence facilitators and barriers

3.1.1. Intrinsic factors

It is reasonable to assume that people recovering from a heart attack will be highly motivated to maintain good health and prevent recurrence of another heart event. The analysis revealed three themes related to intrinsic motivation: willpower, competency, and individual preferences.

3.1.2. Willpower

A theme that was repeatedly articulated by the participants dealt with self-determination. Participants expressed the need for free will in order to be motivated to incorporate modifications in their lifestyle.

67 years (Cardiac rehabilitation) "It's all about will power, you shouldn't panic, it's will power, thinking rationally. I understood that if I will not take care, I will suffer more. I must do something about it. A person must come to the conclusion by himself. Pushing or yelling wouldn't help."

60 years (Cardiac rehabilitation) "I have learned from my experience that everything has a price tag and you will have to pay it in at one point in life. If you don't do what you should do, finally you will pay. If you will not watch your weight, or keep on smoking, something will happen to you. A person must be responsible for his life, to take himself in his own hands."

The participants realized that the most important motivator was their choice to take responsibility for the consequences of their health behaviors. They emphasized that no one else could decide for them.

3.1.3. Self-competency

To be aware of the need to adhere and be determined to act in this direction is insufficient for adherence. A theme raised by the participants was related to feelings of self-competency.

67 years (Cardiac rehabilitation) "I know what I should eat. If it is not good for me, I can only taste one and not five or six. ...If I was able to stop smoking after 40 years three cigarette packages a day, in one second, why shouldn't I be able to stop everything? It's all here (pointed with his finger on his forehead)."

58 years (Cardiac rehabilitation) "This time the doctor told me if I want to live, I must quit smoking cigarettes. I don't want to lie to myself. I can't stop all at once. I will not give my body a punch. I don't feel good about it. I feel that something is missing in my life."

Almost all participants described their difficulties in changing habits. Internalization of the risks of non-adherence and having the willpower to change is very important but not sufficient for action. A sense of competency is needed to turn awareness and willingness into practice.

3.1.4. Personal preferences

All participants shared their efforts to adhere, however, difficulties maintaining certain activities varied and depended on individual preferences.

83 years (Cardiac rehabilitation) "There are things that I can follow and are not tough for me and there are things that are too tough. ... I was told to keep a low salt diet but I do not succeed in doing it. Later on, at night I say to myself that I should behave".

60 years (Cardiac rehabilitation) "There are ups and downs in life, I succeeded to quit smoking, trying to stick to a diet, it is difficult with snacks like nuts and seeds, you know... During the last three years I didn't do much walking, gained weight".

Participants found it most difficult to adhere to recommendations that they disliked (e.g., regular exercise activities), or quit enjoyable activities (e.g., smoking, eating habits). They gave many explanations why it was impossible for them to maintain certain habits and activities. Participants that were engaged in some healthy lifestyle habits before the MI found it easier to maintain those activities.

78 years (Cardiac rehabilitation) "I live by the sea, all the years I used to swim and I kept swimming after the MI, until today. I do sports activities: walking, swimming, sauna and Jacuzzi. I don't know if it helps, it feels good, I love it!"

According to the participants' experiences, adherence can be enhanced when the individuals decide for themselves to adopt behaviors out of their free will; when they feel competent and challenged to carry out those behaviors; and when engaging in healthy behaviors means to do something they prefer as opposed to being pushed to do things they dislike.

3.2. Extrinsic factors

Three extrinsic factors were identified that play a role as facilitators or barriers to adherence: the threat of a recurrent MI event; family and significant others; and health care providers.

3.2.1. The threat of a recurrent MI

All participants remembered their heart attack very vividly as a critical life-threatening event. Most described feelings of pain they had never experienced and some as intolerable pain. The MI became a turning point that propelled the participants into lifestyle changes immediately following the attack. However, the effect of the event diminished over time and people gradually returned to pre-event habits. Interestingly, the impact of a recurrent MI was described as being of a greater magnitude on their everyday behaviors.

58 years (Cardiac rehabilitation) "In the early years after the first attack, let's say two or three years, I kept doing what I was told, then I started eating everything. I did not care what. Life goes on. Shawarma, falafel, all these things. Apparently, it did not do me any good these years. But as soon as I got the other one (nine years later), I got off all this stuff, I threw everything away.... The doctor told me if I want to live longer, I should stop smoking. I have to do these things. I believe this is true. It's up to me."

65 years (Kibbutz) "In the first two or three months, maybe one year at the most, I was careful or tried to be careful with what I ate. At first, I went to the family doctor every month, and then the spaces between visits got longer. Listen! I'd do one follow up with a cardiologist each year then I forget about that too."

67 years (Kibbutz) "The last attack was so strong that I told myself I'd rather die. Everything would change now. Anything that was wrong would turn out to be all right. If it's cigarettes, if it's a concern for my body, everything... Now my health is first. You see, now the thought that if something happens to me, I will not be here... It should be avoided. I must take care of myself. I will not be here. I'll drag myself as much as possible. Seeing my grandchildren grow up, that's my goal. I had this thought even after the first attack, but you disregard. This time it will not happen."

It appears that the first MI was a warning sign that motivated people to look into their everyday lifestyle behaviors. They realized there are factors under their control that can prevent the next attack and save their life. Over time, adherence declined and participants returned to familiar pre-MI habits, with the hope that it would never recur. A second or recurrent attack made them realize that there was a price for their health conduct. At that point, they felt more decisive to make necessary changes in their lives.

3.2.2. Family and significant others

Family members, mainly spouses, were perceived as a major source for instrumental and psychological support.

58 years (Cardiac rehabilitation) "After my first attack I was with my wife, I had family support during the first few years. Everything went well, I stuck to everything, healthy diet, walks on the seashore, she was more into it; I got help and support. Today I live by myself and prepare my own meals, nobody looks after me. I am trying to do what I was told...that's how it is. I think that if I was with a wife it would be easier."

56 years (Kibbutz) "If I didn't have such strong support and a network to lean on, I do not know where I would be today. I think because of my family and all the people around, I'm fine."

78 years (Arab community) "What helped me is my wife. She asks me, for example, about the medications, whether I took from this box and that. She always pays attention to my food and helped me to quit smoking. I think that family support is very important. You're under pressure and you have to remember a lot, and you get confused, when someone is on your side that helps you, that's good."

Participants who live within a supportive family setting and have an organized agenda found it easier to adhere. The structured family framework helped to maintain daily routine activities, including medical regimens and lifestyle habits. Family members, mainly spouses, provided useful adherence reminders and instrumental help. Feeling that people genuinely care about and support you were perceived as critical for adherence.

While the majority of participants valued family's instrumental and emotional support, some participants felt uncomfortable and offended by others' attitudes regarding their adherence.

58 years (Cardiac rehabilitation) "I don't like people telling me what to do. I know what is best for me and what not. I am not a young child. I know exactly what I should do."

65 years (Kibbutz) "My wife's family annoyed me somewhat; they had this attitude that I had to be looked after and helped. It's not my character, I mean, no way. In my family its different, we don't look for support and help."

59 years (Kibbutz) "Only my wife bothers me, trying to buy healthy food. I'm still buying what I want."

Several participants expressed their resentment being patronized or infantilized by others. They opposed stereotypic comments with no caring intentions. They not only perceived these as not

A. Hanna, E.-M. Yael and L. Hadassa et al./International Journal of Nursing Studies 101 (2020) 103416   7

beneficial, but also sometimes described them as annoying and a motivator for contrary reactions. It appears that a crucial factor for adherence is an attitude of caring that respects the participants' values and preferences.

3.2.3. Health care providers

Health care providers were perceived as another source of external support. Participants were asked what kind of medical follow up and cardiac rehabilitation programs they attend and how it affects their adherence. All participants (i.e., Cardiac rehabilitation and community participants) reported lack of regular planned long-term follow-ups with their family physician or other health professionals (e.g., cardiologist, physical therapist, or dietitian). The community participants reported poor participation in cardiac rehabilitation programs. The initiation for a clinic visit came from the patients, mostly for administrative assistance (e.g., prescriptions, lab tests, referrals), or a health problem. Participants expressed good rapport with their family physician, however, couldn't recall planned follow-ups or regular lifestyle education. Being asked by professionals about adherence to medical recommendations or lifestyle habits was exceptional.

> 74 years (Arab community) "I have a good relationship with my family doctor, I go to him every few months. He asks me how I fee. He checks my blood pressure and tells me to do blood tests. Only if I complain about chest pain, he sends me to do E.C.G. He does not refer me to a cardiologist."

Follow-ups by a cardiologist or a cardiac rehabilitation program is part of a hospitals' discharge recommendations for patients after MI. Most participants interviewed in a community setting provided a variety of explanations and excuses for poor participation, such as: lack of time, distance, felt no need to participate, do not think it is interesting or helpful, and feeling they know best what is good for them.

However, the experience of the group of nine participants interviewed during a hospital-based cardiac rehabilitation visit was different. All of them attended the biannual program voluntarily over many years, since their hospital discharge. Those who ceased the follow up for a period of time experienced deterioration in their lifestyle, and felt the need to return back to the program.

> 83 years (Cardiac rehabilitation) "After I was discharged from the hospital the first time (18 years ago), I continued to come every six months to the cardiac rehabilitation in the hospital. I do not visit the family doctor regularly unless I need something. … For a period of two or three years, I was followed by a cardiologist and was not satisfied. After my wife passed away, I went back to the cardiac rehabilitation in the hospital and since then I have been continuing here twice a year."

> 70 years (Cardiac rehabilitation) "I come here to the nurse every six month since 2004 (14 years). I come on my own initiative, no one tells me. I do every test they say. Stress test, blood test, whatever they decide. The family doctor does not see me. I went to a visit maybe once or twice over the years. I enjoy coming here to the nurse and doctor. I feel their support. … I'm always encouraged when I come here. …It's important for me to get this feedback. That's why I make sure to come."

> 60 years (Cardiac rehabilitation) "The framework here (hospital cardiac rehabilitation) held me. But I stopped coming here for two years. … I reduced my walking the past three years, I gained weight, and I did not take care with food. I decided to return to the framework here. Before I come to follow up, I'm putting myself into a regimen so that I will get there in shape and without problems."

The participants described their experience with the cardiac rehabilitation at the hospital as rewarding in a variety of aspects: a source of reinforcements from experts, an organized structure that helps in maintaining adherence, personal caring relationships with the same familiar team; continuity of long-term care, enjoyable interaction, and receiving professional monitoring, treatment, and guidance. Despite the fact that participation in a hospital-based cardiac rehabilitation program meant extra out of pocket money and long-distance travel, compared to community-based cardiac rehabilitation, the participants emphasized the benefits as worth the investment. They emphasized the benefits, as opposed to non-attending participants who looked for excuses not to participate.

In summary, personal and professional environments such as family, relatives and health care services may have an important impact on adherence or non-adherence.

4. Discussion

The findings of this study demonstrate the complexity of the adherence phenomenon and shed some light on the underlying motivators to health-related behaviors. Three intrinsic adherence factors were identified: willpower, sense of competency, and personal preferences. The underlying meaning of the interrelationships was that willpower by itself is insufficient for a person to adhere to a change in life; a sense of competency is required to enable carrying out a change that fits the person's beliefs and preferences. Similarly, the extrinsic factors were interrelated. A person experiencing a stressful event, such as MI, can benefit from support by relatives and health care professionals. Moreover, external and internal attributes are also interrelated, whereby external events and environment can enhance or impede internal attributes and vice versa.

Willpower was identified by the participants as a crucial motivator for behavioral change and supports the importance of inner determination as a major adherence facilitator. This finding is in congruence with the self-determination theory (Ryan and Deci, 2000), and emphasizes the importance of the autonomy of people to choose their own way of life (Bergman and Berterö, 2003). This kind of determination was based primarily on the participants' ability to internalize the consequences of their behavior. Although most participants were knowledgeable and aware of the costs of non-adherence, they still found it difficult to integrate this knowledge into action in their everyday lifestyle.

People with chronic health conditions are often expected to give up personal preferred habits and replace them with less enjoyable, or even unpleasant medical regimens. According to the self-determination theory, the actions of people who are intrinsically motivated depend on whether it gives them pleasure or interest. This explains to some extent why even those who internalize the implications of non-adherence and have a sense of volition, found it difficult to adhere. In light of this understanding, a cardinal question is what differentiates between people who adhere and those who do not?

Findings of the current study suggest that beyond inner-willpower, a sense of self-efficacy (Bandura, 2001) or self-competency along with the ability to tailor behavioral changes according to personal beliefs and preferences, can turn intentions into practice. Participants with high adherence were those who succeeded in integrating all three components. In other words, they had strong will power to live healthy life and felt competent to integrate preferable changes in everyday lifestyle, even though they were not necessarily their most favored choices.

As much as intrinsic motivators play a crucial role in adherence, internalization of extrinsic motivators can strengthen the inner sense of self determination and competency. The threat of a recurrent heart attack, family members, and healthcare

8   *A. Hanna, E.-M. Yael and L. Hadassa et al./International Journal of Nursing Studies 101 (2020) 103416*

professionals were found to be external factors with the potential to affect adherence. Family support, especially spousal support, and structured daily life were identified as factors that encouraged adherence. This finding is consistent with the literature, indicating that people characterized by non-adherence often lived alone, felt socially isolated, or felt controlled and overprotected by their families (Dunbar et al., 2008; Fernandez et al., 2015; Roebuck et al., 2001). Caring relations provided with respect to a person's values, preferences and autonomy supported their basic needs for competence, control, and relatedness (Ryan and Deci, 2000).

All participants (i.e., Cardiac rehabilitation and community participants) reported lack of regular planned long-term follow-up with their family physician or other health professionals (e.g., cardiologist, physical therapist, or dietitian). The community participants reported poor participation in cardiac rehabilitation programs. Those who attended hospital-based cardiac rehabilitation visits regularly emphasized the benefits of their program: routine monitoring, evaluation of health status, feedback and guidance from experts, continuity of care over years, and a personal patient-centered approach. They further emphasized that it filled their needs for reassurance, confidence and trust that was worth the effort and costs required to attend a hospital-based program.

In the current study there were some socioeconomic gaps between Jewish and Arab participants, however, this did not associate with differences in health literacy and adherence perceptions. A possible explanation might be the greater influence of similar social environments and level of education, compared to differences in cultural or religious attributes.

None of the emerged themes was identified as a sole solution to the poor adherence problem. The understanding that the phenomenon of adherence is a complex holistic integration of internal and external motivators and the interrelationships among them could advance theoretical understanding and lead to important practical implications.

4.1. Limitations

Most of the participants in the current study represent normative adherence behaviors. More interviews with non-adherent people would be beneficial to gain a better understanding of non-adherence perspectives. Although the prevalence of MI is higher among men and it was convenient to recruit them, more women should be involved in this research. The interviews were conducted in Hebrew or Arabic and translated into English, which may have misrepresented the laymen language. Transferability should take into consideration socio-cultural differences.

5. Conclusion

The motivational theory was a useful framework to organize the interview data and gain insights to the underlying motivators of the phenomenon of adherence to health-related behaviors. Primary and secondary long-term cardiac care interventions are recommended to incorporate tailored behavior change strategies that would enhance adherence to therapies and healthy lifestyle. Health care practitioners should establish mutually agreed upon plans of care, in cooperation with patients, rather than dictate medical instructions for the patient. In addition, specific objectives should be established with regular planned follow up. Future research should evaluate the effectiveness of interventions designed to strengthen motivation and enhance adherence.

Conflict of interest

None declared.

Funding statement

No funding was obtained for this study.

Acknowledgments

Thanks to the following nursing students from the department of nursing, Yezreel Valley College, for their contribution with data collection: Elena Bukin, Ina Shakayev, Naheel Eghbaryieh, and Yasmin Mohamed.

References

Al-Mallah, M.H., Farah, I., Al-Madani, W., Bdeir, B., Al Habib, S., Bigelow, M.L., Ferwana, M., 2016. The impact of nurse-led clinics on the mortality and morbidity of patients with cardiovascular diseases: a systematic review and meta-analysis. J. Cardiovasc. Nurs. doi:10.1097/JCN.0000000000000224.

Ali, M.A., Yasir, J., Sherwani, R.N., Fareed, M., Arshad, F., Abid, F., Fatima, K., 2017. Frequency and predictors of non-adherence to lifestyle modifications and medications after coronary artery bypass grafting: a cross-sectional study. Indian Heart J. 69 (4), 469–473. doi:10.1016/j.ihj.2017.05.017.

Bansilal, S., Castellano, J.M., Garrido, E., Wei, H.G., Freeman, A., Spettell, C., Fuster, V., 2016. Assessing the impact of medication adherence on long-term cardiovascular outcomes. J. Am. Coll. Cardiol. 68 (8), 789–801. doi:10.1016/j.jacc.2016.06.005.

Bandura, A., 2010. Self-efficacy. Corsini Encyclop. Psychol. 1–3.

Bandura, A., 2001. Social cognitive theory: an agentic perspective. Annu. Rev. Psychol. 52 (1), 1–26.

Barnason, S., Zimmerman, L., Young, L., 2012. An integrative review of interventions promoting self-care of patients with heart failure. J. Clin. Nurs. 21 (3-4), 448–475. doi:10.1111/j.1365-2702.2011.03907.

Bergman, E., Berterö, C., 2003. Grasp life again'. a qualitative study of the motive power in myocardial infarction patients. Eur. J. Cardiovasc. Nurs. 2 (4), 303–310. doi:10.1016/S1474-5151(03)00098-7.

Bergman, E., Malm, D., Karlsson, J.E., Berterö, C., 2009. Longitudinal study of patients after myocardial infarction: sense of coherence, quality of life, and symptoms. Heart Lung: J. Acute Crit. Care 38 (2), 129–140. doi:10.1016/j.hrtlng.2008.05.007.

Campbell, D.J., Ronksley, P.E., Manns, B.J., Tonelli, M., Sanmartin, C., Weaver, R.G.Collaboration, for the I. C. D., 2014. The association of income with health behavior change and disease monitoring among patients with chronic disease. PLoS One 9 (4), e94007. doi:10.1371/journal.pone.0094007.

Choudhry, N.K., Glynn, R.J., Avorn, J., Lee, J.L., Brennan, T.A., Reisman, L., Shrank, W.H., 2014. Untangling the relationship between medication adherence and post-myocardial infarction outcomes: medication adherence and clinical outcomes. Am. Heart J. 167 (1), 51–58. doi:10.1016/j.ahj.2013.09.014, e5.

Colombo, F. (2012). Tackling Inequalities in Health and Health Care in Israel. OECD Reviews of Health Care Quality – Israel. Retrieved from www.oecd.org/health/qualityreviews.

Crowley, M.J., Zullig, L.L., Shah, B.R., Shaw, R.J., Lindquist, J.H., Peterson, E.D., Bosworth, H.B., 2015. Medication non-adherence after myocardial infarction: an exploration of modifying factors. J. Gen. Intern. Med. 30 (1), 83–90. doi:10.1007/s11606-014-3072-x.

Dunbar, S.B., Clark, P.C., Quinn, C., Gary, R.A., Kaslow, N.J., 2008. Family influences on heart failure self-care and outcomes. J. Cardiovasc. Nurs. doi:10.1097/01.JCN.0000305093.20012.b8.

Fernandez, R., Rolley, J.X., Rajaratnam, R., Everett, B., Davidson, P.M., 2015. Reducing the risk of heart disease among Indian Australians: knowledge, attitudes, and beliefs regarding food practices – a focus group study. Food Nutr. Res. 59 (1), 25770. doi:10.3402/fnr.v59.25770.

Giannuzzi, P., Temporelli, P.L., Marchioli, R., Maggioni, A.P., Balestroni, G., Ceci, V., Tavazzi, L., 2008. Global secondary prevention strategies to limit event recurrence after myocardial infarction: results of the gospel study, a multicenter, randomized controlled trial from the Italian cardiac rehabilitation network. Arch. Intern. Med. 168 (20), 2194–2204. doi:10.1001/archinte.168.20.2194.

Graneheim, U.H., Lindgren, B.M., Lundman, B., 2017. Methodological challenges in qualitative content analysis: a discussion paper. Nurse Educ. Today 56 (December 2016), 29–34. doi:10.1016/j.nedt.2017.06.002.

Gregory, S., Bostock, Y., Backett-Milburn, K., 2006. Recovering from a heart attack: a qualitative study into lay experiences and the struggle to make lifestyle changes. Fam. Pract. 23 (2), 220–225. doi:10.1093/fampra/cmi089.

Groleau, D., Whitley, R., Lespérance, F., Kirmayer, L.J., 2010. Spiritual reconfigurations of self after a myocardial infarction: influence of culture and place. Health Place 16 (5), 853–860. doi:10.1016/j.healthplace.2010.04.010.

Guba, E.G., Lincoln, Y.S., 1989. Fourth Generation Evaluation. Sage, Newbury Park, CA.

Israeli Ministry of Health. (2018). Retrieved from https://www.health.gov.il/UnitsOffice/ICDC/Chronic_Diseases/Heart_diseases/Pages/default.aspx (in Hebrew).

Jackevicius, C.A., Li, P., Tu, J.V., 2008. Prevalence, predictors, and outcomes of primary nonadherence after acute myocardial infarction. Circulation 117 (8), 1028–1036. doi:10.1161/CIRCULATIONAHA.107.706820.

A. Hanna, E.-M. Yael and L. Hadassa et al./International Journal of Nursing Studies 101 (2020) 103416   9

Johansson, I., Swahn, E., Strömberg, A., 2007. Manageability, vulnerability and interaction: a qualitative analysis of acute myocardial infarction patients' conceptions of the event. Eur. J. Cardiovasc. Nurs. 6 (3), 184–191. doi:10.1016/J.EJCNURSE.2006.08.003.

Jones, M., Jolly, K., Raftery, J., Lip, G.Y.H., Greenfield, S., 2007. "DNA" may not mean "did not participate": a qualitative study of reasons for non-adherence at home-and centre-based cardiac rehabilitation. Fam. Pract. 24 (4), 343–357. doi:10.1093/fampra/cmm021.

Kotseva, K.EUROASPIRE Investigators, 2017. The Euroaspire surveys: lessons learned in cardiovascular disease prevention. Cardiovasc. Diagn. Ther. 7 (6), 633. doi:10.21037/cdt.2017.04.06.

Kronish, I.M., Ye, S., 2013. Adherence to cardiovascular medications: lessons learned and future directions. Prog. Cardiovasc. Dis. 55 (6), 590–600. doi:10.1016/j.pcad.2013.02.001.

Levin-Zamir, D., Baron-Epel, O.B., Cohen, V., Elhayany, A., 2016. The association of health literacy with health behavior, socioeconomic indicators, and self-assessed health from a national adult survey in Israel. J. Health Commun. 21 (suppl 2), 61–68. doi:10.1080/10810730.2016.1207115.

Li, Y., Pan, A., Wang, D.D., Liu, X., Dhana, K., Franco, O.H., Hu, F.B., 2018. Impact of healthy lifestyle factors on life expectancies in the US population. Circulation 138 (4), 345–355. doi:10.1161/CIRCULATIONAHA.117.032047.

Mohammadpour, A., Rahmati Sharghi, N., Khosravan, S., Alami, A., Akhond, M., 2015. The effect of a supportive educational intervention developed based on the orem's self-care theory on the self-care ability of patients with myocardial infarction: a randomised controlled trial. J. Clin. Nurs. 24 (11–12), 1686–1692. doi:10.1111/jocn.12775.

Piepoli, M.F., Corra, U., Benzer, W., Bjarnason-Wehrens, B., Dendale, P., Gaita, D., Schmid, J.P., 2010. Secondary prevention through cardiac rehabilitation: from knowledge to implementation. A position paper from the cardiac rehabilitation section of the European association of cardiovascular prevention and rehabilitation. Eur. J. Cardiovasc. Prev. Rehabil. 17 (1), 1–17. doi:10.1097/HJR.0b013e3283313592.

Roebuck, A., Furze, G., Thompson, D.R., 2001. Health-related quality of life after myocardial infarction: an interview study. J. Adv. Nurs. 34 (6), 787–794. doi:10.1046/j.1365-2648.2001.01809.x.

Ruano-Ravina, A., Pena-Gil, C., Abu-Assi, E., Raposeiras, S., van't Hof, A., Meindersma, E., González-Juanatey, J.R., 2016. Participation and adherence to cardiac rehabilitation programs. a systematic review. Int. J. Cardiol. doi:10.1016/j.ijcard.2016.08.12010.1006/ceps.1999.1020.

Ryan, R.M., Deci, E.L., 2000. Intrinsic and extrinsic motivations: classic definitions and new directions. Contemp. Educ. Psychol. 25 (1), 54–67. doi:10.1006/ceps.1999.1020.

Sabaté, E., 2003. Adherence to Long-term Therapies: Evidence for Action. World Health Organization https://apps.WHO.int/iris/bitstream/handle/10665/42682/9241545992.pdf;jsessionid=59E16C351D6CA1EEA4E6E71B7D4A5904?sequence=1.

Tong, A., Sainsbury, P., Craig, J., 2007. Consolidated criteria for reporting qualitative research (COREQ): a 32-item checklist for interviews and focus groups. Int. J. Qual. Health Care 19 (6), 349–357. doi:10.1093/intqhc/mzm042.

WHO (World Health Organization) (2018). The top 10 Causes of Death in 2016. Retrieved from https://www.WHO.int/news-room/fact-sheets/detail/the-top-10-causes-of-death.

Wilson, P.W., Douglas, P.S. (2013). Epidemiology of Coronary Heart Disease. UpTo-Date. Gersh BJ, Pellikka PA, Kaski JC (Eds.), Waltham, MA.

Zhang, Y., Kaplan, C.M., Baik, S.H., Chang, C.-C.H., Lave, J.R., 2014. Medication adherence and readmission after myocardial infarction in the medicare population. Am. J. Manag. Care 20 (11), e498–e505. doi:10.1016/j.surg.2006.10.010.

Effect of a Systemwide Approach to a Reduction in Central Line–Associated Bloodstream Infections

Sarah Ferrari, DNP, CNS, CCIM, CPHON; Kristine Taylor, DNP, PCNS-BC, CENP

ABSTRACT

Background: Unit-based initiatives were deployed independently creating silos in practice variability across the system with little impact on reduction of central line–associated bloodstream infections (CLABSI). **Problem:** The goal was to decrease CLABSI systemwide by establishing standardized evidence-based practice (EBP) procedures to advance nursing practice. **Approach:** A new innovative method, the Ferrari Method for Practice Standardization, enhanced the quality infrastructure by merging EBP and lean methodology to translate nursing innovations into practice. Leveraging a culture of shared decision making to support autonomy, as well as collaborating interprofessionally, allowed the organization to standardize and sustain CLABSI prevention. **Outcomes:** The Ferrari Method for Practice Standardization successfully reduced CLABSI rates by 48% over a 1-year improvement cycle. Eight standardized EBP clinical procedures were developed and implemented across the organization. **Conclusion:** The implementation of the Ferrari Method for Practice Standardization swiftly moves new knowledge into clinical practice to improve outcomes. Using standardized improvement methodology, it eases the interprofessional approval processes, maximizes autonomy, and focuses on quality care. **Keywords:** central line–associated bloodstream infections (CLABSI), high reliability, infections, lean methodology, standardization

Author Affiliation: Center for Professional Excellence and Inquiry, Stanford Children's Health, Palo Alto, California.

The authors thank Edward Anthony for his knowledge and encouragement in learning the lean methodology used in this quality improvement project.

The authors declare no conflicts of interest.

Supplemental digital content is available for this article. Direct URL citation appears in the printed text and is provided in the HTML and PDF versions of this article on the journal's Web site (www.jncqjournal.com).

Correspondence: Sarah Ferrari, DNP, CNS, CCIM, CPHON, Center for Professional Excellence and Inquiry, Stanford Children's Health, 725 Welch Rd, Palo Alto, CA 94304 (sferrari@stanfordchildrens.org).

Accepted for publication: March 25, 2019

Published ahead of print: May 27, 2019

DOI: 10.1097/NCQ.0000000000000410

Hospital-acquired conditions (HAC) are a concern across the United States. According to the Centers for Disease Control and Prevention,[1] 1 in every 25 patients will experience at least 1 HAC during hospitalization. Central line–associated bloodstream infections (CLABSI) are recognized as one of the most common HACs in acute care hospitals, and while there has been substantial work to reduce those rates, there remains room for improvement.[1] Increased length of stay, overall cost, and risk of mortality have propelled this serious safety event to an organizational priority.[2] More recently, hospitals have been able to maintain zero or very low rates of infections.[3]

Our large pediatric and obstetric academic organization struggled with maintaining consistent and sustained CLABSI rate reductions. The organization performed an analysis of the problem to identify contributing factors, which highlighted variability in practice, a lack of evidence-based practice (EBP) integration into procedures (procedural integration), and silos of improvement work across the organization. Practice variability was occurring across multiple patient care units and was not consistently evidence-based; dedicated efforts to quality-based improvement work focused on the microsystem's quality outcomes. These microsystems are defined as a group of health care providers consistently working in partnership for the care of a particular patient population.[4] The result of these efforts compromised the systemwide standard of practice to

483

January–March 2020 • Volume 35 • Number 1   www.jncqjournal.com   41

reduce CLABSI rates. Each microsystem created clinical initiatives and practice changes in silos. The bedside nurses within the organization cross-cover to other like microsystems. Therefore, they began to experience challenges in maintaining the knowledge of the various practice methods for central lines due to the variability in each microsystem. The organizational CLABSI rate prior to this intervention was 1.96, mostly attributed to a lack of standardized practice.

LITERATURE REVIEW

Central line catheter use serves an important purpose in the administration of intravenous fluids, nutrition, and medication to support the management of vulnerable patients. In 2009, the Centers for Disease Control and Prevention introduced CLABSI guidelines to help in the reduction of these infections.[1] There has been demonstrated success in the reduction of CLABSI since implementation; however, The Joint Commission[5] has endorsed a plan to eliminate CLABSIs calling for a 50% reduction by 2020. Various studies have shown that when the CLABSI bundle is implemented as a whole, without variation, CLABSI rates decrease.[6-9] Even with the implementation of the CLABSI prevention maintenance bundle, organizations are still witnessing bundle element variation and challenges to sustain the improvement work. Identified organizational barriers to meeting this plan stems from lack of leadership commitment, culture of safety, knowledge, and necessary resources.

A study by Conley[6] identified that nurses, as well as patients, desired evidence-based policies to support a consistent nursing practice specific to CLABSI prevention. Successful adherence to the CLABSI prevention bundle is attributed to knowledge of the bundle as well as engagement of staff to aid in changing behaviors.[7] The success of CLABSI prevention can be influenced by the culture of the organization and peers.[6]

RATIONALE

Achieving zero harm is something that resonates with many organizations as they strive to be a highly reliable organization. As reported by Oster and Deakins,[10] the 5 essential principles of high reliability are sensitivity to operations, preoccupation with failure, deference to expertise, reluctance to simplify, and commitment to resilience. Applying these principles to practice yielded a 33.5% reduction in preventable harm incidents with a cost avoidance of $554 000 for CLABSIs across 4 fiscal years. The implementation of a unit-based safety program grounded by the high reliability framework resulted in a significant reduction of CLABSI rates from 1.95 per 1000 line days to 1.04 per 1000 line days across 6 quarters.[11] Chassin and Loeb[12] suggested that as organizations begin to adopt the framework of high reliability, the incorporation of lean methodology is essential to break the cycles of low reliability.

Lean methodology is a model for continuous improvement where the voice of the end user is highly valued and is vital to the improvement work.[13] It incorporates a set of improvement tools to help address the safety and quality challenges in organizations.[12] Integrating the concepts of lean methodology with EBP, Halm et al[13] addressed a clinical concern by igniting a spirit of inquiry to address standardization of practice. These principles have been associated with sustained improvement of patient outcomes from each contributing member of the health care team. Shared governance serves as a platform to collaborate with bedside nurses within the organization to address quality and safety countermeasures.[14] Shared decision making brings the decision about the practice change to the bedside where the work is going to be done.[15] When it relates to one's practice, involvement in decisions has a positive impact on the improvement work within the environment.[14] Shared governance is a structure that empowers nurses, and when engaged in the process, they actively seek opportunities to improve their practice.[16]

Specific aims

The purpose of this quality improvement (QI) project was to determine whether the development of evidence-based standardized clinical procedures influenced by the combination of lean methodology and shared governance aids in the reduction of CLABSI. The specific aim was to align with organizational strategic goals for HAC reductions.

METHODS
Context

The project setting is a tertiary level 1 trauma, academic, freestanding pediatric and obstetric hospital with 361 patient beds located in California. This organization has a diverse patient population with more than 150 medical specialty services in 6 different clinical groupings or what the organization calls centers of excellence. Inclusion criteria for this QI project were all inpatient units that used central lines from February 2017 to November 2018. The institutional review board at Stanford University deemed this project as QI.

Interventions

Unacceptable CLABSI rates prompted 2 nurses in the Center for Professional Development and Inquiry, experienced in lean methodology and shared governance, to partner with Patient Care Services to implement a new methodology called the Ferrari Method for Practice Standardization (the Ferrari Method). This methodology integrates lean methodology tools with EBP in an effort to streamline and standardize clinical practice. The organization was familiar with each method independently but had never merged these methods together for improvement work. This combination aligned strategic plans, used the shared governance council membership and structure, and incorporated EBP to streamlined approval processes. The Ferrari Method structure involved preplanning activities, work group sessions with the content experts, socialization of recommendations, finalization of the change, and implementation strategies. The team consisted of shared governance bedside nurses from both the inpatient and outpatient areas, members from the Professional Development Council (clinical nurse specialists and nursing professional development specialists), infection prevention and control specialists, a member from the vascular access department, a member from the quality department, providers, a member from supply chain, and the policy program manager as the facilitator. In addition, a lead educator was assigned to assume responsibility for continually assessing the level of education and educational methods throughout the process. Lean methodology served as the basis for the construction of the agenda and charters for each breakout session. These charters served as a tool to guide the team members through the various discussions based on their assigned clinical skill group.

Each workshop consisted of two 4-hour workshops with an overall aim to understand current practice, evaluate the evidence, gain consensus, and construct new standardized clinical house-wide procedures. The first workshop focused on understanding current practice differences across the organization, reviewing the literature, and developing an appraisal table. In between sessions 1 and 2, the team members discussed the ideal best practice proposals with their peers. The second 4-hour workshop focused on revisiting the proposed best practice by weighing the feedback received from peers and constructing the standardized procedures for each identified skill. The educational level was assessed to determine ideal peer-based dissemination and implementation using technology and skill-based education.

Study of interventions

Eight standardized procedures specific to the maintenance of central lines were implemented across the organization over the fiscal year. Over a span of 4 months, organizational consensus was obtained on these 8 evidence-based policies and procedures (see Supplemental Digital Content Table, available at: http://links.lww.com/JNCQ/A590). Once implementation across the organization was complete, the unit's leadership team assessed and gathered feedback from bedside staff with newly implemented procedures and policies. The cyclic evaluation cycles, using the Plan-Do-Study-Act workflow, were deployed 6 months post each new procedure implementation to allow for skill acquisition. To measure the success of the newly implemented standardized procedures, evaluation of CLABSI rates pre- and postimplementation was compared.

Measures

The outcome measure for CLABSI was defined by National Health care Safety Network and reviewed monthly by the infection prevention and control team. The CLABSI rate is calculated by dividing the total number of central line infections per month (numerator) by the total number of central line days (denominator) times 1000 patient days. The cost avoidance calculation is provided by Goudie et al[17] and Goudie et al.[18] The EBP changes were measured by the total number of policy/procedure updates during the implementation time period.

Analysis

The CLABSI rate baseline data were from February 2017 to December 2017 (11 months),

January–March 2020 • Volume 35 • Number 1   www.jncqjournal.com   **43**

and the postdata were from January 2018 to November 2018 (11 months). The pre-/postdata were analyzed using an independent *t* test, effect size, and control chart for mean score and standard deviation. The cost avoidance was evaluated by calculating CLABSI numbers pre- and postimplementation of evidence-based recommendations.[17,18]

RESULTS

The CLABSI rates declined over the 11-month implementation period. The CLABSI rate decreased from 1.96 to 1.02, an overall 48% decrease (Figure). The overall standard deviation narrowed after implementation of 8 new EBP changes. The QI project has a large effect size and was statistically significant at *P* value less than .0005. Because of the overall decrease in number of CLABSI, the organization had a cost avoidance of $1.4 million.[10]

DISCUSSION
Interpretation

An analysis of contributing factors highlighted variability in practice and lack of EBP procedural integration and created silos of improvement work across the organization. This CLABSI reduction project was budget neutral, using existing shared governance structures and organizational clinical experts. Collaborating with

shared governance, the key stakeholders in clinical practice at the bedside provided a platform for success in standardizing practice. Shared governance provided a method for decision making at the system level for standardizing EBP. The implementation of Ferrari Method swiftly moved new knowledge into practice with focus on improving clinical outcomes and patient safety and maximizing autonomy. This process created a strong collaboration across the clinical microsystems using a rapid process improvement method. The participants felt that their voices were heard and valued. In addition, the silos of clinical initiatives ceased, and efforts were standardized through the evidence-based recommendations. Since the implementation of the first rapid process improvement, the organization has now recognized this structure as the method for streamlining and standardizing clinical practice at the bedside.

Limitations

This QI project focused on EBP for the organization, and while the organization supports and encourages a culture of patient safety, the bedside nurses still experienced challenges with peers and leadership during implementation of the procedural changes. First, clinical standardization is difficult to do across an organization with diverse patient populations and clinical

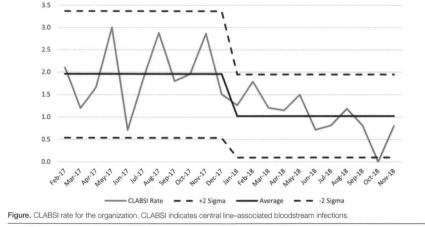

Figure. CLABSI rate for the organization. CLABSI indicates central line–associated bloodstream infections.

needs. This led to the creation of an approved plan for exceptions based on evidence for specific patient populations with various products and/or central line devices. Second, procedural changes were evidence-based, but some patient care units experienced challenges with staff adoption of the change in practice due to disbelief in the evidence. This, therefore, negatively influenced early adopters. Additional education was needed for some areas to better comprehend the evidence. Finally, during the cycles of improvement postimplementation, feedback was provided regarding challenges to obtain the right supplies in a timely fashion. A timed study of the practice changes before and after the change in technique to assess workflow changes or skill acquisition may have helped compliance and understanding of time needed for each practice.

CONCLUSIONS

The specific aim of this project was to decrease CLABSI rates through an organizational focus and standardization of EBP. The creation of Ferrari Method proved to be a valid method for assessing practice, evaluating the evidence, and developing practice standards. Pulling clinical experts from the microsystems established a standard method for the decision making. In conclusion, CLABSI rates decreased after establishing the Ferrari Method for Practice Standardization of organization procedures, supporting high reliability, improving bundle knowledge, and encouraging bedside nurse engagement.

REFERENCES

1. Centers for Disease Control and Prevention. Health care-associated infections (HAIs). https://www.cdc.gov/winnable battles/report/HAIs.html. Published 2017. Accessed November 14, 2018.
2. Medina A, Serratr T, Pelter M, Brancamp T. Decreasing central line-associated bloodstream infections in the non-ICU population. *J Nurs Care Qual*. 2014;29(2):133-140.
3. Cooper MR, Hong A, Beaudin E, et al. Implementing high reliability for patient safety. *J Nurs Regul*. 2016;7(1):46-52.
4. Likosky DS. Clinical microsystems: a critical framework for crossing the quality chasm. *J Extra Corpor Technol*. 2014;46(1):33-37.
5. Rosenberg RE, Devins L, Geraghty G, et al. Engaging front-line staff in central line-associated bloodstream infection prevention practice in the wake of superstorm sandy. *Jt Comm J Qual Patient Saf*. 2015;41(10):462-468.
6. Conley SB. Central line associated bloodstream infection prevention: standardizing practice focused on evidence-based guidelines. *Clin J Oncol Nurs*. 2016;20(1):23-26.
7. Dumyati G, Concannon C, van Wijngaarden E, et al. Sustained reduction of central line-associated bloodstream infections outside the intensive care unit with a multimodal intervention focusing on central line maintenance. *Am J Infect Control*. 2014;42(7):723-730.
8. Savage T, Hodge DE, Pickard K, Myers P, Powell P, Caycae JM. Sustained reduction and prevention of neonatal and pediatric central line-associated bloodstream infection following a nurse-driven quality improvement initiative in a pediatric facility. *J Vasc Access*. 2018;23(1):30-41.
9. Marschall J, Mermel LA, Fakih M, et al. Strategies to prevent central line-associated bloodstream infections in acute care hospitals: 2014 updates. *Infect Control Hosp Epidemiol*. 2014;35(2):89-107.
10. Oster CA, Deakins S. Practical application of high reliability principles in health care to optimize quality and safety outcomes. *J Nurs Adm*. 2018;48(1):50-55.
11. Ritcher JP, McAlearney AS. Targeted implementation of the comprehensive unit-based safety program through an assessment of safety culture to minimize central line-associated bloodstream infections. *Health Care Manage Rev*. 2018;43(1):42-49.
12. Chassin MR, Loeb JM. High reliability health care: getting there from here. *Milbank Q*. 2013;91(3):459-490.
13. Halm MA, Always A, Bunn S, et al. Intersecting evidence-base practice with a lean improvement model. *J Nurs Care Qual*. 2018;33(4):309-315.
14. Graham-Dickerson P, Houser J, Thomas E, et al. The value of staff nurse involvement in decision making. *J Nurs Adm*. 2013;43(5):286-292.
15. Swihart D, Hess RG. *Shared Governance: A Practical Approach to Transforming Interprofessional Health Care*. 3rd ed. Danvers, MA: HCPro; 2014.
16. Clavelle JT, Porter O'Grady T, Drenhard K. Structural empowerment and the nursing practice environment in Magnet organizations. *J Nurs Adm*. 2013;43(11):566-573.
17. Goudie A, Dynan L, Brady PW, Rettiganti M. Attributable cost of length of stay for central line-associated bloodstream infections. *Pediatrics*. 2014;133(6):e1525-e1532.
18. Goudie A, Dynan L, Brady PW, Fieldston E, Brilli RJ, Walsh KE. Costs of venous thromboembolism, catheter-associated urinary tract infection, and pressure ulcer. *Pediatrics*. 2015;136(3):432-439.

INDEX

Page numbers followed by "*f*" indicate figures, "*t*" indicate tables, and "*b*" indicate boxes.